NUTRITION
AND DIET
THERAPY

NUTRITION & DIET THERAPY

Sixth Edition

Carolynn E. Townsend

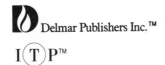

Delmar Publishers Inc.™

I T P™

NOTICE TO THE READER

Delmar publishing team:
Publisher: David C. Gordon
Administrative Editor: Marion Waldman
Developmental Editor: Marjorie A. Bruce
Project Editor: Danya M. Plotsky
Production Coordinator: Jennifer Gaines
Art and Design Coordinator: Mary E. Siener

For information, address

Delmar Publishers Inc.
3 Columbia Circle, Box 15015,
Albany, NY 12212-5015

Printed in the United States of America
Published simultaneously in Canada
by Nelson Canada,
a division of The Thomson Corporation

 2 3 4 5 6 7 8 9 10   XXX   00 99 98 97 96 95 94

Library of Congress Cataloging-in-Publication Data

Townsend, Carolynn E.
     Nutrition and diet therapy / Carolynn E. Townsend. — 6th ed.
          p.   cm.
     Includes bibliographical references and index.
     ISBN 0-8273-5745-1
     1. Diet therapy.   2. Nutrition.   3. Nursing.   I. Title.
RM216.T738   1994
613.2—dc20   93-38517

TABLE OF CONTENTS

LIST OF TABLES

THERAPEUTIC DIETS

PREFACE

Nutrition and Diet Therapy was written for beginning students in health care professions and students enrolled in food service and dietetic technician/assistant programs. This book has proven successful as an introduction to or a review of the fundamentals of nutrition and diet therapy.

This sixth edition has been substantially revised and updated to reflect the increasing awareness of the correlation between nutrition and health, and the latest developments in the nutrition field. The content is organized into four sections to simplify the presentation of nutrition. The complexity increases from Section 1 through Section 3, and is subsequently decreased in Section 4.

Section 1, **Fundamentals of Nutrition,** includes chapters on the relationship of food and health, how the body uses its food, and separate chapters on each of the six nutrients. The chapter on carbohydrates contains expanded discussion of fiber, and the chapter on fats contains additional information including, especially, cholesterol. The chapter on vitamins and the chapter on minerals each contain a table of the specific vitamins and minerals discussed, their sources, functions, and deficiency symptoms. The chapter on water covers electrolytes and acid-base balance.

Section 2, **Maintenance of Health Through Good Nutrition,** includes chapters on meal planning using the Food Guide Pyramid, the basic four food groups, and the U.S. Government's Dietary Guidelines; food customs and their origins; food-related illness, including food allergies; and chapters on nutritional needs during pregnancy and lactation, childhood and adolescence, young and middle adulthood, and late adulthood. Specific nutritional concerns relating to each age group are covered. These

include weight, food for the athlete, anorexia nervosa, bulimia, fast foods, and peer pressure.

Section 3, **Diet Therapy,** has a chapter on nutritional assessment and counseling for the health care professional and one on nutritional care of patients. The latter includes protein-calorie malnutrition in hospitalized patients and long-term care of the elderly. The other seven chapters in this section are devoted to therapeutic diets relevant to the specific disease conditions discussed.

Section 4, **Food Preparation,** contains a chapter devoted to specific concerns of consumers, including irradiated foods, artificial foods, additives, generic brands, and labeling. Also included are chapters on evaluating and preserving food quality, the use of recipes, and cooking equipment and its uses.

As in previous editions, extensive learning aids are provided. Lists of key terms and learning objectives are located at the beginning of each chapter. Chapter summaries, suggested activities, and discussion and review questions reinforce learning. Extensive tables, charts, and photos present important material in a comprehensible and accessible manner. Each chapter in Sections 1 through 3 concludes with two case studies, including case study questions based on the nursing process. These studies are provided to give the students the opportunity to apply theory by deduction and to prepare for state licensing or certification examinations. A bibliography and expanded glossary provide opportunities for further study and research.

The instructor's guide contains answers to the chapter review questions, reproducible section review questions that can be used as test material, and answers to the section review questions.

ACKNOWLEDGMENTS

The author wishes to express her appreciation to the following persons and organizations:

American Diabetes Association

American Heart Association

Marjorie Bruce

Nicholas Castro

Christopher Chien

Marietta Davis

Taylor McLaine Davis

Catherine Eads

Cora Erickson

Food and Drug Administration, U.S. Department of Health and Human Services

Food and Nutrition Board, National Academy of Sciences—National Research Council

Gerber Products Company

Deborah Goldfarb

Lisa and John Houlihan

Mayo Foundation

Metropolitan Life Insurance Company

National Bureau of Standards, U.S. Department of Commerce

National Dairy Council

National Education Association

National Livestock and Meat Board

Lorie Nolan

Parents Magazine

Danya Plotsky

Mary Riederer

Camilla Townsend

Cynthia Townsend

Kenneth Townsend

Marcia Townsend

Tupperware

United Nations Foods and Agricultural Organization

United States Department of Agriculture

Upjohn Company

Marion Waldman

John Wiley & Sons, Inc.

World Health Organization

Reviewers of the fifth edition and the revised manuscript for the sixth edition:

Marsha Cummings
El Paso, Texas

Melissa Ensore
Mobile, Alabama

Lillian Goodman
Granada Hills, California

Pat Huggins
Houston, Texas

Mary Lewin
        Lockport, New York
Linda Mitchell
        Durham, North Carolina
Marva Roddy
        Chula Vista, California
Carole Stacey
        Portage, Michigan
Maryellen Wolfe
        Hayward, California

TO THE STUDENT

In an effort to assist you in making the most efficient use of this book, the author makes the following suggestions.

Read the objectives, discussion topics, review questions, and the words listed under the heading "Vocabulary" before reading the chapter. Then, read the text carefully, noting the various headings and subheadings, which divide the topics into logical sections. Logical breaks in text help you to remember the information presented. When you have finished reading the chapter, re-read the objectives to see if you are able to fulfill them. Then review the discussion topics, special vocabulary, and review questions. Look up those questions you cannot answer or terms you do not remember. Reviewing the text helps to "cement" the information given.

You will also find it useful to understand the following prefixes and suffixes which are commonly found in nutrition.

Prefixes:

a	without
anti	against
cardi	refers to heart
centi	100
endo	within
gastri	refers to stomach
hemo	refers to blood
hyper	abnormally high
hypo	abnormally low
lact	refers to milk
lipid	fat
milli	thousandth
osteo	refers to bone

Suffixes:

. . . emia	in the blood
. . . uria	in the urine
. . . ase	an enzyme

SECTION 1

FUNDAMENTALS OF NUTRITION

The Relationship of Food and Health

OBJECTIVES

After studying this chapter, you should be able to
- Name the essential nutrients and their primary functions
- Recognize common characteristics of well-nourished people
- Recognize symptoms of malnutrition
- Describe ways in which food and health are related

Most people enjoy food. Although they eat primarily because they are hungry, they also find eating pleasant because of the memories it may invoke, the social climate it promotes, and because the taste of the food is pleasing to them. Unfortunately, many people make their food selections only on these bases and are not aware of their bodies' food needs.

ESSENTIAL NUTRIENTS

To function properly, the body must be provided with **nutrients.** Nutrients are chemical substances found in food that are essential to life. They are divided into six basic groups:

- carbohydrates
- fats

- proteins
- vitamins
- minerals
- water

Each nutrient participates in at least one of the following functions (see Table 1-1):

- providing the body with energy and heat
- building and repairing body tissue
- regulating body processes

Carbohydrates and **fats** primarily furnish energy and heat. **Proteins** are used mainly to build and repair body tissues with the help of vitamins and minerals. Proteins also provide energy when carbohydrate and fat reserves are low. **Vitamins, minerals,** and water help regulate the various body processes such as **circulation, respiration, digestion,** and **elimination.**

Each nutrient is essential, but none works alone. For example, carbohydrates and fats are necessary for energy but, to provide it, they need the help of vitamins, minerals, and water. Proteins are essential for the building and repair of body tissue; but without vitamins, minerals, and water, they are ineffective. Foods that contain

Table 1-1 The Six Essential Nutrients and Their Functions

Carbohydrates	Provide energy and heat
Fats	Provide energy and heat
Proteins	Build and repair body tissues Provide energy and heat
Vitamins	Regulate body functions
Minerals	Regulate body functions
Water	Regulate body functions

substantial amounts of nutrients are described as **nutritious** or **nourishing.** Nutrients are discussed in detail in Chapters 3 through 8.

CHARACTERISTICS OF GOOD NUTRITION

Once foods are eaten, the body must process them before they can be used. **Nutrition** is the result of these processes whereby the body takes in and uses food for growth, development, and the maintenance of health. These processes include digestion, absorption, and metabolism. (They are discussed in Chapter 2.) One's physical condition as determined by the diet is called **nutritional status.**

Nutrition helps determine the height and weight of an individual. Nutrition also can affect the body's ability to resist disease, the length of one's life, and the state of one's physical and mental well-being, figure 1-1.

Good nutrition enhances appearance and is commonly exemplified by shiny hair, clear skin, clear eyes, erect **posture** (body position), alert expressions, and firm flesh on well-developed bone structures. Good nutrition aids emotional adjustments, provides **stamina** (resistance to fatigue or illness), and promotes a healthy appetite. It also helps establish regular sleep and elimination habits (see Table 1-2).

MALNUTRITION

Malnutrition (poor nutrition) is a condition that results when the cells do not receive an adequate supply of the essential nutrients because of poor diet or poor utilization of food. Sometimes it occurs because people do not or cannot eat enough of the foods that provide the essential nutrients to satisfy body needs. Other times people may eat full, well-balanced diets, but suffer

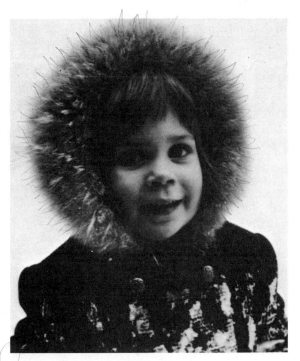 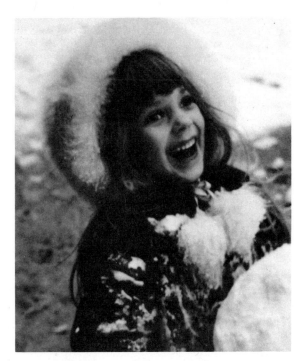

Figure 1-1 Good nutrition shows in the happy faces of these children.

from diseases that prevent normal usage of the nutrients. Drug therapy or surgery sometimes creates changes that prevent food from being used normally.

Some characteristics of malnutrition are: dull, lifeless hair; greasy, pimpled facial skin; dull eyes; slumped posture; fatigue and depression shown in spiritless expressions and behavior, figure 1-2. Malnourished persons may be underweight or overweight and skeletal growth may be stunted. Resistance to disease is reduced, and recovery from disease or surgery may be slower than in well-nourished people. Appetite may be poor or excessive, resulting in underweight or overweight. Sleep may be affected because malnutrition influences the nervous system, just as it affects all body systems. Irritability and nervousness may result. The attention span is reduced. **Constipation** is common. **Mental retardation,** disease, and even death can result from severe malnutrition.

Persons most prone to malnutrition are infants, preschool children, adolescents, the elderly, and pregnant women (especially if they are adolescents). If mothers do not know about proper nutrition, their children will suffer. Infants and preschool children depend on their mothers' selection of foods. Preschool children may face an additional hazard since they tend to be unusually particular about what they eat.

Adolescents may eat often, but at unusual hours. They may miss regularly scheduled meals, become hungry, and satisfy this hunger with snacks of essentially **empty calorie foods** such as potato chips, cakes, sodas, and candy. Empty calorie foods provide an abundance of calories, but the nutrients are primarily carbohydrates and fats and, except for sodium, very limited amounts of proteins, vitamins, and minerals. Adolescents are subject to **peer pressure;** that is, they are easily influenced by the opinions of their friends. If friends favor the empty calorie foods, it is

Health care prof: Needs sound knowledge of nut., aware of food fads etc...
2) May need to assess pt. trays on spec. diets.

Table 1-2 Characteristics of Nutritional Status

Good	Poor
Alert expression	Apathy
Shiny hair	Dull, lifeless hair
Clear complexion with good color	Greasy, blemished complexion with poor color
Bright, clear eyes	Dull, red-rimmed eyes
Pink, firm gums and well-developed teeth	Red, puffy, receding gums and missing or cavity-prone teeth
Firm abdomen	Swollen abdomen
Firm, well-developed muscles	Underdeveloped, flabby muscles
Well-developed bone structure	Bowed legs, "pigeon" breast
Normal weight for height	Over- or underweight
Erect posture	Slumped posture
Emotional stability	Easily irritated; depressed; poor attention span
Good stamina; seldom ill	Easily fatigued; frequently ill
Healthy appetite	Excessive or poor appetite
Healthy, normal sleep habits	Insomnia at night; fatigued during day
Normal elimination	Constipation or diarrhea

difficult for an adolescent to differ with them. Crash diets, which unfortunately are common among adolescents, sometime result in a form of malnutrition. This condition occurs because some essential nutrients are eliminated from the diet when the types of foods allowed are severely restricted.

Pregnancy increases a woman's appetite and the need for certain nutrients, especially proteins, minerals, and vitamins. Pregnancy during adolescence requires extreme care in food selection. The young mother-to-be requires a diet that provides sufficient nutrients for the developing fetus, as well as for her own still-growing body.

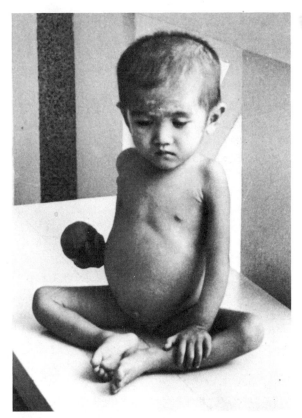

Figure 1-2 The poor quality hair, mottled complexion, dull expression, spindly arms and legs, and bloated stomach of this baby girl exemplify many signs of malnutrition. *(Courtesy of World Health Organization)*

The elderly are often alone and unwell. Their living conditions are not always conducive to forming a healthy appetite. Part of the joy of eating is sharing one's food in pleasant company. Lack of companionship or illness can make eating unpleasant and difficult.

CUMULATIVE EFFECTS OF NUTRITION

There is an increasing concern among health professionals regarding the *cumulative effects* of nutrition. Cumulative effects are the results of something that is done repeatedly over many years. For example, eating excessive amounts of saturated fats (saturated fats are discussed in Chapter 4) for many years is believed to be a major contributor to **atherosclerosis** which leads to heart attacks (see Chapter 20). Years of overeating can, of course, cause **obesity** (excessive weight), but may also contribute to **hypertension** (high blood pressure), diabetes mellitus, gallbladder disease, foot problems, and even personality disorders.

Deficiency Diseases

When essential nutrients are seriously lacking in the diet for an extended period, **deficiency diseases** can occur. The most common form of deficiency disease in the United States is **nutritional anemia,** which is caused by a lack of the mineral **iron** (see Chapter 7). Nutritional anemia is particularly common among children and women of all ages. Iron is a necessary component of the blood and is lost during each menstrual period. In addition, the amount of iron needed during childhood and pregnancy is greater than normal because of the growth of the child or the fetus.

Rickets is another example of deficiency disease. It causes poor bone formation in children and is due to insufficient calcium and vitamin D. These same deficiencies in adults are thought to contribute to **osteoporosis,** a condition that causes bones to become excessively brittle. Too little iodine may cause **goiter,** and a severe shortage of vitamin A can lead to blindness.

Examples of other deficiency diseases (and their causes) are included in Table 1-3. Information concerning these conditions can be found in the chapters devoted to the given nutrients.

That old saying, "You are what you eat," is true, indeed; but one could change it a bit to read, "You are *and will be* what you eat."

Table 1-3 Nutritional Deficiency Diseases and their Causes

Deficiency Disease	Nutrient(s) Lacking
Anemia	Iron
Beriberi	Thiamin
Blindness	Vitamin A
Goiter	Iodine
Kwashiorkor	Protein
Marasmus	All nutrients
Osteomalacia	Vitamin D and Calcium
Osteoporosis	Vitamin D and Calcium
Pellagra	Niacin
Rickets	Vitamin D and Calcium
Scurvy	Vitamin C
Xerophthalmia	Vitamin A

members and friends who know that the health professional has studied nutrition will ask questions. Anyone, in fact, who plans and prepares meals should value and have knowledge of sound nutritional practice and be able to apply the principles of it.

Patients will have questions and complaints about their diets. Their anxieties can be relieved by clear and simple explanations provided by the health professional. Sometimes patients must undergo **diet therapy,** which means their medical treatment includes eating prescribed foods in specified amounts. The health professional must be able to check the patient's tray quickly to see that it contains the correct foods for the diet prescribed. In many cases, diet therapy will have to be a lifelong practice for the patient. In such cases, eating habits will require change and the patient will be especially in need of advice and support from the health professional.

Nutrition is currently a popular subject. It is important to recognize that some of the books and articles in the press concerning nutrition may not be scientifically correct. Also, food ads can be misleading. People with knowledge of sound nutritional practices will not be misled. They will recognize fad and distinguish it from fact.

CONSIDERATIONS FOR THE HEALTH CARE PROFESSIONAL

The practice of good nutritional habits would help eliminate many health problems caused by malnutrition. The health professional is obligated to have a sound knowledge of nutrition. One's personal health, as well as that of one's family, depends on it. Parents must have a good, basic knowledge of nutrition for the sake of their personal health and that of their children. Children learn by imitating their parents. Family

SUMMARY

Nutrition is directly related to health, and its effects are cumulative. Good nutrition is normally reflected by good health, figure 1-3. Poor nutrition can result in poor health and even disease. It is thought that poor nutritional habits contribute to atherosclerosis, osteoporosis, and certain cases of diabetes mellitus in later life.

To be well nourished, one must eat foods that contain the six essential nutrients: carbohydrates, fats, proteins, minerals, vitamins, and wa-

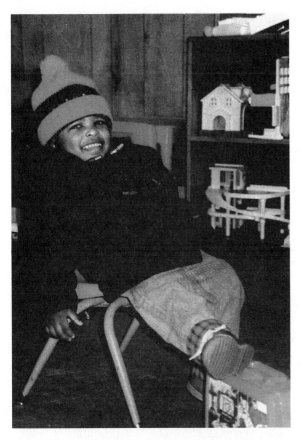

Figure 1-3 Good health radiates from this young man.

ter. These nutrients provide the body with energy and heat, build and repair body tissue, and regulate body processes. When there is a severe lack of specific nutrients, deficiency diseases may develop.

With a sound knowledge of nutrition, the health professional will be a more effective professional and will also be helpful to family, friends, and self.

Prenatal vits = vit, min + Proteins = Needed in preg

Discussion Topics

1. Why is eating pleasant?
2. What is the relationship of nutrition and heredity to each of the following?
   a. the development of physique
   b. the ability to resist disease
   c. the lifespan
3. How may nutritional status affect personality?
4. What health habits, in addition to good nutrition, contribute to making a person healthy?
5. What are the six essential nutrients? What are their three basic functions?
6. Why are women prone to iron deficiency?

7. Why are some foods called empty calorie foods? Give examples of these foods.
8. If anyone in the class has been on a crash diet to lose weight, discuss the diet's effects on the individual and suggest reasons for these effects.
9. What is meant by the saying, "You are what you eat?"
10. Why are people in the following age groups sometimes prone to malnutrition?
    a. young children
    b. adolescents
    c. the elderly
11. Discuss the cumulative effects of nutrition.
12. How could someone be overweight and at the same time suffer from malnutrition?
13. If anyone in class has seen someone suffering from malnutrition, ask for a description. Discuss possible reasons for this malnutrition.
14. Discuss why sales clerks in health food stores may not provide customers nutritionally accurate information concerning the store's products.
15. Discuss why health care professionals should be knowledgeable about nutrition.

Suggested Activities

1. List ten signs of good nutrition and ten signs of poor nutrition.
2. Write an essay discussing your personal nutrition. List possible improvements.
3. List the foods you have eaten in the past 24 hours. Underline the empty calorie foods.
4. Write a brief description of how you feel at the end of a day when you know you have not eaten wisely.
5. Write sentences using all of the words in the vocabulary list correctly. Read them to the class and discuss them.
6. Bring in articles on nutrition that you have found in newspapers and magazines and discuss why they may not be scientifically correct.
7. Find examples of ads for certain foods and explain why they might be misleading as to the nutrient content of the foods.
8. Using information in the chapters that discuss specific nutrients (or using other nutrition textbooks), write brief descriptions of each of the deficiency diseases listed in Table 1-3. Include prevention, symptoms, treatment, and long-term outcome.
9. Browse through the magazines at the local newsstand. Count the number of articles on nutrition. Read one or two and evaluate them.

10. Observe television ads for food products. Keep a log of those that are misleading and/or factually inaccurate.
11. Write the manufacturer of a food product used in your home. Ask for nutrition information on that product.

Review

carb, fats, prot., vits, min, H₂O

preg: Prot., min., vits

A. Multiple choice. Select the *letter* that precedes the best answer.

1. The result of those processes whereby the body takes in and uses food for growth, development, and maintenance of health is called
   a. respiration   c. nutrition
   b. diet therapy   d. digestion

2. Nutritional status is determined by
   a. heredity   c. personality
   b. employment   d. diet

3. To nourish the body adequately, one must
   a. avoid all empty calorie foods   c. include fats at every meal
   b. eat foods containing the six   d. restrict proteins at breakfast
      essential nutrients

4. Nutrients used primarily to provide heat and energy to the body are
   a. vitamins and water   c. proteins and vitamins
   b. carbohydrates and fats   d. vitamins and minerals

5. Nutrients used mainly to build and repair body tissues are
   a. proteins, vitamins, and   c. fats and water
      minerals   d. iron and fats
   b. carbohydrates and fats

6. Foods such as potato chips, cakes, sodas, and candy are called
   a. dietetic foods   c. empty calorie foods
   b. essential nutrient foods d. nutritious foods

7. An inadequate supply of essential nutrients in the diet may result in
   a. stamina   c. indigestion
   b. malnutrition   d. diabetes

8. Nutritional anemia is caused by a lack of → Fe
   a. proteins   c. vitamins
   b. carbohydrates   d. iron

9. The cumulative effect of a high-fat diet could be
   a. iron deficiency   c. heart disease
   b. blindness   d. diabetes mellitus

10. Malnutrition could be caused by
    a. poor posture   c. disease or drug therapy
    b. constipation   d. hypertension

B.   Match the term in Column I with its definition in Column II.

Column I	Column II
e 1. carbohydrates and fats	a. high blood pressure
j 2. proteins	b. with few nutrients
h 3. vitamins and minerals	c. in deficient amounts causes anemia
k 4. fatigue	d. repeated
b 5. empty calories	e. primary source of human energy
d 6. cumulative	f. resistance to disease
a 7. hypertension	g. deficiency disease
g 8. nutritional anemia	h. regulate body functions
c 9. iron	i. peer pressure
f 10. stamina	j. build and repair tissue
	k. possible symptom of malnutrition
	l. iodine

Case Study 1

The Relationship of Food and Health

Joan D. is an 85-year-old widow who has lived alone in her home since her husband, David, died last year. She and David had two children, both of whom live several hundred miles away. She had always been an excellent homemaker and frequently invited friends in for meals.

For the past four to six months, however, she seemed to her friends to be "slipping." She was forgetful and appeared to be losing weight. They also noticed that she sometimes was dressed in her soiled "cleaning day" clothes when they saw her at the local grocery store. She has not invited anyone for a meal since David's funeral.

Her neighbor convinced her to see her doctor. The doctor suggested that Joan D. enter the local "home" for the elderly, but Joan refused. The doctor then told her a public health nurse would visit her and arrange for Meals-on-Wheels to bring a hot meal to her daily. A vitamin was prescribed and Joan agreed to the treatment plan.

A referral was made to the Public Health Agency requesting that the nurse provide nutritional counseling, assessment of the home environment, and a plan for the involvement of support people in Joan's life.

Within a month, Joan's concerned neighbor was assisting Joan in grocery shopping for breakfasts and weekends. The public health nurse filled a seven-day individual compartment pill box with vitamin pills and found Joan only occasionally missed taking a pill. A personal care aide was assisting Joan with grooming and household chores. Joan was less forgetful, her grooming improved, and her weight stabilized.

Case Study Questions Based on the Nursing Process

Assess
1. What are some possible reasons why Joan seemed to be slipping?
2. What questions did the doctor probably ask her?

Plan
3. Why would the doctor suggest Joan participate in Meals-on-Wheels?
4. Why would the doctor prescribe a daily vitamin pill for Joan?

Implement
5. What did the public health nurse do to help Joan follow her medical regimen?

Evaluate
6. What may have contributed to Joan's improvement?
7. What might have been the effects of a nursing home on Joan had she consented to move to one?

Case Study 2

The Need for Nutrition Education

Six-year-old Joey was a lively little boy who lived with his mother and grandfather. His mother was a secretary and was away from home between 8:00 A.M. and 6:00 P.M. Joey did not mind because his grandfather was there, walked him to and from school, and cared for him.

On the way to school, the two of them would stop at the corner convenience store and buy Joey's lunch. His favorite lunch was fruit punch, potato chips, a banana, and a chocolate bar. One hot day, the banana got soft and, since that time, Joey just threw all the bananas in the garbage.

By early October, his teacher called his mother and said Joey was falling asleep in the afternoons and didn't want to play during the play period. The teacher asked the mother to come to school early one morning so they could discuss these problems.

Case Study Questions Based on the Nursing Process

Assess
1.   What may have caused Joey to fall asleep in the afternoons?
2.   Why might the grandfather have purchased such lunches for Joey?

Plan
3.   If you were Joey's teacher, how would you start the discussion with his mother about the lunches?
4.   What written information about nutrition would you review with Joey's mother? What might you suggest regarding his lunches?

Implement
5.   What possible problems could the call from his teacher cause at home? How could they be avoided?
6.   Was it wise for the teacher to suggest a meeting with Joey's mother to discuss the problem rather than discussing it over the telephone? Why?

Evaluate
7.   What would the teacher observe in order to evaluate the effectiveness of the teaching done?

CHAPTER 2

VOCABULARY

absorption	hyperthyroidism
adipose tissue	hypothyroidism
anabolism	ileum
basal metabolic	jejunum
rate (BMR)	kilocalorie (kcal)
bile	kilojoule
body	Krebs cycle
bolus	lactase
caloric density	lacteals
calorie	lean body mass
calorimeter	maltase
capillaries	mechanical digestion
carboxypeptidases	metabolism
catabolism	oxidation
chemical digestion	pancreas
chyme	pancreatic amylase
chymotrypsin	pancreatic lipase
dietary fiber	(steapsin)
digestion	pancreatic proteases
duodenum	pepsin
emulsified fat	peptidases
energy balance	peristalsis
energy requirement	ptyalin
energy value	pylorus
enzymes	rennin
esophagus	resting energy
fatty acids	expenditure (REE)
feces	saliva
food residue	salivary amylase
fundus (of stomach)	sucrase
gastric juices	thyroid gland
gastric lipase	thyroxine (T_4)
gastrointestinal	triiodothyronine (T_3)
(digestive) system	trypsin
hormones	villi
hydrochloric acid	
hydrolysis	

THE BODY'S USE OF NUTRIENTS

OBJECTIVES

After studying this chapter, you should be able to
- Describe the processes of digestion, absorption, and metabolism
- Name the organs in the digestive system and describe their functions
- Name the enzymes or digestive juices secreted by each organ and gland in the digestive system
- Describe the function of the thyroid gland
- Calculate your basal metabolic rate (BMR)

Although the body is infinitely more complex than the automobile engine, it may be compared to the engine because both require fuel to run. The body's fuel is, of course, food. For the body to use its fuel, the food must first be prepared by the body and appropriately distributed. This is done through the processes of digestion and absorption. The actual use of the food as fuel, resulting in energy, is called **metabolism.**

DIGESTION

The body's preparation of its food begins with **digestion.** Digestion is the process whereby food is broken down into smaller parts, chemically changed, and moved through the gastrointestinal system. The **gastrointestinal** or **digestive system** consists of the body structures that participate in digestion. It begins with the mouth and ends with the anus. As the process of digestion is discussed, refer to figure 2-1 and note the locations of the structures that perform the functions of digestion.

Digestion occurs through two types of action—mechanical and chemical. During **mechanical digestion,** food is broken up by the teeth. It is then moved along the gastrointestinal tract through the esophagus, stomach, and intestines. This movement is caused by a rhythmic

mouth = mech + chem dig

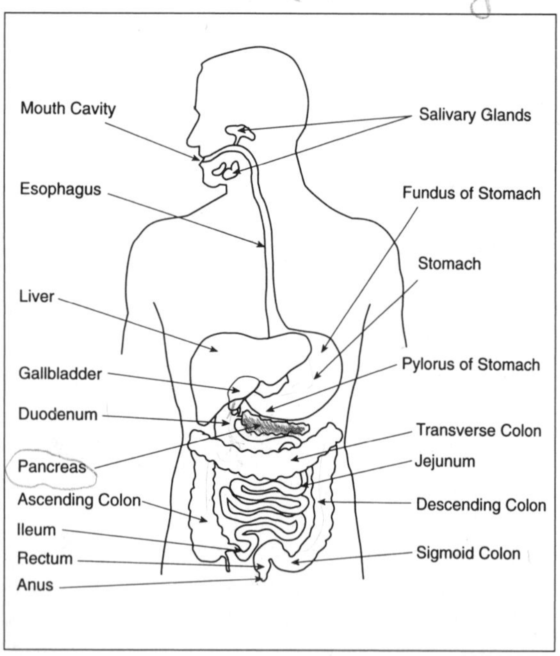

Figure 2-1 The digestive system

contraction of the muscular walls of the tract called **peristalsis.**

During **chemical digestion,** the composition of food is changed. Chemical changes occur through the addition of water, and the resulting splitting, or breaking down of the food molecules. This process is called **hydrolysis.** Food is broken down into nutrients that the tissues can absorb and use. Hydrolysis also involves **enzymes,** which are organic substances that cause chemical changes in other substances. Digestive enzymes are secreted by the mouth, stomach, **pancreas,** and the small intestine (see Table 2-1). An enzyme is often named for the substance on which it acts. For example, the enzyme **sucrase** acts on sucrose, the enzyme **maltase** acts on maltose, and **lactase** acts on lactose.

Enzymes end in ase

Digestion in the Mouth

Digestion begins in the mouth where the food is broken up by the teeth and mixed with saliva, figure 2-2. At this point, each mouthful of food that is ready to be swallowed is called a **bolus. Saliva** is a secretion of the salivary glands that contains a digestive enzyme called **ptyalin** (also called **salivary amylase),** which acts on starch. However, because food is normally held in the mouth for such a short time, little starch is chemically changed there. The final chemical digestion of starch occurs in the small intestine.

in the blood

Digestion in the Stomach

Peristalsis and gravity transfer food from the mouth to the stomach via the esophagus. The **esophagus** is the tube connecting the mouth and the stomach. The stomach has three main functions in digestion. It serves to

- temporarily store food
- mix food with gastric juices
- provide a slow, controlled emptying of food into the small intestine

digst in mouth? Test ??
– mech.
– chem
or
– Both
?

Table 2-1 Enzymes and Foods Acted Upon

Source	Enzyme	Food Acted Upon
Mouth	Ptyalin	Starch
Stomach	Pepsin	Proteins
	Rennin	Proteins in milk
	Gastric lipase	Emulsified fat
Small Intestine	Pancreatic amylase	Starch
	Pancreatic proteases	Proteins
	(trypsin)	
	(chymotrypsin)	
	(carboxypeptidases)	
	Pancreatic lipase	Fats
	(steapsin)	
	Lactase	Lactose
	Maltase	Maltose
	Sucrase	Sucrose
	Peptidases	Proteins

The stomach consists of the upper portion known as the **fundus,** the middle area known as the **body,** and the end nearest the intestine called the **pylorus.**

Food accumulates in the fundus and moves to the body where it mixes with the gastric juices. **Gastric juices** are digestive secretions of the stomach. The gastric juices contain hydrochloric acid and the enzymes, pepsin and gastric lipase. **Hydrochloric acid** breaks the food down so the enzymes can work on the food, helps to dissolve some minerals, and destroys much of the bacteria present on food. **Pepsin** breaks proteins into smaller forms. In children, there is an additional enzyme, **rennin,** which acts on the protein in milk. **Gastric lipase** acts on emulsified fats such as are found in cream and egg yolk. An **emulsified fat** is a fat finely divided and held in suspension by another liquid.

Digestion in the Small Intestine

After the food has been thoroughly mixed with gastric juices, it becomes a semiliquid mass called **chyme** (pronounced kime). In this form it moves through the pylorus by peristalsis into the **duodenum,** the first section of the small intestine. Chyme subsequently passes through the **jejunum,** the midsection of the small intestine, and the **ileum,** the last section of the small intestine.

When food reaches the small intestine, the gallbladder is triggered into releasing a substance called **bile.** Bile is produced in the liver but stored in the gallbladder. Bile emulsifies fat after it is secreted into the small intestine. This action enables the enzymes to digest the fats more easily.

Chyme also triggers the pancreas to secrete its juice into the small intestine. Juice secreted

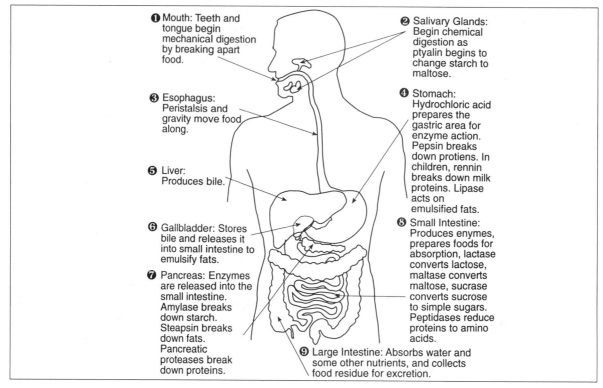

❶ Mouth: Teeth and tongue begin mechanical digestion by breaking apart food.

❷ Salivary Glands: Begin chemical digestion as ptyalin begins to change starch to maltose.

❸ Esophagus: Peristalsis and gravity move food along.

❹ Stomach: Hydrochloric acid prepares the gastric area for enzyme action. Pepsin breaks down protiens. In children, rennin breaks down milk proteins. Lipase acts on emulsified fats.

❺ Liver: Produces bile.

❻ Gallbladder: Stores bile and releases it into small intestine to emulsify fats.

❼ Pancreas: Enzymes are released into the small intestine. Amylase breaks down starch. Steapsin breaks down fats. Pancreatic proteases break down proteins.

❽ Small Intestine: Produces enymes, prepares foods for absorption, lactase converts lactose, maltase converts maltose, sucrase converts sucrose to simple sugars. Peptidases reduce proteins to amino acids.

❾ Large Intestine: Absorbs water and some other nutrients, and collects food residue for excretion.

Figure 2-2 Basic functions of the digestive system

from the pancreas contains the following enzymes:

- **Trypsin, chymotrypsin,** and **carboxypeptidases,** which split proteins into smaller substances. These are called **pancreatic proteases** because they are protein-splitting enzymes produced by the pancreas.
- **Pancreatic amylase,** which converts starches (polysaccharides) to simple sugars.
- **Pancreatic lipase (steapsin),** reduces fats to fatty acids and glycerol.

The small intestine itself produces an intestinal juice that contains the enzymes **lactase, maltase,** and **sucrase.** These enzymes split lactose, maltose, and sucrose, respectively into simple sugars. The small intestine also produces enzymes called **peptidases** that break down proteins into amino acids.

ABSORPTION

After digestion, the next major step in the body's preparation of its food is absorption. **Absorption** is the passage of nutrients into the body fluids and tissues. To be absorbed, nutrients must be in their simplest forms. Carbohydrates must be broken down to the simple sugars (glucose, fructose, and galactose), proteins to amino acids, and fats to fatty acids and glycerol. Most absorption of nutrients occurs in the small intestine, although some occurs in the large intestine. Wa-

Nut = Dig.
Absorb
Metab

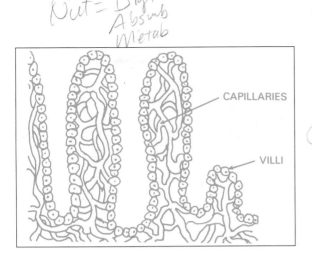

Figure 2-3 Wall of the small intestine

ter is absorbed in the mouth, stomach, small intestine, and large intestine.

Absorption in the Small Intestine

The small intestine is approximately twenty-two feet long. Its inner surface contains many fingerlike projections called **villi,** figure 2-3. Each villus contains numerous blood **capillaries** (tiny blood vessels) and **lacteals** (lymphatic vessels). The villi absorb nutrients from the chyme by way of these blood capillaries and lacteals which eventually transfer them to the bloodstream. Glucose, fructose, galactose, amino acids, minerals, and water-soluble vitamins are absorbed by the capillaries. Fructose and galactose are subsequently carried to the liver where they are converted to glucose. Lacteals absorb glycerol and **fatty acids** (end products of fat digestion), in addition to the fat-soluble vitamins.

Absorption in the Large Intestine

When the chyme reaches the large intestine, most digestion and absorption (except of water) have already occurred. However, some digestive juices are carried into the large intestine in the chyme where they continue their work for a time.

The major tasks of the large intestine are to absorb water and collect **food residue.** Food residue is that part of food which body enzyme action cannot digest and consequently cannot absorb. Such residue is commonly called **dietary fiber.** Examples include the outer hulls of corn kernels and grains of wheat, celery strings, and apple skins. It is important that the diet contain some fiber since it promotes the health of the large intestine by helping to produce softer stools and more frequent bowel movements. (See Chapter 3.)

Undigested food is excreted as **feces** by way of the rectum. In healthy people, 99 percent of carbohydrates, 95 percent of fat, and 92 percent of protein is absorbed.

METABOLISM

build up + break down of substances - Occurs p absorbtion

After digestion and absorption, nutrients are carried by the blood to the cells of the body. Within the cells, nutrients are changed into energy through a complex process called metabolism. During metabolism, nutrients are combined with oxygen within each cell. This is known as **oxidation.** Oxidation ultimately reduces carbohydrates and fats to carbon dioxide and water; proteins are reduced to carbon dioxide, water, and nitrogen. The complete oxidation of carbohydrates, proteins, and fats is commonly called the **Krebs cycle.**

As nutrients are oxidized, energy and its byproduct, heat, are released. When this released energy is used to build new substances from simpler ones, the process is called **anabolism.** *(new)* An example of anabolism is the formation of new body tissues. When released energy is used to reduce substances to simpler ones, the process is called **catabolism.** This building up and breaking down of substances (metabolism) is a continuous process within the body and requires a continuous supply of nutrients.

anabolism + catabolism = metabolism
+ O₂ = Oxidation

Metabolism and the Thyroid Gland

Metabolism is governed primarily by the **hormones** secreted by the **thyroid gland.** These secretions are **triiodothyronine (T_3)** and **thyroxine (T_4).** When the thyroid gland secretes too much of these hormones, a condition known as **hyperthyroidism** may result. In such a case, the body metabolizes its food too quickly, and weight is lost. When too little thyroxine and T_3 are secreted, the condition called **hypothyroidism** may occur. In this case, the body metabolizes food too slowly and the patient tends to become sluggish and accumulates fat.

Beg. dipper for each person.

ENERGY

come from CARBS, Fats ~ Prot.

Energy is constantly needed for the maintenance of body tissue and temperature and for growth (involuntary activity), as well as for voluntary activity. Examples of voluntary activity include walking, swimming, eating, reading, typing, etc. The three groups of nutrients that provide energy to the body are carbohydrates, fats, and proteins. Carbohydrates are and should be the primary energy source. (See Chapter 3.)

Energy Measurement

1 Kcal = 4.2 Kilojoule

The unit used to measure the energy value of foods is the **kilocalorie** or **kcal,** commonly known as the large calorie or **calorie.** In the metric system it is known as the **kilojoule.** One kcal is equal to 4.184 kilojoules, but this may be rounded off to 4.2 kilojoules. A kcal is the amount of heat needed to raise the temperature of one kilogram of water one degree Celsius (C).

Same thing

The number of kcal in a food is its **energy value** or **caloric density.** Energy values of foods vary a great deal because they are determined by the types and amounts of nutrients each food contains.

One gram of carbohydrate yields 4 kcal (17 kilojoules); one gram of protein yields 4 kcal (17 kilojoules); and one gram of fat yields 9 kcal (38 kilojoules). One gram of alcohol yields 7 kcal (29 kilojoules).

The energy values of foods are determined by a device known as a **calorimeter.** The inner part of a calorimeter holds a measured amount of food and the outer part holds water. The food is burned, and its caloric value is determined by the increase in the temperature of the surrounding water. The number of kcal in average servings of common foods are listed in Table A-5 of the Appendix.

Basal Metabolic Rate

(REE 'new' term)
BMR = REE

The rate at which energy is needed only for body maintenance is called the **basal metabolic rate (BMR).** The BMR may be referred to as the **resting energy expenditure (REE).**

Medical tests can determine one's BMR (or REE). When such a test is given, the body is at rest and performing only the essential, involuntary functions. Respiration, circulation, cell activity, and maintenance of temperature are examples of these functions. Voluntary activity is not measured in a BMR test. Factors that affect one's BMR are lean body mass, size, sex, age, heredity, physical condition, and climate.

Lean body mass is muscle as opposed to fat tissue. Because there is more metabolic activity in muscle tissue than in fat or bone tissue, muscle tissue requires more kcal than does fat or bone tissue. People with large body frames require more kcal than do people with small frames because the former have more body mass to maintain and move than do those with small frames.

Men usually require more energy than women. They tend to be larger and to have more lean body mass than women do.

Children require more kcal per pound of body weight than adults because they are growing. As people age, the lean body mass declines and the basal metabolic rate declines according-

1 Kcal = 4.2 Kilojoule

ly. Heredity is also a determining factor. One's BMR may resemble one's parent's, just as one's appearance may. One's physical condition also affects the BMR. For example, women require more kcal during pregnancy and lactation than at other times. The basal metabolic rate increases during fever and decreases during periods of starvation or severely reduced kcal intake. People living and working in extremely cold or warm climates require more kcal to maintain normal body temperature than they would in a more temperate climate.

Estimating BMR

To estimate one's basal metabolic rate or REE:

1. Convert body weight from pounds to kilograms (kg) by dividing pounds by 2.2 (2.2 pounds equal one kilogram).
2. Multiply the kilograms by 24 (hours per day).
3. Multiply the answer obtained in Number 2 above by 0.9 for a woman and by 1.0 for a man.

For example, assume a woman weighs 110 pounds. Divide 110 by 2.2 for an answer of 50 kg. Multiply 50 kg by 24 hours in a day for an answer of 1200 kcal. Then multiply 1200 kcal by 0.9 for an answer of 1080 kcal. This is the estimated basal metabolic energy requirement for that particular woman.

Calculating Total Energy Requirements

An individual's average daily **energy requirement** is the total number of kcal needed in a 24-hour period. Energy requirements of people differ, depending on basal metabolic rate or REE and activities. Someone recuperating from a broken leg requires fewer kcal than normal, largely because of reduced activity. More energy is burned playing soccer than playing the piano. Some examples of energy requirements for various categories of activities are shown in Table 2-2. In this table, the BMR is referred to as the REE.

To determine one's total energy requirement, one must first calculate one's REE, determine the appropriate activity category, and then multiply the REE by the number given for that category. It is important to remember that these are, at best, only estimates.

Energy Balance

A person who takes in fewer nutrients than she or he burns usually loses weight. If someone takes in more nutrients than she or he burns, the body stores them as **adipose tissue** (fat). Some adipose tissue is necessary to protect the body and support its organs. Adipose tissue also helps regulate body temperature, just as insulation helps regulate the temperature of a building. An excess of adipose tissue, however, leads to obesity, which can endanger health because it puts extra burdens on body organs and systems. For the healthy person, the goal is **energy balance.** This means that the number of kcal consumed matches the number of kcal required for body maintenance and activity.

The Food and Nutrition Board of the National Research Council has made recommendations of energy intakes that meet the average needs of people in categories based on age, sex, weight, height, and estimated REE. (See Table 2-3.)

CONSIDERATIONS FOR THE HEALTH CARE PROFESSIONAL

The health care professional probably will find that patients have little factual information

Table 2-2 Approximate Energy Expenditure for Various Activities in Relation to Resting Needs for Males and Females of Average Size[a]

Activity Category[b]	Representative Value for Activity Factor per Unit Time of Activity
Resting Sleeping, reclining	REE × 1.0
Very light Seated and standing activities, painting trades, driving, laboratory work, typing, sewing, ironing, cooking, playing cards, playing a musical instrument	REE × 1.5
Light Walking on a level surface at 2.5 to 3 mph, garage work, electrical trades, carpentry, restaurant trades, house-cleaning, child care, golf, sailing, table tennis	REE × 2.5
Moderate Walking 3.5 to 4 mph, weeding and hoeing, carrying a load, cycling, skiing, tennis, dancing	REE × 5.0
Heavy Walking with load uphill, tree felling, heavy manual digging, basketball, climbing, football, soccer	REE × 7.0

[a] Based on values reported by Durnin and Passmore (1967) and WHO (1985).
[b] When reported as multiples of basal needs, the expenditures of males and females are similar.
Recommended Dietary Allowances 10th Edition.
National Academy Press, Washington, D.C., 1989.

about digestion and metabolism. At the same time, patients may have very strongly held beliefs about these functions.

Many will say, "I can't digest that" regarding specific foods, but will, in fact, not know what occurs during digestion. Some will insist their metabolism is low and is the cause of their extra weight when, in reality, they simply overeat. Others will say they "eat" too many kcal and are, thus, overweight.

The health care professional will need a great deal of patience as he or she educates patients about digestion and metabolism. Creative presentation of the information will motivate patients to learn and remember it.

SUMMARY

The body is comparable to an automobile engine because it too requires fuel. Food acts as the fuel but, to be usable, it must undergo a series of processes which include digestion, absorption, and metabolism. Digestion is the process whereby food is broken down into smaller parts, chemically changed, and moved along the gastrointestinal tract. Mechanical digestion refers to that part of the process performed by the teeth and muscles of the digestive system. Chemical digestion refers to that part of the process wherein food is broken down to nutrients that the blood can absorb. Enzymes are essential for chemical

Table 2-3 Median Heights and Weights and Recommended Energy Intake

Category	Age (years) or Condition	Weight (kg)	Weight (lb)	Height (cm)	Height (in)	REE (kcal/day)	Multiples of REE	Average Energy Allowance (kcal) Per kg	Average Energy Allowance (kcal) Per day
Infants	0.0–0.5	6	13	60	24	320		108	650
	0.5–1.0	9	20	71	28	500		98	850
Children	1–3	13	29	90	35	740		102	1,300
	4–6	20	44	112	44	950		90	1,800
	7–10	28	62	132	52	1,130		70	2,000
Males	11–14	45	99	157	62	1,440	1.70	55	2,500
	15–18	66	145	176	69	1,760	1.67	45	3,000
	19–24	72	160	177	70	1,780	1.67	40	2,900
	25–50	79	174	176	70	1,800	1.60	37	2,900
	51+	77	170	173	68	1,530	1.50	30	2,300
Females	11–14	46	101	157	62	1,310	1.67	47	2,200
	15–18	55	120	163	64	1,370	1.60	40	2,200
	19–24	58	128	164	65	1,350	1.60	38	2,200
	25–50	63	138	163	64	1,380	1.55	36	2,200
	51+	65	143	160	63	1,280	1.50	30	1,900
Pregnant	1st trimester								+0
	2nd trimester								+300
	3rd trimester								+300
Lactating	1st 6 months								+500
	2nd 6 months								+500

Recommended Dietary Allowances 10th Edition.
National Academy Press, Washington, D.C., 1989.

digestion. Following digestion, food is absorbed by the blood, primarily in the small intestine, and then carried to all body tissues. After absorption, food is metabolized. During metabolism, food is combined with oxygen in a process called oxidation. Energy released during oxidation is measured by the kcal or kilojoule. Kcal values of foods vary as do people's energy requirements. Requirements depend on age, size, sex, lean body mass, physical condition, climate, and activity.

Discussion Topics

1. Describe the process of digestion.
2. Of what value are enzymes to digestion? Name five enzymes and the nutrients on which they act.
3. Describe absorption of nutrients.
4. Of what value is fiber in the diet? What are some examples of foods that provide it?
5. Describe metabolism.
6. What is the BMR? If anyone in the class has undergone a BMR test, ask her or him to describe it.
7. Explain why the body requires food even during sleep.
8. Why is it incorrect to say, "He ate 2000 kcal today"? What did he eat? What are kcal? What are kilojoules? How are they comparable?
9. Explain the differences between the terms *energy value* and *energy requirement*.
10. What does it mean to be overweight? What is a common cause of overweight? What reasons do people give for being overweight? How can one prevent excessive weight gain? How might overweight people reduce? How may overweight endanger health?

Suggested Activities

1. Trace figure 2-1. On the traced figure, insert the names of the body structures without referring to the original illustration.
2. Using the method for calculating a person's minimum caloric requirement as given in this chapter, calculate your minimum caloric requirement. Convert it to kilojoules.
3. As a class, use Table 2-3, and Table A-5 (in the Appendix), and plan a menu for one day that would satisfy the caloric requirement of a 40-year-old woman who weighs 138 pounds.
4. Adapt the preceding menu to the needs of a 22-year-old man who weighs 160 pounds.
5. Using Table 2-3, and Table A-5 (in the Appendix), compile a list of foods, especially vegetables, fruits, milk, eggs, and meat, that would satisfy the daily caloric requirement of a woman who is nursing her baby. She is 30 years old and weighs 138 pounds. Compute the grams of protein included.
6. Adapt the preceding menu to the needs of the woman after weaning her baby.
7. Write the definitions for the vocabulary words.

Review

A. Complete the following statements.

1. Food is broken down for body use during the process known as ___ _digestion_ .

2. Food is combined with oxygen during the process called _oxidation_

3. The tube connecting the mouth and the stomach is the _esophagus_

4. The two kinds of digestive action are _mech._ and _chem._ .

5. The rhythmic contraction of the muscular walls of the digestive tract is called _peristalsis_ .

6. Protease, lipase, and amylase are examples of _enzymes_ .

7. Saliva contains the digestive enzyme called _ptalin_ .

8. Hydrochloric acid, pepsin, and rennin are all secretions of the _stomach_ .

9. The semiliquid mass of food that has been mixed with gastric juices is called _chyme_ .

_p.J.18_   10. The passage of nutrients into the body fluids and tissues is called _absorption_ .

11. Metabolism is primarily governed by the secretions of the ___ _(Hormones T3 T4) thyroid gland_ .

12. The unit used to measure the fuel value of food is the _Kcal_ or the _Kilojoule_ .

✳13. The average daily total of kcal needed by an individual is called the _energy requirement_ .

✳14. The number of kcal in a food is its _energy value OR caloric density_ .

✳15. The rate of energy that is needed just for body maintenance is called the _BMR or REE_ .

Digest → Absorb → metabolize

chem. digestion + H₂O = Hydrolysis
Hydrolysis involves ENZYMES

Enzymes secreted by mouth, stomach, pancreas, sml. intest.

digest starch 1ST mouth THEN sml. intest.
(+ absorbed by blood.)

1 gm carb = 4 kcal
1 gm Prot = 4 kcal
1 gm fat = 9 kcal !
1 gm alcohol = 7 kcal

B.   Label the structures on the following diagram.

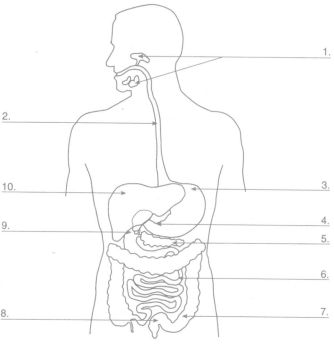

1.

2.

10.

3.

9.

4.

5.

6.

8.

7.

C.   In the space opposite each enzyme or secretion, name the structure that secretes it.

1.   ptyalin   _____

2.   hydrochloric acid   _____

3.   pepsin   _____

4.   rennin   _____

5.   trypsin   _____

6.   steapsin   _____

7.   lactase   _____

8.   maltase   _____

9.   peptidases   _____

10. bile   _____

D.   Briefly answer the following questions.

1.   Name the three steps in estimating an individual's BMR.

2.   Where does most absorption of nutrients take place?

3.   What is energy balance?

Case Study 1

Abnormal Metabolic Rate

Sally K. is a 5′6″ 35-year-old secretary who spends most of her time at her desk. She knows that her sedentary job is not conducive to good health, so she normally exercises three times a week at a health club. In addition, she eats healthfully and has easily maintained her weight at 120 pounds since she was 18.

Recently, however, she has begun to notice her waistbands growing tight, and her weight has crept up to 130 pounds. In addition, she has felt unusually tired and has sometimes skipped her exercise sessions after work. The only change in her eating habits is that she sometimes falls asleep in her easy chair after work, not waking until midnight or after and thus, skips dinner.

After visiting her physician, she learned that she has a glandular problem that can be treated with medication.

Case Study Questions Based on the Nursing Process

Assess
1. What gland is probably directly involved in Sally's condition?
2. Is this gland probably underactive or overactive?
3. Describe a "sedentary" job.

Plan
4. According to the height-weight chart on page 23, was Sally's weight of 120 pounds appropriate for her height and age?
5. What might cause Sally to gain weight even though she sometimes skips dinner?

Implement
6. Will she continue to gain weight after she starts taking medication?

Evaluate
7. What blood work will the doctor periodically order to monitor Sally's glandular problem?
8. Will her energy and activity level change after she takes her medication? Explain.

Case Study 2

On New Year's Day, Marion promised herself that she would lose 15 pounds before July 4. She was 15 years old, 5'4" tall, and weighed 120 pounds. She had learned how to estimate her resting energy expenditure (REE) in her nutrition class and decided she would lose those pounds by simply limiting her daily kcal intake to the amount of her REE, as she had determined it to be.

Case Study Questions Based on the Nursing Process

Assess
1. Was this a wise decision? Explain.
2. If Marion had weighed 135 pounds, would this have been a wise decision? Explain.

Plan
3. If Marion, at 120 pounds, were your friend and asked for your opinion of her plan, what would you tell her? Why?
4. How would you advise Marion if she weighed 150 pounds and asked for your opinion of her plan?

Implement
5. You have given Marion, at 120 pounds, your opinion of her plan. She states that she still is going to start limiting her intake. What could you take as a next step to help your friend?

Evaluate
6. If Marion, at 150 pounds, started limiting her diet and weighed 140 pounds by July 4, would she be using the REE appropriately? Explain.

CHAPTER 3

VOCABULARY

acidosis	pancreas
adipose (fatty) tissue	polysaccharides *complex sugar*
bran	refined foods
carbohydrates	residue
cellulose	roughage
curd	starch
dextrins	sucrose
diabetes mellitus	synthesis
dietary fiber	whey
disaccharides	
endosperm	
flatulence	
fructose	
galactose	
germ	
glucagon	
glucose (dextrose)	
glycogen	
hyperglycemia *↑ gluc*	
hypoglycemia *↓ gluc*	
insulin	
islets of Langerhans	
ketones	
ketosis	
lactose	
lactose intolerance	
maltose	
monosaccharides *simple*	

CARBOHYDRATES

OBJECTIVES

After studying this chapter, you should be able to
- Identify the functions of carbohydrates
- Name the primary sources of carbohydrates
- Describe the classification of carbohydrates

1 gm = 4 Kcal

Carbs = ↓ $, major energy source
50-55%/d Kcal.

Carbs = Carbon, Hydrogen, O₂ (chem elements)

DESCRIPTION

Energy foods are those that can be rapidly oxidized by the body to release energy and its byproduct, heat. Carbohydrates, fats, and proteins provide energy for the human body, but carbohydrates are the primary source. They are the least expensive and most abundant of the energy nutrients. Foods rich in carbohydrates grow easily in most climates. They keep well and are generally easy to digest.

Carbohydrates provide the major source of energy for people all over the world, figure 3-1.

They provide approximately half the kcal for people living in the United States. In some areas of the world, where fats and proteins are scarce and expensive, carbohydrates provide as much as 80 to 100 percent of kcal. Carbohydrates are named for the chemical elements they are composed of—carbon, hydrogen, and oxygen.

Carbon, Hydrogen, + O₂

FUNCTIONS

Providing energy is the major function of carbohydrates. Each gram of carbohydrate pro-

eat for body

50%-55% of total intake
should be carb
Majority of calories

29

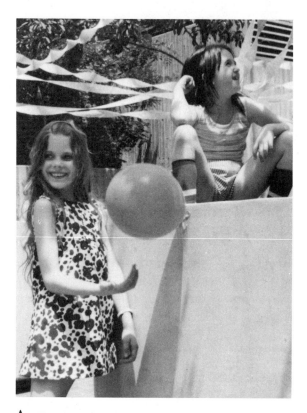

A.

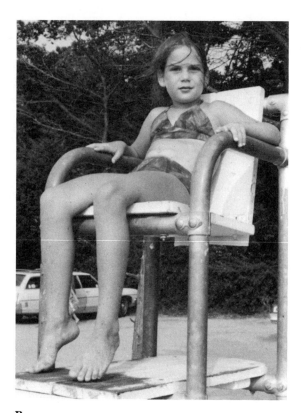

B.

Figure 3-1 The need for carbohydrates is constant, whether at play (A) or at rest (B).

vides 4 kcal (17 kJ). The body needs to maintain a constant supply of energy. Therefore, it stores approximately half a day's supply of carbohydrate in the liver and muscles for use as needed. In this form, it is called **glycogen.**

Protein sparing action also is an important function of carbohydrates. When carbohydrates provide sufficient energy for the body, they spare proteins for their primary function of building and repairing body tissues.

Normal fat metabolism requires an adequate supply of carbohydrates. If there is too little carbohydrate to fulfill the energy requirement, an abnormally large amount of fat is metabolized. This results in an increase of **ketones,** an inter-

mediate product of fat metabolism, in the body. Some ketones are used for energy but the excess accumulate in the blood and urine. Ketones are acids and can upset the acid-base balance, causing **acidosis** or **ketosis.** In this condition, large amounts of water and sodium are excreted and body tissue breaks down. This may result from diabetes mellitus (see Chapter 19), from starvation, or from extremely low-carbohydrate diets.

Providing fiber in the diet is another important function of carbohydrates. Dietary fiber is found in the indigestible parts of plants, such as skins and seeds. It provides no kcal, but it absorbs water in the large intestine. This helps create a soft, bulky stool that moves quickly through the large intestine. Some fiber is believed to bind cholesterol in the colon, thus reducing the risk of heart attack. (See Chapter 20.)

FOOD SOURCES

The principal sources of carbohydrates are plant foods: cereal grains, vegetables, fruits, nuts, and sugars, figure 3-2. The only substantial animal source of carbohydrates is milk.

Cereal grains and their products are dietary staples in nearly every part of the world. Rice is the basic food in Latin America, Africa, Asia, and many sections of the United States. Wheat and the various breads, pastas, and breakfast cereals made from it are basic to American and European diets. Rye and oats are commonly used in breads and cereals in the United States and Europe. Cereals also contain vitamins, minerals, and some proteins. During processing, some of

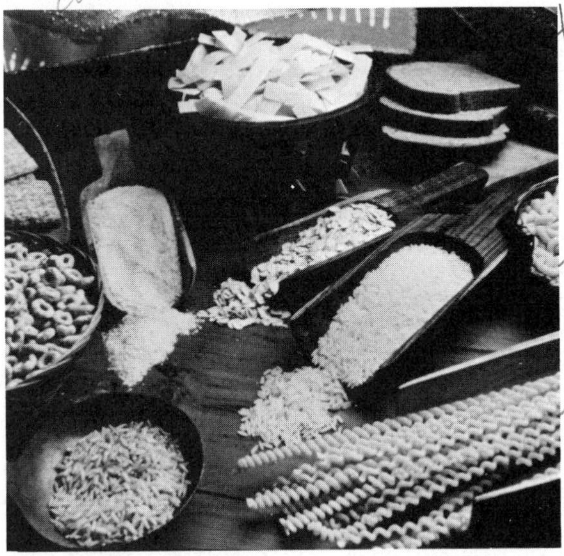

Figure 3-2 Good sources of carbohydrates. *(Courtesy of Tupperware)*

these nutrients are lost. To compensate for this loss, three of the B vitamins, thiamin, riboflavin, and niacin, plus the mineral, iron, are commonly added to the final product in the United States. The product is then called *enriched*.

Vegetables such as potatoes, carrots, beets, turnips, peas, lima beans, and corn provide substantial amounts of starch. Green, leafy vegetables provide dietary fiber. All of them also provide vitamins and minerals.

Fruits provide sugar, fiber, and vitamins.

Sugars such as table sugar, syrup, honey, and sugar-rich foods such as desserts and candy provide carbohydrates in the form of sugar with few other nutrients except for fats. Therefore, the foods in which they predominate are commonly called *empty calorie foods*.

CLASSIFICATION

Carbohydrates are divided into three groups: monosaccharides, disaccharides, and polysaccharides (see Table 3-1).

Monosaccharides (also known as simple or single sugars) are the simplest form of carbohydrates. They are sweet, require no digestion, and can be absorbed directly into the bloodstream from the small intestine. They include glucose, fructose, and galactose.

Glucose, also called **dextrose,** is the form of carbohydrate to which all other forms are converted for eventual metabolism. It is found naturally in corn syrup and some fruits and vegetables.

Fructose, also called levulose or fruit sugar, is found with glucose in many fruits and vegetables and in honey. It tastes especially sweet.

Galactose is a product of the digestion of milk. It is not found naturally.

Disaccharides are sometimes called double sugars. They are sweet and must be changed to

Table 3-1 Carbohydrates

Type	Source	Functions	Deficiency Symptoms
Monosaccharides (Simple Sugars)			
Glucose	carrots grapes berries corn syrup sweet corn	Furnish energy Spare proteins Prevent ketosis	fatigue weight loss

Fructose	ripe fruits vegetables
	honey soft drinks
		Fruits and vegetables
		  provide vitamins,
		  minerals, and fiber	

Galactose	lactose		
Disaccharides (Double Sugars)			

Sucrose	sugar cane
	sugar beets
	  granulated sugar
	  confectioner's sugar
	  brown sugar
	  molasses
	maple syrup
	pineapple
	carrots
	candy
	jams and jellies
		Furnish energy
		Spare proteins
		Prevent ketosis
		Fruits and vegetables
		  provide vitamins,
		  minerals, and fiber
			fagitue
			weight loss

Maltose	digestion of starch		
Lactose	milk		
Polysaccharides (Complex Carbohydrates)			

Starch	cereal grains and their products
	  cereals breads
	  rice flour
	  pastas crackers
	potatoes lima beans
	corn navy beans
	yams green bananas
	sweet potatoes
		Furnish energy
		Prevent ketosis
		Fruits and vegetables
		  provide vitamins,
		  minerals, and fiber
			fatigue
			weight loss

Dextrins	starch hydrolysis		
Glycogen	liver and muscles		
Cellulose	bran, whole grain cereals green and leafy vegetables, fruits, especially apples, pears, oranges, grapefruit, grapes	Provide fiber	possible constipation

32

chg to simple sugars by hydrolysis

simple sugars by hydrolysis before they can be absorbed. Disaccharides include *sucrose, maltose,* and *lactose.*

Sucrose is composed of glucose and fructose. It is the form of carbohydrate present in granulated, powdered, and brown sugar, and in molasses. It is one of the sweetest and least expensive sugars. Its sources are sugar cane, sugar beets, and the sap from maple trees.

Maltose is a disaccharide that is an intermediary product in the hydrolysis of starch. It is produced by enzyme action during the digestion of starch in the body, and commercially, by adding water to cereal grains. It can be found in some infant formulas, malt beverage products, and beer. It is considerably less sweet in taste than glucose or sucrose.

Lactose is the sugar found in milk. It is distinct from most other sugars because it is not found in plants. It helps the body absorb calcium. Lactose is less sweet than the other single or double sugars.

Many adults are unable to digest lactose and suffer from abdominal cramps and diarrhea after drinking milk. This is called **lactose intolerance.** It is caused by insufficient lactase, the enzyme required for digestion of lactose. There are special low-lactose milk products available that can be used instead of regular milk.

During the process of making hard cheese, milk separates into **curd** (solid part from which hard cheese is made) and **whey** (liquid part). Lactose becomes part of the whey and not the curd. Therefore, lactose is not a component of natural cheese. However, manufacturers can add milk or milk solids to process cheese, so it is important that those allergic to lactose check the labels on cheese products.

Polysaccharides are commonly called *complex carbohydrates* because they are compounds of single sugars. The digestible polysaccharides include starch, glycogen, and dextrins. The indigestible polysaccharides include cellulose, hemicellulose, pectins, gums, and mucilages.

Starch is a polysaccharide found in grains and vegetables. Vegetables contain less starch than grains because vegetables have a higher moisture content. The starch in grain is found mainly in the **endosperm** (center part of the grain). This is the part from which white flour is made. The tough outer covering of grain kernels is called the **bran,** figure 3-3. The bran is used in coarse cereals and whole wheat flour. The **germ** is the smallest part of the cereal grain and is a rich source of vitamin B complex, vitamin E,

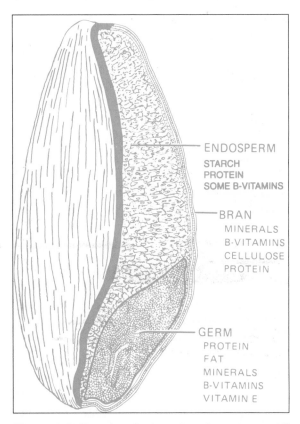

Figure 3-3 A grain of wheat has three parts. All parts are used in whole wheat flour; only the endosperm is used in white flour.

minerals, and protein. Wheat germ is included in products made of whole wheat. It also can be purchased and used in baked products or as an addition to breakfast cereals.

Before the starch in grain can be used for food, the bran must be broken down. The heat and moisture of cooking break this outer covering, making the food more flavorful and more easily digested. Although bran itself is indigestible, it is important that some be included in the diet because of the fiber it provides.

Glycogen is sometimes called *animal starch* because it is the form in which carbohydrates are stored in the body. In the healthy adult, approximately one half day's supply of energy is stored as glycogen in the liver and muscles. The hormone, **glucagon,** helps the liver convert glycogen to glucose as needed. (See page 208–209 about information on glycogen loading.)

Dextrins are the intermediate products of hydrolysis of starch by enzymes during digestion or cooking. They form, for example, during the toasting of bread.

Dietary Fiber, Table 3-2, is the indigestible polysaccharide that has been called **roughage or residue. Cellulose** is a primary source of dietary fiber. It is found in the skins of fruits, the leaves and stems of vegetables, and the bran of cereal grains. Highly processed or **refined foods** such as white bread, macaroni products, and pastries contain little if any cellulose because it is removed during processing. Because humans cannot digest cellulose, it has no energy value. It is useful because it provides bulk for the stool, thus stimulating peristalsis.

Other *nondigestible* complex carbohydrates include *hemicellulose, pectins, gums,* and *mucilages.* They are soluble in water and form a gel that helps provide bulk for the intestines. They are useful also because they bind cholesterol, thus reducing the amount the blood can absorb.

Fiber is considered helpful to patients with diabetes mellitus because it lowers blood glucose levels. It may prevent some colon cancers by moving waste materials through the colon faster than would normally be the case. This reduces the colon's exposure time to potential carcinogens. Fiber helps prevent constipation, hemorrhoids, and diverticular disease by softening and increasing the size of the stool.

Although there is no officially recommended intake for dietary fiber, it is thought that 15 to 20 grams a day may be advisable. The normal American diet is thought to contain approximately 11 grams. An increase should be made over time. Too much in a short time can produce discomfort, **flatulence** (abdominal gas), and diarrhea. Fiber can bind the minerals, calcium, iron, and magnesium, so excessive intake should be avoided. The type of fiber consumed should be from natural food sources rather than from commercially prepared fiber products because the foods contain vitamins and minerals as well as fiber.

DIGESTION AND ABSORPTION

The monosaccharides, **glucose, fructose,** and **galactose,** are single or simple sugars that may be absorbed from the intestine directly into the bloodstream. They are subsequently carried to the liver where fructose and galactose are changed to glucose. The blood then carries glucose to the cells.

The disaccharides, sucrose, maltose, and lactose, require an additional step of digestion. They must first be converted to the simple sugar, glucose, before they can be absorbed into the bloodstream. This is accomplished by the enzymes, sucrase, maltase, and lactase, which were discussed in Chapter 2.

Table 3-2 Dietary Fiber Content of Selected Foods

	Grams Per Serving				
	0.5 or less	0.5–1.0	1.1–2.0	2.1–3.0	3.0 or greater ‡

Fruit*†	banana
	cherries
	coconut
	  shredded
	currants
	  (dried)
	dates
	fruit juice
	plums (ckd)
	pomegranate
	prunes
	raisons
	rhubarb (raw)
	watermelon
		apricots, raw or
		  dried
		apple (peeled or
		  dried)
		applesauce
		blueberries
		cantaloupe
		coconut, raw, ½
		  cup
		cranberries,
		  relish, ½ cup
		honeydew
		kiwifruit
		mango
		nectarine
		orange
		peach, raw or
		  dried
		pear, dried
		pineapple
		plums (raw)
		prunes
		rhubarb, raw (1
		  cup) & ckd
		strawberries
		tangerine
		watermelon
			apple skin
			cranberries,
			  raw (1 cup)
			figs
			papaya
				blackberries
				boysenberries
				gooseberries
				kumquats
				pears
					blackberries (4)
					elderberries (5)
					guava (5)
					raspberries (4)

(continued)

The polysaccharides are more complex and their digestibility varies. After the cellulose wall is broken down, starch is changed to an intermediate product called dextrin; it is then changed to maltose and finally to glucose. Cooking can change starch to dextrin. For example, when bread is toasted, it turns golden brown and tastes sweeter because the starch has been changed to dextrin.

The digestion of starch begins in the mouth where the enzyme ptyalin begins to change starch to dextrin. The second step occurs in the stomach where the food is mixed with gastric juices. The final step occurs in the small intestine where the digestible carbohydrates are changed to simple sugars by enzyme action and subsequently absorbed by the blood.

Table 3-2 (*Continued*)

	Grams Per Serving				
	0.5 or less	0.5–1.0	1.1–2.0	2.1–3.0	3.0 or greater‡
Vegetables*†	bamboo shoots	artichoke hearts	artichoke, Jerusalem		
	bean sprouts, cooked or canned	asparagus	broccoli (ckd)		
	cabbage, cooked	bean sprouts, raw	Brussels sprouts		
	celery	beans (string)	chicory		
	eggplant	beets	mushrooms		
	endive	broccoli (raw)	pumpkin		
	lettuce	cabbage, raw	rutabagas		
	onions	carrots	sauerkraut		
	radishes	cauliflower	soybean sprouts, raw		
	summer squash	cucumber	spaghetti sauce		
	vegetable juice	green pepper	tomato paste		
	water chestnuts	greens	turnips, raw		
	watercress	beet			
		collard			
		dandelion			
		kale			
		mustard			
		spinach			
		swiss chard			
		turnip			
		kohlrabi			
		mushrooms			
		okra			
		parsley			
		soybean sprouts, cooked			
		summer squash, raw			
		tomato puree			
		turnips, cooked			

(*continued*)

METABOLISM AND ELIMINATION

All carbohydrates are changed to the simple sugar glucose before metabolism can take place in the cells. After glucose has been carried by the blood to the cells, it can be oxidized. Frequently, the volume of glucose that reaches the cells exceeds the amount the cells can use. In these cases, some glucose is converted to glycogen and is stored in the liver and muscles. (Glycogen is subsequently broken down and released as glucose is needed for energy.) When more glucose is

Table 3-2 (Continued)

	Grams Per Serving				
	0.5 or less	0.5–1.0	1.1–2.0	2.1–3.0	3.0 or greater‡
Starches*	Cornflakes	bread, white	black-eyed	beans, dried	All-Bran (9)
	corn grits	Cheerios	peas	40%	Bran Buds (8)
	cream of	corn	bread, whole	Branflakes	100% Bran (6)
	wheat or	flour, white	wheat	bulgur	bran muffin (3.5)
	rice	granola	flour, whole	lentils	wheat bran (9)
	farina	oatmeal (ckd)	wheat	parsnips	bulgur (3.5)
	graham	roll or bun, white	Grapenuts	peas, dried	
	crackers	spaghetti &	green peas	Raisin Bran	
	Maltomeal	macaroni from	lima beans	Rykrisp	
	plantain	whole wheat	popcorn	Shredded	
	potato chips	flour	pumpkin	Wheat	
	potatoes		Ralston	wheat germ	
	puffed cereals		(cooked		
	rice, white		cereal)		
	Rice Krispies		rice, brown or		
	saltines		white		
	spaghetti,		sesame seed		
	refined		kernels		
			soybeans		
			squash, winter		
			sweet		
			potatoes		

* Based on the content of one diabetic exchange for each item listed.
† Includes all forms (raw, dried, cooked) for fruits and vegetables except where noted.
‡ Actual dietary fiber content listed in parentheses.
Courtesy of Mayo Clinic, Rochester, Minnesota.

ingested than the body can either use immediately or store in the form of glycogen, it is converted to fat and stored as **adipose (fatty) tissue.**

The process of glucose metabolism is controlled mainly by the hormone **insulin,** which is secreted by the **islets of Langerhans** in the **pancreas.** When the secretion of insulin is impaired or absent, the glucose level in the blood becomes excessively high. This condition is called **hyper-**glycemia and is usually a symptom of **diabetes mellitus.** In such cases insulin, or a hypoglycemic agent that stimulates the production of insulin in the pancreas, must be provided. When insulin is given, the diabetic patient's intake of carbohydrates must be carefully controlled to balance the prescribed dosage of insulin. (See Chapter 19.) When blood glucose levels are unusually low, the condition is called **hypoglycemia.** A mild form of hypoglycemia may occur if one waits too long between meals or because the pancreas secretes too much insulin. Symptoms include fatigue and headache.

Oxidation of glucose results in energy. With the exception of cellulose, the only waste products of carbohydrate metabolism are carbon dioxide and water. It is a very efficient nutrient.

DIETARY REQUIREMENTS

While there is no specific daily dietary requirement for carbohydrates, the Food and Nutrition Board of the National Research Council recommends that half of one's energy requirement come from carbohydrates. For example, assume that one's total energy requirement is 2000 kcal. One half of this is 1000. Divide 1000 kcal by 4 kcal (the number in each gram of carbohydrate), for an estimated carbohydrate requirement of 250 grams per day. It is estimated that current American diets contain only 45 percent of their kcal from carbohydrates.

A mild deficiency of carbohydrates can result in weight loss and fatigue. A diet seriously deficient in carbohydrates could cause ketosis and dehydration. To prevent this, one needs a minimum of 50 to 100 grams of carbohydrates each day.

Because overweight is a major health problem in the United States, it should be noted that eating an excess of carbohydrates is one of the most common causes of obesity. Although some of the surplus carbohydrate is changed to glycogen, the major part of any surplus becomes adipose tissue. Also, an excess of carbohydrate in the form of sugar can spoil an appetite for other nutrients that are more important. Too many carbohydrates may cause tooth decay, may irritate the lining of the stomach, or cause **flatulence** (gas in the colon).

CONSIDERATIONS FOR THE HEALTH CARE PROFESSIONAL

The role of the health care professional in teaching about carbohydrates may be complicated. Carbohydrates have been considered "fattening" by many people who have not received nutrition education. Some will have to be taught the nutritional differences between a baked potato and potato chips; between whole wheat toast and Danish pastry; between a fresh peach and canned fruit cocktail. Many will need to learn what dietary fiber is, where it can be found, and why it is needed. Some will need to learn that sugar can be used in moderation; others that it cannot be used in excess. All will require acceptance, understanding, and patience on the part of the health care professional.

SUMMARY

Energy foods are those that can be rapidly oxidized by the body to release energy. Carbohydrates are and should be the major source of energy. They are composed of carbon, hydrogen, and oxygen. One gram of carbohydrate provides 4 kcal (17 kilojoules). Carbohydrates are the least expensive and the most abundant nutrient. The principal sources of carbohydrates are plant products such as cereals and their products, vegetables, fruits, legumes, and sugars. In addition to providing energy, carbohydrates spare proteins, maintain normal fat metabolism, and provide fiber. Digestion of carbohydrates begins in the mouth, continues in the stomach, and is completed in the small intestine. While they are obviously essential to the health and well-being of the body, eating an excess of carbohydrates can cause dental caries, digestive disturbances, and overweight.

Discussion Topics

1. What are the three basic groups of carbohydrates? Name several foods in each group. *mono., di., poly.)*
2. Discuss the effects of regularly eating an excess of carbohydrates.
3. Which polysaccharides (starches) might be considered a dietary staple for the following nationalities? Explain why this may be so.
   - Italian
   - Mexican
   - Chinese
   - American Indian
   - French
4. Why should one's diet contain dietary fiber? Name three sources of dietary fiber. *Beans, grains, bran, seeds, skins, ↑ bulk - moves stool - stim. peristal.*
5. Describe the digestion and metabolism of carbohydrates.
6. What could develop from eating too few carbohydrates?
7. Discuss the following menus. Which foods contain carbohydrates? (Refer to Table A-5 in the Appendix.)

Orange Juice	Baked Chicken	Cheese Sandwich
Cereal	Baked Potato	on Whole Wheat Bread
Milk—Sugar	Green Beans	with Lettuce and Tomato
Toast	Coleslaw	Carrot and Celery Sticks
Butter—Jelly	Bread—Butter	Fresh Fruit
Milk	Raspberry Sherbet	Cookies
(Coffee for Adults)	Milk	Milk

8. Why are complex carbohydrates preferable to single sugars? To double sugars?
9. Discuss *enrichment*. What does it mean? Why is it done? Which foods are typically enriched in the United States? Would you recommend that one purchase enriched foods? Why?
10. Is it true as many people say that "carbos are fattening?" Explain your answer. *yes + no*
11. In what way can an inadequate intake of carbohydrates result in serious fluid loss to the body?

Suggested Activities

1. Hold a soda cracker in your mouth until you notice the change in flavor as the starch changes to dextrin.
2. Toast a slice of bread and describe the changes in appearance and flavor that occurred in the carbohydrate.
3. Make a chart of the monosaccharides and the disaccharides and their sources.
4. Visit a grocery store. Compare the costs of six foods that are good sources of complex carbohydrates with six foods that are good sources of

monosaccharides or disaccharides. Using Table A-5 in the Appendix, compare their energy values.

5. Make a list of the foods you have eaten in the past 24 hours. Circle the carbohydrate-rich foods and underline the complex carbohydrates. Approximately what percentage of your calories were in the form of carbohydrate? In the form of complex carbos? Could your diet be improved? If so, how?

6. Trace figure 2-1 in Chapter 2. Use it to explain the digestion of carbohydrates using words and arrows.

7. Role play a situation between a diet counselor and a teenage girl who has placed herself on an extremely low-kcal diet. She refuses to eat anything that she believes contains carbohydrates. Explain to her the functions of carbohydrates in the human body.

8. Write a short essay on the value of dietary fiber.

Review

A. Multiple choice. Select the *letter* that precedes the best answer.

1. The three main groups of carbohydrates are
   a. fats, proteins, and minerals
   b. glucose, fructose, and galactose
   c. monosaccharides, disaccharides, and polysaccharides
   d. sucrose, cellulose, and glycogen

2. Galactose is a product of the digestion of
   a. milk   c. breads
   b. meat   d. vegetables

3. A simple sugar to which all forms of carbohydrates are ultimately converted is
   a. sucrose   c. galactose
   b. glucose   d. maltose

4. Wheat germ is a source of vitamins
   a. B complex and D   c. B complex and E
   b. B complex and C   d. none of these

5. A fibrous form of carbohydrate that cannot be digested is
   a. glucose   c. cellulose
   b. glycogen   d. fat

6. Glycogen is stored in the
   a. heart and lungs   c. pancreas and gallbladder
   b. liver and muscles   d. small and large intestines

7. Glucose is metabolized
   a. by combining it with fat
   b. in all body cells
   c. exclusively in the liver
   d. in the form of glycogen

8. Refined foods normally
   a. do not contain cellulose
   b. are excellent sources of fiber
   c. contain large amounts of cellulose
   d. contain no carbohydrates

9. Glucose, fructose, and galactose
   a. are polysaccharides
   b. are disaccharides
   c. are enzymes
   d. are monosaccharides

10. Before carbohydrates can be metabolized by the cells, they must
    a. be converted to glycogen
    b. be converted to glucose
    c. be converted to polysaccharides
    d. be converted to sucrose

B. Match the definition in column I with its term in column II.

	Column I	Column II
C	1. least expensive energy nutrient	a. body fat
a	2. adipose tissue	b. endosperm
i	3. carbohydrate as stored in the liver	c. carbohydrate
j	4. disaccharide	d. four
b	5. center part of grain	e. six
h	6. outer covering of grain	f. nine
d	7. number of calories per gram of carbohydrate	g. glucose
		h. bran
n	8. carbohydrate in milk	i. glycogen
l	9. sugar found in fruit	j. sucrose
k	10. secretion of the islets of Langerhans in the pancreas	k. insulin
		l. fructose
		m. molasses
		n. lactose

Case Study 1

Abnormal Metabolism of Carbohydrates

Mary G. is a 60-year-old bookkeeper who spends most of her working day sitting at a desk. Because she had been feeling increasingly tired in the past few weeks, she visited her doctor.

After examining her and testing her blood and urine, Mary's doctor asked her if anyone in her family has diabetes mellitus. In fact, Mary's aunt had had it from the time she was 45 until she died. The doctor told Mary she was overweight and had a form of diabetes mellitus. She was advised to lose 30 pounds at a rate that did not exceed two to three pounds a week, to limit the carbohydrates in her diet, and to exercise daily—preferably by swimming or walking. The doctor told her most carbohydrates were found in breads, pastas, rich desserts, and concentrated sweets such as candy and sodas. She was to return in two weeks.

Mary thought she had followed the doctor's advice and did, in fact, lose four pounds in the intervening two weeks. But when the doctor tested her blood and urine during her second visit, the blood sugar remained elevated at 220 mg/dl. The doctor asked Mary to write a list of the foods she had eaten during the past 24 hours. This is what the doctor read:

Breakfast	Lunch	Snack	Dinner
1 medium glass orange juice	1 cup cream of chicken soup	1 cup fruit yogurt	Meat Loaf (two ½-inch slices)
1 fried egg	Cheese sandwich made		Baked potato (1 medium)
1 slice whole wheat toast	with 1 slice bread, 1 pat butter, 2 leaves		Steamed broccoli (two stalks)
1 pat margarine	lettuce, and 3 slices		Gelatin salad with canned fruit
1 Tbsp. jelly	tomato		½ cup rice pudding
Coffee with skim milk	Fresh apple		1 cup skim milk
	1 cup milk		

Case Study Questions Based on the Nursing Process

Assess
1. Why did the doctor want Mary to reduce the amount of carbohydrates in her diet?
2. What were the hidden carbohydrates in Mary's diet?

Plan
3. What might Mary substitute for these foods?

Implement
4. Should the doctor have told Mary to eliminate all carbohydrates in her diet?

Evaluate
5. Do you think it might be difficult for Mary to continue on this diet for an indefinite period? Why?

Case Study 2

The Need for Dietary Fiber

David was recently widowed and his only child, a daughter, lives 500 miles away. She worries that he is not eating properly. He prepares his own breakfast of orange juice, dry cereal, and coffee. At noon, he usually goes for a short walk and buys a slice of pizza or a hot dog along the way and, occasionally, a beer. In the evening, he goes to the corner coffee shop where he orders one of their daily specials that includes soup, entree, rolls, and dessert. He doesn't feel as well as he used to, and he suffers from constipation.

Case Study Questions Based on the Nursing Process

Assess
1. What form of carbohydrate is grossly lacking in David's diet? How could it be included? *needs fruits + vegies*

Plan
2. If you were David's daughter, what improvements would you recommend about his eating habits? How would you suggest doing this?

Implement
3. What possible changes in his lifestyle might help to improve his eating habits and his feelings of well-being? How might these changes be accomplished?

Evaluate
4. David lives in a small town. How might this help Mary to check on his condition?

Call
Pat →
① will she give case study examples on quizes?
② Math

CHAPTER 4

FATS

OBJECTIVES

After studying this chapter, you should be able to
- State the functions of fats in the body
- Identify sources of dietary fats
- Explain common classifications of fats
- Describe disease conditions with which excessive use of fats is associated

Fats, also called **lipids,** are oily substances that are not soluble in water. They are soluble in some solvents, such as ether and alcohol. They provide a more concentrated form of energy than carbohydrates as each gram of fat contains nine kilocalories. This is slightly more than twice the kcal content of carbohydrates. Fat-rich foods are generally more expensive than carbohydrate-rich foods. Like carbohydrates, fats are composed of carbon, hydrogen, and oxygen, but with a substantially lower proportion of oxygen.

FUNCTIONS

In addition to providing energy and heat, fats are essential for the functioning and structure of body tissues, Table 4-1. Fats are a necessary part of **cell membranes** (cell walls). Fats act as carriers of essential fatty acids and fat-soluble vitamins. The fat stored in body tissues provides energy when one cannot eat, as may occur during illness. **Adipose** (fatty) **tissue** protects organs and bones from injury by serving as protective pad-

Table 4-1 Fats

Functions	Deficiency Symptoms	Sources
Provide energy and heat	Eczema Weight loss	*Animal* Fatty meats
Carry fat-soluble vitamins	Retarded growth	Lard Butter
Supply essential fatty acids		Cheese Cream
Protect and support organs and bones		Whole milk Egg yolk *Plant* Vegetable oils
Insulate from cold		Nuts Chocolate
Provide satiety to meals		Avocados Olives Margarine

ding and support. Body fat also serves as insulation from cold. In addition, fats provide a feeling of **satiety** (satisfaction) after meals. This is due partly to the flavor fats give other foods and partly to their slow rate of digestion, which delays hunger.

FOOD SOURCES

Fats are present in both animal and plant foods. The animal foods that provide the richest sources of fats are meats, especially fatty meats such as bacon, sausage, and luncheon meats; whole milk, one- and two-percent milk; cream; butter; cheeses made with cream, whole, or one- or two-percent milk; egg yolks (egg white contains no fat; it is almost entirely protein and water); and fatty fish such as tuna and salmon.

The plant foods containing the richest sources of fats are cooking oils made from sunflower, safflower, or sesame seeds, or from corn, peanuts, soybeans, or olives; margarine (which is made from vegetable oils); nuts; avocados; coconut; and chocolate.

Visible and Invisible Fats

Sometimes fats are referred to as visible or invisible, depending on their food sources.

Fats that are purchased and used as fats such as butter, margarine, lard, and cooking oils, are called **visible fats.** Hidden or **invisible fats** are those found in other foods such as meats, cream, whole milk, cheese, eggs, fried foods, pastries, avocados, and nuts, figure 4-1.

It is often the invisible or hidden fats that can make it difficult for patients on limited-fat diets to regulate their fat intake. For example, one three-inch doughnut may contain 12 grams of fat, whereas one three-inch bagel contains only 2 grams of fat. One fried chicken drumstick may contain 11 grams of fat, whereas one roasted drumstick may contain only 2 grams of fat.

It is essential that the health care professional confirm that patients on limited fat diets are carefully educated about sources of hidden fats.

CLASSIFICATION

The components of dietary fats are **fatty acids** and **glycerol.** The fatty acids **linoleic, linolenic,** and **arachidonic** are needed by the body, but only linoleic acid is considered essential in the diet. Corn, sunflower, and safflower oils are excellent sources of linoleic acid. The other fatty acids can be synthesized by the body. Most natural fats are composed of three fatty acids combined with glycerol. They are called **triglycerides.** Triglycerides are found in body cells and circulate in the blood.

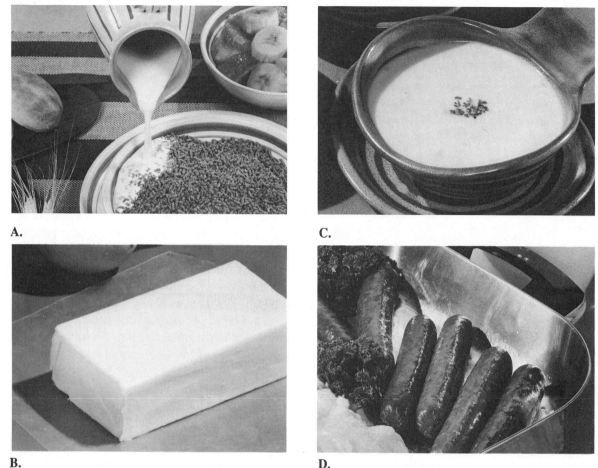

A.

C.

B.

D.

Figure 4-1 A fat may be hidden in other foods or used as a food itself. (A) Cream (B) Margarine (C) Creamed Soup (D) Sausage

Fats are commonly described and thus classified as being saturated, monounsaturated, or polyunsaturated, depending on the hydrogen content of the fatty acids that predominate in their makeup.

Saturated Fats

worst

When a fatty acid is **saturated,** each of its carbon atoms carries all the hydrogen atoms possible. Generally, animal foods contain more saturated fatty acids than unsaturated. Examples include meat, poultry, egg yolks, whole milk, whole milk cheeses, cream, ice cream, and butter. Although plant foods generally contain more polyunsaturated fatty acids than saturated fatty acids, chocolate, coconut, and palm oil are exceptions. They contain substantial amounts of saturated fatty acids. Foods containing a high proportion of saturated fats are usually solid at room temperature.

Monounsaturated Fats

If a fat is **monounsaturated,** there is one place among the carbon atoms of its fatty acids where there are fewer hydrogen atoms attached than in saturated fats. Examples of foods containing monounsaturated fats are olive oil, avocados, and cashew nuts.

Polyunsaturated Fats

If a fat is **polyunsaturated,** there are two or more places among the carbon atoms of its fatty acids where there are fewer hydrogen atoms attached than in saturated fats. Linoleic fatty acid is polyunsaturated. Examples of foods containing polyunsaturated fats include cooking oils made from sunflower, safflower, or sesame seeds, or from corn or peanuts; soft margarines whose major ingredient is *liquid* vegetable oil; fish; and peanuts. Foods containing high proportions of polyunsaturated fats are usually soft or oily.

Hydrogenated Fats

Poly + Hydrogen = Sat.

Hydrogenated fats are polyunsaturated vegetable oils to which hydrogen has been added commercially to make them resemble butter. This process, called *hydrogenation,* turns polyunsaturated vegetable oils into saturated fats. Margarine is made in this way. (Soft margarine contains less saturated fat than firm margarine.)

CHOLESTEROL

Cholesterol is a fat-like substance that exists in animal foods and body cells. It does not exist in plant foods. It is a precursor of steroid hormones and is essential for the production of vitamin D and bile acids. The body **synthesizes** (manufactures) it in the liver so it is not essential in the diet.

However, cholesterol is a common **constituent** (part) of one's daily diet because it is found so abundantly in egg yolk, fatty meats, shellfish, butter, cream, cheese, whole milk, and **organ meats** (liver, kidneys, brains, sweetbreads.) (See Table 4-2.)

Cholesterol is thought to be a contributing factor in heart disease because **high serum cholesterol,** also called **hypercholesterolemia,** (abnormally high amounts of cholesterol in the blood), is common in patients with **atherosclerosis.** Atherosclerosis is a cardiovascular disease in which **plaque** (fatty deposits containing cholesterol and other substances) forms on the inside of artery walls, reducing the space for blood flow. When the blood cannot flow through an artery near the heart, a heart attack occurs. When this is the case near the brain, stroke occurs. (See Chapter 20.) It is considered advisable that blood cholesterol levels not exceed 200 mg/dl (200 milligrams of cholesterol per one deciliter of blood). A reduction in the amount of total fat, saturated fats, and cholesterol, and an increase in the amount of polyunsaturated fats in the diet, weight loss, and exercise all help to lower serum cholesterol levels. Dietary fiber also is considered helpful in lowering blood cholesterol because wheat and oat fiber bind to the cholesterol, eliminating some of it via the feces and thus preventing it from being absorbed in the small intestine. In some cases, medication may be prescribed if diet, weight loss, and exercise do not sufficiently lower serum cholesterol.

Since the development of plaque is cumulative, the preferred means of avoiding or at least limiting its development is to limit cholesterol intake throughout life. If children are not fed high-cholesterol foods on a regular basis, their chances of overusing them as adults are reduced. Thus, their risk of heart attack and stroke is also reduced.

Table 4-2 Fat and Cholesterol Content of Some Common Foods

Food	Amount	Saturated Fat (g)	Cholesterol (mg)	Total Fat (g)	Total kcal
Creamed Cottage Cheese (4% fat)	1 cup	6.4	34	10	235
Uncreamed Cottage Cheese (0.5% fat)	1 cup	0.4	10	1	125
Cream Cheese	1 oz	6.2	31	10	100
Swiss Cheese	1 oz	5.0	26	8	105
American Process	1 oz	5.6	27	9	105
Half & Half	1 Tbsp	1.1	6	2	20
Heavy Cream	1 Tbsp	3.5	21	6	54
Non-dairy Creamer	1 Tbsp	1.4	0	1	20
Whole Milk	1 cup	5.1	33	8	150
2% Milk	1 cup	2.9	18	5	120
1% Milk	1 cup	1.6	10	3	100
Skim Milk	1 cup	0.3	4	trace	85
Chocolate Milk Shake	10 oz	4.8	30	8	335
Ice Cream (11% fat)	½ cup	8.9	59	14	270
Soft Ice Milk	1 cup	2.9	13	5	225
Egg	1	1.7	274	6	80
Butter	1 Tbsp	7.1	31	11	100
Margarine	1 Tbsp	2.2	0	11	100
Corn Oil	1 Tbsp	1.8	0	14	125
Crabmeat (canned)	1 cup	0.5	135	3	135
Salmon (canned)	3 oz	0.9	34	5	120
Shrimp (canned)	3 oz	0.2	128	1	100

It is recommended that daily cholesterol intake not exceed 300 mg. Current estimates of average daily cholesterol intake by Americans is 400 to 700 mg.

DIGESTION AND ABSORPTION

Although 95 percent of **ingested** (eaten) fats are digested, it is a complex process. The chemical digestion of fats occurs mainly in the small intestine. Fats are not digested in the mouth. They are digested only slightly in the stomach where gastric lipase acts on emulsified fats such as those found in cream and egg yolk. Fats must be mixed well with the gastric juices before entering the small intestine. In the small intestine, bile emulsifies the fats and the enzyme steapsin (pancreatic lipase) reduces them to fatty acids and glycerol, which the body subsequently absorbs.

Lipoproteins

Fats are insoluble in water, which is the main component of blood. Because of this, special carriers must be provided for the fats to be

Carb 50%   Fats 30%

Fats-

Chol   300mg/d or less

~ Carb 50
- Prot 15-20
- Fat 30

CHAPTER 4   FATS   49

Table 4-2 (*Continued*)

Food	Amount	Saturated Fat (g)	Cholesterol (mg)	Total Fat (g)	Total kcal
Tuna					
Water pk	3 oz	0.3	48	1	135
Oil pk	3 oz	1.4	55	7	165
Avocado	½	2.2	0	15	150
Banana	1	0.2	0	1	105
Orange	1	trace	0	trace	60
Bagel	1	0.3	0	2	200
Doughnut	1	2.8	20	12	210
English Muffin	1	0.3	0	1	140
Coconut (raw)	2" × 2" × ½"	13.4	0	15	160
Peanuts (dry roasted)	1 oz	2.0	0	15	170
Ground Beef (lean)	3 oz	6.2	74	16	230
Roast Beef (lean)	4.4 oz	7.2	100	18	300
Leg Lamb (lean)	5.2 oz	4.8	130	12	280
Leg Lamb (lean and fat)	6 oz	11.2	156	26	410
Bacon	3 sl.	3.3	16	9	110
Pork Chop (lean)	5 oz	5.2	142	16	330
Frankfurter	1.5 oz	4.8	23	13	145
Chicken Leg, Fried (meat and skin)	5 oz	6.0	124	22	390
Chicken Leg, Roasted (meat only)	3.2 oz	1.4	82	4	150

Adapted from *Nutritive Value of Foods*, U.S.D.A. Home & Garden Bulletin No. 72. 1981.

absorbed and transported by the blood to body cells. In the initial stages of absorption, bile joins with the products of fat digestion to carry fat. Later, protein combines with the final products of fat digestion to form special carriers called **lipoproteins.** The lipoproteins subsequently carry the fats to the body cells by way of the blood.

Lipoproteins are classified as **very-low-density lipoproteins (VLDL), low-density lipoproteins (LDL),** and **high-density lipoproteins (HDL),** according to their mobility and density.

VLDL carry triglycerides and are converted in the liver to LDL. LDL carry most of the blood cholesterol to the cells. Elevated blood levels of LDL are thought to be contributing factors in atherosclerosis. LDL is sometimes termed *bad cholesterol* or *bad fat.*

HDL carry cholesterol from the tissues to the liver for eventual excretion. They are thought to reduce the risk of heart disease. HDL are sometimes called *good fat* or *good cholesterol.*

METABOLISM AND ELIMINATION

The liver controls fat metabolism. It hydrolyzes triglycerides and forms new ones from this hydrolysis as needed. Ultimately, the metabolism of fats occurs in the cells, where fatty acids are broken down to carbon dioxide and water, releasing energy. The portion of fat that is not needed for immediate use is stored as adipose tissue. Carbon dioxide and water are waste products that are removed from the body by the circulatory, respiratory, and excretory systems.

FATS AND THE CONSUMER

Fats continue to be of particular interest to the consumer. Most people know fats are high-calorie foods and that they are related to heart disease. But people who are not in the health field may not know *how* fats affect health. Consequently, they may be easily duped by clever ads for or salespersons of nutritional supplements or new "health food" products.

It is important that the health care professional carefully evaluate any new dietary "supplement" for which a nutritional claim is made. If the item is not included in the Recommended Dietary Allowances, it is safe to assume that medical research has not determined that it is essential. Ingestion of dietary supplements of unknown value could, ironically, be damaging to one's health.

Lecithin

Lecithin is a fatty substance that is found in both plant and animal foods. It is synthesized in the liver. It is a natural emulsifier that helps transport fat in the bloodstream. It is used commercially to make food products smooth.

Lecithin supplements have been promoted by some health food salespersons as being able to prevent cardiovascular disease. To date, this has not been scientifically proven.

Omega-3 Fatty Acids

Research has indicated that the amount of coronary artery disease is less than normal in areas where the amount of fish oil in the diet is higher than normal. Fish oil contains the polyunsaturated fatty acids, *eicosapentaenoic* (EPA) and *docosahexaenoic* (DHA). They are generally termed **omega-3 fatty acids** because of their chemical structure.

Consequently, fish oil capsules are selling well. However, until research provides a definitive answer about the total effects on health of omega-3 fatty acids, it would be wise to include fatty fish in the diet but to avoid supplementary fish oil capsules.

Artificial Fats

Artificial fats are a relatively new product, and their number continues to grow. One is available made from egg white or milk protein; another from sucrose and another from corn starch. They contain little or no natural fats, and their caloric contents are correspondingly low. Their long-term effects on human health and nutrition are unknown. If they are used similar to the way the American population uses artificial sweeteners, they probably will not reduce the actual fat content in the diet. They may simply be additions to it. One concern among nutritionists is that they will be used in place of nutritious food that, in addition to fat, also provides vitamins, minerals, proteins, and carbohydrates.

DIETARY REQUIREMENTS

Although no specific dietary requirement for fats is included in the RDAs (Appendix Table A-1), deficiency symptoms do occur when fats provide less than 10 percent of the total daily kcal requirement. When **gross deficiency** (severe) occurs, **eczema** (inflamed and scaly skin condition) can develop. This has been observed in infants who were fed formulas lacking the essential fatty acid, linoleic acid, and in patients maintained for long periods on intravenous feedings that lack linoleic acid. Also, growth may be retarded, and weight loss can occur when diets are seriously deficient in fats.

On the other hand, excessive fat in the diet can lead to overweight or heart disease. In addition, studies point to an association between high-fat diets and cancers of the colon, breast, uterus, and prostate.

The Food and Nutrition Board's Committee on Diet and Health recommends that people reduce their fat intake to 30 percent of total kcal. No more than 10 percent of total kcal should be provided by saturated fats. The National Research Council in its 1989 edition of the RDAs states that 36 percent of kcal in current American diets are derived from fats.

CONSIDERATIONS FOR THE HEALTH CARE PROFESSIONAL

Because of the attention fats receive in the media and the common concern about heart dis-ease and overweight, many patients have opinions on them. Some are factually correct; many are not. Obviously, it is especially important that the health care professional be able to explain accurately, but simply, the possible damage from too much fat in the diet.

To accomplish dietary change, it is important that patients' usual diets be reviewed *with* them. Changes then can be introduced clearly, sensitively, and with the patients' active participation. Unless patients understand *why* dietary changes are needed and want to make them, it is unlikely they will do so.

SUMMARY

In addition to providing an important source of energy, fats carry essential fatty acids and fat-soluble vitamins, protect organs and bones, insulate from cold, and provide satiety to meals. They are composed of carbon, hydrogen, and oxygen and are found in both animal and plant foods. Each gram of fats provides 9 kcal. Digestion of fats occurs mainly in the small intestine where they are reduced to fatty acids and glycerol. An excess of fat in the diet can result in obesity and possibly heart disease or cancer.

Discussion Topics

1. Why are fats considered a more concentrated form of energy than carbohydrates? *9 kcal vs 4 kcal*
2. Of what value are fats to the body? List some foods rich in fats. Identify them as animal foods or plant foods. Identify them as saturated or polyunsaturated.
3. Discuss adipose tissue. Is it good? Is it bad? Explain.
4. Describe atherosclerosis. It is said that its effects are cumulative. Explain.
5. Discuss saturated fats and cholesterol. Point out the differences and explain why patients are often confused by them.
6. What are organ meats? Why might it be unwise to eat them several times a week?

7. Describe the digestion and metabolism of fats. What are the end products of fat digestion?
8. Why might a patient on a low-fat diet complain? How might the health care professional be helpful in such a case?
9. What are hydrogenated fats? Are they polyunsaturated? Explain.
10. Why is there a greater danger of excess fat in the American diet than a deficiency of fat?
11. Discuss hidden fats and their potential impact on low-fat diets.
12. What are the probable reasons that omega-3 fatty acid capsules and lecithin have become so popular with the general public?
13. How might the health care professional convince a patient recovering from a first heart attack that omega-3 fatty acid capsules may not prevent a second attack?

Suggested Activities

1. Make a list of foods rich in fats. Make another list of carbohydrate-rich foods. Check their costs at the supermarket and compare. Using Table A-5 in the Appendix, compare the kcal values of these foods. Compare their cholesterol contents.
2. Write one or two paragraphs about dietary fats, using as many of the words in the chapter vocabulary list as possible. Ask a friend to read and evaluate it.
3. Make a list of foods containing saturated fats. Make a parallel list of foods containing large amounts of cholesterol. Compare them. Suggest substitutes for those containing large amounts of saturated fats and/or cholesterol.
4. Fry an egg in a pan that has been coated to prevent foods sticking to it, using no fat. Fry another egg, using fat. Taste and compare them for flavor and appearance.
5. Role play a situation between a health care professional and a teenage girl who refuses to eat anything she thinks contains fats.
6. List the foods you ate yesterday. Circle those containing visible fats. Underline those containing invisible fats. Explain why some foods are both circled and underlined. Revise it, making it appropriate for someone on a limited-fat diet.
7. Role play a scene in which a cantankerous patient, who is recovering from a heart attack, is complaining to the nurse about her or his low-fat diet, saying she or he "can't eat anything good anymore."
8. Visit a health food store and ask for brochures and descriptions of their products intended to prevent heart disease. Evaluate them in class.

9. Using a cookbook, review recipes for baked products and answer the following questions about them.
   a. Why do bagels contain no cholesterol?
   b. Why does angel cake contain no cholesterol?
   c. Why does a doughnut contain cholesterol when an English muffin does not?
   d. Why does French toast contain cholesterol when the white bread it is made from may not?
   e. Why does lemon meringue pie filling contain cholesterol when apple pie filling does not?
   f. Why does a cheeseburger contain more cholesterol than a hamburger?

Review

A. Multiple choice. Select the *letter* that precedes the best answer.

1. Fats provide the most concentrated form of
   a. carbon
   b. oxygen
   c. lipase
   d. energy

2. Fats are essential because they are carriers of
   a. water-soluble vitamins
   b. fatty acids
   c. bile
   d. plaque

3. Adipose tissue is useful because it
   a. can synthesize triglycerides
   b. prevents eczema
   c. provides satiety
   d. protects and insulates

4. Atherosclerosis is thought to contribute to
   a. cancer
   b. plaque
   c. heart attacks
   d. hypercholesterolemia

5. A diet grossly deficient in fats may be deficient in
   a. lipase
   b. linoleic acid
   c. cholesterol
   d. all of the above

6. Invisible fats can be found in
   a. cake and cookies
   b. orange and tomato juice
   c. egg white and skim milk
   d. lettuce and tomatoes

7. Plant foods that contain saturated fats are
   a. olives and avocados
   b. coconut and chocolate
   c. corn and soybeans
   d. none of the above

8. When a polyunsaturated vegetable oil is changed to a saturated fat, the process is called
   a. hydrolysis
   b. hypercholesterolemia
   c. hydrogenation
   d. none of the above

9. Linoleic acid is the only fatty acid that is known to be
    a. a triglyceride
    b. polyunsaturated
    c. monounsaturated
    d. essential to the human diet
10. Cholesterol
    a. is not essential to the human diet
    b. is thought to contribute to atherosclerosis
    c. is not found in animal foods
    d. may be described as all of the above

B. Match the definition listed in Column I with its term in Column II.

fats = lipids

1gm fat = 9 Kcal

	Column I	Column II
f	1. Number of kcal per gram of fat ⁹	a. 4
e	2. can be caused by gross deficiency of fat *eczema*	b. carbohydrates
i	3. another name for fats *Lipids*	c. adipose tissue
j	4. to manufacture in the body *synthetize*	d. monounsaturated fats
l	5. combinations of three fatty acids and glycerol *Triglyceride*	e. eczema
m	6. examples of saturated fats	f. 9
h	7. examples of polyunsaturated fats	g. cholesterol
o	8. special carriers of fats in the blood *Lipoproteins*	h. corn and sunflower seed oils
g	9. substance found in animal fats that is essential to the body, but not in the diet *chol.*	i. lipids
c	10. body fat *Adipose*	j. synthesize
		k. hydrolize
		l. triglycerides
		m. cream and egg yolk
		n. 6
		o. lipoproteins

pg. 47 –
p. 45 –

oils →

fats cannot mix by itself – blood is H₂O base

Case Study 1

Diet and Atherosclerosis

Jim Burns is a 45-year-old business executive who plays squash about three times a week. He visited his doctor recently because he had experienced chest pains the last time he played squash. After the examination, his doctor told him he appeared to have a mild form of angina pectoris. The doctor explained that this was his heart's way of telling him it was short of oxygen at times because it was not receiving sufficient blood during periods of exertion. The doctor tested Jim's blood and told him he would be called with the results in two days. In the meantime, the doctor suggested he cut down on the amount of fats in his diet. He was advised to be particularly careful to avoid foods containing saturated fats and cholesterol.

Case Study Questions Based on the Nursing Process

Assess
1. What may be causing Jim's shortage of oxygen?
2. Is this condition a recent development? Why or why not? *cumulative*
3. Why did the pains occur during a period of exercise and not while Jim sat at his desk?
4. Why did the doctor test Jim's blood?

Plan
5. What specific foods did the doctor probably advise Jim to avoid? Why?

Implement
6. That night Jim and his family had roast beef, baked potatoes with sour cream, green beans with butter, lettuce with mayonnaise dressing, bread and butter, milk, and apple pie for dessert. Which of these foods should Jim avoid? Why? What could he easily substitute for them without disrupting the entire family dinner menu?

Evaluate
7. What could occur if Jim ignores the doctor's advice?
8. What would a moderate reduction of Jim's weight mean to the doctor?

Case Study 2

Weight Loss Requires Professional Advice

After Ellen had a heart attack at the age of 59, her doctor advised her to limit the fats in her diet. She read all the articles on heart and diet that she found in magazines, newspapers, and pamphlets in the local health food store. She became convinced that by lowering her fat intake to less than 10 percent of her total kcal she would avoid a second attack. Within one month after beginning the regimen, she had lost 8 pounds, her skin had become unusually dry and scaly in spots, and she felt tired most of the time.

At her next scheduled visit to her doctor, she was asked about the weight loss. On learning of her plan, the doctor insisted that she increase the fat content of her diet to 30 percent of total kcal, with no more than 10 percent of the fat coming from saturated fats.

Case Study Questions Based on the Nursing Process

Assess
1. Why was Ellen's decision unwise?
2. Why is it essential that decisions about diet be based on the advice of a health professional trained in nutrition and not on the advice of salespeople in health food stores?
3. What may have caused Ellen's weight loss? Her fatigue? Her scaly skin?

Plan
4. What specific foods should Ellen limit if she is to keep her saturated fat intake to 10 percent of her total daily kcal?

Implement
5. Plan a one day menu for Ellen.

Evaluate
6. What might have been the long-term effects if Ellen kept her fat intake at less than 30 percent of total kcal?

CHAPTER 5

PROTEINS

OBJECTIVES

After studying this chapter, you should be able to
• State the functions of proteins in the body
• Identify the elements of which proteins are composed
• Describe the effects of protein deficiency
• State the energy yield of proteins
• Identify at least six food sources of complete proteins and six food sources of incomplete proteins

carbs, fats, Protein, vits, min, H₂O

Body cells are constantly wearing out. As a result, they are continuously in need of replacement. Of the six nutrient groups, only proteins can make new cells and rebuild tissue.

Proteins are the basic material of every body cell. By the age of four years, body protein content reaches the adult level of about 18 percent of body weight. Obviously, an adequate supply of proteins in the daily diet is essential for normal growth and development and for the maintenance of health. Proteins are appropriately named. The word **protein** is of Greek derivation and means "of first importance."

COMPOSITION

Like carbohydrates and fats, proteins contain carbon, hydrogen, and oxygen, but in different proportions. In addition, and most importantly, they are the only nutrient group that contains **nitrogen** (chemical element essential to the body). Many also contain sulphur, phosphorus, iron, and copper, as well as other mineral elements. (See Chapter 7.)

Proteins are composed of chemical compounds called **amino acids.** Amino acids are sometimes called the building blocks of protein because they are combined to form the thousands of proteins in the human body. Heredity determines the specific types of proteins within each person.

CLASSIFICATION

The quality and classification of a protein depend on the number and types of amino acids it contains. There are 22 amino acids, but only 9 are considered essential to humans. (See Table 5-1.) Essential amino acids are necessary for normal growth and development and must be provided in the diet. Proteins containing all the essential amino acids are of high biologic value and

Table 5-1 Amino Acids

Essential	Nonessential
Histidine	Alanine
Isoleucine	Arginine
Leucine	Asparagine
Lysine	Aspartic acid
Methionine	Cysteine
Phenylalanine	Cystine
Threonine	Glutamic acid
Tryptophan	Glutamine
Valine	Glycine
	Hydroxyproline
	Proline
	Serine
	Tyrosine

Table 5-2 Examples of Complementary Protein Foods

Corn	and	Beans
Rice	and	Beans
Bread	and	Peanut Butter
Bread	and	Split Pea Soup
Bread	and	Cheese
Bread	and	Baked Beans
Macaroni	and	Cheese
Cereal	and	Milk

(animal) all essential amino acid

are called **complete proteins.** The nonessential amino acids can be produced in the body if an adequate supply of nitrogen is provided in the diet. *(plant)* **Incomplete proteins** are those that lack one or more of the essential amino acids. Consequently, incomplete proteins cannot build tissue without the help of other proteins. The value of each is increased when it is eaten in combination with another incomplete protein at the same meal. In this way, one incomplete protein food can provide the essential amino acids the other lacks. The combination may thereby provide all nine essential amino acids. When this occurs, the proteins are called **complementary proteins.** (See Table 5-2.)

FUNCTIONS

Proteins build and repair body tissue, play major roles in regulating various body functions, and provide energy if there is insufficient carbohydrate and fat in the diet.

Building and Repairing Body Tissue

The primary function of proteins is to build and repair body tissues. This is made possible by the provision of the correct type and number of amino acids in the diet. Also, as cells are broken down during metabolism (catabolism), some

Fat 9 Kcal / Cal (handwritten)

amino acids released into the blood plasma are recycled to build new and repair other tissue (anabolism). The body uses the recycled amino acids as efficiently as those obtained from the diet.

Regulating Body Functions

Proteins are important components of hormones and enzymes that are essential for the regulation of metabolism and digestion. Proteins help maintain fluid balance in the body and thus prevent **edema** (abnormal retention of body fluids). Proteins also are essential for the development of antibodies and, consequently, for a healthy immune system.

Providing Energy

Proteins can provide energy if and when the supply of carbohydrates and fats in the diet is insufficient. Each gram of protein provides four kcal. This is not a good use of proteins, however. Generally, they are more expensive than carbohydrates, and most of the complete proteins also contain saturated fats and cholesterol.

1 gm protein = 4 Kcal (handwritten)

FOOD SOURCES OF PROTEINS

Proteins are found in both animal and plant foods, Table 5-3. The animal food sources provide the highest quality, or complete proteins. They include meats, fish, poultry, eggs, milk, and cheese.

Despite the high biologic value of proteins from animal food sources, they also provide saturated fats and cholesterol. Consequently, complete proteins should be carefully selected from low-fat animal foods such as fish, lean meats, and low-fat dairy products. Eggs should be limited to two or three per week.

Table 5-3 Rich Sources of Proteins	
Complete Proteins	**Incomplete Proteins**
Meats	Corn
Fish	Peanuts
Poultry	Peas
Eggs	Navy beans
Milk	Soybeans
Cheese	Grains
	Nuts
	Sunflower seeds
	Sesame seeds

Proteins found in plant foods are incomplete proteins and are of a lower quality than those found in animal foods. Even so, plant foods are important sources of protein. Examples of plant foods containing protein are corn, grains, nuts, sunflower seeds, sesame seeds, and **legumes** such as soybeans, navy beans, pinto beans, split peas, chick peas, and peanuts.

Plant proteins can be used to produce **textured protein** products, also called **analogues.** These products are made by extracting the protein from plants (usually soybeans), and spinning it into fibers of nearly pure protein. The fibers are colored, flavored, and shaped into a product that resembles and tastes like meat. Textured protein can be used as a filler in other foods, such as ground meat. Textured protein increases the protein content of the food to which it is added. It can be used as an economical meat replacement.

DIGESTION AND ABSORPTION

The mechanical digestion of protein begins in the mouth where the teeth grind the food into small pieces. Chemical digestion begins in the stomach. Hydrochloric acid prepares the stomach so the enzyme **pepsin** can begin its task of reducing proteins to **polypeptides** (partially digested proteins). In young children, the enzyme **rennin coagulates** (thickens) milk in the stomach, which prevents the milk from passing through the stomach too quickly. Adults do not produce rennin.

After the polypeptides reach the small intestine, three pancreatic enzymes (**trypsin, chymotrypsin,** and **carboxypeptidase**) continue chemical digestion. Intestinal peptidases finally reduce the proteins to amino acids.

After digestion, the amino acids in the small intestine are absorbed by the blood and carried to all body tissues. There, they are used to form needed proteins.

METABOLISM AND ELIMINATION

All essential amino acids must be present to build and repair the cells as needed. Surplus amino acids are sent back to the liver where they are dismantled by splitting off the nitrogen. The remaining parts are used for energy or converted to carbohydrate or fat and stored as glycogen or adipose tissue. The end products of the metabolism of amino acids are carbon dioxide, water, and nitrogen. The excess nitrogen is sent to the kidneys and excreted in **urea.**

nitrogen → kidneys → UREA

DIETARY REQUIREMENTS

∅ use for energy + heat - hard to digest

One's protein requirement is determined by size, age, sex, and physical and emotional conditions. A large person has more body cells to maintain than a small person. A growing child, a pregnant woman, or a woman who is breastfeeding needs more protein per pound of body weight than the average adult. When digestion is inefficient, fewer amino acids are absorbed by the body, consequently raising the protein requirement. This is sometimes thought to be the case

Daily req. { Fats - 30% >10% sat fat (only)
Carbs - 50%
Prot - 15 - 20%

with the elderly. Extra proteins are usually required after surgery, severe burns, or during infections in order to replace lost tissue and manufacture antibodies. In addition, **emotional trauma** (stressful situations) can cause the body to excrete more nitrogen than it normally does, thus increasing the need for protein foods.

The National Research Council of the National Academy of Sciences considers the average adult's daily requirement to be 0.8 grams of protein per kilogram of body weight. To determine your requirement:

1. divide body weight by 2.2 (the number of pounds per kilogram)
2. multiply the answer obtained in Number 1 above by 0.8 (grams of protein per kilogram of body weight)

The National Research Council's 1989 chart of Recommended Daily Allowances (RDA) of protein for average groups of people is shown in Table 5-4. Table 5-5 provides an idea of the amount of protein in an average day's diet. (For specific amounts of protein in other foods, refer to Table A-5 in the Appendix.) It is obviously easy for people living in the developed parts of the world to ingest more proteins than the body requires. However, because of the saturated fats and cholesterol often found in complete protein foods, an excess may contribute to heart disease and provide more kcal than are desirable. Additionally, excess proteins may put more demands on the kidneys than they are prepared to handle and possibly contribute to **osteoporosis** (deterioration of the bones after the age of 50; see Chapter 7). Therefore, the National Research Council recommends that protein intake represent no more than 15 to 20 percent of one's daily kcal intake and not exceed double the amount given in the table of Recommended Dietary Allowances. (See Table 5-4.)

Prot = 15 % DAILY

Table 5-4 Recommended Daily Allowances of Protein

Category	Age (years) or Condition	Weight (kg)	Weight (lb)	Height (cm)	Height (in)	Protein (g)
Infants	0.0–0.5	6	13	60	24	13
	0.5–1.0	9	20	71	28	14
Children	1–3	13	29	90	35	16
	4–6	20	44	112	44	24
	7–10	28	62	132	52	28
Males	11–14	45	99	157	62	45
	15–18	66	145	176	69	59
	19–24	72	160	177	70	58
	25–50	79	174	176	70	63
	51+	77	170	173	68	63
Females	11–14	46	101	157	62	46
	15–18	55	120	163	64	44
	19–24	58	128	164	65	46
	25–50	63	138	163	64	50
	51+	65	143	160	63	50
Pregnant						60
Lactating	1st 6 months					65
	2nd 6 months					62

Source: Food & Nutrition Board, National Academy of Sciences, Washington, DC, 1989

Protein requirements may be discussed in terms of **nitrogen balance.** This occurs when nitrogen intake equals the amount of nitrogen excreted. **Positive nitrogen balance** exists when nitrogen intake exceeds the amount excreted. This indicates new tissue is being formed and occurs during pregnancy, during children's growing years, when athletes develop additional muscle tissue, and when tissues are rebuilt after **physical trauma** such as illness or injury. **Negative nitrogen balance** indicates protein is being lost. It may be caused by fevers, injury, surgery, burns, starvation, or immobilization.

Protein Deficiency

When people are unable to obtain an adequate supply of protein for an extended period, muscle wasting will occur and arms and legs become very thin. At the same time, **nutritional edema** may develop, resulting in an extremely swollen appearance. This water is excreted when sufficient protein is eaten. People may lose appetite, strength, and weight, and wounds may heal very slowly. Patients suffering from nutritional edema become lethargic and depressed. This is seen in grossly neglected children or in the elderly poor or incapacitated.

Protein Calorie Malnutrition (PCM)

People suffering from **protein calorie malnutrition (PCM)** lack both protein and energy-rich foods. Such a condition is not uncommon in third-world countries where there are long-term shortages of both protein and energy foods. Chil-

Table 5-5 Protein in an Average Diet for One Day

	Serving Size	Protein (Grams)	kcal
Breakfast			
Orange Juice	½ cup	1	45
Cornflakes	¾ cup	1	75
with sugar	2 tsp.		30
Toast	2 slices	4	140
Butter	1 Tbsp.		65
Jelly	1 Tbsp.		60
Skim Milk	½ cup	4	50
Lunch			
Grapefruit Juice	½ cup	1	50
Tuna Salad Sandwich	⅔ cup tuna salad	20	220
on Bread	2 slices (bread)	4	140
c/ lettuce			
Carrot Sticks	1 carrot	1	25
Canned Pears	½ cup	1	100
Oatmeal Cookies	2	1	160
Skim Milk	1 cup	8	100
Dinner			
Chicken Breast	½ (3 oz.)	26	160
Baked Potato	1	4	145
Asparagus	½ cup		25
Sliced Tomato Salad	1 tomato	1	25
Roll	1	1	100
with butter	1 Tbsp.		65
Ice Cream	⅔ cup	3	200
Skim Milk	1 cup	8	100
		89	2080

dren who lack sufficient protein do not grow to their potential size. Infants born to mothers eating insufficient protein during pregnancy can have permanently impaired mental capacities.

There are two **deficiency diseases** caused by a grossly inadequate supply of protein that affect children. **Marasmus,** a condition resulting from severe malnutrition, afflicts very young children who lack both protein and energy foods. The infant with marasmus appears emaciated, but does not have edema. Hair is dull and dry,

and the skin is thin and wrinkled, figure 5-1. The other protein deficiency disease that affects children is **kwashiorkor,** figure 5-2. Kwashiorkor causes fat to accumulate in the liver and results in edema, painful skin **lesions** (sores), and changes in the pigmentation of skin and hair. The mortality rate for kwashiorkor patients is high. Those who do survive these deficiency diseases may suffer from permanent **mental retardation.** The ultimate cost of **food deprivation** (lack) among young children is high, indeed.

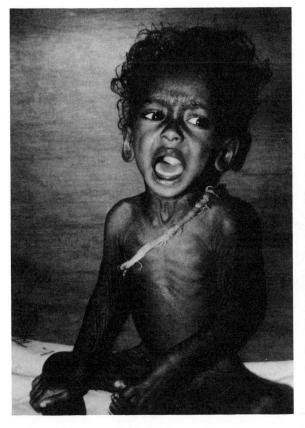

A. Visible signs of marasmus include extreme wasting, wrinkled skin, and irritability.

B. After 4 1/2 months of nutritional therapy, the same child shows great improvement.

Figure 5-1 A child with marasmus may not recover completely but is greatly helped by nutritional therapy. *(Courtesy of the World Health Organization)*

CONSIDERATIONS FOR THE HEALTH CARE PROFESSIONAL

Proteins have acquired an unfairly high value among the general public in the United States. Also, many people think proteins are found only in animal food sources. As a result, complete proteins tend to be overused in most diets.

Research about the cumulative effects of the overuse of proteins in the diet is beginning to suggest that excessive use of protein could damage kidneys and possibly contribute to osteoporosis and cancer and cause overweight and heart disease.

The health care professional may find that reeducating patients about the need to reduce their protein intake to 15 to 20 percent of total kcal is a challenging task. Humor and patience combined with suggestions for menus and recipe alterations will all be needed.

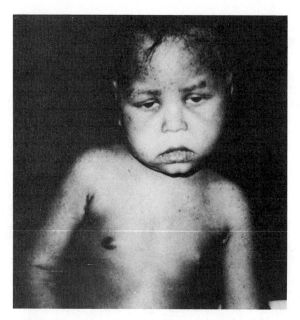

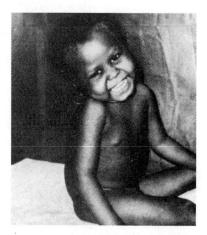

A. Edema, skin lesions (sores), and hair changes are common signs of kwashiorkor.

B. Only one month after receiving a proper diet, hunger, discomfort, and visible signs of disease are greatly reduced.

Figure 5-2 Effects of kwashiorkor can be partly eliminated by putting protein back into the diet. *(Courtesy of the World Health Organization)*

SUMMARY

Proteins contain nitrogen, an element that is necessary for growth and the maintenance of health. In addition to building and repairing body tissues, proteins regulate body processes and can supply energy. Each gram of protein provides 4 kcal (17 kJ). Proteins are composed of amino acids, nine of which are essential for growth and repair of body tissues.

Complete proteins contain all of the essential amino acids and can build tissues. The best sources of complete proteins are animal foods such as meat, fish, poultry, eggs, milk, and cheese. Incomplete proteins do not contain all of the essential amino acids and two or more of

these proteins must be combined in order to build tissues. The best sources of incomplete proteins are legumes, corn, grains, and nuts. The nutritional value of incomplete protein foods can be increased by eating two or more incomplete protein foods at the same meal. Chemical digestion of proteins occurs in the stomach and small intestine. Proteins are reduced to amino acids and ultimately absorbed into the blood through the small intestine.

A severe deficiency of protein in the diet can cause marasmus or kwashiorkor in children, and can result in impaired physical and mental development.

Discussion Topics

1. Why are proteins especially important to children, pregnant women, and people who are ill?
2. Of which elements are proteins composed? *Carbon, Hydrogen, O₂, Nitrogen*
3. What functions do proteins perform in the body?
4. Discuss why it may be unwise to use protein foods as energy foods.
5. Discuss the effects of protein deficiency.
6. Describe the digestion of proteins.
7. Describe the metabolism of proteins.
8. Tell what amino acids are and explain their importance. Tell where they are found.
9. Describe textured protein products. If anyone in class has eaten textured protein, ask her or him to describe the taste, color, appearance, and cost of the food.
10. Discuss why foods rich in complete proteins are usually more expensive than foods containing incomplete proteins.
11. Why are protein-rich foods typically more expensive than carbohydrate-rich foods? *from animal sources vs plant (meat, cheese)*
12. Describe complete and incomplete protein foods and name several of each type.
13. Why are complete protein foods also generally rich in saturated fats? *from Animals*
14. What determines protein requirements? *age, sex, size, phys + emotional condt*
15. Why might someone with a broken hip develop negative nitrogen balance in the hospital? *need protein for healing - built repair tiss.*

Suggested Activities

1. Cook an egg at a low temperature and another at a high temperature. Observe, taste, and discuss the differences. Do the same with two portions of ground meat. What characteristics of protein foods do these demonstrations indicate?
2. Keep a record of the foods you eat in a 24-hour period. Using Table A-5 in the Appendix, compute the grams of protein consumed. Did your diet provide the recommended amount of protein as indicated in Table 5-4 of this chapter?
3. Make a chart for display in the classroom showing complete and incomplete protein foods.
4. Add 1 teaspoon of lemon juice to $\frac{1}{2}$ cup of milk. Observe, taste, and discuss the result.

5. Plan a day's menu for yourself. Include foods especially rich in complete proteins.
   a. Alter your planned menu; replace some of the complete protein foods with those containing incomplete proteins.
   b. Visit a local supermarket and compute the cost of the menu that contains complete proteins. Compute the cost of the menu that contains incomplete proteins. Which is less expensive? Why?
   c. Adapt the planned menu to suit a 30-year-old pregnant woman.
6. Role play a situation in which a diet counselor attempts to convince a pregnant teenager that she should eat at least two servings of meat, fish, or poultry each day.
7. Write a speech that could be made to a class of nine-year-old children, explaining what proteins are and why they should eat foods containing them every day.
8. Invite a registered nurse with experience in caring for badly burned patients to discuss the dietary needs of these patients and their reactions to food.

Review

A. Multiple choice. Select the *letter* that precedes the best answer.
   1. The building blocks of proteins are
      a. ascorbic acids
      b. amino acids
      c. nitrogen and sulphur only
      d. meat and fish
   2. Proteins are essential because they are the only nutrient that contains
      a. nitrogen
      b. niacin
      c. hydrochloric acid
      d. carbon
   3. Corn, peas, and beans
      a. are complete protein foods
      b. are incomplete protein foods
      c. contain no protein
      d. lose proteins during cooking
   4. A person's daily protein requirement
      a. may be met by use of complementary proteins
      b. can be met only by complete proteins
      c. is not affected by one's age
      d. is difficult to fulfill in the U.S.

5.   Protein deficiency may result in
    a. beriberi   **c.** nutritional edema
    b. goiter   d. leukemia

6.   Good sources of complete protein foods are
    a. eggs and ground beef   c. butter and margarine
    b. breads and cereals   d. legumes and nuts

7.   One gram of protein provides
    a. 4 kcal   c. · 19 kilojoules
    b. 9 kcal   d. 37.8 kilojoules

— 8.   The chemical digestion of protein occurs in
    a. the mouth and stomach
    b. the mouth and small intestine   *stomach + sml intest*
    c. the stomach and small intestine
    d. all of these

9.   Complete proteins contain all the essential
    a. nutrients   **c.** amino acids
    b. ascorbic acids   d. kcalories

10.   The *primary* function of protein is to
    a. build and repair body cells   c. digest minerals and vitamins
    b. provide heat and energy   d. none of these

B.   Arrange the following foods into two lists, one containing those that are the best sources of complete proteins and one containing those that are the best sources of incomplete proteins.

    c scrambled eggs C
    I lima beans   I
    I corn on the cob I
    C hot chocolate milk C
    I chick peas and rice I
    C skim milk C
Animal C beefburgers C
    I baked navy beans I
Animal C filet of sole C
Animal C fried chicken C
    I peanuts   I
Animal C Swiss cheese C

C.   Match the term in column I with its definition in column II.

Column I	Column II
_____ 1. rennin	a. chemical element in amino acids
__g__ 2. amino acids *g*	b. disease of severe protein deficiency
_____ 3. marasmus *k*	c. reduces proteins to smaller substances in the stomach
_____ 4. pepsin	d. coagulates milk
__i__ 5. roast beef *i*	e. retention of body fluids
__h__ 6. legumes *h*	f. carbohydrate
_____ 7. kwashiorkor *b*	g. building blocks of protein
__e__ 8. edema *e*	h. example of incomplete protein
__a__ 9. nitrogen *a*	i. example of complete protein
_____ 10. textured protein	j. meat substitute
	k. lack of proteins and calories

peas/beans (handwritten note pointing to legumes)

Case Study 1

Insufficient Protein

Milly had always loved visiting her grandmother in her city apartment. Everything was spotless, there was lots of good food, and her grandmother was peppy and fun to be around. Unfortunately, Milly noticed changes during her last visit. Despite the fact that her grandmother appeared to have gained weight, there was little to eat in the apartment other than crackers and canned soup. Her grandmother seemed lethargic and cranky, and complained about the cost of food. Milly was particularly concerned because she had to leave on a week-long business trip the next day. She bought some of her grandmother's favorite foods—canned peaches, coffee cake, fresh strawberries, and vanilla ice cream—and left them in the refrigerator. When she returned from her trip, the food was gone, but her grandmother seemed worse, so she took her to her doctor.

After examining her grandmother and questioning both of them, the doctor prescribed a one-a-day vitamin, coordinated dietary counseling with the local dietitian, and advised Milly to contact Meals-on-Wheels on her grandmother's behalf.

Milly and her grandmother met with the dietitian. Together, they reviewed the foods her grandmother liked, her budgetary constraints, and planned a balanced diet for her.

Milly's grandmother was pleased with the diet plan. Meals-on-Wheels would provide one hot meal a day, and Milly would work with her grandmother to plan and prepare the rest of the meals. In the following weeks, her grandmother lost her puffiness and regained her old personality.

Case Study Questions Based on the Nursing Process

Assess
1. What questions did the doctor probably ask the grandmother?
2. What questions did the doctor probably ask Milly?
3. Is it possible that the doctor asked Milly about her grandmother in her grandmother's presence? Why?
4. What was a possible cause of her grandmother's puffiness? Crankiness?
5. What might have initiated this problem?

Plan
6. Did any foods Milly put in her grandmother's refrigerator help alleviate the problem? Why?

Implement
7. Is it important for Milly's grandmother to agree with the diet plan? Why?
8. Plan a week's menu for Milly's grandmother.
9. What organizations exist in your neighborhood that would be helpful in a situation such as this?

Evaluate
10. What solutions might there be if Milly's grandmother lived in a small town?

Case Study 2

Too Much of a Good Thing

When Donald was a rising football star in high school, his coach advised him and his teammates to eat "lots" of protein. Donald did. He had either a minute steak or three to six scrambled eggs for breakfast. At lunch he favored cheeseburgers and milk shakes and dinner always centered on a roast. His mother served homogenized (whole) milk because it had all of nature's ingredients. Donald disliked fish—except for fried shrimp. Over the years, Donald felt rather virtuous because he seldom touched desserts.

He retained this eating pattern until he had heart problems at the age of 55. He is recovering well and, at his doctor's urging, is making changes in his eating habits.

Case Study Questions Based on the Nursing Process

Assess

1. How might Donald's perceived need for protein have contributed to his subsequent heart problems?
2. What did the doctor probably tell Donald about his eating habits? About his actual protein requirement?

Plan

3. Suggest some alternative menus for Donald that the doctor would probably approve.

Implement

4. Is Donald's new menu likely to affect his family's eating habits? Explain.

Evaluate

5. How would you react if your son were told to eat as much protein as possible? Explain your reaction.

CHAPTER 6

alpha-tocopherol
amenorrhea
antibiotic therapy
anticoagulant
antioxidant
ascorbic acid
avitaminosis
beriberi
biotin
carotene
catalysts
cheilosis
cholecalciferol
coagulation
cobalamin
coenzymes
collagen
dermatitis
enriched
ergocalciferol
fat soluble
folic acid
fortified
gingivitis
glossitis
hemolysis
hemorrhage
hormone
hypervitaminosis
hypocalcemia
International Units
   (IU)
intracranial
   hemorrhage
intrinsic factor
iron enhancer
leukocytes
megadoses
megaloblastic
   anemia
menadione
menaquinone
mucous membranes
myelin

niacin
niacin equivalents
   (NE)
norepinephrine
opaque
osteomalacia
osteoporosis
pallor
panacea
pantothenic acid
pellagra
pernicious anemia
phylloquinone
pigmentation
precursor
prohormone
prothrombin
provitamin
pyridoxal
pyridoxamine
pyridoxine
RDA
restored
retinol
retinol equivalents
   (RE)
riboflavin
rickets
scurvy
synthesize
synthetic
tachycardia
tetany
thiamin
tocopherols
tocotrienols
toxic
tryptophan
vascular dilation
vitamers
vitamin
vitamin supplements
water soluble
xerophthalmia

VITAMINS

OBJECTIVES

After studying this chapter, you should be able to
- State one or more functions of each of the 13 vitamins discussed
- Identify at least two food sources of each of the vitamins discussed
- Identify some symptoms of, or diseases caused by, deficiencies of the vitamins discussed

living

Vitamins are organic compounds containing carbon, oxygen, and other elements that are essential for body processes. Vitamins themselves do not provide energy. They enable the body to use the energy provided by fats, carbohydrates, and proteins. The name **vitamin** implies their importance. *Vita* in Latin, means life. They do not, however, represent a **panacea** (universal remedy) for physical or mental illness, or a way to alleviate the stress of modern life. They should not be overused—more is not necessarily better.

they themselves do NOT do the work

Protein Defic.
Marsusus
Kwashorkor

Vits = carbon + O₂
Vits. allow, Carb. fats + Prot to do work!

Table 6-1 Vitamins *B + C*	
Fat Soluble (4)	**Water Soluble (9)**
Vitamin A *A D C K*	Vitamin B Complex
Vitamin D	includes:
Vitamin E	Thiamin
Vitamin K	Riboflavin
	Niacin
	Vitamin B_6
	Folacin
	Vitamin B_{12}
	Pantothenic Acid
	Biotin
	Vitamin C

In fact, **megadoses** (extraordinarily large amounts) can be **toxic** (poisonous). Normally, a healthy person eating a balanced diet (see Chapter 9) will obtain all the nutrients—including vitamins—needed. *Otherwise flushed down toilet + toxicity*

The existence of vitamins has been known since early in the twentieth century. It was discovered that animals fed diets of pure proteins, carbohydrates, fats, and minerals did not thrive as did those fed normal diets that included vitamins.

Vitamins were originally named by letter. Subsequent research has shown that many of the vitamins that were originally thought to be a single substance are actually groups of substances doing similar work in the body. Vitamin B proved to be more than one compound—B_1, B_6, B_{12}, and so on—and consequently is now known as "B complex." Many of the 13 known vitamins are currently named according to their chemical composition or function in the body. (See Table 6-1.)

Vitamins are found in minute amounts in natural foods. The specific amounts and types of vitamins in foods vary.

Vits; many they must not made in body take In

HUMAN REQUIREMENTS

The Food and Nutrition Board, National Academy of Sciences—National Research Council has prepared a list of **RDA** (recommended dietary allowances) for those eleven vitamins for which it considers current scientific research adequate for such determinations. (See Table 6-2.) In addition, the Board also has prepared a list of estimated safe and adequate daily dietary intakes of two additional vitamins for which current research is inadequate to allow them to propose RDA. (See Table 6-3.)

Vitamin allowances are given by weight—milligrams (mg) or micrograms (mcg or μg)—in most cases as in the tables, but sometimes, on labels, amounts of A, D, and E are listed as **IU (International Units). IU** represent the measurement used in early experiments with animals.

Vitamin deficiencies can occur and can result in disease. Those inclined to vitamin deficiencies because they do not eat balanced diets include alcoholics, the poor and incapacitated elderly, patients with serious diseases that affect appetite, mentally retarded persons, and young children who receive inadequate care.

The term **avitaminosis** means "without vitamins." This word followed by the name of a specific vitamin is used to indicate a serious lack of that particular vitamin. **Hypervitaminosis** is the excess of one or more vitamins. Either a lack or excess of vitamins can be detrimental to a person's health.

Vitamins taken in addition to those received in the diet are called **vitamin supplements.** These are available in concentrated forms in tablets, capsules, and drops. Vitamin concentrates are sometimes termed natural or **synthetic** (manufactured). Some people believe a meaningful difference exists between the two types and that the natural are far superior in quality to the synthetic.

Table 6-2 Recommended Dietary Vitamin Allowances

Category or Condition	Age (years)	Weight (kg)	Weight (lb)	Height (cm)	Height (in)	Protein (g)	Fat-Soluble Vitamins Vita-min A (µg RE)	Vita-min D (µg)	Vita-min E (mg α-TE)	Vita-min K (µg)	Water-Soluble Vitamins Vita-min C (mg)	Thia-min (mg)	Ribo-flavin (mg)	Niacin (mg NE)	Vita-min B6 (mg)	Fo-late (µg)	Vita-min B12 (µg)
Infants	0.0–0.5	6	13	60	24	13	375	7.5	3	5	30	0.3	0.4	5	0.3	25	0.3
	0.5–1.0	9	20	71	28	14	375	10	4	10	35	0.4	0.5	6	0.6	35	0.5
Children	1–3	13	29	90	35	16	400	10	6	15	40	0.7	0.8	9	1.0	50	0.7
	4–6	20	44	112	44	24	500	10	7	20	45	0.9	1.1	12	1.1	75	1.0
	7–10	28	62	132	52	28	700	10	7	30	45	1.0	1.2	13	1.4	100	1.4
Males	11–14	45	99	157	62	45	1,000	10	10	45	50	1.3	1.5	17	1.7	150	2.0
	15–18	66	145	176	69	59	1,000	10	10	65	60	1.5	1.8	20	2.0	200	2.0
	19–24	72	160	177	70	58	1,000	10	10	70	60	1.5	1.7	19	2.0	200	2.0
	25–50	79	174	176	70	63	1,000	5	10	80	60	1.5	1.7	19	2.0	200	2.0
	51+	77	170	173	68	63	1,000	5	10	80	60	1.2	1.4	15	2.0	200	2.0
Females	11–14	46	101	157	62	46	800	10	8	45	50	1.1	1.3	15	1.4	150	2.0
	15–18	55	120	163	64	44	800	10	8	55	60	1.1	1.3	15	1.5	180	2.0
	19–24	58	128	164	65	46	800	10	8	60	60	1.1	1.3	15	1.6	180	2.0
	25–50	63	138	163	64	50	800	5	8	65	60	1.1	1.3	15	1.6	180	2.0
	51+	65	143	160	63	50	800	5	8	65	60	1.0	1.2	13	1.6	180	2.0
Pregnant						60	800	10	10	65	70	1.5	1.6	17	2.2	400	2.2
Lactating	1st 6 months					65	1,300	10	12	65	95	1.6	1.8	20	2.1	280	2.6
	2nd 6 months					62	1,200	10	11	65	90	1.6	1.7	20	2.1	260	2.6

Source: Food and Nutrition Board, National Academy of Sciences—National Research Council Recommended Dietary Allowances, Revised 1989

73

Table 6-3 Estimated Safe and Adequate Daily Dietary Intakes of Selected Vitamins and Minerals

Category	Age (years)	Vitamins	
		Biotin (μg)	Pantothenic Acid (mg)
Infants	0–0.5	10	2
	0.5–1	15	3
Children and adolescents	1–3	20	3
	4–6	25	3–4
	7–10	30	4–5
	11+	30–100	4–7
Adults		30–100	4–7

Source: Food and Nutrition Board, National Academy of Sciences—National Research Council Recommended Dietary Allowances.

However, according to the United States Food and Drug Administration (FDA), the body cannot distinguish between a vitamin of plant or animal origin and one manufactured in a laboratory since once they have been dismantled by the digestive system, both types of the same vitamin are chemically identical.

Synthetic vitamins are frequently added to foods during processing. When this is done, the foods are described as **enriched** or **fortified.** Examples of these foods are enriched breads and cereals to which thiamin, niacin, riboflavin, and the mineral iron have been added. Vitamins A and D are added to milk and fortified margarine.

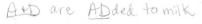
A+D are ADded to milk

Preserving Vitamin Content in Food

Occasionally, vitamins are lost during food processing. In most cases, food producers can replace these vitamins with synthetic vitamins, making the processed food nutritionally equal to the natural, unprocessed food. Foods in which vitamins are replaced are called **restored** foods.

Because some vitamins are easily destroyed by light, air, heat, and water, it is important to know how to preserve the vitamin content of food during its preparation and cooking. To avoid vitamin loss, it is advisable to:

- Buy the freshest, unbruised vegetables and fruits and use them raw whenever possible.
- Prepare fresh vegetables and fruits just before serving.
- Heat canned vegetables quickly and in their own liquid.
- Follow package directions when using frozen vegetables or fruit.
- Use as little water as possible when cooking and have it boiling when adding vegetables. Or, preferably, steam them.
- Cover the pan (except for the first few minutes when cooking strongly flavored vegetables such as broccoli and cauliflower), and cook as short a time as possible.
- Save the cooking liquid for later use in soups, stews, and gravies.

- Store fresh vegetables and most fruits in a cool, dark place.

CLASSIFICATION

Vitamins are commonly grouped according to solubility. A, D, E, and K are **fat soluble,** and B complex and C are **water soluble.** In addition, vitamin D is sometimes classified as a **hormone** (substance that produces specific biological effects) and the B complex group may be classified as **catalysts** or **coenzymes.** (Catalysts and enzymes are substances that cause chemical changes in other substances. A coenzyme is the active part of an enzyme.) When a vitamin has different chemical forms but serves the same purpose in the body, these forms are sometimes called **vitamers.** Vitamin E is an example of this. Sometimes a **precursor,** or a **provitamin** is found in foods. This is a substance from which the body can **synthesize** (manufacture) a specific vitamin. Carotene is an example of this.

FAT-SOLUBLE VITAMINS

The fat-soluble vitamins A, D, E, and K are chemically similar. They are not lost easily in cooking, but are lost when mineral oil is ingested. Mineral oil is not absorbed by humans. Consequently, it is sometimes used in salad dressings to avoid the kcal of vegetable oils. It is also commonly used as a laxative by the elderly. Its use should be discouraged because it picks up and carries with it fat-soluble vitamins that are then lost to the body. After absorption, fat-soluble vitamins are transported through the blood by means of carriers because they are not soluble in water. Excess amounts can be stored in the liver. Therefore, deficiencies of fat-soluble

vitamins are slower to appear than those caused by a lack of water-soluble vitamins. Because of the body's ability to store them, megadoses of fat-soluble vitamins should be avoided as they can reach toxic levels.

Vitamin A

Vitamin A consists of two basic dietary forms: preformed vitamin A, **retinol,** and provitamin A, **carotene.**

Functions

Vitamin A is essential for maintaining healthy eyes and skin, for normal growth and reproduction, and for a healthy immune system. In addition, it aids in the prevention of infections by helping to maintain healthy **mucous membranes** (the lining of the nose and throat, the gastrointestinal tract, and genitourinary tract).

Some carotene is converted into retinol during absorption in the intestines. Some is converted in the liver, after being carried there by the blood, and some is stored in adipose tissue.

Sources

Preformed vitamin A or retinol is found in fat-containing animal foods such as fish liver oils, liver, butter, cream, whole milk, whole milk cheeses, and egg yolk. It is also found in foods such as margarine, lowfat milk products, and cereals that have been fortified with vitamin A. Provitamin A or beta-carotene is found in yellow and dark green leafy vegetables, in yellow fruits, and products fortified with vitamin A.

Requirements

A well-balanced diet is the preferred way to obtain the required amounts of vitamin A. Vitamin A values are commonly listed as IU on commercial food products in the United States, but the term **retinol equivalents (RE)** is recommended by the Food and Nutrition Board. A retinol equivalent is equal to 3.33 IU of retinol, 1 μg retinol or 6 μg beta carotene (a particular type of carotene).

See Table 6-2 for the recommended dietary allowances as prescribed by the Food and Nutrition Board, National Academy of Sciences—National Research Council.

Hypervitaminosis A

The use of vitamin supplements should be discouraged as an excess of vitamin A can have serious consequences. Hypervitaminosis A has been noted in adults ingesting over 50,000 IU a day for sustained periods. In children, 20,000 IU per day for some months have produced toxic effects. Symptoms may include hair loss, dry skin, headaches, nausea, dryness of mucous membranes, liver damage, and bone and joint pain. Generally, these symptoms tend to disappear when excessive intake is discontinued.

Deficiency Symptoms

Deficiency symptoms of vitamin A include night blindness, figure 6-1; dry, rough skin; and increased susceptibility to infections. Avitaminosis A can result in blindness or **xerophthalmia,** a condition characterized by dry, lusterless, mucous membranes of the eye.

Vitamin D

Vitamin D exists in two forms—D_2 (**ergocalciferol**) and D_3 (**cholecalciferol**). Each is formed from a provitamin when irradiated with (exposed to) ultraviolet light. They are equally effective in human nutrition, but D_3 is the one that is formed in humans from cholesterol in the skin. D_2 is formed in plants. Vitamin D is considered a **prohormone** because it is converted to a hormone in the human body.

Vitamin D is heat stable and not easily oxidized so it is not harmed by storage, food processing, or cooking.

Functions

The major function of vitamin D is the promotion of calcium and phosphorus absorption in the body. By contributing to the absorption of these minerals, it helps to raise their concentration in the blood so that normal bone and tooth mineralization can occur and **tetany** (involuntary muscle movement) can be prevented. (Tetany can occur when there is too little calcium in the blood. This condition is called **hypocalcemia.**)

Vitamin D is absorbed in the intestines and is chemically changed in the liver and kidneys. Excess amounts of vitamin D are stored in the liver and in adipose tissue.

Sources

The best source of vitamin D is the sun which, as noted previously, changes a provitamin to vitamin D_3 in humans. It is sometimes referred to as "the sunshine vitamin." The amount of vitamin D that is formed depends on the individual's **pigmentation** (coloring matter in the skin) and the amount of sunlight available. The best food sources of vitamin D are fish liver oils, egg yolk, butter, and fortified margarine. Because of the rather limited number of food sources of vitamin D and the unpredictability of sunshine, health authorities decided that the vitamin should be added to a common food. Milk was selected. Consequently, most milk available in the United States today has had 400 IU (10 mcg) of vitamin D concentrate added per quart.

Requirements

While the vitamin D requirement has not been established, the Food and Nutrition Board, National Academy of Sciences—National Re-

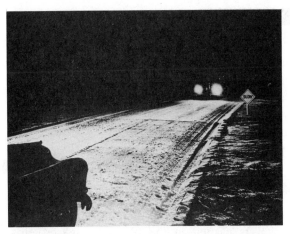

A.

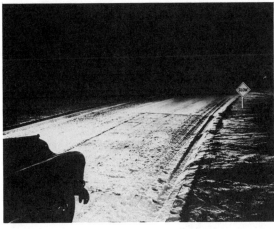

B.

Figure 6-1 Both the normal individual and the person suffering from a deficiency of vitamin A see the headlights of the approaching car (A). After the car has passed, the normal individual sees a wide stretch of road (B). The vitamin-A deficient person cannot see the road at all (C). This reaction to the contrast of light and dark at night is termed "night blindness." *(Courtesy of the Upjohn Company, Kalamazoo, Michigan)*

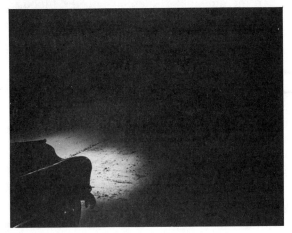

C.

search Council has recommended dietary allowances. (See Table 6-2.) It is believed that the needs of most adults can be met by an average exposure to sunlight. People who are seldom outdoors should use dietary sources also. Drinking one quart of irradiated milk each day fulfills the recommended daily dietary allowance for people from birth to 25 years of age and pregnant and lactating women, and more than fulfills the RDA for all others.

Vitamin D has commonly been measured in IU, but scientists are currently expressing its values in weight, specifically, micrograms of cholecalciferol. One IU equals .025 mcg (μg) cholecalciferol.

Hypervitaminosis D

Hypervitaminosis D must be avoided because it can cause calcium and phosphorous deposits in soft tissues, kidney and heart damage, and bone fragility.

Deficiency

The deficiency of vitamin D inhibits the absorption of calcium and phosphorus in the intes-

↑ vit D = cal + phos deposits

tine and results in poor bone and tooth formation. Young children suffering vitamin D deficiency may develop **rickets** (skeletal deformities), figure 6-2, and their teeth may be poorly formed, late in appearing, and particularly subject to decay. Adults lacking sufficient vitamin D may develop **osteomalacia** (softening of the bones because of a loss of calcium). And it is thought that a deficiency of vitamin D may contribute to **osteoporosis,** a disease characterized by brittle, porous bones, which is common in people over 50 years of age, especially women.

↓ vit D = rickets

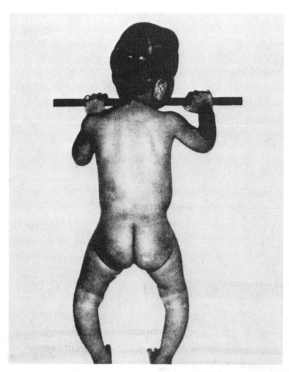

Figure 6-2 One of the symptoms of rickets is bowed legs, a symptom appearing after the child has learned to walk. *(Courtesy of the Upjohn Company and Dr. R. L. Nemir)*

Vitamin E

Vit E = antioxidant = protects cell membranes!

↓ Vit E = Hemolysis

Vitamin E consists of two groups of chemical compounds. They are the **tocopherols** and the **tocotrienols.** The most active of these is **alpha-tocopherol.**

Functions

Vitamin E is an **antioxidant.** This means it protects cell membranes and other substances from oxidation. It is aided in this process by vitamin C and the mineral, selenium. (See Chapter 7.) It is carried in the blood by lipoproteins. When the amount of vitamin E in the blood is low, the red blood cells become vulnerable to a higher than normal rate of **hemolysis.** It has been found helpful in a form of anemia among premature infants. It also has been associated with a reduced risk of cancer. Because of its antioxidant properties, it is commonly used in commercial food products to retard spoilage.

Sources

Vit E / wheat germ, nuts

Cooking oils made from corn, soybean, safflower, and cottonseed and products made from them, such as margarine, are the best sources of vitamin E. Wheat germ, nuts, and green leafy vegetables also are good sources. Animal foods, fruits, and most vegetables are poor sources.

Requirements

Research indicates that the vitamin E requirement increases if the amount of PUFA (polyunsaturated fatty acids) in the diet increases. Generally, however, the American diet is thought to contain sufficient vitamin E. Vitamin E was previously measured in IU, but it is now given as α-TE (alpha-tocopherol equivalents). One mg of this is the equivalent of 1 IU.

Hypervitaminosis

Although vitamin E appears to be relatively nontoxic, it is a fat-soluble vitamin and the excess is stored in adipose tissue. It would seem advisable to avoid long-term megadoses of vitamin E.

Deficiency

A deficiency of vitamin E has been detected in premature, low birth weight infants and in patients who are unable to absorb fat normally. Malabsorption can cause serious neurological defects in children but, in adults, it takes five to ten years before deficiency symptoms occur.

Vitamin K   *Blood Klotting*

Vitamin K is made up of several compounds that are essential to blood clotting. Vitamin K_1, commonly called **phylloquinone,** is found in dietary sources, especially green leafy vegetables such as cabbage, and in animal tissue. Vitamin K_2, called **menaquinone,** is synthesized in the intestine by bacteria and is also found in animal foods. In addition, there is a synthetic vitamin K, called **menadione.** Vitamin K is destroyed by light and alkalis.

Vitamin K is absorbed like fats, mainly from the small intestine and slightly from the colon. Its absorption requires a normal flow of bile from the liver, and it is improved when there is fat in the diet.

Function

Vitamin K is essential for the formation of **prothrombin,** which permits the proper clotting of the blood. It may be given to newborns immediately after birth because human milk contains little vitamin K and the intestines of newborns contain few bacteria. With insufficient vitamin K, newborns may be in danger of **intracranial hemorrhage** (bleeding within the head).

Vitamin K may be given to patients who suffer from faulty fat absorption; to patients after extensive **antibiotic therapy** (ingestion of antibiotic drugs to combat infection) because these drugs destroy the bacteria in the intestines; as an antidote for an overdose of **anticoagulant** (blood thinner); or to treat cases of **hemorrhage** (bleeding).

Sources   *Vit K = Kale, Kabbige, Spinick*

The best dietary sources of vitamin K are green leafy vegetables such as cabbage, spinach, or kale. Dairy products, eggs, meats, fruits, and cereals also contain some vitamin K. Cow's milk is a much better source of vitamin K than human milk. The synthesis of vitamin K by bacteria in the small intestine does not provide a sufficient supply by itself. It must be supplemented by dietary sources.

Requirements

Vitamin K is measured in micrograms. The RDA for vitamin K is one mcg/kg of body weight from the age of one year through the senior years. This is not increased during pregnancy or lactation. Infants up to six months should have 5 mcg per day. Those between six months and one year should receive 10 mcg per day.

Deficiency   *↓ Vit K = ↓ blood koagul.*

The only major symptom of a deficiency of vitamin K is defective blood **coagulation** (clotting). This increases clotting time, making the patient more prone to hemorrhage. Human deficiency may be caused by faulty fat metabolism, antibiotic therapy, inadequate diet, or anticoagulants (blood thinners).

Hypervitaminosis

Ingestion of excessive amounts of synthetic vitamin K can be toxic and cause a form of anemia.

WATER-SOLUBLE VITAMINS

Water-soluble vitamins include B complex and C. These vitamins dissolve in water and are easily destroyed by air and cooking. They are not stored in the body to the extent that fat-soluble vitamins are stored.

Vitamin B Complex

Beriberi is a disease that affects the nervous, cardiovascular, and gastrointestinal systems. The legs feel heavy, there is burning of the feet and muscle degeneration. The patient is irritable and suffers from headaches, depression, anorexia, constipation, **tachycardia** (rapid heart rate), edema, and heart failure.

very rare — seen in alcoholics (vit B12 Inj!)

Toward the end of the nineteenth century, a doctor in Indonesia discovered that chickens that were fed table scraps of polished rice developed symptoms much like those of his patients suffering from beriberi. When these same chickens were later fed brown (unpolished) rice, they recovered.

Some years later, this mysterious component of unpolished rice was recognized as an essential food substance and named vitamin B. Subsequently, it was named vitamin *B complex* because the vitamin was found to be composed of several compounds. The B complex vitamins include thiamin (B_1), riboflavin (B_2), niacin, B_6, cobalamin (B_{12}), folic acid, pantothenic acid, and biotin.

Thiamin

Thiamin, a coenzyme, was originally named vitamin B_1. It is partially destroyed by heat and alkalies, and is lost in cooking water.

Functions

Thiamin is essential for the metabolism of carbohydrates and some amino acids. It is absorbed in the small intestine.

Sources

Thiamin is found in many foods, but generally in small quantities. (See Table A-5 in the Appendix.) Some of the best natural food sources of thiamin are unrefined and enriched cereals, dry yeast, wheat germ, lean pork, organ meats, and legumes.

Requirements

Thiamin is measured in milligrams. The daily thiamin requirement for the average adult female is 1.1 mg a day, and for the average adult male it is 1.5 mg a day. The requirement is not thought to increase with age. Generally, however, an increase in kcal increases the need for thiamin.

Most breads and cereals in the United States are enriched with thiamin so that the majority of people can and do easily fulfill their recommended dietary requirements (see Table 6-2).

Deficiency

Symptoms of thiamin deficiency include loss of appetite, fatigue, nervous irritability, and constipation. An extreme deficiency causes beriberi. Its deficiency is rare, however, occurring mainly among alcoholics whose diets include reduced amounts of thiamin while their requirements of it are increased and their absorption of it is decreased. Others at risk include renal patients undergoing long-term dialysis; patients fed intravenously for long periods; and patients with chronic fevers.

Because some raw fish contain thiaminase, an enzyme that inhibits the normal action of thiamin, frequent consumption of large amounts of raw fish could cause thiamin deficiency. Cooking inactivates this enzyme.

Riboflavin

Riboflavin is sometimes called B_2. It is sensitive to light and unstable in alkalies.

Functions

Riboflavin is essential for carbohydrate, fat, and protein metabolism. It is also necessary for tissue maintenance, especially the skin around the mouth, and for healthy eyes. Riboflavin is absorbed in the small intestine.

Sources

Riboflavin is widely distributed in animal and plant foods but in small amounts. Milk, meats, poultry, fish, and enriched breads and cereals are some of its richest sources. Some green vegetables such as broccoli, spinach, and asparagus are also good sources.

Requirement

Riboflavin is measured in milligrams. The average adult female daily requirement is thought to be 1.3 mg and the adult male is 1.7 mg. The riboflavin requirement appears to increase with increased energy expenditure. Therefore, the requirement seems to diminish with age.

Deficiency

Because of the small quantities of riboflavin in foods and its limited storage in the body, deficiencies of riboflavin can develop. The generous use of skim milk in the diet is a good way to prevent deficiency of this vitamin. It is important, however, that milk be stored in **opaque** containers (prevent light penetration) because riboflavin can be destroyed by light. It appears that fiber laxatives can reduce riboflavin absorption, and their use over long periods should be discouraged.

A deficiency of riboflavin can result in **cheilosis,** a condition characterized by sores on the lips and cracks at the corners of the mouth; **glossitis** (inflammation of the tongue); dermatitis; and eye strain in the form of itching, burning, and eye fatigue. Its toxicity is unknown.

Niacin

Niacin is the generic name for nicotinic acid and nicotinamide.

Niacin is fairly stable in foods. It can withstand reasonable amounts of heat and acid and is not destroyed during food storage.

Functions

Niacin serves as a coenzyme in energy metabolism and consequently is essential to every body cell. In addition, niacin is essential for the prevention of **pellagra.** Pellagra is a disease characterized by sores on the skin, and by diarrhea, anxiety, confusion, irritability, poor memory, dizziness, and untimely death if left untreated.

Sources

The best sources of niacin are meats, poultry, and fish. Peanuts and other legumes are also good sources. Enriched breads and cereals also contain some. Milk and eggs do not provide niacin per se, but they are good sources of its precursor, **tryptophan** (an amino acid). Vegetables and fruits contain little niacin.

Requirements

Niacin is measured in **niacin equivalents (NE).** One NE equals one milligram of niacin or 60 milligrams of tryptophan. The general recommendation is a daily intake of 15 mg/NE for adult women and 19 mg/NE for adult men. Because excessive amounts of niacin have caused flushing due to **vascular dilation** (expansion of blood vessels), self-prescribed doses of niacin concentrate should be discouraged.

Deficiency

A deficiency of niacin is apt to appear if there is a deficiency of riboflavin. Symptoms of niacin deficiency include weakness, anorexia, indigestion, anxiety, and irritability. In extreme cases, pellagra may occur.

Vitamin B$_6$

Vitamin B$_6$ is composed of three vitamers—**pyridoxine, pyridoxal,** and **pyridoxamine.** It is stable to heat, but sensitive to light and alkalies.

Functions

Vitamin B$_6$ is essential for protein metabolism and affects the conversion of tryptophan to niacin. It is absorbed in the small intestine.

Sources

Some of its best sources are poultry, fish, liver, kidney, pork, eggs, unmilled rice, whole wheat, oats, and legumes.

Requirements

Vitamin B$_6$ is measured in milligrams and the need increases as the protein intake increases. For adult females, the daily requirement is 1.6 mg and for males, 2.0 mg. Oral contraceptives interfere with the metabolization of vitamin B$_6$ and can result in a deficiency.

Deficiency

A deficiency of vitamin B$_6$ is usually found in combination with deficiencies of other B vitamins. Symptoms include convulsions, dermatitis, and anemia. In infants, its deficiency can cause various neurological symptoms and abdominal problems. Although rare, its toxicity can cause neurological problems.

Folic Acid

Folic acid, folate, and folacin are compounds that are chemically similar. Their names are often used interchangeably. Some forms of folic acid are destroyed by storage, processing, heat, oxidation, and light, and others are not.

Function

Folic acid is necessary for protein metabolism and the formation of hemoglobin.

Sources

Folic acid is found in many foods, but the best sources are green leafy vegetables, legumes, liver, and fruits.

Requirements

Folic acid is measured in micrograms. The average daily requirement for the adult female is 180 mcg and for the adult male, 200 mcg. During pregnancy and periods of growth, there is an increased need for folic acid because of the increased production of red blood cells. These additional red blood cells are needed for the increased production of hemoglobin, which is needed to provide sufficient oxygen and nutrients for the new tissue. Since the folic acid requirement also increases with increased metabolic activity, this, too, contributes to the increased need during pregnancy as well as during lactation and periods of stress, when metabolic activity is increased. Consequently, obstetricians can prescribe a folic acid supplement for the pregnant or lactating woman and pediatricians may prescribe it for some infants.

Deficiency

A deficiency of folic acid can impair cell division, affect protein synthesis, and cause **megaloblastic anemia.** Megaloblastic anemia is a condition wherein red blood cells are large and immature, and cannot carry oxygen properly.

Vitamin B₁₂

Vitamin B_{12} (**cobalamin**) is a compound that contains the mineral cobalt. It is slightly soluble in water and fairly stable to heat, but is damaged by strong acids or alkalies, and light. It can be stored in the human body for three to five years.

Functions

Vitamin B_{12} is involved with metabolism of amino acids and is essential for healthy red blood cells and nerve tissue. In order for vitamin B_{12} to be absorbed, it must be joined with a form of protein called **intrinsic factor.** Intrinsic factor is secreted by the stomach mucosa. It carries vitamin B_{12} to the small intestine for absorption.

Sources

The best food sources of B_{12} are animal foods, especially liver, kidney, lean meat, seafood, eggs, and dairy products.

Requirements

Vitamin B_{12} is measured in micrograms. The RDA for adults is 2 mcg per day, but increases during pregnancy and lactation.

Deficiency

Fortunately, a vitamin B_{12} deficiency is rare and is thought to be caused by congenital problems of absorption, which inhibit the body's ability to absorb or synthesize sufficient amounts of vitamin B_{12}. It may also be due to years of a strict vegetarian diet that contains no animal foods.

When the amount of B_{12} is insufficient, megaloblastic anemia may result. If there is a deficiency of intrinsic factor, this anemia is called pernicious anemia. **Pernicious anemia** is a severe blood disease characterized by immature red blood cells. In this case, vitamin B_{12} is given (by intramuscular injections).

Vitamin B_{12} deficiency may also result in inadequate **myelin** synthesis. Myelin is a lipoprotein essential for the protection of nerves. This deficiency causes damage to the nervous system. Symptoms of vitamin B_{12} deficiency include anorexia, glossitis, sore mouth and tongue, pallor, neurological upsets such as depression and dizziness, and weight loss.

Pantothenic Acid

Pantothenic acid is appropriately named as the word *pantothenic* is of Greek derivation and means "from many places." It is fairly stable, but can be damaged by acids and alkalies.

Functions

Pantothenic acid is involved in metabolism of carbohydrates, fats, and proteins. It is also essential for the synthesis of acetylcholine (which is necessary for the transmission of nerve impulses) and steroid hormones.

Sources

This vitamin is found extensively in foods, especially animal foods such as meats, poultry, fish, and eggs. It is also found in whole grain cereals and legumes. In addition, it is thought to be synthesized by the body.

Requirements

There is no RDA for this vitamin, but the Food and Nutrition Board has provided an estimated intake of 4 to 7 mg per day for normal adults. (See Table 6-3.)

Deficiency

Natural deficiencies are unknown. However, deficiencies have been produced experimentally and include weakness, fatigue, and a burning sensation in the feet. Toxicity from excessive intake has not been confirmed.

Biotin

Function and Sources

Biotin participates as a coenzyme in human metabolism. Some of its best dietary sources are liver, egg yolk, soy flour, cereals, and yeast. Biotin is also synthesized in the intestine by microorganisms, but the amount that is available for absorption is unknown.

Requirements

Biotin is measured in micrograms. Although RDA have not been established, the Food and Nutrition Board has provided suggested daily dietary intakes of 30 to 100 mcg for normal adults. (See Table 6-3.)

Deficiency

Deficiency symptoms include nausea, anorexia, depression, **pallor** (paleness of complexion), **dermatitis** (inflammation of skin), and an increase in serum cholesterol. Toxicity from excessive intake is unknown.

Vitamin C

Vitamin C is also known as **ascorbic acid.** It has antioxidant properties and protects foods from oxidation. It is readily destroyed by heat, air, and alkalies, and is easily lost in cooking water.

Functions

Vitamin C is known to prevent **scurvy.** This is a disease characterized by **gingivitis** (soft, bleeding gums, and loose teeth); flesh that is easily bruised; tiny, pinpoint hemorrhages of the skin; poor wound healing; sore joints and muscles; and weight loss. In extreme cases, scurvy can result in death. Scurvy used to be common among sailors who lived for months on bread, fish, and salted meat, with no fresh fruits or vegetables. During the middle of the eighteenth century, it was discovered that the addition of limes or lemons to their diets prevented this disease.

Vitamin C also has an important role in the formation of **collagen,** a protein substance that holds body cells together, making it necessary for wound healing. Therefore, the requirement for vitamin C is increased during trauma, fever, and periods of growth. Tiny, pinpoint hemorrhages are symptoms of the breakdown of collagen.

Vitamin C aids in the absorption of iron from the small intestine when both nutrients are ingested at the same time. Because of this, it is called an **iron enhancer.**

Vitamin C also appears to have several other functions in the human body that are not well understood. For example, it may be involved with the formation and/or functioning of **norepinephrine** (a neurotransmitter and vasoconstrictor that helps the body cope with stressful conditions), some amino acids, folic acid, **leukocytes** (white blood cells), the immune system, and allergic reactions.

It is believed to reduce the number and severity of colds, and can reduce the cancer risk in some cases by reducing nitrites in foods.

Vitamin C is absorbed in the small intestine.

Sources

The best sources of vitamin C are citrus fruits, melon, strawberries, tomatoes, potatoes, red and green peppers, cabbage, and broccoli.

Requirements

Vitamin C is measured in milligrams with the average adult in the United States requiring 60 milligrams per day under normal circumstances. In times of stress, this need is increased. Regular cigarette smokers are advised to ingest 100 mg per day.

It is generally considered non-toxic, but this has not been confirmed. It is known that an excess can cause diarrhea, nausea, cramps, and an excessive absorption of food iron.

Deficiency

Know

Deficiencies of vitamin C are indicated by bleeding gums, loose teeth, tendency to bruise easily, poor wound healing and, ultimately, scurvy.

CONSIDERATIONS FOR THE HEALTH CARE PROFESSIONAL

Vitamins are a popular subject about which many people have strong beliefs. Some beliefs are based on fact; many are incorrect. Today's magazines and newspapers frequently contain articles about vitamins, but they are not always factual. Those patients having no other source of nutrition information tend to believe the statements in these articles. It is important that the patient/client have correct information about vitamins. Both continuation of a poor diet or continued abuse of vitamin supplements are potential dangers to the patient.

Health care professionals will need a solid knowledge of vitamins, a convincing manner, and enormous patience to re-educate patients as may be needed. Some will believe that vitamin E will prevent heart attack; that the only source of vitamin C is orange juice; that codliver oil is essential for all young children; that megadoses of vitamin A will prevent cancer; that a one-a-day vitamin pill is necessary for nearly everyone. Others will confuse milligrams with grams.

Patient education about vitamins may be difficult until the health care professional gains the confidence of the patient. Simple and clear written materials with pictures to reinforce the information will be helpful to the patient.

SUMMARY

Vits work $\equiv$ other compounds

Vitamins are organic compounds that regulate body functions and promote growth. Each vitamin has a specific function or functions within the body. Food sources of vitamins vary, but generally a well-balanced diet provides sufficient vitamins to fulfill body requirements. Vitamin deficiencies can result from inadequate diets or from the body's inability to utilize vitamins. (See Table 6-4.) Vitamins are available in concentrated forms, but their use should be carefully monitored because overdoses can be detrimental to health. Vitamins A, D, E, and K are fat-soluble. Vitamin B complex and Vitamin C are water-soluble. Water-soluble vitamins can be destroyed during food preparation. It is important that care is taken during the preparation of food to preserve its vitamin content.

Table 6-4 Sources, Functions, and Deficiency Symptoms of Vitamins

Vitamins	Best Sources	Functions	Deficiency Symptoms
Fat-Soluble Vitamins Vitamin A	Fish liver oils Liver Butter, margarine (fortified) Whole milk, cream, cheese Egg yolk Vegetables (leafy green and yellow) Fruits (yellow)	Growth Health of eyes and skin Structure and functioning of the cells of the skin and mucous membranes Immune system	Functional disorders of the eye (night blindness) Increased susceptibility to infections Changes in skin and membranes Xerophthalmia Blindness
Vitamin D	Sunshine Fish liver oils Milk (irradiated) Egg yolk Fortified margarine Butter	Growth Regulating absorption of calcium and phosphorus Building and maintaining normal bones and teeth Prevention of tetany	Rickets Poor tooth and bone development Osteomalacia Osteoporosis
Vitamin E	Wheat germ and wheat germ oils Vegetable oils Margarine Nuts Dark green, leafy vegetables	Considered essential for protection of cell structure, especially of red blood cell	Increased rate of hemolysis of the red blood cells
Vitamin K	Spinach Kale Cabbage	Normal clotting of blood	Defective blood clotting
Water-Soluble Vitamins Thiamin (B_1)	Wheat germ Lean pork Yeast Legumes Whole grain and enriched cereal products Liver Heart Kidney	Metabolism of carbohydrates and some amino acids	Loss of appetite Irritability Fatigue Constipation Beriberi
Riboflavin	Milk, cheese Enriched bread and cereals Green, leafy vegetables Liver, kidney, heart	Carbohydrate, fat, and protein metabolism Health of the mouth tissue Healthy eyes	Cheilosis Eye sensitivity Dermatitis

Table 6-4 (*Continued*)

Vitamins	Best Sources	Functions	Deficiency Symptoms
Niacin	Meats (especially organ meats) Poultry and fish Enriched breads and cereals Legumes	Prevention of pellagra Carbohydrate, fat, and protein metabolism	Skin eruptions Diarrhea Nervous disorders Anorexia Pellagra
Vitamin B_6	Fish Poultry Whole grain cereals Liver, kidney Pork Eggs Legumes	Metabolism of proteins	Anemia Dermatitis Confusion Depression Convulsions Nausea
Vitamin B_{12}	Liver, kidney Muscle meats Milk, cheese Eggs Poultry Fish	Metabolism Healthy red blood cells Treatment of pernicious anemia	Anemia Sore mouth and tongue Anorexia Neurological disorders Pernicious anemia
Folic Acid	Dark green, leafy vegetables Liver Legumes Fruits	Metabolism Formation of hemoglobin	Anemia Impaired cell division and protein synthesis
Pantothenic Acid	Meats Poultry Eggs Fish Whole-grain cereals	Metabolism of carbohydrates, fats, and proteins	Weakness Fatigue Burning sensation of the feet
Biotin	Organ Meats Egg yolk Cereals Legumes	Metabolism	Nausea Anorexia Dermatitis Increased serum cholesterol
Vitamin C (Ascorbic Acid)	Citrus fruits, pineapple Melons Berries Tomatoes Cabbage Broccoli Green Peppers	Maintaining collagen Healthy gums Aids in wound healing Aids in absorption of iron	Sore gums Tendency to bruise easily Scurvy

1. How do vitamins help to provide energy to the body?
2. Discuss possible times when avitaminosis of one or more vitamins may occur.
3. Discuss any vitamin deficiencies that class members have observed. What treatments were prescribed?
4. Discuss why it may be unwise for anyone but a physician to prescribe vitamin supplements.
5. Discuss the terms *enriched, fortified,* and *restored.* What do they mean in relation to food products? Name foods that are enriched, fortified, or restored.
6. Discuss the proper storage and cooking of foods to retain their vitamin content.
7. If any member of the class has experienced night blindness ask her or him to describe it. Discuss how this condition occurs and how it can be prevented.
8. Ask if any class member has observed a child with rickets. Discuss the appearance of a child with rickets. Discuss how this disease can be prevented.
9. Why is it advisable to use liquids left over from vegetable cooking? How might these be used?
10. Why are fewer vitamins lost during cooking when the vegetables are cooked whole than when they are cooked in smaller pieces?
11. Explain the role of vitamin C in collagen formation and wound healing.
12. The addition of baking soda (an alkali) to green vegetables during cooking helps to maintain their color. Why is this not advisable?
13. If anyone in the class has taken concentrated vitamin C, ask why. If it was useful, ask why.
14. Why are some vitamins being called prohormones? Coenzymes? Give examples.
15. What is a precursor? Give an example.
16. Discuss appropriate nutritional advice for a 60-year-old woman whose doctor has suggested she drink one quart of milk per day, and she says she cannot.
17. Discuss appropriate nutritional advice for a young mother who is giving her four-year-old 50 mcg of vitamin D each day.
18. What are some possible reasons for vitamin K deficiency?
19. If only part of the daily vitamin K requirement is supplied by the diet, how is the other part obtained?
20. What nutrients are commonly added to breads and cereals in the United States?

21. What is beriberi, and how can it be prevented?
22. Why should milk be sold in opaque containers?
23. Discuss appropriate nutritional advice for a young woman who has been on a very strict vegetarian diet for six months and says she intends to continue.

Suggested Activities

1. Prepare two packages of a frozen vegetable. Cook one package according to the directions on the package and the other in 2 cups of water for 30 minutes. Compare them for palatability. Discuss their probable vitamin and mineral content.
2. Many foods are described as enriched, fortified, and restored. Visit a supermarket and make lists of foods described by each term.
3. Write a menu for one day that is especially rich in the B-complex vitamins. Underline the foods that are the best sources of these vitamins.
4. Organize a "spelldown," asking the functions and sources of vitamins. Organize another, using chapter vocabulary terms.
5. List the foods you have eaten in the past 24 hours. Write the names of the vitamins supplied by each food. What percentage of your day's food did *not* contain vitamins? Could this diet be nutritionally improved? How?
6. Plan a day's menu for a person who has been instructed to eat an abundance of foods rich in vitamin A.
7. Cut two slices of a peach. Leave one slice exposed to the air and pour lemon juice on the other. Set aside for five minutes. Describe what happened (or did not happen) to each slice and explain why.
8. Using other sources, write a short history of one of the vitamins.
9. Review the names and costs of legumes and dietary sources of vitamins. Write a paragraph on the value of legumes.

Review

A. Multiple choice. Select the *letter* that precedes the best answer.
   1. The daily vitamin requirement is best supplied by
      a. eating a well-balanced diet
      b. eating one serving of citrus fruit for breakfast
      c. taking one of the many forms of vitamin supplements
      d. eating at least one serving of meat each day

2. All of the following measures preserve the vitamin content of food except
   a. using vegetables and fruits raw
   b. preparing fresh vegetables and fruits just before serving
   c. adding raw, fresh vegetables to a small amount of cold water and heating to boiling
   d. storing fresh vegetables in a cool place

3. Fat-soluble vitamins
   a. cannot be stored in the body
   b. are lost easily during cooking
   c. are dissolved by water
   d. are slower than water-soluble vitamins to exhibit deficiencies

4. Night blindness is caused by a deficiency of
   a. vitamin A   c. niacin
   b. thiamin   d. vitamin C

5. Good sources of thiamin include
   a. citrus fruits and tomatoes   c. carotene and fish-liver oils
   b. wheat germ and liver   d. nuts and milk

6. Water-soluble vitamins include
   a. A, D, E, and K
   b. A, B_6, and C
   c. thiamin, niacin, and retinol
   d. thiamin, riboflavin, niacin, B_6, B_{12}

7. Injections of vitamin B_{12} are given in the treatment of
   a. scurvy   c. pellagra
   b. pernicious anemia   d. beriberi

8. Blindness can result from a severe lack of
   a. vitamin K   c. thiamin
   b. vitamin A   d. vitamin E

9. Organ meats are good sources of the vitamins
   a. thiamin, riboflavin, B_{12} c. vitamins E and K
   b. biotin, vitamin C   d. all of these

10. Irradiated milk is a good source of
    a. vitamin E   c. vitamin K
    b. vitamin D   d. vitamin C

11. Good sources of vitamin C are
    a. meats   c. breads and cereals
    b. milk and milk products   d. citrus fruits

12. The vitamin that aids in the prevention of rickets is
    a. vitamin A   c. vitamin C
    b. thiamin   d. vitamin D

13. The vitamin that is necessary for the proper clotting of the blood is
   a. vitamin A   c. vitamin D
   b. vitamin K   d. niacin
14. The three vitamins commonly added to breads and cereals are
   a. vitamins A, D, and K
   b. thiamin, riboflavin, and niacin
   c. vitamins E, B_6, and B_{12}
   d. ascorbic acid, pantothenic acid, and folic acid
15. The vitamin known to prevent scurvy is
   a. vitamin A   c. vitamin C
   b. vitamin B complex d. vitamin D

B. Match the vitamins listed in column I with their characteristics listed in column II.

Column I	Column II
f 1. vitamin A	a. also called vitamin C
h (B₁) 2. thiamin beriberi	b. also called amino acids
l 3. riboflavin	c. appears essential to the structure of red blood cells
j 4. niacin	
c 5. vitamin E	d. substance the body converts to vitamin A
i 6. vitamin D	e. primarily found in polished rice
g 7. vitamin B_{12}	f. deficiency causes night blindness
a 8. ascorbic acid	g. best-known treatment for pernicious anemia
k 9. vitamin K	h. extreme deficiency can cause beriberi
d 10. carotene	i. severe deficiency can result in rickets
	j. deficiency can cause pellagra
	k. essential for proper clotting of the blood
	l. deficiency can cause cheilosis

C. Briefly answer the following quesitons.
   1. Which vitamins are fat soluble? Name three characteristics of fat-soluble vitamins.
   2. Which vitamins are water soluble? Name three characteristics of water-soluble vitamins.

Case Study 1

Hypervitaminosis

Milagros R. considered herself lucky. She and her husband were young and happy together. They both had good jobs, and now they were expecting their first child. Except for her acne, her world couldn't have been better. After reading a magazine article in which the author said vitamin A had cured her acne and her aunt's cancer as well, Milagros decided to take vitamin A. The label on the bottle of vitamin A she bought said that each capsule provided 200% of the RDA for adults. She took two capsules, three times a day for a week—until the day her sister came to visit. When her sister learned what Milagros was taking, she insisted she stop immediately and tell her doctor what she had been doing. When Milagros asked why, her sister told her. Milagros did as her sister advised.

Case Study Questions Based on the Nursing Process

Assess
1. Was the magazine article Milagros read reliable? Why?
2. Is it possible that vitamin A could relieve acne? Why?
3. If vitamin A "cured" cancer, is it likely Milagros would have learned of it in some obscure magazine article?

Plan
4. Why was it unwise of Milagros to take such excessive amounts of vitamin A?
5. If Milagros had not been pregnant, would these amounts have been acceptable? Why?

Implement
6. What did Milagros' sister probably tell her about excessive ingestion of vitamin A?

Evaluate
7. Is it likely that Milagros' baby was harmed by her indiscriminate use of vitamin A for one week?
8. Would there have been no cause for alarm if Milagros had taken vitamin D rather than vitamin A? Explain.

Case Study 2

Hypervitaminosis C

Shirley's three-year-old twins started nursery school in early September. By Thanksgiving, both the children and Shirley had had four colds. After reading an article on vitamin C in a current magazine, Shirley decided to take 7,000 milligrams of vitamin C daily. Although she did not get a cold in the next two months, she began to have gastrointestinal (GI) problems involving flatulence and diarrhea. She visited her doctor because of the gastrointestinal problems but failed to mention the vitamin C she was continuing to take. She was put through the usual battery of gastrointestinal tests and, fortunately, nothing serious was found.

Following the tests, her doctor quizzed her again about her diet and about any medicines or vitamins she was taking. On learning of her self-prescribed megadose of vitamin C, the doctor told her this was foolish and that it was probably causing the GI problems. The doctor advised her to stop taking the vitamin C gradually over the next two weeks. She stopped the vitamin C abruptly, however. The GI problems were relieved soon but, although she had had no colds during the total of three months on the megadose of vitamin C, she caught another cold two weeks after stopping the vitamin C.

Case Study Questions Based on the Nursing Process

Assess
1. What was probably causing Shirley to catch colds so frequently? Might the frequency of these colds have been reduced in time?

Plan
2. Discuss why Shirley was vulnerable to the incorrect advice in the magazine article.

Implement
3. Why did the doctor advise gradual withdrawal from the megadose of vitamin C?

Evaluate
4. What might have caused Shirley to catch cold again?

CHAPTER 7

acidosis	iron-deficiency
alkaline	anemia
alkalosis	iron enhancer
antioxidant	Keshan disease
bone marrow	major minerals
cardiovascular	membrane
cerebrospinal fluid	permeability
cretinism	myoglobin
dehydration	myxedema
demineralization	natural foods
diuretics	nonheme iron
edema	nutritional anemia
electrolytes	osmosis
enriched foods	osteomalacia
erythrocytes	osteoporosis
etiology	parenteral nutrition
extracellular	periodontal
goiter	rickets
heme iron	tetany
hemochromatosis	toxicity
hemoglobin	trace elements
hyperkalemia	
hypertension	
hypogonadism	
hypokalemia	
intracellular	
iodized salt	
ions	

MINERALS

OBJECTIVES

After studying this chapter, you should be able to

* List at least two food sources of given mineral elements
* List one or more functions of given mineral elements
* Describe the recommended method of avoiding mineral deficiencies

Chemical analysis shows that the human body is made up of specific chemical elements. Four of these elements—oxygen, carbon, hydrogen, and nitrogen—make up 96 percent of body weight. All the remaining elements, called *mineral elements* or just *minerals,* represent only four percent of body weight. Nevertheless, these minerals are essential for good health.

A *mineral* is an *inorganic* (nonliving) element that is necessary for the body to build tissues, regulate body fluids, or assist in various body functions. Minerals are found in all body tissues. They cannot provide energy by themselves, but in their role as body regulators, they contribute toward the production of energy within the body.

Minerals are found in water and in **natural** (unprocessed) **foods,** together with proteins, carbohydrates, fats, and vitamins. Minerals in the soil are absorbed by growing plants. Humans obtain minerals by eating plants grown in mineral-rich soil, or by eating animals that in turn have eaten such plants. The specific mineral content of food is determined by burning the food and then chemically analyzing the remaining ash.

Highly processed or refined foods such as sugar and white flour contain almost no minerals. Iron and calcium together with the vitamins, thiamin, riboflavin, and niacin, are commonly added to some flour and cereals, which are then labeled **enriched.**

Most minerals in food occur as salts, which are soluble in water. Therefore, the minerals leave the food and remain in the cooking water. Foods should be cooked in as little water as possible and the cooking liquid saved to be used in soups, gravies, and white sauces. Using this liquid improves the flavor of foods to which it is added. If there is fat in the liquid, it should be chilled until the fat solidifies on the top. The fat can then be easily removed.

Table 7-1 Major Minerals and Trace Elements	
Major Minerals	**Trace Elements**
Calcium	Iron
Phosphorus	Copper
Magnesium	Iodine
Sodium	Manganese
Potassium	Zinc
Chlorine	Fluoride
Sulfur	Chromium
	Molybdenum
	Selenium

CLASSIFICATION

Minerals are divided into two groups. One groups consists of the **major minerals,** which are required in amounts greater than 100 mg a day. The second group consists of the **trace elements,** which are needed in much smaller amounts. Table 7-1 lists both.

Some minerals can be referred to as **electrolytes.** Electrolytes are substances that break up into separate particles in water. These separate particles are called **ions** (electrically charged atoms). Sodium, potassium, and chloride are often called electrolytes.

Scientists lack exact information on some of the trace elements although they do know trace elements are essential to good health. The study of these elements continues to discover their specific relationships to human nutrition. A balanced diet is the only safe way of including minerals in the amounts necessary to maintain health.

The Food and Nutrition Board, National Academy of Sciences—National Research Council (hereafter "NRC") has recommended dietary allowances for minerals where research indicates knowledge is adequate to do so. See Table 7-2.

For those minerals where there remains some uncertainty as to amounts of specific human requirements, the Board has provided a table of Estimated Safe and Adequate Daily Dietary Intakes of Selected Minerals, Table 7-3. The Board recommends that the upper levels of listed amounts not be habitually exceeded. (Table 7-6 on pages 106–08 lists the best sources, functions, and deficiency symptoms of minerals.)

TOXICITY

Because it is known that minerals are essential to good health, charlatans and would-be nutritionists sometimes make claims that "more is better." Ironically, more can be hazardous to one's health when it comes to mineral elements. In a healthy individual eating a balanced diet, there will be some normal mineral loss through perspiration and saliva, and amounts in excess of body needs will be excreted in urine and feces. However, when concentrated forms of minerals are taken on a regular basis, over a period of time, they become more than the body can handle, and **toxicity** (poisonous condition) develops. An excessive amount of one mineral can sometimes cause a deficiency of another mineral. In addition, excessive amounts of minerals can

Table 7-2 Recommended Dietary Allowances

Category	Age (years) or Condition	Weight (kg)	Weight (lb)	Height (cm)	Height (in)	Calcium (mg)	Phosphorus (mg)	Magnesium (mg)	Iron (mg)	Zinc (mg)	Iodine (µg)	Selenium (µg)
Infants	0.0–0.5	6	13	60	24	400	300	40	6	5	40	10
	0.5–1.0	9	20	71	28	600	500	60	10	5	50	15
Children	1–3	13	29	90	35	800	800	80	10	10	70	20
	4–6	20	44	112	44	800	800	120	10	10	90	20
	7–10	28	62	132	52	800	800	170	10	10	120	30
Males	11–14	45	99	157	62	1,200	1,200	270	12	15	150	40
	15–18	66	145	176	69	1,200	1,200	400	12	15	150	50
	19–24	72	160	177	70	1,200	1,200	350	10	15	150	70
	25–50	79	174	176	70	800	800	350	10	15	150	70
	51+	77	170	173	68	800	800	350	10	15	150	70
Females	11–14	46	101	157	62	1,200	1,200	280	15	12	150	45
	15–18	55	120	163	64	1,200	1,200	300	15	12	150	50
	19–24	58	128	164	65	1,200	1,200	280	15	12	150	55
	25–50	63	138	163	64	800	800	280	15	12	150	55
	51+	65	143	160	63	800	800	280	10	12	150	55
Pregnant						1,200	1,200	320	30	15	175	65
Lactating	1st 6 months					1,200	1,200	355	15	19	200	75
	2nd 6 months					1,200	1,200	340	15	16	200	75

Source: Food and Nutrition Board, National Academy of Sciences—National Research Council, 1989.

				Trace Elements		
Category	Age (years)	Copper (mg)	Manganese (mg)	Fluoride (mg)	Chromium (μg)	Molybdenum (μg)
Infants	0–0.5	0.4–0.6	0.3–0.6	0.1–0.5	10–40	15–30
	0.5–1	0.6–0.7	0.6–1.0	0.2–1.0	20–60	20–40
Children and	1–3	0.7–1.0	1.0–1.5	0.5–1.5	20–80	25–50
adolescents	4–6	1.0–1.5	1.5–2.0	1.0–2.5	30–120	30–75
	7–10	1.0–2.0	2.0–3.0	1.5–2.5	50–200	50–150
	11+	1.5–2.5	2.0–5.0	1.5–2.5	50–200	75–250
Adults		1.5–3.0	2.0–5.0	1.5–4.0	50–200	75–250

Table 7-3 Estimated Safe and Adequate Daily Dietary Intakes of Selected Minerals

Source: Food and Nutrition Board, National Academy of Sciences—National Research Council, 1989

cause hair loss, and changes in the blood, hormones, bones, muscles, blood vessels, and nearly all tissues. Concentrated forms of minerals should be used only on the advice of a physician.

MAJOR MINERALS

Calcium (Ca)

The human body contains more calcium than any other mineral. The body of a 154-pound person contains approximately four pounds of calcium. All but about one percent of that calcium is found in the skeleton and teeth. The remaining one percent is found in body fluids and soft tissues.

Functions

Calcium, in combination with phosphorus, is a component of bones and teeth, giving them strength and hardness. Bones, in turn, provide storage for calcium. Calcium is needed in the soft tissues for normal nerve and muscle action, blood clotting, heart function, **membrane permeability** (the passage of substances through cell walls), and to activate enzymes. Because the body is continually building and repairing tissue, the blood constantly carries calcium to and from bones and other tissue.

Sources

The best sources of calcium are milk and milk products. They provide large quantities of calcium in small servings. For example, one cup of milk provides 300 milligrams of calcium, figure 7-1. One ounce of cheddar cheese provides 250 milligrams of calcium.

Calcium is also found in some dark green, leafy vegetables. However, when the vegetable contains oxalic acid, as spinach and Swiss chard do, the calcium remains unavailable because the oxalic acid binds it and prevents it from being absorbed. It is unwise to use calcium-rich foods at the same time as high-fiber foods as the calcium binds to the fiber and the mineral cannot be absorbed. Factors that are believed to enhance the absorption of calcium include adequate vitamin D, a calcium-to-phosphorus ratio that includes no more phosphorus than calcium, and the presence of lactose. A lack of physical activity reduces the amount of calcium absorbed.

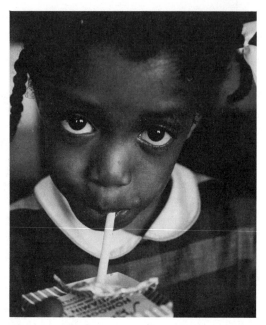

Figure 7-1 Milk is an important source of calcium and phosphorus. These minerals are essential for the normal growth and development of bones and teeth. *(Courtesy of the National Education Association)*

Requirements

After the age of 24 and except during pregnancy and lactation, the recommended allowance of calcium and phosphorus is 800 milligrams for both sexes. Until the age of 24, and during pregnancy and lactation, calcium and phosphorus requirements are higher.

Deficiency

Calcium deficiency may result in **rickets.** This is a disease that occurs in early childhood and results in poorly formed bone structure, figure 7-2. It causes bowed legs, "pigeon breast," and enlarged wrists or ankles. Severe cases can result in stunted growth. Insufficient calcium can also cause "adult rickets" (**osteomalacia**), a con-

dition in which bones become soft. And, although the precise **etiology** (cause) of **osteoporosis** is not known, it is thought that long-term calcium deficiency is a contributing factor. Other factors contributing to osteoporosis include deficiency of vitamin D and certain hormones.

Insufficient calcium in the blood can cause a condition characterized by involuntary muscle movement, known as **tetany.** Excessive intake may cause constipation or kidney stones, or inhibit the absorption of iron and zinc.

Phosphorus (P)

Phosphorus, together with calcium, is necessary for the formation of strong, rigid bones and teeth. Phosphorus is also important in the metabolism of carbohydrates, fats, and proteins. Phosphorus is a constituent of all body cells. It is

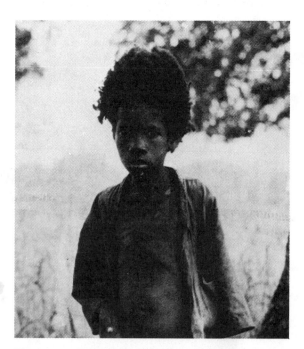

Figure 7-2 Calcium deficiency can cause bone malformation, as seen in this child's chest. *(Courtesy of the World Health Organization)*

Hypocalcemia - def. of Calcium

necessary for a proper acid-base balance of the blood, and is essential for the effective action of several B vitamins. Like calcium, phosphorus is stored in bones and its absorption is increased in the presence of vitamin D.

Sources

Although phosphorus is widely distributed in foods, its best sources are protein-rich foods such as milk, cheese, meats, poultry, and fish. Cereals, legumes, and nuts are also good sources.

Requirements

The RDA for phosphorus is the same as for calcium after the first year of life. During a child's first 12 months, the RDA for phosphorus is slightly less than for calcium. (See Table 7-2.) Nature made this need very clear. The calcium-to-phosphorus ratio in breast milk is 2.3 to 1. In cow's milk, it is 1.3 to 1.

Because of the high phosphorus content of carbonated soft drinks, there is some concern that people who consume large quantities of these drinks take in too much phosphorus. This could cause the calcium-to-phosphorus ratio to become unbalanced and, ultimately, reduce the amount of calcium available. This could then contribute to rickets in children and osteoporosis in adults.

Deficiency

Because phosphorus is found in so many foods, its deficiency is rare. Excessive use of antacids can cause it, however, because they affect its absorption. Symptoms of phosphorus deficiency include bone **demineralization** (loss of minerals), fatigue, and anorexia.

Magnesium (Mg)

Magnesium is vital to both hard and soft body tissues. It is essential for metabolism, and to nerve and muscle tissue. It is stored in bone.

Sources

Like phosphorus, magnesium is widely distributed in foods, but it is found primarily in plant foods. Green leafy vegetables, legumes, nuts, whole grains, and some fruits such as avocados and bananas are very good sources. Milk is also a good source if taken in sufficient quantity. For example, two cups of skim milk, which is the amount recommended for normal adults, provide about 60 mg of magnesium.

Magnesium is lost during commercial food processing and in cooking water so it is preferable to use vegetables and fruits raw rather than cooked.

Requirements

The RDA for magnesium is 280 mg for adult women and 350 mg for adult men. During pregnancy or lactation the RDA is increased slightly.

Deficiency

Because of the wide availability of magnesium, its deficiency among people on normal diets is unknown. When deficiency was experimentally induced, the symptoms included nausea and mental, emotional, and muscular disorders.

Sodium (Na)

Sodium is an **electrolyte** whose primary function is the control of water balance in the body. It controls the **extracellular** fluid (fluid outside of cells) and is essential for **osmosis** (the passage of fluids through body cell walls). Sodium is also necessary to maintain the acid-base balance in the body. In addition, it participates in the transmission of nerve impulses essential for normal muscle function.

Sources

The primary dietary source of sodium is table salt (sodium chloride), which is 40 percent

Table 7-4 Estimated Sodium, Chloride, and Potassium Minimum Requirements of Healthy Persons				
Age	Weight (kg)	Sodium (mg)	Chloride (mg)	Potassium (mg)
Months				
0–5	4.5	120	180	500
6–11	8.9	200	300	700
Years				
1	11.0	225	350	1,000
2–5	16.0	300	500	1,400
6–9	25.0	400	600	1,600
10–18	50.0	500	750	2,000
>18	70.0	500	750	2,000

Source: Food and Nutrition Board, National Academy of Sciences—National Research Council, 1989

sodium. (One teaspoon of table salt contains 2300 mg sodium.) It is also naturally available in animal foods. Salt is typically added to commercially prepared foods because it enhances flavor and helps to preserve some foods by controlling growth of microorganisms. Fruits and vegetables contain little or no sodium. Drinking water contains sodium, but in varying amounts. "Softened" water has a much higher sodium content than "hard" or unsoftened water.

Requirements

Although no RDA has been established for sodium, the NRC has suggested an estimated minimum requirement for adults of 500 mg per day. (See Table 7-4.) However, studies indicate that the average dietary intake of sodium in the United States may be 4 grams (4000 mg) or more.

Deficiency or Excess

Either deficiency or excess of sodium can cause upsets in the body's fluid balance. Although rare, a deficiency of sodium can occur after severe nausea, diarrhea, or heavy perspira-

tion. In such cases, **dehydration** (loss of body fluids) can result. A sodium deficiency also can upset the acid-base balance in the body. Cells function best in a neutral or slightly **alkaline** (base) medium. If too much acid is lost (which can happen during severe nausea), tetany due to **alkalosis** (too little acid) may develop. If the alkaline reserve is deficient as a result of starvation or faulty metabolism as in the case of diabetes, **acidosis** (too much acid) may develop.

An excess of sodium is a more common problem and may cause **edema.** This edema (excess fluid) adds pressure to artery walls that can cause **hypertension** (high blood pressure). Thus, an excess of sodium is frequently associated with **cardiovascular** (heart) conditions such as hypertension and congestive heart failure. In such cases, sodium-restricted diets may be prescribed.

Potassium (K)

Potassium is an electrolyte found primarily in **intracellular** (within the cells) fluid. Like sodium, it is essential for water balance and osmosis. Potassium holds the water that belongs there *in* the cell and sodium keeps the water that belongs there *outside* the cell. Osmosis moves the water in and out of cells as needed to maintain electrolyte (and water) balance. There is normally more potassium than sodium inside the cells and more sodium than potassium outside the cells. If this balance is upset, and the sodium inside the cell increases, the water within the cell also increases, swelling it and causing edema. If the sodium level outside the cell drops because the body has lost sodium, water enters the cell to dilute the potassium level there, and extracellular water is reduced. This can cause blood pressure to drop.

Potassium is also necessary for maintaining normal acid-base balance, transmitting nerve impulses for muscle action, and regulating the release of insulin from the pancreas.

Sources

Potassium is found in many foods, but fruits, especially melons, oranges, bananas, and peaches, and vegetables, notably mushrooms, Brussels sprouts, potatoes, winter squash, lima beans, and carrots are particularly rich sources of it.

Deficiency or Excess

Potassium deficiency (**hypokalemia**) can be caused by diarrhea, vomiting, diabetic acidosis, severe malnutrition, or excessive use of laxatives or **diuretics** (medication promoting excretion of urine). Nausea, anorexia, fatigue, muscle weakness, and heart abnormalities (tachycardia) are symptoms of its deficiency. **Hyperkalemia** (high blood levels of potassium) can be caused by dehydration, renal failure, or excessive intake. Cardiac failure can result.

Chloride (Cl)

Chloride is an electrolyte that is essential for osmosis, maintenance of fluid, and acid-base bal-

ance in the body. Like sodium, it is a constituent of extracellular fluid. It is also a component of gastric juices, where, in combination with hydrogen, it is found in hydrochloric acid; **cerebrospinal** (of the brain and spinal cord) **fluid;** and muscle and nerve tissue. It helps the blood carry carbon dioxide to the lungs and contributes to potassium conservation.

Sources

Chloride is found almost exclusively in table salt (sodium chloride), or in foods containing sodium chloride.

Requirements

Although there is no RDA for chloride, the estimated minimum requirement for normal adults is 750 mg per day.

Deficiency

Because chloride is found in salt, deficiency is rare. It can occur, however, following severe vomiting, diarrhea, or excessive use of diuretics, and alkalosis can result. Also, it could occur in patients who must follow long-term sodium-restricted diets. In such cases, patients can be provided with an alternative source of chloride.

Sulfur (S)

Sulfur is necessary to all body tissue and is found in all body cells. It contributes to the characteristic odor of burning hair and tissue. It is necessary for metabolism.

Sources

Sulfur is a component of some amino acids and consequently is found in protein-rich foods.

Requirements

Neither the amount of sulfur required by the human body nor its deficiency is known.

TRACE ELEMENTS

Iron (Fe)

The principal role of iron is to deliver oxygen to body tissues. It is a component of **hemoglobin,** the coloring matter of red blood cells (**erythrocytes**). Hemoglobin allows red blood cells to combine with oxygen in the lungs and carry it to body tissues.

Iron is also a component of **myoglobin,** a protein compound in muscles that provides oxygen to cells, and it is a constituent of other body compounds involved in oxygen transport.

Sources   Vit C goes to Fe

Red meats, especially liver, egg yolk, chicken, turkey, legumes, dark green vegetables, potatoes, dried fruits, and enriched breads and cereals are among the best sources of iron. Milk is one of the poorest sources. (See Table A-5 in the Appendix.)

Approximately half of the iron from animal foods is actually part of the hemoglobin molecule and as such is called **heme iron.** The part of iron from animal foods that is not part of the hemoglobin molecule and all of the iron in plant foods is called **nonheme iron.** Heme iron is much better absorbed than nonheme iron.

For iron to be absorbed, it must be chemically changed from ferric to ferrous iron. Both hydrochloric acid in the stomach and ascorbic acid (vitamin C) can accomplish this change. This is why vitamin C is known as an **iron enhancer.** Bran, tea, and antacids can decrease iron absorption.

Requirements

The National Research Council has determined that men lose approximately 1 mg of iron a day, and that women lose 1.5 mg a day. Assuming that only 10 percent of ingested iron is ab-

sorbed, the RDA for men has been set at 10 mg, and for women from the age of 11 through the childbearing years, at 15 mg. This is doubled during pregnancy and cannot be met by diet alone. Consequently, an iron supplement is commonly prescribed during pregnancy. Women should make a special effort to include iron-rich foods in their diets at all times. (See Table 7-5.) The rapid growth periods of infancy and adolescence also produce a heavy need for iron.

Table 7-5 Iron Content in Average Day's Menus	
Breakfast	
½ cup orange juice	0.1 mg
2 slices whole wheat toast	2.0
1 tablespoon margarine	trace
1 tablespoon jelly	trace
1 ounce corn flakes	1.0
½ cup whole milk	0.5
2 teaspoons sugar	0
black coffee	0
Lunch	
roast beef sandwich on white bread with lettuce and mayonnaise	3.7 mg
apple	0.2
1 brownie	0.6
1 cup skim milk	0.1
Dinner	
1 cup baked macaroni and cheese	1.8 mg
½ cup cooked green peas	1.2
lettuce and tomato salad	0.9
1 roll	0.8
1 tablespoon margarine	trace
1 cup skim milk	0.1
1 cup ice cream	0.1
2 sugar cookies	0.4
Total iron	13.5 mg

Deficiency

Because the need for iron, particularly of women, is so high, iron deficiency continues to be a problem. Such a condition is called **iron-deficiency anemia** or **nutritional anemia.** When such a condition exists, the body lacks hemoglobin. The bloodstream, in turn, becomes unable to carry enough oxygen to the cells, and the anemic person can suffer from dizziness, fatigue, weakness, and shortness of breath.

Some people suffer from **hemochromatosis.** This is a condition due to an inborn error of metabolism and causes excessive absorption of iron. Unless treated, this condition can damage the liver.

Copper (Cu)

Copper is found in all tissues, but its heaviest concentration is in the liver, kidneys, heart, and brain. As an essential component of several enzymes, it helps in the formation of hemoglobin; aids in the transport of iron to **bone marrow** (soft tissue in bone center) for the formation of red blood cells; and participates in energy production.

Sources

Copper is available in many foods, but its best sources include organ meats, shellfish, legumes, nuts, and whole grain cereals. Human milk is a good source of copper, but cow's milk is not.

Requirements

Although there is no RDA for copper, the NRC's estimated safe intake for adults is 1.5 to 3 mg per day.

Deficiency

Copper deficiency is extremely rare among adults, occurring only in people with malabsorption conditions and in cases of gross protein deficiency, such as kwashiorkor. It is apparent sometimes in premature infants fed only modified cow's milk and in infants on long-term **parenteral nutrition** (feeding via a vein) programs lacking copper. Anemia, bone demineralization and impaired growth may result.

Iodine (I)

Iodine is a component of the thyroid hormones, thyroxine (T_4), and triiodothyronine (T_3). It is necessary for the normal functioning of the thyroid gland, which determines the rate of metabolism.

Sources

The primary sources of iodine are **iodized salt,** seafood, and some plant foods grown in soil bordering the sea. Iodized salt is common table salt to which iodine has been added in an amount that, if used in normal cooking, provides sufficient iodine.

Requirements

The RDA for adults is 150 mcg per day. Additional amounts are needed during pregnancy and lactation.

Deficiency

When the thyroid gland lacks sufficient iodine, the manufacture of thyroxine and triiodothyronine is retarded. The gland, in its attempt to produce T_4 and T_3, grows, forming a lump on the neck called a **goiter** (see figure 7-3). Goiter appears to be more common among women than among men. A thyroid gland that doesn't function properly causes **myxedema** (hypothyroidism) in adults. The children of mothers lacking sufficient iodine may suffer from **cretinism** (retarded physical and mental development).

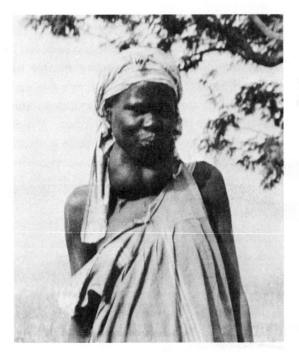

Figure 7-3 In goiter, which results primarily from iodine deficiency, the thyroid gland enlarges. *(Courtesy of the Food and Agriculture Organization of the United Nations)*

Manganese (Mn)

Manganese is a constituent of several enzymes involved in metabolism.

Sources

The best sources of manganese are whole grains and tea. Vegetables and fruits also contain moderate amounts.

Requirements

The estimated safe and adequate daily dietary intake for adults is 2.0 to 5.0 mg.

Deficiency or Excess

Its deficiency has not been documented. Toxicity from excessive ingestion of manganese is unknown. However, people who have inhaled high concentrations of manganese dust have developed neurological problems.

Zinc (Zn)

Zinc is a component of several enzymes. Consequently, it affects many body tissues. It appears to be essential for growth, wound healing, taste acuity, glucose tolerance, and the mobilization of vitamin A within the body.

Sources

The best sources of zinc are protein foods, especially meat, fish, eggs, and dairy products.

Requirements

The RDA for zinc in normal adult males is 15 mg and for adult females, 12, mg with increased requirements during pregnancy and further increases during lactation.

Deficiencies

Decreased appetite and taste acuity, delayed growth, dwarfism, **hypogonadism** (subnormal development of male sex organs), poor wound healing, anemia, changes in the skin, and impaired immune response are all symptoms of zinc deficiency.

Fluoride (F)

Fluoride increases one's resistance to dental caries. It also can help protect against osteoporosis and **periodontal** (gum) disease. It appears to strengthen bones and teeth by making the bone mineral less soluble and thus less inclined to being reabsorbed.

Sources

The principal source of fluoride is fluoridated water (water to which fluoride has been added). In addition, fish and tea contain fluoride. Commercially prepared foods in which fluoridated water has been used during the preparation process also contain fluoride.

Requirements

There is no RDA for fluoride, but the estimated safe and adequate daily dietary intake for adults is 1.5 to 4.0 mg.

Deficiency or Excess

The deficiency of fluoride can result in increased tooth decay and may also contribute to osteoporosis. Excessive amounts of fluoride in drinking water have been known to cause discoloration or mottling of children's teeth.

Chromium (Cr)

Chromium is associated with glucose metabolism. Chromium levels decrease with age except in the lungs where chromium accumulates.

Sources

The best sources of chromium include cheese, yeast, calves liver, and wheat germ.

Requirements

Although there is as yet no RDA for chromium, the estimated safe and adequate daily intake for adults is 50 to 200 mcg. There appears to be no difficulty fulfilling this when one has a balanced diet.

Deficiency

Chromium deficiency appears related to disturbances in glucose metabolism.

Molybdenum (Mo)

Molybdenum is a constituent of enzymes.

Function

Molybdenum is thought to play a role in metabolism.

Sources

The best sources of molybdenum include milk, legumes, and cereals.

Requirements

The estimated safe and adequate daily intake for adults is 75 to 250 mcg. This is normally fulfilled with a balanced diet.

Deficiency or Excess

Effects of molybdenum deficiency can involve metabolism. Excessive intake can cause gout-like symptoms.

Selenium (Se)

Selenium is a constituent of most body tissues, but the heaviest concentration of the mineral is in the liver, kidneys, and heart.

Functions

Selenium is a component of an enzyme that acts as an **antioxidant** (substance that protects another against breakdown from oxygen). In this way, it protects cells against oxidation and spares vitamin E.

Sources

The best sources of selenium are seafood, kidney, liver, and muscle meats.

Requirements

The RDA for selenium for an adult male is 70 mcg and for an adult female, 55 mcg.

Deficiency

Symptoms of selenium deficiency are unclear, but selenium supplements appear effective

Table 7-6 Sources, Functions, and Deficiency Symptoms of Minerals

Minerals	Best Sources	Functions	Deficiency Symptoms
Calcium	Milk Cheese Some dark green, leafy vegetables	Normal development and maintenance of bones and teeth Clotting of the blood Nerve irritability Normal heart action Normal muscle activity Activates enzymes	Retarded growth Poor tooth and bone formation Rickets Slow clotting time of blood Tetany
Phosphorus	Milk and cheese Lean meat Poultry Fish Whole grain cereals Legumes Nuts	Normal development and maintenance of bones and teeth Maintenance of normal acid-base balance of the blood Constituent of all body cells Necessary for effectiveness of some vitamins Metabolism of carbohydrates, fats, and proteins	Poor tooth and bone formation Rickets Weakness Anorexia Pain in bones General malaise
Magnesium	Avocados Nuts Milk Whole grains Green, leafy vegetables Legumes Bananas	Constituent of bones, muscles, and red blood cells Necessary for healthy muscles and nerves Metabolism	Mental, emotional, and muscle disorders
Sodium	Salt Meat Poultry Eggs Milk and cheese	Fluid balance Acid-base balance Osmosis Regulates muscle and nerve irritability Glucose absorption	Nausea Exhaustion Muscle cramps
Potassium	Vegetables Fruits, especially oranges, bananas, and prunes	Osmosis Fluid balance Regular heart rhythm Cell metabolism	Muscle weakness Apathy Abnormal heartbeat

Table 7-6 (Continued)

Minerals	Best Sources	Functions	Deficiency Symptoms
Chloride	Salt Meat Milk Eggs Seafood	Osmosis Fluid balance Acid-base balance Formation of hydrochloric acid	Nausea Exhaustion
Sulfur	Meat Poultry Fish Eggs	For building hair, nails, and all body tissues Constituent of all body cells Metabolism	Unknown

Trace Minerals
Iron
	Liver
	Muscle meats
	Legumes
	Dried fruits
	Whole grain or enriched
	  breads and cereals
	Dark green and leafy
	  vegetables
	Potatoes
		Essential for formation of
		  hemoglobin of the red blood
		  cells and provision of
		  oxygen to cells
		Constituent of cellular enzymes
			Anemia characterized by
			  weakness, dizziness,
			  loss of weight, and
			  pallor

Copper	Liver
	Kidney
	Shellfish
	Legumes
	Nuts
	Whole grain cereals
		Essential for formation of
		  hemoglobin and red blood
		  cells
		Component of enzymes
			Anemia
			Bone disease

Iodine	Seafood
	Foods grown in soil
	  bordering salt water
	Iodized salt
		Formation of hormones in
		  thyroid gland
			Goiter
			Myxedema
			Cretinism

Manganese	Whole grains Nuts Vegetables Fruits	Component of enzymes	Unknown

Table 7-6 (Continued)

Minerals	Best Sources	Functions	Deficiency Symptoms
Zinc	Seafood, especially oysters Liver Meat Eggs Milk	Component of insulin and enzymes Wound healing Taste acuity Essential for growth	Dwarfism, hypogonadism, anemia Loss of appetite Skin changes Impaired wound healing Decreased taste acuity
Fluoride	Fluoridated water Seafood	Increases resistance to tooth decay	Tooth decay Possibly osteoporosis
Chromium	Yeast Calves liver Cheese Wheat germ	Associated with glucose metabolism	Possibly disturbances of glucose metabolism
Molybdenum	Milk Cereal Legumes	Enzyme functioning Metabolism	Unknown
Selenium	Seafood Kidney Liver Muscle meats	Constituent of most body tissue	Unclear, but related to Keshan's disease

in treating **Keshan disease** (causes abnormalities in the heart muscle).

CONSIDERATIONS FOR THE HEALTH CARE PROFESSIONAL

Second to vitamins, minerals are of great interest to the general public. They often are given mythic powers in current articles. A patient may continue to take her or his self-prescribed dosage of a favorite mineral while in the hospital. This could be contraindicated, depending on the patient's condition.

It is imperative that the health care professional be aware of the dangers of megadoses of minerals and be able to translate this information in a meaningful way to the patients.

SUMMARY

Minerals are necessary to promote growth and regulate body processes. They originate in soil and water, and are ingested via food and drink. Deficiencies can result in conditions such as anemia, rickets, and goiter. A well-balanced diet can prevent mineral deficiencies. Concentrated forms of minerals should be taken only on the advice of a physician. Excessive amounts of minerals can be toxic, causing hair loss and changes in nearly all body tissues.

Discussion Topics

1. Discuss the special importance of calcium and phosphorus to children and to pregnant women.
2. List ways of supplying an adequate amount of calcium in the diet of an adult who dislikes milk. Plan a day's menu for this adult.
3. Ask if any member of the class has suffered from anemia. If so, ask the class member to describe the symptoms and treatment. What kind of anemia was it? If it's preventable, what measures are being taken to prevent a recurrence of the condition?
4. What is a goiter? Has anyone observed a goiter? If so, describe it. What causes goiter?
5. If a person is to decrease sodium in her or his diet, should animal foods be increased or decreased?
6. Why does the NRC recommend that the upper limits of RDAs for minerals not be habitually exceeded?
7. Why might the following luncheon menu be inadvisable for a pregnant woman?
   Spinach/bacon/mushroom salad, whole wheat rolls, milk, and vanilla ice cream
8. Evaluate the following breakfast menu for a pregnant woman:
   Orange juice, honey-bran muffin, bran flakes, milk
9. In addition to their high sugar content, why are carbonated drinks ill-advised for children or pregnant women?
10. If anyone in class knows someone with osteoporosis, ask for a description of the patient including sex, age, physical appearance, physical complaints, life-long dietary habits, and medical treatment.
11. Explain the relationship of sodium and edema.
12. Why is it recommended that patients on sodium-restricted diets have the mineral content of their local water supply evaluated?
13. Explain the relationship of sodium and potassium.
14. Why would a doctor prescribe potassium at the same time a diuretic is prescribed?
15. Although rare, why does chloride deficiency sometimes occur in patients on long-term sodium-restricted diets?
16. Discuss the differences between heme and nonheme iron.
17. What is an "iron enhancer"? Name one.
18. Why is iron commonly prescribed for pregnant women?
19. What might cause the hair of children with kwashiorkor to change color?
20. Why is selenium said to spare vitamin E?

Suggested Activities

1. Ask a biology teacher to demonstrate the process of osmosis. Discuss its function in the body.

2. Ask a chemistry teacher to explain the properties of acids and alkalies to the class. Have the teacher relate these properties to the body's use of minerals.

3. Using outside sources, prepare a report on how sodium and potassium regulate the body's fluid balance.

4. Plan a day's menu. List the minerals found in the foods included.

5. List the foods you have eaten in the past 24 hours. Using Table A-5 in the Appendix, list the minerals in these foods. Note whether there appear to be mineral deficiencies. Make a list of foods that could be added to your diet to make up for the mineral deficiencies.

6. Name four foods rich in at least three minerals.

7. Using other sources, write a report on at least one of the following:
   Rickets
   Tetany
   Nutritional anemia
   Goiter
   Hypothyroidism
   Hyperthyroidism
   Diabetes
   Edema
   Dwarfism
   Hypogonadism
   Cretinism
   Dehydration
   Myxedema
   Osteoporosis
   Osteomalacia
   Periodontal disease
   Parenteral nutrition

8. Check four or five varieties of bread at the local supermarket. Using the labels on the breads, evaluate their mineral content.

9. Cut an apple and leave it open to the air for 24 hours. Cut a second apple 24 hours later. Compare them. Explain the role of oxygen in this experiment.

10. List five good sources of heme iron and five sources of nonheme iron. Compare their costs.

11. Describe possible uses for the water in which fresh vegetables have been cooked.

12. Spend five or ten minutes observing customers at a drugstore display of various vitamin and mineral compounds. Write a short report on which minerals were most frequently purchased. Include your opinion as to why this was the case.

13. Write a short essay on why iodized salt is a better choice than plain salt.

14. Revise the menu in Table 7-5 so that it includes the appropriate RDA of iron for a 40-year-old woman.

15. List the minerals available over-the-counter at the local drugstore or health food store.

16. List the minerals richly supplied in legumes.

Review

A. Multiple choice. Select the *letter* that precedes the best answer.

1. Minerals are inorganic elements that
    a. help to build and repair tissues
    b. are found only in bones
    c. provide energy when carbohydrates are lacking
    d. can substitute for proteins

2. The trace elements in the human body are defined as
    a. those minerals that cannot be detected in laboratory tests
    b. those essential minerals found in very small amounts
    c. those minerals that are not essential to health
    d. only those minerals that are found in the blood

3. Calcium is necessary for
    a. healthy bones and teeth
    b. normal red blood cells
    c. preventing goiter
    d. energy

4. Phosphorus is found in
    a. poultry   c. vegetable oils
    b. common table salt   d. leafy vegetables

 5. The coloring matter of the blood is
    a. hemoglobin   c. marrow
    b. lymph   d. plasma

6. Some of the common symptoms of nutritional anemia are
    a. muscle spasms and pain in the liver
    b. bowed legs and an enlarged thyroid gland
    c. edema and loss of vision
    d. dizziness and weakness

7. Iodine is essential to health because it
    a. is necessary for red blood cells
    b. strengthens bones and teeth
    c. helps the blood to carry oxygen to the cells
    d. affects the rate of metabolism

8. Sodium is often restricted in cardiovascular and nephritic conditions because it
    a. causes the heart to beat slowly
    b. encourages the growth of the heart
    c. contributes to edema
    d. raises the blood sugar

9. Iron is known to be a necessary component of
    a. thyroxin   c. hemoglobin
    b. adipose tissue   d. amino acids

10. Liquid from cooking vegetables should be used in preparing other dishes because
    a. mineral salts are soluble in water
    b. the hydrogen and oxygen in water aid the digestion of minerals
    c. the amino acids are soluble in water
    d. none of the above

B. Complete the following statements.
    1. This mineral is essential for healthy bones and teeth. Its best sources are milk and cheese. It works closely with phosphorus. It is

        _____ .

    2. This mineral is essential for the formation of hemoglobin. Some of its best sources are meats, legumes, and whole grain cereals. It works closely with copper. It is _____ .

    3. This mineral is essential for a healthy thyroid gland. Its best natural sources are seafood and foods grown in soil bordering the sea. It is

        _____ .

    4. This mineral is essential for osmosis, maintenance of body neutrality, and water balance. It is sometimes restricted in cardiovascular conditions. It works closely with chloride. It is _____ .

    5. This trace mineral increases resistance to tooth decay. It is _____ .

    6. This mineral is essential for healthy muscles and nerves. It is found in milk, cereal grains, and fresh green vegetables. Its deficiency can result in mental, emotional, and muscular disorders. It is _____ .

    7. This mineral is essential for regular heart rhythm. Good sources include oranges, bananas, and peaches. Its deficiency can result in an abnormal heartbeat. It is _____ .

8. This mineral is essential in the production of red blood cells. It works closely with iron. It is found in organ meats. Its deficiency can result in anemia. It is _____ .

9. This mineral is essential for healthy bones and teeth. It is found in milk and meats. It works closely with calcium. It is _____ .

10. This mineral, along with sodium and potassium, is essential for normal osmosis. It is found in table salt, meat, milk, and eggs. It is

_____ .

C. Match the item in column I with its description in column II.

	Column I		Column II
e	1. nutritional anemia	a.	red coloring matter in blood
h	2. bone marrow	b.	the passing of materials through cell walls
a	3. hemoglobin	c.	involuntary muscle movement
k	4. goiter	d.	disease resulting in poorly formed bones
j	5. iodized salt	e.	lack of iron
b	6. osmosis	f.	dry from loss of water
c	7. tetany	g.	essential mineral needed in very small amounts
d	8. rickets	h.	soft tissue filling bone cavity
g	9. trace element	i.	salt with iodine removed
f	10. dehydrated	j.	salt with iodine added
		k.	enlarged thyroid gland

Case Study 1

Diet and Hypertension

Ella T. was a 65-year-old woman who suffered from hypertension. Her physician had told her to stop adding salt to any foods she cooked, and to cut her table consumption of salt in half. She had followed this advice, but her blood pressure still remained higher than the doctor thought it should be. After quizzing her carefully concerning her dietary habits, the physician learned that she frequently—at least five or six nights a week—ate TV dinners and was extremely fond of cheese and crackers with milk at bedtime. In addition, she often ate lunch in restaurants.

Case Study Questions Based on the Nursing Process

Assess

1. What factors contributed to the physician's advice that Ella change her diet?

Plan

2. What did the physician probably advise Ella about eating TV dinners?
3. Was Ella's bedtime snack affecting her sodium intake? Explain.

Implement

4. What suggestions might be given Ella as substitutes for cheese, crackers, and milk at bedtime?
5. When given dietary instructions, what foods should Ella be told to avoid?
6. What steps might Ella take in restaurants to reduce her sodium intake?
7. Suggest a day's menu for Ella, assuming she had lunch in a restaurant and dinner at home.

Evaluate

8. What should Ella do if she is invited to a friend's for dinner and she is served baked ham?
9. If Ella follows her new diet regimen, what physical changes might her physician note about her on her next visit to the physician's office?

Case Study 2

Pregnancy and Nutrition

Jonetta's first pregnancy at the age of 25 was uneventful. She ate, drank, and smoked as she pleased, refusing the recommended quart of milk a day. The same rules prevailed during her second pregnancy two years later. This second child was fine, but broke her arm when she tripped on a rug at the age of two. Her third baby, which she delivered when she was 29, did not develop baby teeth and, when he was four, broke his femur when he fell out of the lower bunk bed.

Case Study Questions Based on the Nursing Process

Assess

1. What mineral was most probably lacking in Jonetta's diet?

Plan

2. How might Jonetta have obtained the necessary calcium without drinking milk?
3. Is it possible that given the lack of milk in her diet during her pregnancy, Jonetta may have shortchanged herself on other minerals as well? Explain your answer.

Implement

4. If you were Jonetta's diet counselor, what would you tell her about her total lack of milk during pregnancy? Do you think this would convince her? Why or why not?
5. Jonetta's children also have a poor intake of milk. What would you teach Jonetta about children's calcium needs?

Evaluate

6. When Jonetta brings the children to the doctor's office for checkups, what will the doctor evaluate to determine whether their intake of calcium is adequate?
7. What may possibly happen to Jonetta's teeth?

VOCABULARY

ADH
acid-ash foods
acid-base balance
acidosis
aldosterone
alkaline-ash foods
alkalosis
blood plasma
buffer
cellular edema
dehydration
extracellular fluid
homeostasis
hypoproteinemia
hypothalamus
interstitial fluid
intracellular fluid
osmosis
pH
positive water balance
solute
solvent
vasopressin

WATER

OBJECTIVES

After studying this chapter, you should be able to
- Describe the functions of water in the body
- Explain water balance and its maintenance
- Name causes and consequences of water depletion
- Give causes and consequences of positive water balance
- Describe the acid-base balance of the human body

FUNCTIONS OF BODY WATER

Although humans can live three to four weeks without food, it is possible to live only a few days without water. Water is a component of all body cells, and comprises from 50 to 60 percent of body weight of normal adults. The percentage is higher in males than females because men usually have more muscle tissue than women. The water content of muscle tissue is higher than in fat tissue. Percentage of water content is highest in newborns (75 percent) and decreases with age.

Body water is divided into two basic compartments—intracellular and extracellular. **Intracellular fluid** (ICF) is water within the cells and accounts for about 45 percent of total body weight. **Extracellular fluid** (ECF) is water outside the cells and accounts for about 20 percent of total body weight. Extracellular water is found in **blood plasma** (fluid part of the blood), **interstitial fluid** (between tissues), and in glandular secretions.

While it is a component of all body tissues, water is the major component of blood plasma. It is a **solvent** (liquid part of solution) for nutrients and waste products, and helps transport both to and from body cells by way of the blood. It is necessary for the hydrolysis of nutrients in the cells, making it essential for metabolism. It functions as a lubricant in joints and in digestion. In addition, it cools the body through perspiration and may, depending on its source, provide some mineral elements. (See Table 8-1.)

Although the best sources of water are beverages of all types, a considerable amount is also found in foods, especially fruits, vegetables, soups, milk, and gelatin deserts. In addition, energy metabolism also produces water. When carbohydrates, fats, and proteins are metabolized, their end products include carbon dioxide and water.

WATER AND ELECTROLYTE BALANCE

For optimum health there must be **homeostasis** (internal stability). For this to exist, the body must be in *water and electrolyte balance.* This means the water lost through urination, feces, perspiration, and the respiratory tract, must be replaced both in terms of volume and electrolyte content (see Chapter 7).

Water moves through cell walls by **osmosis.** It flows from the side with the lesser amount of **solute** (substance dissolved in solution) to the side with the greater solute concentration. The electrolytes, sodium, chloride, and potassium, are the solutes that maintain the balance between intracellular and extracellular fluids. Potassium is the principal electrolyte in intracellular fluid. Sodium is the principal electrolyte in extracellular fluid.

When the electrolytes in the extracellular fluid are *increased,* ICF moves to the ECF in an

Table 8-1 Functions of Water
Component of all body tissues
Solvent for nutrients and body wastes
Provides transport for nutrients and wastes
Essential for hydrolysis and thus metabolism
Lubricant of joints and in digestion
Cools the body

attempt to equalize the concentration of electrolytes on both sides of the membrane. This reduces the amount of water in the cells. The cells of the **hypothalamus** (area at the base of the brain; regulates appetite and thirst) then become dehydrated, as do those in the mouth and tongue, and the body experiences thirst. The hypothalamus then alerts the pituitary gland to excrete **ADH** (antidiuretic hormone, also called **vasopressin**) which causes the kidneys to conserve fluid. At such times, thirst causes the healthy person to drink fluids, thereby providing the water and electrolytes needed by the cells.

When the sodium in the ECF is reduced, water flows from the ECF into the cells, causing them to swell (**cellular edema**). When this occurs, the adrenal glands secrete **aldosterone,** which triggers the kidneys to increase the amount of sodium reabsorbed. When the missing sodium is replaced in the ECF, the excess water that has been drawn from the ECF into the cells, moves back to the ECF, and the edema is relieved. If the water in the extracellular fluid is not replaced, such a condition can result in a loss of blood volume and, ultimately, reduced blood pressure.

The amount of water used and thus needed each day varies, depending on age, size, activity, environmental temperature, and physical condition. The average adult water requirement is approximately 1 ml per kcal for adults. Youth, fever, diarrhea, unusual perspiration, and hyperthyroidism increase the requirement.

Dehydration

neg. H₂O balance [handwritten]

Test [handwritten]

When the amount of water in the body is inadequate, **dehydration** can occur. It can be caused by inadequate intake or abnormal loss. Such loss can occur from severe diarrhea, vomiting, hemorrhage, burns, excessive perspiration, or excessive urination. Symptoms of dehydration include low blood pressure, thirst, dry skin, fever, and mental disorientation. As water is lost, electrolytes are also lost. Thus, treatment includes replacement of electrolytes and fluids. Electrolyte content must be checked and corrections made if necessary. A loss of ten percent of body water can cause serious problems. Blood volume and nutrient absorption are reduced, and kidney function is upset. A loss of 20 percent of body water can cause circulatory failure and death.

(10%) Know [handwritten]

Excessive Water Accumulation

pos [handwritten]

Know! [handwritten]

Some conditions cause an excessive accumulation of fluid in the body. This is called **positive water balance.** It occurs when more water is taken in than is used and excreted, and edema results, figure 8-1. Hypothyroidism, congestive heart failure, **hypoproteinemia** (low amounts of protein), some infections, some cancers, and some renal conditions can cause such water retention because sodium is not being excreted normally. Fluids and sodium may then be restricted.

ACID-BASE BALANCE

In addition to maintaining water and electrolyte balance, the body must also maintain **acid-base balance.** This is the regulation of hydrogen ions in body fluids (**pH** balance).

In a water solution, an acid gives off hydrogen ions and a base picks them up. Hydrochloric acid is an example of an acid found in the body.

ph 7 = neutral [handwritten]

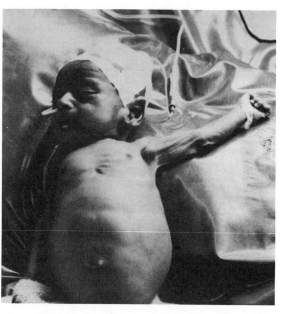

Figure 8-1 This child is suffering from cellular edema. *(Courtesy of the World Health Organization)*

It is secreted by the stomach and is necessary for the digestion of proteins. Ammonia is a base produced in the kidneys from amino acids.

Acidic substances run from 1 to 7, with the lowest numbers representing the most acidic (which contain the most hydrogen ions). Alkaline substances run from 7 to 14, with the alkalinity increasing with the number (as the number of hydrogen ions decrease). A "pH 7" is considered neutral. Blood plasma runs from pH 7.35 to 7.45. Intracellular fluid has a pH of 6.8.

Acid-Ash and Alkaline-Ash Foods

The minerals available to the cells from the extracellular fluid affect the pH of the cells. The minerals chlorine, sulfur, and phosphorus form acids when dissolved in water. They are called *acid-forming elements.* The groups of foods in which they predominate are protein-rich foods, specifically, meats, fish, poultry, eggs, and cereal products. These foods are called **acid-ash foods** because they leave an acid ash after metabolism. (See Table 8-2.)

Calcium, sodium, potassium, and magnesium are basic in solution. They predominate in fruits and vegetables. (See Table 8-3.) Fruits and vegetables are referred to as **alkaline-ash foods.** Despite popular belief and their slightly acidic taste, fruits generally are not acid forming, because chlorine, sulfur, and phosphorus are not predominant minerals in fruits. The sometimes sour taste comes from mild, organic acids. Except for cranberries and plums, fruits do not leave an acid ash. Cranberries and plums contain organic acids that the body does not metabolize. Eating them causes an increase of acidity in body fluids. Milk is neutral because its base-forming calcium is balanced by its acid-forming phosphorus content. Pure carbohydrates and fats do not affect acid-base balance because they contain almost no minerals.

Buffer Systems

The body has **buffer** (protective) systems which regulate hydrogen ion content in body fluids. Such a system is a mixture of a weak acid

Table 8-2 Acid-forming Elements and Acid-ash Foods

Acid-forming Elements	Acid-ash Foods
Chlorine	Meats
Sulfur	Fish
Phosphorus	Poultry
	Eggs
	Cereals
	Cranberries
	Plums

Table 8-3 Base-forming Elements and Alkaline-ash Foods

Base-forming Elements	Alkaline-ash Foods
Calcium	Fruits
Sodium	Vegetables
Potassium	
Magnesium	

and a strong base which reacts to protect the nature of the solution in which it exists. In a normal buffer system, the ratio of base to acid is 20:1. For example, when a strong acid is added to a buffered solution, the base takes up the hydrogen ions of the strong acid, thereby weakening it. When a strong base is added to a solution, the acid of the buffer system combines with this base and weakens it.

A mixture of carbonic acid and sodium bicarbonate forms the body's main buffer system. This is because they are easily accessed and amounts are easily adjusted by the lungs and kidneys. For example, the end products of metabolism are carbon dioxide and water, and together they can form carbonic acid. The hemoglobin in the blood carries carbon dioxide to the lungs where the excess is excreted. If the amount of carbon dioxide is more concentrated than it should be, the medulla oblongata in the brain causes the breathing rate to increase. This increases the rate at which the body rids itself of carbon dioxide. Excess sodium bicarbonate is excreted via the kidneys. The kidneys can excrete urine from pH 4.5 to pH 8. The pH of average urine is 6.

Acidosis and Alkalosis

The healthy person eating a balanced diet does not normally have to think about acid-base balance. Upsets can occur in some disease conditions, however. Renal failure, uncontrolled diabetes mellitus, starvation, or severe diarrhea can cause **acidosis.** This is a condition in which the body is unable to balance the need for bases with the amount of acids it is retaining. **Alkalosis** can occur when the body has suffered a loss of hydrochloric acid from severe vomiting, or ingested too much alkali, such as too many antacid mints.

CONSIDERATIONS FOR THE HEALTH CARE PROFESSIONAL

Patients who are required to limit both their salt and liquid intake will probably be unhappy with their diets. In such cases, it is helpful when the health care professional can discuss realistic ways of planning menus for them and *with* them. These menus should be based, of course, on good nutrition, but they also must be based on the patient's normal habits and desires as much as is possible. Review a patient's former diet with the patient. Point out the high-salt and high-liquid foods and suggest alternative foods in a positive manner.

SUMMARY

Water is a component of all tissues. It is a solvent for nutrients and body wastes, and provides transport for both. It is essential for hydrolysis, lubrication, and maintenance of normal temperature. Its best sources are beverages, fruits, vegetables, soups, and water-based desserts. Water balance and electrolyte balance are dependent upon one another. An upset in one can cause an upset in the other. An inadequate supply of water can result in dehydration, which can be caused by severe diarrhea, vomiting, hemorrhage, burns, or excessive perspiration or urination. Symptoms include thirst, dry skin, fever, lowered blood pressure, and mental disorientation. Dehydration can result in death. Positive water balance is an excess accumulation of water in the body. It causes edema. Acid-base balance is the regulation of hydrogen ions in the body. Excessive acids or inadequate amounts of base can cause acidosis. Excessive base or inadequate amounts of acids can cause alkalosis. Healthy people eating a balanced diet need not be concerned about water, electrolyte, or acid-base balance, as the body has intricate maintenance systems for all.

Discussion Topics	
1.	Why can people live longer without food than without water?
2.	Why does water comprise a larger proportion of man's body weight than a woman's?
3.	Describe homeostasis.
4.	Why might the following holiday dinner cause one to need an antacid after the meal? Deviled eggs, roast turkey, green peas, rice, whole wheat rolls, cranberry sauce, plum pudding.
5.	Are fruits acid-forming? Explain your answer?
6.	Describe a buffer system. Why is it needed?
7.	How do the lungs help to prevent excess acid from developing in the body?

8. What happens to the skin when it touches a red-hot pan? How might such developments on a large scale upset the body's water and electrolyte balance?

9. What is alkalosis? What causes it?

10. Explain how dehydration is dangerous in adults and in infants and children.

11. Can water be a source of minerals? Explain.

12. What does "pH" mean? How does it relate to the homeostasis of the body?

13. Is milk an acid-ash food? An alkaline-ash food? Explain.

14. Which minerals must predominate in a food for it to be an acid-ash food? An alkaline-ash food?

15. Explain why pure carbohydrates and fats are neutral.

Suggested Activities

1. Ask the biology teacher to demonstrate osmosis.

2. Pour a cup of coffee and add a spoonful of sugar. Explain which is the solute, which is the solvent, which is the solution.

3. Visit a supermarket and make a list of 50 products that are good sources of water.

4. Ask a nurse to describe what happens to body tissue when it is badly burned, and the treatment of burn patients, including diet.

5. Ask a nurse to describe a diabetic coma, explaining what causes it, why it can be life threatening, and treatment of it.

6. Write a five-minute speech to be given to 12-year-olds, explaining electrolytes and their roles in the body.

7. List the functions of water in the human body.

8. Role-play a situation in which a nurse tries to convince an elderly woman with edema due to heart failure to follow her prescribed sodium-restricted diet.

9. Role play a situation in which a nurse attempts to convince a patient that orange juice does not create "acidic blood."

Review

A. Multiple choice. Select the *letter* that precedes the best answer.

1. Water within the cells is called
   a. interstitial fluid
   b. extracellular fluid
   c. intracellular fluid
   d. none of the above

2. Blood plasma contains
   a. interstitial fluid
   b. extracellular fluid
   c. intracellular fluid
   d. none of the above

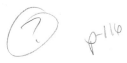

3. In a mixture of sugar and water, water is the
   a. solvent
   b. solute
   c. solution
   d. none of the above

4. Water
   a. is essential for hydrolysis
   b. causes hydrogenation
   c. reduces hypoproteinemia
   d. is produced by hypothyroidism

5. Good sources of water include
   a. oranges and melon
   b. seafood and meats
   c. baked desserts and rice
   d. all of the above

6. The solute in the extracellular fluid principally responsible for maintaining fluid balance is
   a. potassium
   b. phosphorus
   c. calcium
   d. sodium

7. The solute in the intracellular fluid principally responsible for maintaining fluid balance is
   a. potassium
   b. phosphorus
   c. calcium
   d. sodium

8. The hormone, vasopressin, causes the kidneys to
   a. conserve fluid
   b. reabsorb additional sodium
   c. release additional sodium
   d. excrete increased amounts of urine

9. The amount of water needed by individuals
   a. varies from day to day
   b. is not affected by one's activities
   c. decreases with fever
   d. all of the above

10. Positive water balance
    a. means one's intake is equal to output
    b. can cause hydrogenation
    c. may cause edema
    d. is a good thing

B. Completion. Complete the following sentences.
   1. In osmosis, water moves from the side with the _most_ amount of solute to the side with the _least_ amount of solute.
   2. Intracellular fluid is water _within_ cells.
   3. Extracellular fluid is water _outside_ cells.
   4. Interstitial fluid is water _____ cells.
   5. Hydrolysis is the _____ of water with the resulting _____ of remaining substances.
   6. The end products of metabolism are _____ and water.
   7. _____ is a word meaning "internal stability."
   8. The area at the base of the brain that regulates the appetite and thirst is the _____ .

9. ADH is also called _____ , and is a(n) _____ hormone.
10. When there is a serious lack of body water, _____ can occur.
11. Acid-base balance is the regulation of _____ ions in body fluids.
12. The systems that protect the body against acidosis and alkalosis are called _____ systems.

Case Study 1

Dehydration

Mr. B. planned to spend Saturday afternoon cleaning the beach near his summer home. It was a very hot day, but there was a brisk wind. He took a jar of water with him, but when he went to drink it, it had become too warm to drink, and he barely wet his tongue.

By 3:00 P.M., he was extremely thirsty and even felt a bit light-headed, so he walked to the house for a cold drink. When he stepped inside, however, he fainted. Fortunately, his wife was there and when she felt his hot, dry skin, and noticed how weak his pulse was, she called their next door neighbor who was a physician. After quickly checking Mr. B., the doctor called an ambulance and took him to the hospital right away. The doctor administered intravenous fluids in the ambulance. Later, when Mr. B. felt better, he couldn't understand why he hadn't realized what was happening to him. He said he hadn't perspired much although the thermometer had registered 95° that day.

Case Study Questions Based on the Nursing Process

Assess
1. What did Mr. B's symptoms indicate?
2. Why did Mr. B. faint?
3. Why hadn't he noticed much perspiration on such a hot day?

Plan
4. What mineral would the doctor probably replace? Why?
5. What would you teach Mr. B. to prevent further episodes?

Implement
6. Why did the doctor provide intravenous fluids rapidly?
7. While the fluids are being replaced, what will the nurse monitor?

Evaluate
8. Mr. B. states he feels much better. What laboratory reports will confirm that Mr. B. is out of danger?
9. What could have happened to Mr. B. if he had fainted at the beach?

Case Study 2

Water

Mrs. Johnson was 75 years old and having increasing trouble with edema, particularly around her ankles. After examining her, her doctor prescribed a diuretic and a potassium supplement, and suggested she avoid salty foods.

Case Study Questions Based on the Nursing Process

Assess
1. Why did the doctor prescribe a diuretic for Mrs. Johnson?
2. Why was supplemental potassium prescribed?

Plan
3. What would you teach Mrs. Johnson about eating salty foods?

Implement
4. Make a list of salty foods that Mrs. Johnson should avoid.

Evaluate
5. Would it be correct to say Mrs. Johnson was in positive water balance? Explain.
6. What are the goals of treatment for the patient in positive water balance?

SECTION 2

Maintenance of Health Through Good Nutrition

CHAPTER 9

DIET GUIDELINES AND MENU PLANNING

OBJECTIVES

After studying this chapter, you should be able to

- Define a balanced diet
- List the U.S. government's Dietary Guidelines for Americans and explain the reasons for each
- Identify the food groups and their placement on the Food Guide Pyramid
- Identify the Basic Four Food Groups and the chief nutrients provided by each
- State and define criteria for planning appetizing meals

The statement "eat a balanced diet" has been repeated so often that its importance may have been overlooked. The value of this statement is so great, however, that it deserves serious consideration by people of all ages. A **balanced diet** includes all the essential nutrients, as well as kcal, in amounts that preserve and promote good health.

A BALANCED DIET

Daily review of the RDA (see Table A-1 in the Appendix) would provide enough informa-tion to plan balanced diets. However, ordinary meal planning would be cumbersome and time-consuming if these tables had to be consulted each time a meal was planned. Fortunately, the United States Department of Agriculture (USDA) and the U.S. Department of Health and Human Services developed a simple method to help with the selection of healthful diets. It is called the Dietary Guidelines for Americans. In addition, the Food Guide Pyramid was developed by the USDA as an outline for daily food choices based on the Dietary Guidelines. The Basic Four Food Groups devised by the USDA in the 1950s is clear and simple and also can be useful in food selection.

DIETARY GUIDELINES FOR AMERICANS

1. Eat a variety of foods.
2. Maintain a healthy weight.
3. Choose a diet low in fat, saturated fat, and cholesterol.
4. Choose a diet with plenty of vegetables, fruits, and grain products.
5. Use sugars only in moderation.
6. Use salt and other forms of sodium only in moderation.
7. If you drink alcoholic beverages, do so in moderation.

Eat a Variety of Foods

There are over 40 nutrients needed by the body. Because no one food contains all of these nutrients, eating a variety of foods is the best way to ensure a healthy diet. Additionally, if some foods contain toxins, such as residue of insect repellants or additives that behave as allergens, variety would reduce the amount ingested.

As one selects foods, it's important to choose those with high **nutrient density.** These are foods that provide many nutrients but few kcal. For example, tuna fish salad made with an oil dressing and served with tomatoes and mixed greens has high nutrient density. A meal consisting of a hamburger with french fries has low nutrient density.

Maintain a Healthy Weight

Overweight increases the risk of developing high blood pressure and diabetes (disorders asso-ciated with increased risk of heart attacks and strokes) and possibly some cancers. (See Table A-2 in the Appendix for acceptable body weights.) As discussed in Chapter 2, energy needs of people differ, depending on basal metabolism, age, size, sex, physical condition, and activity. However, the bottom line remains this: the number of kcal taken in must not exceed the number of kcal burned by the body each day if the current weight is to be maintained.

If there is need to lose weight, it should be done on a gradual basis of no more than one to two pounds per week. This may seem slow, but in fact 26 to 52 pounds can be lost in a six-month period. This is the most effective method of weight loss because it is most conducive to effecting genuine change in eating habits, which helps to maintain the reduced weight afterward. This is also the safest method of weight loss. Diets of less than 1,000 calories per day (crash diets) tend to limit the varieties of foods to such an extent that the nutrient intake may be reduced below the recommended daily allowances. This can damage one's health and, in extreme cases, cause death.

Because one pound of body fat contains 3,500 Kcal, 3,500 Kcal must be burned to lose one pound. If, for example, a person takes in 500 calories less than is burned each day, there will be a one-pound weight loss at the end of the week. One way to speed weight loss is to increase physical activity, causing additional calories to be burned.

Conversely, it is important that weight loss does not continue beyond the acceptable range. Extreme weight loss can contribute to nutrient deficiencies, menstrual irregularities, infertility, hair loss, skin changes, intolerance to cold, constipation, psychological disturbances, and even death. If there is unexplained weight loss, a physician should be consulted because it can be an indication of underlying disease.

Choose a Diet Low in Fat, Saturated Fat, and Cholesterol

Because fats contain slightly more than twice the kcal of carbohydrates or proteins, they contribute to obesity and, thus, heart disease, diabetes, and some forms of cancer. (See Chapter 4.) In addition, large amounts of saturated fats generally tend to raise blood cholesterol levels, which also increases the risk of heart disease. It is considered advisable to limit one's total fat intake to 30 percent of total daily kcal intake. Blood cholesterol levels in adults should be kept to 200 mg/dl or less. Both may be done without sacrificing necessary nutrients or flavor:

- Lean meats, fish, poultry, and **legumes** (various beans and peas) can be substituted for fatty meats.
- The fat on meats can be trimmed.
- The skin on poultry should not be eaten.
- Skim milk can be substituted for whole milk.
- Whenever possible, water-packed canned goods should be used instead of oil-packed.
- Eggs, organ meats, butter, margarine, and cream can be used in moderation, and foods can be baked, broiled, or boiled rather than fried.

Choose a Diet with Plenty of Vegetables, Fruits, and Grain Products

In this guideline, adults are advised to eat a minimum of three servings of vegetables, two fruits, and six servings of grain products each day. These foods provide numerous vitamins, minerals, complex carbohydrates, and dietary fiber. With the exception of avocado, they are very low in fat. Also, by eating this number of these foods, a person probably will eat fewer fat-rich foods.

Use Sugars Only in Moderation

Sugar serves as a preservative and thickener in jellies and jams, and adds color and flavor to numerous foods. However, the foods in which it is commonly found, such as desserts and candies, tend to have few other nutrients except for fats. Thus, if one eats sugar-rich foods in place of other foods, the total nutrient intake will be inadequate but the kcal content will be high. Additionally, sugar causes tooth decay (dental caries).

Use Salt and Sodium Only in Moderation

Excessive amounts of sodium can contribute to **hypertension** (blood pressure over 140/90), which is known to increase the risk of coronary heart disease (see Chapter 20). It is recommended that little, if any, salt be added during cooking or at the table. Canned and frozen foods generally have had salt added, so fresh foods are preferred.

If You Drink Alcoholic Beverages, Do So in Moderation

One ounce of gin, rum, vodka, or whiskey contains approximately 80 kcal and only traces of a few nutrients. In moderate drinkers, alcohol tends to increase the appetite, which can contribute to weight gain. Conversely, heavy drinkers can lose their appetites, not eat, and subsequently suffer nutritional deficiencies. The use of alcohol by pregnant women can cause birth defects. Heavy drinking can cause cirrhosis of the liver, brain damage, and increase the risk of cancer of the throat and neck. One drink per day for a woman and two for a man is considered moderate drinking. Twelve ounces of beer, 5 ounces of wine, or $1\frac{1}{2}$ ounces of 80-proof liquor all count as *one* drink.

FOOD GUIDE PYRAMID

The **Food Guide Pyramid** was introduced in 1992, and is intended as an outline to aid the consumer in meal planning. It is hoped that the Pyramid will promote healthful food habits among both adults and children. (See Figure 9-1.)

The Pyramid consists of six food groups that are presented in proportions appropriate for a healthful diet:

- Bread, Cereal, Rice, and Pasta Group
- Vegetable Group
- Fruit Group
- Milk, Yogurt, and Cheese Group
- Meat, Poultry, Fish, Dry Beans, Eggs, and Nuts Group
- Fats, Oils, and Sweets

Bread, Cereal, Rice, and Pasta Group

The largest section of the Pyramid is made up of the Bread, Cereal, Rice, and Pasta Group.

Food Guide Pyramid
A Guide to Daily Food Choices

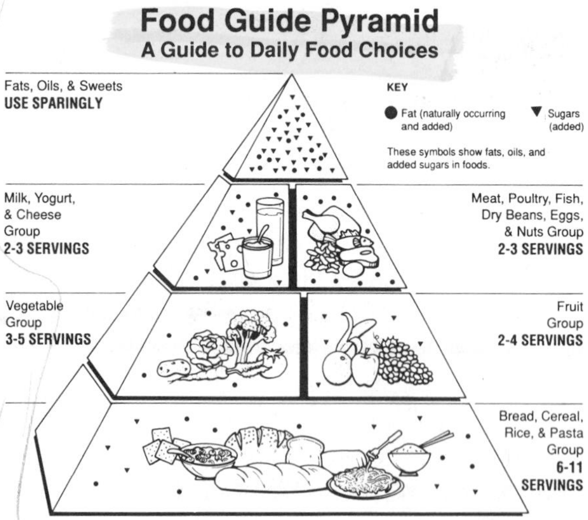

Figure 9-1 Food Guide Pyramid: A Guide to Daily Food Choices

Table 9-1 Breads, Cereals, Rice, and Pasta Group	
Breads	**Cereals**
whole wheat	whole wheat
dark rye	rolled oats
enriched	brown rice
Cornmeal, whole	converted rice
grain or enriched	other cereals, if
Rolls or biscuits made	whole grain or
with whole wheat or	restored
enriched flour	noodles, spaghetti,
Flour, enriched	macaroni
whole wheat, other	
whole grain	
oatmeal bread	
grits, enriched	

(See Table 9-1.) These foods are rich in complex carbohydrates and should make up 50 to 55% of one's diet. In addition, when they are made from whole grains, these foods provide dietary fiber, B vitamins, iron, and magnesium. Enriched or fortified products also contain B vitamins, iron, and magnesium plus calcium, but if they are not made from whole grains, they contain little dietary fiber.

It is recommended that one have from 6 to 11 servings of these foods each day. One serving is considered one slice of bread; one-half an English muffin; one ounce dry cereal; or one-half cup cooked cereal, pasta, or rice.

Vegetable Group

All vegetables are included in this group: green and leafy, yellow, starchy, and legumes. (See Table 9-2.) This group provides carbohydrates; dietary fiber; vitamins A, B-complex, C, E, and K; and iron, calcium, phosphorus, potassium, magnesium, copper, manganese and, sometimes, molybdenum and iodine.

It is recommended that one have from three to five servings of these foods each day. One-half

Table 9-2 Vegetable Group

Sources of Vitamin A	Sources of Vitamin C
Carrots	Raw or lightly
Squash	cooked cabbage
Spinach	Green peppers
Kale	Turnip greens
Other greens	Broccoli
Pumpkin	Potatoes
Sweet potatoes	Brussels sprouts
Corn	Tomatoes
Broccoli	Red peppers
Chard	Asparagus
	Spinach

cup of cooked or chopped raw vegetables or one cup of uncooked, leafy vegetables is considered one serving.

Fruit Group

All fruits are included in this group. They provide vitamins A and C, potassium, magnesium, iron, and carbohydrates, including dietary fiber. (See Table 9-3.)

Table 9-3 Fruit Group

Souces of Vitamin A	Sources of Vitamin C	
Bananas	Oranges	Cantaloupe
Cantaloupe	Lemons	Kiwi Fruit
Avocadoes	Grapefruit	Honeydew Melon
Apricots	Limes	Watermelon
Mangoes	Raspberries	Mangoes
	Strawberries	Papaya
	Pineapple	

It is recommended that two to four servings be included in the diet each day, at least one being an especially rich source of vitamin C. One serving is $\frac{3}{4}$ cup fruit juice; $\frac{1}{2}$ grapefruit; one whole raw apple, orange, peach, pear, or banana; $\frac{1}{2}$ cup canned or cooked fruit; and $\frac{1}{4}$ cup dried fruit.

Milk, Yogurt, and Cheese Group

Milk, yogurt, and cheese are excellent sources of carbohydrate (lactose, calcium, phosphorus, and magnesium; proteins; riboflavin, vitamins A, B_{12} and, if the milk is fortified, vitamin D. Unfortunately, whole milk and whole milk products also contain sodium, saturated fats, and cholesterol. Skim milk has had the fats removed.

It is recommended that two to three servings of these foods be included in one's daily diet. The serving size is one 8-ounce glass of milk or the equivalent in terms of calcium content.

Children	2 servings
Adolescents	3 servings
Adults	2 servings
Pregnant or Lactating Women	3 servings
Pregnant or Lactating Teens	4 servings

The following dairy foods contain calcium equal to that found in one 8-ounce cup of milk:

- $1\frac{1}{2}$ ounces of cheddar cheese
- $1\frac{1}{2}$ cups of cottage cheese
- $1\frac{3}{4}$ cups of ice cream or ice milk
- 1 cup yogurt

Milk used in making cream sauces, gravies, or baked products fulfills part of the calcium requirement. A cheese sandwich would fulfill one of the serving requirements, and a serving of ice cream or milk could fulfill half of one of the serving requirements. Obviously, drinking milk is not the only way to fulfill the calcium requirement.

Some patients suffer from lactose intolerance and cannot digest milk or milk products. If they eat or drink foods containing untreated lactose, they experience abdominal cramps and diarrhea. This condition is caused by a deficiency of lactase. (See Chapter 3.) In such cases, milk that has been treated with lactase can be used, or commercial lactase can be added to the milk.

Meat, Poultry, Fish, Dry Beans, Eggs, and Nuts Group

All meats, poultry, fish, eggs, soybeans, dry beans and peas, lentils, nuts and seeds are included in this group. (See Table 9-4.) These foods provide proteins, iron, copper, phosphorus, zinc, sodium, iodine, B vitamins, fats, and cholesterol.

Caution must be used so the foods selected from this group are low in fat and cholesterol. Many meats contain large amounts of fats, and egg yolks and organ meats have very high cholesterol content.

It is recommended that one have two to three servings from this group each day.

Fats, Oils, and Sweets

use sparingly

This group contains butter, margarine, cooking oils, mayonnaise and other salad dressings, sugar, syrup, honey, jam, jelly, and sodas. All of these foods have a low nutrient density, meaning they have few nutrients other than fats and carbohydrates and a high kcal content. There are no serving recommendations except that items from this group should be used sparingly because of their low nutrient content and high kcal content.

THE BASIC FOUR FOOD GROUPS

obsolete

The **Basic Four Food Groups** represent the simplest method of planning a balanced diet. Foods are divided into the following four groups:

- Vegetables and fruits
- Milk and milk products
- Breads and cereals
- Meats and meat alternates

The nutrients provided and servings suggested are shown in Table 9-5. When the minimum number of servings is used, the kcal count will be too low for adults. Thus, extra servings should be included when planning diets. However, it is important that these extra servings not include excessive amounts of meats or whole milk products because of the fats and cholesterol they contain.

MEAL PLANNING

A knowledge of basic nutrition must be combined with artistry and imagination when planning meals. Appetite appeal is as important as nutritive value in meal planning because the

Table 9-4 Meats, Poultry, Fish, Dry Beans, Eggs, and Nuts	
Beef	Dried beans
Lamb	Dried peas
Veal	Lentils
Pork, except bacon	Nuts
Organ meats, such as heart, liver, kidney, brain, tongue, sweetbread	Peanuts Peanut butter Soybean flour
Poultry, such as chicken, duck, goose, turkey	Soybeans
Fish, shellfish	

Table 9-5 Basic Four Food Groups

Group	Number of Servings		Nutrients Provided
Vegetables and Fruits		4+	Carbohydrates, including dietary fiber, Vitamin A, B vitamins, Vitamin C, Vitamin K, Calcium, Phosphorus, Magnesium, Iron, Potassium, possibly Iodine, Manganese, & Molybdenum
Milk and Milk Products	Children Adolescents Adults Pregnant women Lactating women	3+ 4+ 2+ 4+ 4+	Proteins, Fats, Carbohydrates, Calcium, Magnesium, Phosphorus, Sodium, Vitamin A, Vitamin D (if irradiated), Riboflavin, B_{12}
Breads and Cereals		4+	Carbohydrates, including dietary fiber, Thiamin, Niacin, Riboflavin, B_6, Pantothenic acid, Calcium (if enriched), Phosphorus, Iron, Magnesium
Meats and Meat Alternates		2+	Proteins, Fats, Iron, Copper, Phosphorus, Sodium, Iodine, Zinc, and B vitamins

best food is nutritious only when it is eaten. Although nutrient and kcal requirements must guide meal planning, the following criteria must also be considered: variety, appearance, flavor and aroma, texture, satiety, and individual likes and dislikes.

Variety

Even favorite foods lose their appeal when they are prepared day after day without variation. The finest cut of steak is no longer appetizing if it is served seven days a week. Variety improves both appetite and nutrient value of meals.

Appearance

Because the initial reaction to food is based on its appearance, it is essential to consider the colors and shapes of food when planning meals. Colors and shapes should vary and blend in a harmonious way, figure 9-2. Although a meal of tomato soup, corned beef, red cabbage, beets, and raspberry sherbet is nutritious, it lacks variety in color. Melon balls, fish balls, small boiled potatoes, brussels sprouts, and cherries lack variety in shape.

Flavor and Aroma

Flavor and aroma are so closely related that they should be considered together. Imagine eating a meal of onion soup, spiced sausage, mustard, sauerkraut, and hot peppers. Compare it, in terms of flavor and aroma, with a meal of chicken consomme, unspiced veal, mashed potatoes, and custard. Neither menu is appetizing. The first has too many foods with strong flavor and aroma, and the second has an excess of bland foods. **Bland** foods have mild flavors.

Texture

The **texture** (**consistency** or feel) of foods must also vary. For example, cream soup, baked

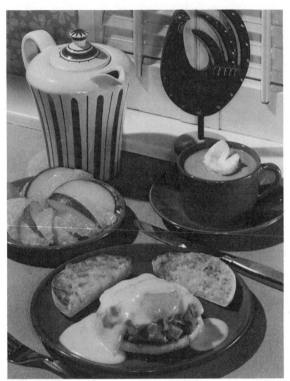

Figure 9-2 Breakfast can stimulate the appetite by a pleasing variety of shapes and colors of foods. *(Courtesy of the National Dairy Council)*

fish, mashed potatoes, squash, and rice pudding would make a dull meal. On the other hand, jaws would tire while eating a meal in which all of the foods required considerable chewing.

Satiety

A feeling of **satiety,** or satisfying fullness in the stomach, should linger after the meal, but the individual should not feel as if he or she has overeaten. One reason meals should include some protein and fat is that these nutrients stay in the stomach longer than carbohydrates, thus giving satiety value to the meal. Carbohydrate is necessary, however, to satisfy taste and provide quick energy.

Individual Likes and Dislikes

It is especially important to consider the individual likes and dislikes of various family members. If a particular food is disliked by everyone, it may be possible to substitute its nutritional equal. When a particular food is disliked by only one member of the family, it is advisable to serve it during that person's absence. Naturally, family and religious customs are respected when planning meals.

THE MENU PATTERN

A menu pattern, as shown in figure 9-3, simplifies meal planning. Evaluate the menu patterns shown in figure 9-3 in terms of nutritional adequacy.

The actual menus in figure 9-4 are based on the menu patterns in figure 9-3. Evaluate them in terms of nutritional adequacy, attractiveness, and economy.

Adapting the Menu Pattern

Sometimes there are family members such as young children, elderly people, or the ill, who are unable to conform to the family meal plan. In such circumstances, the menu should be adapted to suit the person with the particular needs. Minor changes must then be made in the basic plan. Individual variations in the menu should require little or no extra preparation. Suppose the sample menu was planned for a family that included a young couple, a 3-year-old boy, and an 80-year-old grandmother. The foods served should appeal to everyone and be easy for the elderly woman and the child to chew and digest.

In figure 9-4, breakfast is especially adaptable because a variety of ready-to-eat cereals can be served. The remaining foods on the menu

Breakfast	Lunch	Dinner
Fruit	Meat or Substitute	Meat or Substitute
Cereal	Fruit or Vegetable	2 or 3 Vegetables
Bread	Bread	Pasta or Rice
Milk	Fruit Juice	Bread
		Milk

Figure 9-3 A day's menu pattern based on the Food Guide Pyramid

Breakfast	Lunch	Dinner
Orange Juice	Tuna Sandwich on Whole Wheat	Baked Chicken
Cereal	Bread with Lettuce and Tomato	Noodles
Milk—Sugar	Carrot and Celery Sticks	Green Beans
2 slices Toast	Fresh Fruit	Coleslaw
Margarine—Jelly	Cookies	Bread—Margarine
Skim Milk	Pineapple Juice	Raspberry Sherbet
(Coffee for Adults)		Skim Milk

Figure 9-4 These three meals demonstrate how foods are selected from menu patterns.

should be suitable for everyone. The coleslaw on the sample dinner menu might present a problem, but a substitution of a cooked vegetable for the grandmother and the little boy could solve it. For lunch or supper, the tuna sandwiches might be made with enriched white bread instead of whole wheat, and a cooked vegetable could be substituted for the fresh vegetable sticks. If fresh fruit is served for dessert, it should be something easily chewed and digested, such as a banana, or a variety of fruit might be offered.

If a member of the family is ill, that person may require a special diet prescribed by the doctor. Even in such cases, the family menu should be adapted whenever possible to save time and expense in preparation and to make the patient feel that he or she is not causing extra work. (See Chapter 25.)

Efficient Planning

Efficiency in planning is increased by planning meals for several days or a week at one time. It is also economical to plan several meals at one time to allow for adequate use of leftovers. **Convenience foods** can be used provided they are nutritionally adequate. Convenience foods are partially prepared foods such as frozen foods, baking mixes, TV dinners, etc. Meals that can be prepared in the oven are both efficient and economical.

CONSIDERATIONS FOR THE HEALTH CARE PROFESSIONAL

Meal plans develop over time, and depend on a person's background, environment, economic and social status, and activities. For example, a mother who works outside the home as a highly paid professional might hire a cook or occasionally bring restaurant food home for dinner. A mother who works outside the home in a lower paying profession will probably have to prepare her family's dinner. These mothers may or may not consider their families' nutritional needs when they plan meals. If health needs require nutritional improvements in a family's meal plans, the health care professional will find it helpful to learn about the family's situation before beginning to teach the patients how to make the required changes.

SUMMARY

The Food Guide Pyramid is useful in planning nutritionally sound menus. The groups include breads, cereals, rice, and pasta; vegetables; fruits; milk, yogurt, and cheese; and meats, poultry, fish, dry beans, eggs, and nuts; and fats, oils, and sweets. Each group has a recommended number of servings. Other foods can be added as desired if they do not raise the total kcal value of the diet above the recommended amount.

The seven Dietary Guidelines developed by the U.S. government are important tools in the maintenance of good health through good nutrition. Essentially, they recommend a balanced diet.

To stimulate appetites, meals should provide satiety value and variety in color, flavor, aroma, texture, and shape. Menus should be flexible so they can be easily adapted to the special needs of individual family members. This flexibility helps save time and money. Planning several meals at one time is efficient and economical. The use of leftovers, convenience foods, and oven meals should be considered in weekly planning.

Discussion Topics

1. Define a balanced diet.
2. Describe the Food Guide Pyramid, including number of servings recommended per group.
3. How does careful use of the Food Guide Pyramid eliminate the need to check menus with a chart of the recommended dietary allowances?
4. What criteria, in addition to nutrient value of foods, should be considered when planning family meals? Why?
5. Discuss the difference between nutrient content and kcal value.
6. What groups of nutrients are provided by the vegetable group? The fruit group? The milk group? The meat group? The bread, cereal, rice and pasta groups?
7. How can one minimize the amount of fat in meats?
8. How might one include milk in the diet of a four-year-old who refuses to drink it?
9. Why would yogurt be a good snack or dessert for a pregnant woman?
10. List the Dietary Guidelines and state the reasons for them.
11. Alcohol is not considered a food so why is there a Dietary Guideline devoted to it?
12. Of what use is fiber in the diet?

13. Why is it advisable to adapt the family meal to suit the special needs of the patient rather than prepare a separate meal for the patient?

14. Why should "crash" or "fad" reducing diets be avoided? What is a better alternative? Why?

15. What would you advise your best friend if she or he was about to begin an 800-calorie reducing diet? Why would you give such advice?

16. Discuss the advantages and disadvantages of convenience foods for a family. For an individual.

17. Evaluate the menu in figure 9-4 in terms of its appetite appeal. List possible changes and discuss their effects on nutrient and kcal content.

18. Evaluate a menu consisting of macaroni and cheese, soft rolls, bananas, milk, and custard. Suggest improvements.

19. Discuss the sale of empty calorie foods in school cafeterias. Is it a good policy? If so, why? If not, why not? What would your position be on this subject if you were principal of an elementary school? Of a junior or senior high school?

20. Discuss how the following family dinner menu might be adapted to the needs of a family member on a reducing diet:

Fried Hamburgers
Boiled Potatoes with Butter
Steamed Broccoli
Lettuce with Mayonnaise
Rolls with Butter
Angel Cake with Whipped Cream
Whole Milk

21. How might the foregoing menu be adapted to the needs of someone who must limit intake of saturated fats?

Suggested Activities

1. Visit a market and identify the various meat group sources (sweetbreads, muscle meats, shellfish, etc.). What essential nutrients does each of these foods provide? Price these foods at the store. Look up a recipe for one and explain its preparation to the class. If possible, prepare it for the class.

2. Organize a campaign to educate your fellow students in regard to the Food Guide Pyramid. Consider using classroom and lunchroom bulletin boards, flyers, assembly programs with speakers, or a short play and lunchroom demonstrations of foods and their preparation.

3. Buy some fruits and vegetables that are new to you. Bring these to class and prepare and sample them. Share ideas as to their potential uses. Perhaps these might be added to home menus.

4. Using a restaurant menu, choose breakfast, lunch, and dinner. Check the selection of foods used with the Food Guide Pyramid. Are they balanced meals? Discuss the problems that people who eat all their meals in restaurants might have in maintaining a well-balanced diet.

5. Using the following table, fill in the "Menus" column with the foods eaten in the past two days. In the "Food Groups Used" column list the groups to which each food belongs. To evaluate personal dietary habits, fill in the "Food Groups Not Used" column. Compare the table with those of the rest of the class and discuss how eating habits may be improved.

	MENUS	FOOD GROUPS USED	FOOD GROUPS NOT USED
Breakfast			
Lunch			
Dinner			
Snacks			

6. Visit a local supermarket and make a list of the various convenience foods available. Compare their prices to the same foods that have not been partially prepared.

7. Look up recipes that use leftover roast beef. Present them to the class.

8. Check labels on sour cream and yogurt containers. Which would be preferable for someone on a fat-restricted diet? Why? How does the calcium content compare?

9. Using Table A-5 in the Appendix, adapt the meals in figure 9-4 for someone on a 1500-kcal diet.

10. Plan a week's menu for a family of four whose members have no special dietary needs. Use the menu pattern as a guide for listing the foods in proper order. Consider each of the following criteria in planning the menu:

nutritive quality   attractiveness
economy   efficiency of preparation

11. Select a menu for one day from the planned menu in activity 10. Adapt it for a visiting grandmother who has difficulty chewing.

Review

A. Multiple choice. Select the *letter* that precedes the best answer.

1. A balanced diet is one that includes
   a. equal amounts of carbohydrates and fats
   b. no animal products
   c. all of the essential nutrients
   d. more vegetables than fruits

2. When a food lends satiety to meals, it
   a. is always fattening
   b. provides enormous amounts of bulk
   c. gives satisfaction
   d. is chewy

3. When planning meals
   a. the nutrient content of meals is the main consideration
   b. both nutrient content and kcal value must be considered
   c. only the kcal value need be considered
   d. none of the above is true

4. Fruits and vegetables are rich sources of
   a. vitamins   c. proteins
   b. fats   d. all of these

5. Teenagers should have a serving of milk (or its substitute)
   a. not more than twice a day
   b. three times a day
   c. not more than four times a week
   d. not at all if they are overweight

6. Milk products are made from milk and include
   a. butter and margarine
   b. yogurt and cottage cheese
   c. bean curd and coconut milk
   d. all of the above

7. Milk and its products are the best dietary source of
   a. proteins and fats   b. carbohydrates
   c. calcium   d. all of the above

8. Breads, cereals, rice, and pasta are rich sources of
   - a. vitamin D
   - b. fats
   - c. carbohydrates
   - d. all of these

9. Foods from the meat group should be served
   - a. once a day
   - b. 2–3 times a day
   - c. 6–11 times a day
   - d. 3–5 times a day

10. Foods from the meat group are rich sources of
    - a. proteins
    - b. carbohydrates
    - c. vitamin C
    - d. all of these

11. An example of a meal plan that lacks variety is preparing
    - a. two vegetables for dinner every day
    - b. various dishes using meat each day
    - c. a fried egg with cinnamon toast each morning
    - d. fruit for lunch and dinner on the same day

12. Food products that are partially prepared commercially are called
    - a. empty calorie foods
    - b. convenience foods
    - c. bland foods
    - d. brand name foods

13. The appearance of food refers to the way it
    - a. tastes
    - b. smells
    - c. looks
    - d. all of these

14. The flavor of food refers to its
    - a. taste
    - b. smell
    - c. satiety value
    - d. cost

15. The aroma of food refers to its
    - a. appearance
    - b. smell
    - c. taste
    - d. satiety value

16. The texture or consistency of food refers to its
    - a. appearance
    - b. feel
    - c. aroma
    - d. satiety value

17. Menus should be evaluated in terms of
    - a. nutritional adequacy
    - b. kcal content only
    - c. efficiency of preparation
    - d. all of the above

18. Changing a menu to meet the special needs of a family member is called
    - a. planning the menu
    - b. adapting the menu
    - c. the pattern of the menu
    - d. varying the menu

19. Two examples of bland foods are
    a. grapefruit and oranges
    b. mashed potatoes and custard
    c. Italian sausage and salami
    d. all of the above
20. Foods that provide satiety value
    a. also provide large amounts of vitamin C
    b. give a lasting feeling of satisfying fullness in the stomach
    c. are those that all family members like
    d. are sugars and starches

B. Plan two dinners, selecting menus from the foods listed below.
Consider variety in color, texture and flavor. Adapt the steak menu
to suit an 80-year-old woman who finds it difficult to chew.
Baked halibut, broiled steak, creamed corn, stewed tomatoes, jellied vegetable salad, tossed green salad, mashed potatoes, baked potatoes, cherry upside-down cake, rice pudding with pineapple.

Case Study 1

Nutritional Deficiencies

George H. is a widower in his eighties. He lives alone and has so many complaints that few of his neighbors listen to him. After not having seen him in several weeks, one neighbor did listen because he appeared to be markedly thinner than the last time she had seen him. He also had visible sores at the corners of his mouth.

He complained that he was always tired, but couldn't sleep; that food had no taste; that the sores at the corner of his mouth hurt; and that his teeth felt loose. When she was able to break into his soliloquy, she asked what he ate.

George said he had canned pears, buttered white toast, and tea with milk at breakfast. At lunch he fried minced garlic and a little chopped onion in oil and cooked a hamburger in it. This he ate on a white roll with a glass of milk. At dinner he boiled a potato, opened a small can of tuna fish to which he added some mayonnaise, and had applesauce for dessert.

His neighbor contacted his son. The son took George to the doctor who recommended that George either have someone cook one meal a day for him, or that the son contact the city's Meals-on-Wheels program so that George would be brought one hot meal each weekday and have someone help him plan and learn to prepare weekend meals. In addition, the doctor told George to drink at least half a cup of orange juice every day, and to take one 500-mg. calcium tablet and a multiple vitamin supplement with iron each day.

The doctor's advice was followed, and within a month George both looked and felt better. He even began to seem slightly less unhappy.

Case Study Questions Based on the Nursing Process

Assess

1. What was it about George's diet that concerned the neighbor enough to contact George's son?
2. From what nutritional deficiencies did George probably suffer?
3. What may have caused George's teeth to feel loose?

Plan

4. What factors may have caused George to prepare the same meals every day?
5. What nutrients were probably added to George's diet by the new meal plan?

Implement

6. How might the new diet plan have contributed to the improvement of George's spirits?
7. Plan a weekend day's meals for George that he can prepare for himself.

Evaluate

8. George's story is not unusual among elderly people who live alone. Why is this the case?
9. What might have happened to George had his neighbor failed to notice George's condition and take action?

Case Study 2

Cholesterol Count

Myrna thought she was a great cook. She enjoyed food and having friends visit. One of her favorite breakfast treats was "Auntie Nina's Wonderful Frozen Waffles" topped with canned blueberry pie filling and a frozen whipped nondairy "cream." For her famous chicken casserole, she combined canned chicken, undiluted cream of celery soup, and sliced olives, topped with crushed potato chips. She also liked to serve brownies from the local bakery, but topped with canned chocolate icing and slivered salted peanuts. Occasionally, she would prepare TV dinners, but she always topped the veggies with melted American cheese.

After a recent physical examination, her physician told her that her cholesterol count was 275 and that she should bring it down. The doctor asked her to describe her meals.

Case Study Questions Based on the Nursing Process

Assess

1. What is the doctor probably going to tell Myrna about her favorite breakfast?

Plan

2. Is the doctor likely to suggest any changes in Myrna's chicken casserole? If yes, what?
3. What will the doctor probably say about the brownies? The addition to the TV dinners?

Implement

4. Are these changes going to be easy for Myrna? Why?
5. If you were to help Myrna change her diet to reduce her cholesterol count, what would you suggest?
6. How would you involve Myrna in the plans for her dietary changes?

Evaluate

7. When discussing Myrna's diet at the next office visit, what will convince the doctor that Myrna understands and is following the low-cholesterol diet?

FOOD CUSTOMS

OBJECTIVES

After studying this chapter, you should be able to
- Describe the development of food customs
- List some food customs of various cultural groups
- Identify at least three nutritionally poor food habits
- Adapt menus to suit a cultural or religious group with strict dietary laws

The guidelines for good nutrition discussed in Chapter 9 are more easily recited than practiced. It is important not only to know these guidelines, but to follow them daily. It is much easier to help other people correct their eating habits after evaluating and correcting your own eating habits.

Some common bad eating habits include eating an excess of foods containing fats and carbohydrates, attempting to control weight gain by crash reducing diets, and skipping meals. Obesity and malnutrition can be caused by an excess of carbohydrates or fats in the diet. Such malnutri-

tion can develop if foods containing primarily these two nutrients are substituted for foods containing the other essential nutrients. **Crash reducing diets** typically consist of only a narrow selection of foods, thus limiting the types of nutrients obtained. Skipping meals also can limit the variety of nutrients eaten. Ironically, this can also cause an increase in the total daily caloric intake because a person is likely to overeat after being without food for a long period.

Although habits are not easily changed, the key to change rests on understanding the reasons eating habits develop.

DEVELOPMENT OF FOOD CUSTOMS

People from each country have favorite foods. Frequently, there are distinctive **food customs** originating in just a small section of a particular country. People of a particular area favor the foods that are produced in that area. They are available and economical. Some religions have **dietary laws** that require particular food practices. Because most people prefer the foods they were accustomed to while growing up, food habits are often based on nationality and religion. One's **economic** and **social status** also contribute to food habits. For example, the poor do not grow up with a taste for caviar, while the wealthy may at least be accustomed to it—whether or not they like it. Those in a certain social class will be apt to use the same foods as others in their class. And the foods they choose will probably depend on the work they do. For example, people doing hard, physical labor will require higher calorie foods than those in sedentary jobs.

When people move from one country to another, or from one area to another, their economic status may change. They can be introduced to new foods and new food customs. Although their original food customs may have been nutritionally adequate, their new **environment** may cause them to change their eating habits. For example, if milk was a **staple** (basic) **food** in their diet before moving and is unusually expensive in the new environment, milk may be replaced by a cheaper, nutritionally inferior beverage such as soda, coffee, or tea. Candy, a luxury in their former environment, can be inexpensive and popular in their new environment. As a result, a family might increase consumption of soda or candy, and reduce purchases of more nutritious foods. Someone who is not familiar with the nutritive values of foods can easily make such mistakes in their food selection.

The meal patterns of national and religious groups different from one's own may seem strange. However, the diet may well be nutritionally adequate. When a patient's eating habits need to be corrected, such corrections are more easily made if the food customs of the patient are known and understood by the health care professional. To gain this knowledge, it is advisable to talk with the patient and learn about her or his background. This knowledge can be used to plan nourishing menus consisting of foods that appeal to the patient. The necessary adjustments in the diet can then be made gradually and effectively.

FOOD PATTERNS BASED ON CULTURE

American **cuisine** (cooking style) is a marvelous composite of countless national, regional, **cultural** (sociological background), and religious food customs. Consequently, it can be difficult to categorize a patient's food habits. Nevertheless, it is sometimes helpful to be able to do so to a certain extent. When people are ill, it is not uncommon for them to have little interest in food, and sometimes foods that were familiar to them during their childhood and youth are more apt to tempt them than other types. The following section briefly discusses some food patterns typical of various cultures, regions, and countries. It is important to remember that there can be and usually are enormous variations within any one classification.

Native American

It is thought that approximately half of the edible plants commonly eaten in the United States today originated with the Native Americans. Examples are corn, potatoes, squash, cranberries, pumpkins, peppers, beans, wild rice, and cocoa beans. In addition, they used wild fruits, game, and fish. Foods were commonly prepared as soups and stews, and dried. The original Native American diets were probably more nutritionally adequate than their current diets, which frequently consist of too high a proportion of sweet and salty, snack-type, empty calorie foods. Native American diets today may be deficient in calcium, vitamins A, C, and riboflavin.

U.S. Southern

Hot breads such as corn bread and baking powder biscuits are common in the U.S. South because the wheat grown in the area does not make good quality yeast breads. Grits and rice are also popular carbohydrate foods. Favorite vegetables include sweet potatoes, squash, green beans, and lima beans. Green beans cooked with pork are commonly served. Watermelon, oranges, and peaches are popular fruits. Fried fish is served often, as are barbecued and stewed meats and poultry. There is a great deal of carbohydrate and fat in these diets and limited amounts of protein in some cases. Iron, calcium, and vitamins A and C may sometimes be deficient.

Mexican

Mexican food is a combination of Spanish and Native American foods. Beans, rice, chili peppers, tomatoes, and corn meal are favorites. Meat is often cooked with the vegetable as in chili con carne. Corn meal is used in a variety of ways to make **tortillas** and **tamales,** which serve as bread. The combination of beans and corn makes a complete protein. While tortillas filled with cheese (called enchiladas) provide some calcium, the use of milk should be encouraged. Additional green and yellow vegetables and vitamin C-rich foods would also improve these diets.

Puerto Rican

Rice is the basic carbohydrate food in Puerto Rican diets. Vegetables commonly used include beans, plantains, tomatoes, and peppers. Bananas, pineapple, mangoes, and papayas are popular fruits. Favorite meats are chicken, beef, and pork. Milk is not used as much as would be desirable from the nutritional point of view.

Italian

Pastas with various tomato or fish sauces, and cheese are popular Italian foods. Fish and highly seasoned foods are common to Southern Italian cuisine while meat and root vegetables are common to northern Italy. The eggs, cheese, tomatoes, green vegetables, and fruits common to Italian diets provide excellent sources of many nutrients, but additional milk and meat would improve the diet.

Northern and Western European

Northern and Western European diets are similar to those of the U.S. Midwest, but with a greater use of dark breads, potatoes, and fish, and fewer green vegetable salads. Beef and pork are popular as are various cooked vegetables, breads, cakes, and dairy products.

Central European

Citizens of Central Europe obtain the greatest portion of their calories from potatoes and grain, especially rye and buckwheat. Pork is a popular meat. Cabbage cooked in many ways is a popular vegetable as are carrots, onions, and turnips. Eggs and dairy products are used abundantly.

Middle Eastern

Grains, wheat, and rice provide energy in these diets. Chickpeas in the form of **homous** are popular. Lamb and yogurt are commonly used as are cabbage, grape leaves, eggplant, tomatoes, dates, olives, and figs. Black, very sweet coffee is a popular beverage.

Chinese

The Chinese diet is varied. Rice is the primary energy food and is used in place of bread. Foods are generally cut into small pieces. Vegetables are lightly cooked and the cooking water is saved for future use. Soybeans are used in many ways, and eggs and pork are commonly served. Soy sauce is extensively used, but it is very salty and could present a problem with patients on low-salt diets. Tea is a common beverage, but milk is not. This diet may be low in fat.

Japanese

Japanese diets include rice, soybean paste and curd, vegetables, fruits, and fish. Food is frequently served **tempura** style, which means fried. Soy sauce (**shoyu**) and tea are commonly used. Current Japanese diets have been greatly influenced by Western culture.

Southeast Asian

Many Indians are vegetarians who use eggs and dairy products. Rice, peas, and beans are frequently served. Spices, especially curry, are popular. Indian meals are not typically served in courses as Western meals are. They generally consist of one course with many dishes. Eating with one's fingers is considered acceptable.

Thailand, Vietnam, Laos, and Cambodia

Rice, curries, vegetables, and fruit are popular in Thailand, Vietnam, Laos, and Cambodia. Meat, chicken, and fish are used in small amounts. The **wok** (a deep, round fry pan) is used for sautéing many foods. A salty sauce made from fermented fish is commonly used.

FOOD PATTERNS BASED ON RELIGION OR PHILOSOPHY

Jewish

Interpretations of the Jewish dietary laws vary. Those who adhere to the Orthodox view consider tradition important and always observe the dietary laws. Foods prepared according to these laws are called *kosher*. Conservative Jews are inclined to observe the rules only at home. Reform Jews consider their dietary laws to be essentially ceremonial and so minimize their significance. Essentially the laws require the following:

- Slaughtering must be done by a qualified person, in a prescribed manner. The meat or poultry must be drained of blood, first by severing the jugular vein and carotid artery, then by soaking in brine before cooking.
- Meat or meat products may not be prepared or eaten with milk or milk products.
- The dishes used in the preparation and serving of meat dishes must be kept separate from those used for dairy foods.
- A specified time, six hours, must elapse between consumption of meat and milk.
- The mouth must be rinsed after eating fish and before eating meat.

- There are prescribed fast days—Passover Week, Yom Kippur, and Feast of Purim.
- No cooking is done on the Sabbath—from sundown Friday to sundown Saturday.

These laws forbid the eating of the following:

- the flesh of animals without cloven (split) hooves or that do not chew their cud
- hind quarters of any animal
- shellfish or fish without scales or fins
- fowl that are birds of prey
- creeping things and insects
- **leavened** (contains ingredients that cause it to rise) **bread** during the Passover

Generally, the food served is rich. Fresh smoked and salted fish, and chicken are popular, as are noodles, egg, and flour dishes. These diets can be deficient in fresh vegetables and milk.

Roman Catholic

Although the dietary restrictions of the Roman Catholic religion have been liberalized, meat is not allowed its adherents on Ash Wednesday and Fridays during Lent.

Eastern Orthodox

Followers of this religion include Christians from the Middle East, Russia, and Greece. Although interpretations of the dietary laws vary, meat, poultry, fish, and dairy products are restricted on Wednesdays and Fridays and during Lent and Advent.

Seventh Day Adventist

Generally, Seventh Day Adventists are **ovo-lacto-vegetarians,** which means they use milk products and eggs, but no meat, fish, or poultry. They may also use nuts, legumes, and **meat analogues** (substitutes) made from soybeans. They consider coffee, tea, and alcohol to be harmful.

Mormon (Latter Day Saints)

The only dietary restriction observed by the Mormons is the prohibition of coffee, tea, and alcoholic beverages.

Islamic

Adherents of Islam are called Muslims. Their dietary laws prohibit the use of pork and alcohol, and other meats must be slaughtered according to specific laws. During the month of Ramadan, Muslims do not eat or drink during daylight hours.

Hindu

To the Hindus, all life is sacred and small animals contain the souls of ancestors. Consequently, Hindus are usually vegetarians. They do not use eggs as they represent life.

OTHER FOOD PATTERNS

Vegetarians

There are several vegetarian diets. The common factor among them is that they do not include red meat. Some include eggs, some fish, some milk, and some even poultry. When carefully planned, these diets can be nutritious. They can even contribute to a reduction of obesity, high blood pressure, heart disease, some cancers, and possibly diabetes. They must be carefully planned, of course, so they include all the needed nutrients.

Lacto-Ovo Vegetarians

Lacto-ovo vegetarians use dairy products and eggs but no meat, poultry, or fish.

Lacto-Vegetarians

Lacto-vegetarians use dairy products but no meat, poultry, or eggs.

Vegans

Vegans avoid all animal foods. They use soybeans, chick peas, and meat analogues made from soybeans. It is important that their meals be carefully planned to include appropriate combinations of the nonessential amino acids to provide the needed amino acids. For example, beans served with corn or rice, or peanuts eaten with wheat, are better in such combinations than any of them would be if eaten alone. Vegans can show deficiencies of calcium, zinc, vitamins A, D, and B_{12} and, of course, proteins.

Zen-Macrobiotic Diets

The macrobiotic diet is a system of ten diet plans, developed from Zen Buddhism. Adherents progress from the lower number diet to the higher, gradually giving up foods in the following order: desserts, salads, fruits, animal foods, soups, and ultimately vegetables, until only cereals—usually brown rice—are consumed. Beverages are kept to a minimum and only organic foods (see Chapter 27) are used. Foods are grouped as Yang (male) or Yin (female). A ratio of 5:1 Yang to Yin is considered important. Most macrobiotic diets are nutritionally inadequate. As the adherents give up foods according to plans, their diets become increasingly inadequate. These diets can be especially dangerous because avid adherents promise medical cures from the diets that cannot be attained, and so medical treatment may be delayed when needed.

CONSIDERATIONS FOR THE HEALTH CARE PROFESSIONAL

It is particularly important that the health care professional view patients' normal diets with an open mind. Often, diets different from one's own are, in fact, nutritionally balanced. To correctly evaluate the nutritional status of an unfamiliar diet, one must determine the ingredients of the various foods. This can involve discussions with members of the patients' families; reading recipes in cookbooks that include recipes favored by a particular nationality or region; and visiting markets that sell the ingredients used in these recipes. Only at this point can improvements in a patient's diet begin.

SUMMARY

Food habits have many diverse origins. Nationality, religion, and economic and social status all affect their development. When such customs result in inadequate diets, corrections should be made gradually. Corrections are easier and more effectively made when the reasons for the food habits are understood.

Discussion Topics

1. Discuss the reasons why nurses and homemakers should practice the rules of good nutrition themselves.
2. How do food habits originate?

3. What effects does environment have on particular food habits? When do the effects of a new environment improve diets and when do they impair them?

4. From personal experience, explain why certain foods are enjoyed more than others that are commonly available in the local area.

5. Discuss the dangers of skipping meals and explain how this habit can result in an *increased* caloric intake.

6. Ask if anyone in class has been on a crash reducing diet. Ask that person to describe the diet and its ultimate result. Would that person recommend this diet? Why?

7. Why are hot breads more popular with people from the U.S. South than yeast breads?

8. Would a banker or a bricklayer be more apt to choose a chef's salad for lunch? Explain.

9. Why might Scandinavians be more inclined to like fish than Hungarians?

10. Why are Zen-macrobiotic diets dangerous?

11. Discuss vegetarian diets. Are they safe? Explain.

12. Why is it difficult to convince someone to change her or his food habits? Discuss.

Suggested Activities

1. Give a series of short reports on food customs. Each student should select a different country or area within a country for study. After the reports have been presented, hold a class discussion on whether climate, availability of food, economic, or other factors determine the food customs of the countries studied. Include answers to the following in the reports— What is the climate of the country? What type of crops are grown there? Are modern methods of agriculture used? Does the country depend on imports for much of its food supply? If so, what foods are imported? Is the majority of the citizenry poor? What types of foods are popular? Expensive? Which of these foods are produced in the country? Which are imported? What is the prevalent religion?

2. Plan a Good Friday menu for a patient of the Roman Catholic faith.

3. Investigate the lunch program of a local school. Have a panel discussion on its purpose, limitations, favorable characteristics, and suggested improvements.

4. Make attractive posters for the school lunchroom or cafeteria in which the improvement of eating habits is stressed.

5. Role-play a situation in which a nurse tries to persuade a patient to use more milk.

Review

A. Multiple choice. Select the *letter* that precedes the best answer.

1. Food customs mean one's
   a. food nutrients
   b. food habits
   c. food requirements
   d. all of the above

2. A bad eating habit that is common is
   a. skipping meals
   b. eating protein at every meal
   c. using reducing diets
   d. following religious dietary laws

3. Food customs
   a. may be based on religion or nationality
   b. are always nutritious
   c. are easily changed
   d. are not affected by one's social status

4. Moving to a new environment or experiencing a change in salary
   a. rarely changes established food habits
   b. usually influences established food habits
   c. always reduces the amount of food eaten
   d. never reduces the quality of food eaten

5. Crash reducing diets
   a. may limit the types of nutrients obtained
   b. are an acceptable way to control weight gain
   c. contain a wide selection of foods
   d. are usually recommended by nutritionists

6. Hot breads are common to diets of people from
   a. Mexico
   b. the Midwest
   c. China
   d. the U.S. South

7. Rice is a popular carbohydrate food in
   a. Puerto Rico
   b. Central Europe
   c. Northern Europe
   d. all of the above

8. Sedentary jobs include those of
   a. physical education teachers
   b. bricklayers
   c. dancers
   d. secretaries

9. Generally, the diets of U.S. Southerners, Mexicans, Puerto Ricans, and Italians would be improved by the addition of more
   a. rice
   b. corn
   c. milk
   d. pasta

10. A diet of dried beans, corn, and chili peppers would most likely be used by a(n)

a. Mexican family

b. Italian family

c. Armenian family

d. Orthodox Jewish family

B.   Adapt the following menu for a person of the Orthodox Jewish faith.

Baked Ham
Scalloped Potatoes
Buttered Peas
Bread and Butter
Fresh Fruit
Milk or Coffee

C.   Matching.

Write "B" for Breads and Cereals, "M" for Meats and Meat Substitutes, "V" for Vegetables and Fruits, and "D" for Dairy Foods. Some foods may fit into more than one group.

_____ 1. Yogurt

_____ 2. Cornbread

_____ 3. Grits

_____ 4. Collard greens

_____ 5. Yams

_____ 6. Buttermilk

_____ 7. Pizza

_____ 8. Tofu made from Soybeans

_____ 9. Caviar

_____ 10. Tortillas

Case Study 1

Altered Food Customs

When Maria's husband died, her brother Roberto brought her and her five-year-old daughter Carmen to New York City to live with him. Maria had lived her entire 25 years in a small town in Mexico, and had a very limited knowledge of English. Her brother worked long hours to support the three of them. He had little time or energy to help her. In her loneliness and fear of the city, Maria fell into a state of apathy for several months. Carmen adapted quickly however, and soon learned to love the "gringo" food—especially the sweet sodas. When Carmen refused to drink milk, instead of arguing with her, Maria simply stopped buying it. Although the school nurse sent a notice home saying that Carmen needed to see a dentist, Maria ignored it. She was making some money as a seamstress by that time, but she didn't have enough for a dentist. She was ashamed to ask Roberto for any more. Eventually, the cavities reached the nerves and Carmen was in pain. Maria took Carmen to a dentist who repaired her decayed teeth and then discussed Carmen's diet with both of them.

Case Study Questions Based on the Nursing Process

Assess
1. What probably contributed to the decay in Carmen's teeth?

Plan
2. What advice might the dentist have given Carmen and Maria?
3. Is it likely that in the future Maria will let Carmen make choices she is not yet prepared to make? Why?

Implement
4. What can Maria do if Carmen simply refuses to drink milk?
5. What factors may have contributed to Maria's apathy in New York?

Evaluate
6. How might the lack of milk in the house have affected Maria?
7. In your area, identify support groups available to help Maria adjust to the new culture.
8. What other physical problems might Carmen have as a result of her limited calcium intake?

Case Study 2

Anemia during Pregnancy

Sara, at the age of 30, was pregnant for the first time and was excited about the prospect of having a baby. She suffered little from morning sickness but was frequently light-headed and tired.

She looked forward eagerly to the arrival of the baby. She hoped to teach the child to respect other people and animals, and hoped she could influence the child to become a vegetarian as she had been since her freshman year at college.

She was crushed when her obstetrician told her she was anemic and must eat meat during her pregnancy and the period of lactation. The obstetrician also prescribed a multivitamin capsule and an iron supplement.

Case Study Questions Based on the Nursing Process

Assess
1. What may have been the cause of Sara's light-headedness? Of her fatigue?

Plan
2. Why did the obstetrician prescribe an iron supplement?
3. Why was a multivitamin prescribed at the same time?

Implement
4. What might Sara do to increase the absorption of this iron?
5. Why would the obstetrician prescribe iron during lactation?
6. If Sara refuses to eat meat, what food alternatives to gain more iron would you recommend?

Evaluate
7. How will Sara feel physically when her anemia is under control?

CHAPTER 11

FOOD-RELATED ILLNESSES AND ALLERGIES

OBJECTIVES

After studying this chapter, you should be able to
- Identify diseases caused by contaminated food, their symptoms, and the means by which they are spread
- List signs of food contamination
- State precautions for protecting food from contamination
- Describe allergies, elimination diets, and their uses

ILLNESSES CAUSED BY MICROORGANISMS IN FOOD

The most nutritious food can cause illness if it is contaminated with harmful **microorganisms** (microscopic plants and animals such as bacteria, viruses, worms, and molds), or chemical poisons. Fortunately, in the United States there are strict federal, state, and local laws regulating the commercial production of food. Dairies, canneries, bakeries, and meat-packing houses are all subject to government inspection. The commercial pro-cessing of foods is regularly checked so that these foods are wholesome and safe to eat. Nevertheless, people do sometimes become sick because of something they ate. With few exceptions, such illnesses occur because of the ignorance or carelessness of people who handle food in the kitchen.

There are always microorganisms in the **environment** (surroundings). Sometimes they are present in the food because its animal-source contained them. When foods are undercooked these microbes may be carried to consumers and make them sick. Microorganisms may be introduced to food by a carrier. A **carrier** is a person (or animal) capable of transmitting an **infectious** (disease-causing) organism. Often the carrier suffers no effects from the organism and therefore is unaware of the danger. A food handler may have a cut on the hand, a cold, or a skin infection, or simply fail to wash her or his hands after using the toilet, and microorganisms from this person can easily spread to the food. Insects, dust, and animals may contaminate the food if it is improperly stored, and food from contaminated water can carry microbes.

Foods are generally moist and soft, and provide an excellent place for microorganisms to grow. When foods are not stored at proper temperatures, these microorganisms multiply rapidly. Foods should be handled, stored, and cooked in ways that best control the growth of these organisms.

Salmonella

Salmonellosis (commonly called **salmonella**) is an infection caused by the Salmonella bacteria (see Table 11-1). Salmonella can be found in raw meats, poultry, fish, milk, and eggs. It is transmitted by eating contaminated food or by contact with a carrier. Salmonellosis is characterized by headache, vomiting, **diarrhea** (loose, frequent bowel movements), abdominal cramps, and fever. In severe cases, it can result in death. Those who suffer the most severe cases are typically the very young, the very old, and the weak or incapacitated.

Refrigeration at 7.2°C (45°F) or below inhibits the growth of these bacteria. However, bacteria can remain alive in the freezer and in dried foods. Salmonella bacteria are destroyed by heating to at least 60°C (140°F) for a minimum of ten minutes. One species of Salmonella causes typhoid fever.

Perfringens

Perfringens poisoning is caused by the *Clostridium perfringens* bacteria. It is commonly found in soil, on food, and in the intestinal tracts of warm-blooded animals. It is transmitted by eating heavily contaminated food. It is characterized by **nausea,** diarrhea, and inflammation of the stomach and intestines. These are spore-forming bacteria that grow without oxygen and are difficult to destroy. The spores can survive most cooking temperatures. The best method of controlling them is to refrigerate meats quickly at 4.4°C (40°F) or below.

Staph

Staphylococcal poisoning, commonly called **staph,** is caused by the *Staphylococcus aureus* bacteria. These bacteria are found on the skin and in the respiratory passages. They grow in meats, poultry, fish and egg dishes, in salads such as potato, egg, macaroni, and tuna, and in cream-filled pastries. This poisoning is transmitted by carriers and by eating food that contains the toxin. It is characterized by vomiting, diarrhea, and abdominal cramps. It is considered a mild illness. The growth of these bacteria is inhibited if foods are kept at temperatures above 60°C (140°F) or below 4.4°C (40°F). The toxin can be destroyed by boiling the food for several hours, or by heating it in a pressure cooker at 115.6°C (240°F) for 30 minutes. In most cases, long periods of high-temperature cooking would reduce the appeal and nutritional value of food. It is more practical to discard foods suspected of being contaminated.

Botulism

Botulism is caused by the toxin produced by the *Clostridium botulinum* bacteria. This is perhaps the rarest but most deadly of all food poisonings. It is characterized by double vision, speech difficulties, inability to swallow, respiratory paralysis, and sometimes death. The fatality rate in the United States is about 65 percent. The spores of this bacteria can divide and produce **toxin** without oxygen. This means that toxin can be produced in sealed containers such as cans and jars. The spores are extremely heat resistant. They must be boiled for six hours before they will be destroyed. The toxin, however, can be destroyed by boiling for twenty minutes.

Great care must be taken to prevent botulism when canning foods at home. The FDA and USDA report five deaths from botulism traced to commercially canned foods in the United States between 1925 and 1974, and 700 deaths from home-canned foods during that same time period.

Trichinosis

Trichinosis is a disease caused by the parasite *Trichinella spiralis*. A **parasite** is a life form that depends completely on another life form without making any contribution toward the needs of the host. **Trichinosis** is transmitted by eating inadequately cooked pork from pigs that are infected with the *Trichinella spiralis* parasite. Symptoms include vomiting, fever, chills, and muscle pain. Cooking all pork to an internal temperature of at least 58.3°C (137°F) kills the organism and prevents this disease. The parasite can also be destroyed by freezing.

Dysentery

Dysentery is a disease caused by a **protozoa** (a tiny, one-celled animal). The protozoa is transmitted through food by carriers or by **contaminated water.** It causes severe diarrhea that

can occur intermittently until the patient is properly treated.

PREVENTION OF FOOD-BORNE ILLNESS

All of the foregoing illnesses are caused by contaminated food or water. Except for trichinosis, food becomes contaminated because of poor **sanitation** on the part of the food handler or from improper storage.

To prevent contamination, persons preparing food must have clean hands that are not cut or infected in any way, clean clothes, and clean cooking equipment. They should touch the food as little as possible. After handling uncooked food, people should wash their hands and all utensils carefully and discard protective gloves. Cutting boards used in the preparation of uncooked meats should be washed thoroughly and not used in the preparation of any cooked foods; wood is porous and can retain microorganisms such as salmonella. Tests should be made regularly of people working as professional food handlers to ascertain that they are not carriers of infectious organisms.

Food poisons cannot be seen, but sometimes there are telltale signs of their existence. If a can bulges, if its contents appear different than usual, or if the food has an unusual odor, it should be discarded in a place where animals and children cannot reach it. CAUTION: The food should never be tasted in these circumstances because *Clostridium botulinum* might be present, and can be fatal. A good rule of thumb is: "If in doubt, throw it out."

Cooking and Storage of Food

Proper food storage is extremely important in inhibiting the growth of microorganisms. Al-

Table 11-1 Bacterial Food-borne Illnesses: Causes, Symptoms, and Prevention

Name of Illness	What Causes It	Symptoms	Characteristics of Illness	Preventive Measures
Salmonellosis Examples of foods involved: Poultry, red meats, eggs, dried foods, dairy products.	**Salmonellae.** Bacteria wide-spread in nature, live and grow in intestinal tracts of human beings and animals.	Severe headache, followed by vomiting, diarrhea, abdominal cramps, and fever. Infants, elderly, and persons with low resistance are most susceptible. Severe infections cause high fever and may even cause death.	Transmitted by eating contaminated foods, or by contact with infected persons or carriers of the infection. Also transmitted by insects, rodents, and pets. Onset: Usually within 12 to 36 hours. Duration: 2 to 7 days	Salmonellae in food are destroyed by heating the food to 140°F and holding for 10 minutes or to higher temperatures for less time, for instance, 155°F for a few seconds. Refrigeration at 40°F inhibits the increase of Salmonellae, but they remain alive in foods in the refrigerator or freezer, and even in dried foods.
Perfringens poisoning Examples of foods involved: Stews, soups, or gravies made from poultry or red meat.	**Clostridium perfringens.** Spore-forming bacteria that grow in the absence of oxygen. Temperatures reached in thorough cooking of most foods are sufficient to destroy vegetative cells, but heat-resistant spores can survive.	Nausea (without vomiting), diarrhea, acute inflammation of the stomach and intestines.	Transmitted by eating food contaminated with abnormally large numbers of the bacteria. Onset: Usually within 8 to 20 hours. Duration: May persist for 24 hours.	To prevent growth of surviving bacteria in cooked meats, gravies, and meat casseroles that are to be eaten later, cool foods rapidly and refrigerate promptly to 40°F or below or hold them above 140°F.

Table 11-1 (*Continued*)

Name of Illness	What Causes It	Symptoms	Characteristics of Illness	Preventive Measures
Staphylococcal poisoning (frequently called staph) Examples of foods involved: Custards, egg salad, potato salad, chicken salad, macaroni salad, ham, salami, cheese	**Staphylococcus aureus.** Bacteria fairly resistant to heat. Bacteria growing in food produce a toxin that is extremely resistant to heat.	Vomiting, diarrhea, prostration, abdominal cramps. Generally mild and often attributed to other causes.	Transmitted by food handlers who carry the bacteria and by eating food containing the toxin. Onset: Usually within 3 to 8 hours. Duration: 1 or 2 days.	Growth of bacteria that produce toxins is inhibited by keeping hot foods above 140°F and cold foods at or below 40°F. Toxin is destroyed by boiling for several hours or heating the food in a pressure cooker at 240°F for 30 minutes.
Botulism Examples of foods involved: Canned low-acid foods, smoked fish	**Clostridium botulinum.** Spore-forming organisms that grow and produce toxin in the absence of oxygen, such as in a sealed container.	Double vision, inability to swallow, speech difficulty, progressive respiratory paralysis. Fatality rate is high, in the United States about 65 percent.	Transmitted by eating food containing the toxin. Onset: Usually within 12 to 36 hours or longer. Duration: 3 to 6 days.	Bacterial spores in food are destroyed by high temperatures obtained only in the pressure canner. More than 6 hours is needed to kill the spores at boiling temperature (212°F). The toxin is destroyed by boiling for 10 to 20 minutes; time required depends on kind of food.

Adapted from USDA Home and Garden Bulletin No. 162, 1975, and 242, 1986

though freezing does not necessarily kill microbes, it does prevent their growth. Because bacteria grow best at temperatures between 15.6° and 51.7°C (60° and 125°F), it is important to keep food refrigerated, that is, below 15.6°C (60°F); or to keep it hot, above 51.7°C (125°F).

It is essential that meat and poultry be cooked thoroughly, and to the proper temperature (see figure 11-1 and Table 11-2). A meat thermometer is a good investment.

Leftover food should *always* be refrigerated as soon as the meal is finished, and covered after it is cold. *It should not be allowed to cool at room temperature before being refrigerated.* Frozen foods should either be cooked from the frozen state or thawed in the refrigerator. (When cooked from the frozen state, cooking time will be increased by at least 50 percent.) Frozen foods should not be thawed at room temperature. Food must *always* be protected from dust, insects, and animals since all of these can spread contamination.

MISCELLANEOUS FOOD POISONINGS

Occasionally, food poisoning is caused by ingesting certain plants or animals that contain poison. Examples are plants such as poisonous mushrooms, rhubarb leaves, and fish from polluted water.

Poisoning also can result from ingesting cleaning agents, **insecticides,** or excessive amounts of a drug. Children may swallow cleaning agents or medicines. The cook may mistakenly use a poison instead of a cooking ingredient. Sometimes insecticides cling to fresh fruits and vegetables. It is essential that all potential poisons be kept out of the reach of young children and kept separate from all food supplies. Fresh fruits and vegetables should be thoroughly washed before being stored.

FOOD ALLERGIES

An **allergy** is an altered reaction of the tissues of some individuals to substances that, in similar amounts, are harmless to other people. The substances causing **hypersensitivity** (abnormal, adverse reaction) are called **allergens.** Some common allergens are pollen, dust, animal dander (bits of dried skin), drugs, cosmetics, and certain foods. This discussion will be limited to allergic reactions to foods. Food allergens are usually proteins.

Allergies to specific substances are not inherited, but the tendency to develop allergies is inherited. Therefore, although children frequently outgrow their sensitivities, it is wise to delay the introduction of typical food allergens to young children, particularly if their parents suffer from allergies.

Types of Allergic Reactions

Sometimes allergic reactions are immediate and sometimes several hours elapse before symptoms occur. Allergic individuals seem most prone to allergic reactions during periods of stress. Typical symptoms of food allergies include hay fever, **urticaria** (hives), edema, headache, **dermatitis** (inflammation of skin), nausea, dizziness, and asthma (which causes breathing difficulties).

Allergic reactions are uncomfortable, can be detrimental to health and, when breathing difficulties are severe, life threatening.

Allergic reactions to the same food can differ in two individuals. For example, the fact that someone gets hives from eating strawberries does not mean that an allergic reaction to strawberries will appear as hives in another member of

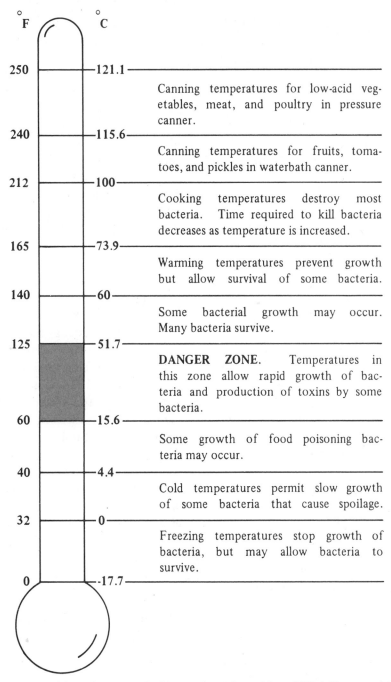

Figure 11-1 Temperatures of food for control of bacteria *(Adapted from USDA Home and Garden Bulletin No. 247, 1990)*

Table 11-2 Appropriate Internal Temperatures to Which Meats Should be Cooked

Fresh Beef	Fahrenheit
Rare	140*
Medium	160
Well Done	170
Ground Beef	160
Fresh Veal	170
Fresh Lamb	
Medium	160
Well Done	170
Fresh Pork	170
Poultry	
Chicken	180
Turkey	180
Boneless	
Turkey Roasts	170
Stuffing	
(Inside or outside the bird)	165
Cured Pork	
Ham, Raw	
(Cook before eating)	160
Ham, Fully cooked	
(Heat before serving)	140

*Rare beef is popular, but cooking it to only 140°F means some food poisoning organisms may survive.
Adapted from USDA Home and Garden Bulletin No. 248, 1990.

the same family. Allergic reactions can even differ from time to time with the same individual.

Treatment of Allergies

The simplest treatment for allergies is to remove the item that causes the allergic reaction. However, because of the variety of allergic reactions, finding the allergen can be difficult.

When food allergies are suspected, it is wise for the patient to keep a food diary for several days and record all food and drink ingested as well as allergic reactions and the time of their onset. Such records can help pinpoint specific allergens. Some common food allergens are listed in Table 11-3. It is common for other foods in the same class as the allergens to cause allergic reactions as well. Cooking sometimes alters the foods and can eliminate allergic reactions in some people.

Skin tests (application of a common allergen to a small area of skin) may be used to detect allergies. Because food allergies are difficult to determine from skin tests, elimination diets often are prescribed to find the food or foods causing the allergic reaction.

Elimination diets are composed of specific foods that are not common allergens. The patient is kept on an elimination diet for one week. If symptoms persist, a more stringent diet is planned, eliminating additional suspect foods. Sometimes, these diets allow only a limited number of foods and can be nutritionally inadequate. If that is the case, vitamin and mineral supplements may be prescribed during the time the diets are used. Examples of four elimination diets, devised by Rowe, are given in Table 11-4.

When and if relief is found from the allergic symptoms, the patient is continued on the diet and, gradually, other foods are added to the diet at a rate of only one every four to seven days. Those foods most likely to produce allergic reactions are added last until an allergic reaction occurs. The allergy can then be pinpointed, and the

Table 11-3 Common Food Allergens

Milk	Chocolate
Wheat	Legumes
Eggs	Strawberries
Citrus fruit	Nuts
Tomatoes	Soybeans
Fish	Pork

Table 11-4 Elimination Diets

Diet 1	Diet 2	Diet 3	Diet 4
Rice	Corn	Tapioca	Milk†
Tapioca	Rye	White potato	Tapioca
Rice biscuit	Corn pone	Breads made of any	Cane sugar
Rice bread	Corn-rye muffins	combination of soy, potato	
	Rye bread	starch, and tapioca flours	
Lettuce	Ry-Krisp		
Chard		Tomato	
Spinach	Beets	Carrot	
Carrot	Squash	Lima beans	
Sweet potato or yam	Asparagus	String beans	
Lamb	Artichoke	Peas	
Lemon	Chicken (no hens)	Beef	
Grapefruit	Bacon	Bacon	
Pears	Pineapple	Lemon	
	Peach	Grapefruit	
Cane sugar	Apricot	Peach	
Sesame oil	Prune	Apricot	
Olive oil*	Cane or beet sugar	Cane sugar	
Salt	Mazola	Sesame oil	
Gelatin, plain or	Sesame oil	Soybean oil	
flavored with lime or	Salt	Gelatin, plain, or flavored	
lemon	Gelatin, plain or	with lime or lemon	
Maple syrup or syrup	flavored with	Salt	
made with cane	pineapple	Maple syrup or syrup made	
sugar flavored with	Karo corn syrup	with cane sugar flavored	
maple	White vinegar	with maple	
Royal baking powder	Royal baking powder	Royal baking powder	
Baking soda	Baking soda	Baking soda	
Cream of tartar	Cream of tartar	Cream of tartar	
Vanilla extract	Vanilla extract	Vanilla extract	
Lemon extract		Lemon extract	

* Allergy to it may occur with or without allergy to olive pollen. Mazola may be used if corn allergy is not present.

† Milk should be taken up to 2 or 3 quarts a day. Plain cottage cheese and cream may be used. Tapioca cooked with milk and milk sugar may be taken.

Source: Rowe, A. H. *Elimination Diets and the Patient's Allergies* ed. 2, Philadelphia: Lee & Febiger, 1944

offending foods eliminated from the diet. Knowing the cause of the allergy enables the patient to lead a healthy, normal life, provided that eliminating these foods does not affect her or his nutrition.

If the elimination of the allergen results in a diet deficient in certain nutrients, suitable substitutes for these nutrients must be found. For example, if a patient is allergic to citrus fruits, other foods rich in vitamin C to which the patient is not allergic must be found. If the allergy is to milk, soybean milk may be substituted.

The patient must be taught the food sources of the nutrient or nutrients lacking so that other foods can be substituted that are nutritionally equal to those causing the allergy. It is essential that the patient be taught to read the labels on commercially prepared foods, and to check the ingredients of restaurant foods carefully. Baked products, mixes, meatloaf, or pancakes may contain egg, milk, or wheat that may be responsible for the allergic reaction.

Sometimes, however, the allergies require such a restriction of foods that the diet does become nutritionally inadequate. As in all cases of allergy, and particularly in such cases, it is hoped that the patient can become **desensitized** (made less sensitive) to the allergens so that a nutritionally balanced diet can be restored. To desensitize the patient, a minute amount of food allergen is given after a period of complete **abstinence** (avoidance) from it. The amount of the allergen is gradually increased until the patient can tolerate it.

CONSIDERATIONS FOR THE HEALTH CARE PROFESSIONAL

Some patients will need simple instructions from the health care professional about avoiding microbial contamination of food supplies at home. Many, if not most, should be warned not to thaw frozen protein foods at room temperature. Others should be reminded that leftover foods should *not* be cooled at room temperature before being refrigerated.

Patients with food allergies will require careful training to avoid their specific allergens. They must be taught to read food labels carefully and to ask the ingredients of foods in restaurants and at friends' homes. Role-playing is an effective way to help such patients.

SUMMARY

Infection or poisoning traced to food is usually caused by human ignorance or carelessness. The serving of safe meals is essentially the responsibility of the cook. Food should not be prepared by anyone who has or carries a contagious disease. All fresh fruits and vegetables should be washed before being eaten. Meats, poultry, fish, eggs, and dairy products should be refrigerated. Pork should always be cooked to the well-done stage. Food should be covered to prevent contamination by dust, insects, or animals. Garbage should also be covered so that it does not attract insects. Hands that prepare foods should be clean and free of cuts or wounds. Kitchen equipment should be spotless. Finally, the food itself should be safe. People should avoid foods containing natural poisons.

Food allergies can cause many different and unpleasant symptoms. To determine their causes, elimination diets are used. Some of the most common food allergens have been found to be milk, chocolate, eggs, tomatoes, fish, citrus fruit, legumes, strawberries, and wheat.

Discussion Topics

1. Name four types of food poisoning. If any class member has suffered from food poisoning, ask the person to describe the symptoms.
2. How may food become contaminated?

3. How can insects contaminate food?
4. How can food be kept free of insect and animal contamination?
5. Why should foods be refrigerated?
6. Discuss appropriate storage of cleaning agents in a home with young children.
7. What are allergies? What may cause them?
8. What are some common allergic reactions to food? How can they be avoided?
9. Do people inherit allergies? Explain.
10. Of what use is a food diary in relation to allergies? What are elimination diets and when are they used?
11. What is the most difficult part of treating food allergies?
12. How may an allergic patient be desensitized?
13. Is an elimination diet always nutritious? Explain.
14. Explain how eggs, wheat, or milk may be hidden in each of the following foods: mayonnaise, bread, rye crackers, potato salad, gravy, meatloaf, breaded veal cutlet, bologna, malted milk.

Suggested Activities

1. Using outside sources, present a committee report on diseases that can be carried in food. Include the agent of transmission, mode of transmission, symptoms, and treatment.
2. Visit a restaurant kitchen. Look for practices that may lead to potential food poisoning. Note the practices and uses of equipment designed to prevent food poisoning.
3. Visit a local supermarket and look for the ingredients wheat, eggs, and milk in frozen prepared meals, baked products, and baking mixes.
4. Find recipes that are suitable for diets in which eggs, wheat, or milk must be eliminated.
5. Plan a luncheon for a patient who is allergic to wheat.
6. Ask a doctor or registered nurse to explain skin tests to the class. Discuss these tests after the lecture.
7. Write the menus of the meals eaten yesterday. Adapt one meal to a wheat-free diet. Adapt another to an egg-free diet. Adapt a third meal to a milk-free diet.
8. Ask someone with food allergies to speak to the class. Follow this talk with questions from the audience.

9.   Adapt the following menu for someone who is allergic to milk.

Cream Soup
Roast Beef
Mashed Potatoes
Buttered Peas
Baker's Bread
Butter
Ice Cream
Black Coffee

Review

A.   Multiple choice. Select the *letter* that precedes the best answer.

1.   A microorganism is a(n)
   a. unit of measurement   c. component of a microscope
   b. tiny animal or plant   d. individual human cell

2.   Salmonella bacteria are destroyed by heating foods to 60°C (140°F) for a minimum of
   a. 2 minutes   c. 30 minutes
   b. 10 minutes   d. 2 hours

3.   Someone who is capable of spreading an infectious organism but is not sick is called a
   a. food handler   c. transport
   b. carrier   d. fomite

4.   When an organism is infectious, it is
   a. disease-causing   c. not contagious
   b. prone to infections   d. always fatal

5.   Most cases of food poisoning in the United States are caused by
   a. careless processing in commercial factories
   b. lack of government inspection
   c. careless handling of food in the kitchen
   d. house pets

6.   Generally, food poisoning symptoms include
   a. joint pain   c. abdominal upset and
   b. constipation   headache
                                   d. none of the above

7.   Salmonella infection and staphylococcal poisoning are caused by
   a. virus   c. protozoa
   b. bacteria   d. worms

8. The deadliest of the bacterial food poisonings is
   a. Staphylococcus
   b. Salmonella
   c. botulism
   d. perfringens poisoning

9. The disease caused by a parasite sometimes found in pork is
   a. tularemia
   b. dysentery
   c. avitaminosis
   d. trichinosis

10. The disease caused by a protozoa and characterized by severe diarrhea is
    a. Salmonella
    b. botulism
    c. dysentery
    d. infectious hepatitis

11. Foods may be contaminated by
    a. people
    b. overcooking them
    c. refrigeration
    d. all of these

12. The temperatures in the danger zone that encourage bacterial growth are between
    a. 0 to 32°F (−18 to 0°C)
    b. 32 to 60°F (0 to 16°C)
    c. 60 to 125°F (16 to 52°C)
    d. 125 to 212°F (52 to 100°C)

13. Leftover foods should be
    a. put in the refrigerator immediately after meals
    b. cooled to room temperature before refrigerating
    c. cooled in the refrigerator for at least an hour before freezing
    d. stored unwrapped in the refrigerator

14. Frozen foods should be
    a. thawed at room temperature
    b. refrozen if not used immediately after thawing
    c. thawed in the refrigerator
    d. any of the above

15. An adverse physical reaction to a food is called a food
    a. refusal
    b. allergy
    c. symptom
    d. allergen

16. Substances that cause altered physical reactions are called
    a. symptoms
    b. allergies
    c. allergens
    d. abstinence

17. One of the typical symptoms of food allergies is
    a. diabetes mellitus
    b. colitis
    c. hives
    d. atherosclerosis

18. The simplest treatment for a food allergy is
    a. a skin test
    b. avoiding all fruit
    c. elimination of the allergen
    d. the use of penicillin

19. In cases of food allergy, an elimination diet may be prescribed to
   a. desensitize the patient   c. avoid surgery
   b. avoid medication   d. find the allergen
20. Some foods that frequently cause an allergic reaction are
   a. milk, eggs, and wheat   c. canned pears and tapioca
   b. lamb, rice, and sugar   d. rice and pears

Case Study 1

Food Allergy

At the age of 35, Carrie T. began to suffer severe and frequent headaches. After seeing several doctors, she was advised that her headaches were common migraine. After much urging, she visited an allergist. Skin tests were made, and she was found to be allergic to several environmental substances, but no food allergies were discovered. The doctor gave her a list of foods (chocolate, tomatoes, oranges, red wine, fish, strawberries), however, to which many people are allergic. She ignored it, saying she did not "believe in" allergies. She had heard too often about her parents' allergies and considered them to be "just a state of mind."

Finally, after an extremely severe and long-lasting headache, she began to wonder if she was wrong about allergies and if there were certain foods to which she was allergic. She considered the foods she had eaten the day before this last headache. She had had orange juice and eggs at breakfast, chocolate cake and milk in the afternoon, and wine and shrimp at dinner. All of these foods were common allergens. Although she remained somewhat skeptical, she did begin to record her diet. The next day she had another slice of chocolate cake. The day after that, she suffered another headache. The next time she suffered a headache, she realized she had had red wine the previous evening. There were as yet no headaches after she had eaten tomatoes, oranges, or fish. However, after a period of family stress during which Carrie had two and three migraines a week, she began to suspect fish, certain ice creams, and some raw fruits, as well as chocolate. When the family situation was resolved and the stress was relieved, the frequency of Carrie's headaches was reduced. Except for chocolate, eating foods she had begun to suspect as allergens did not always result in headache.

Now, since Carrie has learned to cope more comfortably with stressful situations and to avoid known food allergens, the frequency of her headaches has been greatly reduced.

Case Study Questions Based on the Nursing Process

Assess

1. Was it surprising that the allergist did not discover Carrie's food allergies with the skin tests? Explain.
2. Carrie's parents both suffer from allergies that affect their nasal passages. Is it not rather strange that Carrie's allergies were from foods? Explain.
3. Why did the headaches increase in frequency during periods of stress?

Plan

4. Why did Carrie begin to keep a food diary? How can that be useful in a situation such as Carrie's?
5. Carrie discovered that she could not eat raw apples but that she could eat applesauce. Explain.

Implement

6. Later on, Carrie did develop an allergy to oranges. Do you think she would be wise to eat grapefruit instead? Why?
7. Carrie's husband suffers from asthma. Do you think Carrie's daughter may develop allergies? Explain.
8. Carrie is expecting a second child soon. How would you advise her about introducing solid foods to the baby?

Evaluate

9. Carrie has discovered that she cannot eat chocolate, fish, oranges, raw apples, nuts, and coconut. Is she likely to develop nutritional deficiencies because of her allergies? Why?
10. Would you counsel Carrie to read nutritional and ingredient labels on products she purchases? Why?

Case Study 2   *Salmonella*

Arnold and his wife, Flora, were both 75 years old and proud to be living without help. Arnold knew that he was the primary homemaker, but he didn't mind. He enjoyed cooking and loved surprising Flora with an occasional batch of his homemade cookies.

Recently, he mixed a new recipe containing fresh eggs, margarine, and chocolate chips. He refrigerated the dough, intending to bake the cookies the next day. When he was out that afternoon, Flora saw the fresh dough in the refrigerator and ate some of it. It was good, and she ate several spoons full.

Early the next morning, she awoke with a fever and stomach pains so severe that Arnold took her to the hospital. After tests, the doctor told Arnold that Flora had a serious case of salmonella, and asked what she had eaten recently.

Flora was quite ill for a week, but she recovered.

Case Study Questions Based on the Nursing Process

Assess
1. What may have given Flora salmonella?
2. What other symptoms might Flora have experienced?

Plan
3. Do all fresh eggs carry salmonella?

Implement
4. What should Arnold do with the remainder of the cookie dough?
5. Why is it inadvisable to give young children raw cookie dough?

Evaluate
6. What would you tell Arnold and Flora to help prevent the recurrence of the illness?

DIET DURING PREGNANCY AND LACTATION

OBJECTIVES

After studying this chapter, you should be able to
- Identify nutritional needs of adults during pregnancy and lactation
- Describe nutritional needs of pregnant adolescents
- Modify the normal diet to meet the needs of pregnant and lactating women

THE IMPORTANCE OF GOOD NUTRITION DURING PREGNANCY

Good nutrition during pregnancy is essential to both the mother-to-be and the child. In addition to her normal nutritional requirements, the pregnant woman must provide nutrients and kcal for the **fetus** (infant developing in the mother's uterus), **amniotic fluid** (fluid surrounding the fetus in the uterus), the **placenta** (organ in the uterus linking the blood supplies of mother and infant to deliver nutrients and oxygen to and re-

171

move wastes from the infant), and for increased blood volume and breast, uterine, and fat tissue.

The pregnant woman who follows a nutritionally appropriate diet is more apt to feel better, to retain her health, and to bear a healthy infant than one who chooses her foods thoughtlessly.

Studies have shown a relationship between the mother's diet and the health of the baby at birth. It is also thought that the woman who consumed a nutritious diet before pregnancy is more apt to bear a healthy infant than one who did not. Malnutrition of the mother is believed to cause growth **retardation** in the fetus. Low birth weight infants have a higher **mortality** (death) **rate** than those of normal birth weight. Also, a relationship is suspected between maternal nutrition and the subsequent mental development of the child.

WEIGHT GAIN DURING PREGNANCY

Weight gain during pregnancy is natural and necessary so the infant develops normally and the mother retains her health. In addition to the developing infant, the mother's uterus, breasts, placenta, blood volume, body fluids, and fat must all increase to accommodate the infant's needs. (See Table 12-1.)

The average weight gain during pregnancy is 24 to 30 pounds (11 to 14 kg). During the first **trimester** (three-month period) of pregnancy, there is an average weight gain of only two to four pounds. Most of the weight gain occurs during the second and third trimesters of pregnancy, when it averages about one pound per week. This is because there is a substantial increase in maternal tissue during the second trimester, and the fetus grows a great deal during the third trimester.

Table 12-1 Components of Weight Gain During Pregnancy With Approximate Amounts of Gain	
Fetus	7.5 pounds
Placenta	1 pound
Amniotic fluid	2 pounds
Uterus	2 pounds
Breasts	1–3 pounds
Blood volume	4 pounds
Maternal fat	4+ pounds

Weight gain varies, of course. A pregnant **adolescent** who is still growing will gain more weight than a mature woman of the same size. Underweight women should gain more than a woman of average weight. Women of average weight should avoid excessive weight gain and try to stay within the 24 to 30 pound average gain. Obese women can afford to gain less than the average woman, but not less than 15 pounds. No one should lose weight during pregnancy because it could cause nutrient deficiencies for both mother and infant. On average, a pregnant adult requires no additional kcal during the first trimester of pregnancy and only an additional 300 kcal per day during the second and third trimesters. (See Table 12-2.)

NUTRITIONAL NEEDS DURING PREGNANCY

Some of the specific nutrient requirements are increased dramatically during pregnancy, as can be seen in Table 12-3. These figures are recommended for the general U.S. population; the physician may suggest alternative figures based on the patient's nutritional status, age, and activities.

Table 12-2 Median Heights and Weights and Recommended Energy Intake for Pregnant and Lactating Women Compared With Those Who Are Neither Pregnant Nor Lactating

Category	Age (years) or Condition	Weight (kg)	Weight (lb)	Height (cm)	Height (in)	REE (kcal/day)	Multiples of REE	Average Energy Allowance (kcal) Per kg	Average Energy Allowance (kcal) Per day
Females	11–14	46	101	157	62	1,310	1.67	47	2,200
	15–18	55	120	163	64	1,370	1.60	40	2,200
	19–24	58	128	164	65	1,350	1.60	38	2,200
	25–50	63	138	163	64	1,380	1.55	36	2,200
	51+	65	143	160	63	1,280	1.50	30	1,900
Pregnant	1st trimester								+0
	2nd trimester								+300
	3rd trimester								+300
Lactating	1st 6 months								+500
	2nd 6 months								+500

Source: Food and Nutrition Board, National Academy of Sciences—National Research Council, Washington, DC, 1989

The protein requirement is increased by 20 percent for the pregnant woman over 25 and by 25 percent for the pregnant adolescent. Proteins are essential for tissue building, and protein-rich foods are excellent sources of many other essential nutrients, especially iron, copper, zinc, and the B vitamins.

Current research indicates there is no need for increased vitamin A during pregnancy, and the need for vitamin K is increased only for those 24 years and younger. However, the vitamin D requirement is doubled for the pregnant woman 25 and older and the vitamin E requirement is increased by 25 percent.

The requirements for all the water-soluble vitamins are increased during pregnancy. Additional vitamin C is needed for collagen development and for its role as an iron enhancer. The B vitamins are needed in greater amounts because of their roles in metabolism and the development of red blood cells.

The requirements for the minerals calcium, phosphorus, magnesium, iron, zinc, iodine, and selenium are all increased during pregnancy. Calcium is, of course, essential for the development of the infant's bones and teeth as well as for blood clotting and muscle action. The need for iron increases because of the increased blood volume during pregnancy. Additionally, the fetus increases its **hemoglobin** level to 20 to 22 g per 100 ml of blood. This is nearly twice the normal human hemoglobin level of 13 to 14 mg per 100 ml of blood. The infant's hemoglobin level is reduced to normal shortly after birth as the extra hemoglobin breaks down. The resulting iron is stored in the liver and is available when needed during the infant's first few months of life when the diet is essentially milk. Therefore, an iron supplement is commonly prescribed during pregnancy. However, if the pregnant woman's hemoglobin remains at an acceptable level without a supplement, the physician will not prescribe one.

Table 12-3 RDAs During Pregnancy and Lactation

		Weight (kg)	Weight (lb)	Height (cm)	Height (in)	Protein (g)	Fat-Soluble Vitamins Vita-min A (µg RE)	Vita-min D (µg)	Vita-min E (mg α-TE)	Vita-min K (µg)
11–14 years	Not pregnant	46	101	157	62	46	800	10	8	45
	Pregnant					60	800	10	10	65
	Lactating	1st 6 months				65	1,300	10	12	65
		2nd 6 months				62	1,200	10	11	65
15–18 years	Not pregnant	55	120	163	64	44	800	10	8	55
	Pregnant					60	800	10	10	65
	Lactating	1st 6 months				65	1,300	10	12	65
		2nd 6 months				62	1,200	10	11	65
19–24 years	Not pregnant	58	128	164	65	46	800	10	8	60
	Pregnant					60	800	10	10	65
	Lactating	1st 6 months				65	1,300	10	12	65
		2nd 6 months				62	1,200	10	11	65
25 years+	Not pregnant	63	138	163	64	50	800	5	8	65
	Pregnant					60	800	10	10	65
	Lactating	1st 6 months				65	1,300	10	12	65
		2nd 6 months				62	1,200	10	11	65

Source: Food and Nutrition Board, National Academy of Sciences—National Research Council, Washington, DC, 1989

FULFILLMENT OF NUTRITIONAL NEEDS DURING PREGNANCY

To meet the nutritional requirements of pregnancy, the diet should be based on the Food Guide Pyramid. Special care should be taken in the selection of food so that the necessary additional nutrients and not just additional kilocalories are provided (see Table 12-4).

One of the best ways of providing these nutrients is by drinking additional milk each day, or using appropriate substitutes. The extra milk will provide additional protein, calcium, phosphorus, thiamin, riboflavin, and niacin. If **whole milk** is used, it will also contribute saturated fat and cholesterol and provide 175 kcal per eight ounces of milk. **Skim milk** contributes no fat or cholesterol, and provides only 80 kcal per eight-ounce serving.

To be sure that the vitamin requirements of pregnancy are met, **obstetricians** often prescribe a vitamin supplement in addition to an iron supplement. However, it is not advisable for the mother to take any unprescribed nutrient supplement, as an excess of vitamins or minerals can be toxic to mother and infant. Excessive vitamin A, for example, can cause birth defects.

The unusual cravings for certain foods during pregnancy do no harm unless eating them interferes with the normal balanced diet or causes excessive weight gain.

CONCERNS DURING PREGNANCY

Nausea

Sometimes **nausea** (the feeling of a need to vomit) may occur during the first trimester

Table 12-3 (Continued)

Water-Soluble Vitamins							Minerals						
Vitamin C (mg)	Thiamin (mg)	Riboflavin (mg)	Niacin (mg NE)	Vitamin B$_6$ (mg)	Folate (μg)	Vitamin B$_{12}$ (μg)	Calcium (mg)	Phosphorus (mg)	Magnesium (mg)	Iron (mg)	Zinc (mg)	Iodine (μg)	Selenium (μg)
50	1.1	1.3	15	1.4	150	2.0	1,200	1,200	280	15	12	150	45
70	1.5	1.6	17	2.2	400	2.2	1,200	1,200	320	30	15	175	65
95	1.6	1.8	20	2.1	280	2.6	1,200	1,200	355	15	19	200	75
90	1.6	1.7	20	2.1	260	2.6	1,200	1,200	340	15	16	200	75
60	1.1	1.3	15	1.5	180	2.0	1,200	1,200	300	15	12	150	50
70	1.5	1.6	17	2.2	400	2.2	1,200	1,200	320	30	15	175	65
95	1.6	1.8	20	2.1	280	2.6	1,200	1,200	355	15	19	200	75
90	1.6	1.7	20	2.1	260	2.6	1,200	1,200	340	15	16	200	75
60	1.1	1.3	15	1.6	180	2.0	1,200	1,200	280	15	12	150	55
70	1.5	1.6	17	2.2	400	2.2	1,200	1,200	320	30	15	175	65
95	1.6	1.8	20	2.1	280	2.6	1,200	1,200	355	15	19	200	75
90	1.6	1.7	20	2.1	260	2.6	1,200	1,200	340	15	16	200	75
60	1.1	1.3	15	1.6	180	2.0	800	800	280	15	12	150	55
70	1.5	1.6	17	2.2	400	2.2	1,200	1,200	320	30	15	175	65
95	1.6	1.8	20	2.1	280	2.6	1,200	1,200	355	15	19	200	75
90	1.6	1.7	20	2.1	260	2.6	1,200	1,200	340	15	16	200	75

(three-month period) of pregnancy. This type of nausea is commonly known as **morning sickness.** It typically passes as the pregnancy proceeds to the second trimester. Dry crackers or dry toast eaten before rising, eliminating some of the fat in the diet, and avoiding liquids at mealtimes may help to reduce it.

In rare cases, the nausea persists and becomes so severe that it is life threatening. This condition is called **hyperemesis gravidarum.** The mother may be hospitalized and given **parenteral nutrition.** This means the patient is given nutrients via a vein. This is discussed more fully in Chapter 24. Such cases are difficult, and the patients need support and optimism from those who help them.

Excessive Weight Gain

If weight gain becomes excessive, the pregnant woman should reevaluate her diet and eliminate foods (except for the extra pint of milk) that do not fit within the Food Guide Pyramid. Examples of these include candy, cookies, rich desserts, potato chips, salad dressings, and sweet beverages. In addition, she might substitute skim milk for whole milk, which would reduce her kcal intake, but not her intake of proteins, vitamins, and minerals. Except in cases where the woman cannot tolerate lactose (the sugar in milk), it is not advisable to substitute calcium pills for milk because this reduces the protein, vitamin, and mineral content of the diet.

A bowl of clean, crisp, raw vegetables such as broccoli or cauliflower tips, carrots, celery, cucumber, zucchini sticks, and radishes can provide interesting snacks that are nutritious, filling, satisfying, and low in kcal. Fruits and custards made with skim milk make nutritious satisfying desserts that are not high in kcal. Broiling, baking, or boiling foods instead of frying can further reduce the caloric content of the diet.

Table 12-4 Suggested 2400-kcal Menu for Pregnant Women

Breakfast	kcal	Lunch	kcal	Dinner	kcal
½ cup orange juice	50	¾ cup citrus fruit cup	60	¾ cup tomato juice	30
1 egg scrambled with		Roast Beef Sandwich with		3 oz. calves' liver	185
1 tsp. margarine	110	3 oz. beef with lettuce	205	1 small baked potato	100
2 slices rye toast	150	and 1 tbsp. mayonnaise	100	with 1 tbsp. margarine	100
with 1 tbsp peanut butter	100	on 2 slices whole wheat		¾ cup baked squash	60
1 cup skim milk	85	bread	150	with 1 tbsp. margarine	100
Black coffee	0	½ cup vanilla pudding	150	1 cup spinach salad	10
		1 cup skim milk	85	with 2 tbsp oil and	
				vinegar dressing	140
				⅔ cup ice milk	120
				1 cup skim milk	85
	495		**750**		**930**

Snacks: 1 small apple   80
           1 plain, low-fat yogurt   145

Pregnancy-Induced Hypertension

Pregnancy-induced hypertension was formerly called toxemia or **preeclampsia.** It is a condition that sometimes occurs during the third trimester of pregnancy. It is characterized by high blood pressure, the presence of albumin in the urine (**proteinuria**), and edema. The edema causes a somewhat sudden increase in weight. If the condition persists and reaches the **eclamptic** (convulsive) stage, convulsions and coma may occur. The cause of this condition is not known, but it occurs more frequently among pregnant women on inadequate diets (particularly when the diets are inadequate in protein) than among pregnant women on good diets. Sodium is not prohibited, but it should be used in moderation.

Pica

Pica is the **craving** for nonfood substances such as starch or clay (soil). The reasons why people do this are not clear. While both men and women indulge in the practice, it is most common among pregnant women. Some believe it relieves nausea. Others think the practice is based on cultural heritage. It should be discouraged as it can cause blockage of the colon and create nutritional deficiencies. If the soil binds with minerals, the body cannot absorb them. If these substances take the place of nutrient-rich foods in the diet, there can also be multiple nutritional deficiencies. Eating laundry starch in addition to a regular diet will add unwanted calories.

Anemia

Anemia is a condition caused by an insufficiency of red blood cells, hemoglobin, or blood volume. The patient suffering from it does not receive sufficient oxygen from the blood, and consequently feels weak and tired, has a poor appetite, and appears pale. *Iron-deficiency anemia* is its most common form. During pregnancy, the increased volume of blood creates the need for additional iron for the hemoglobin of this blood. When this need is not met by the diet or by the iron stores in the mother's body, iron-deficiency anemia develops. This may be treated with a daily iron supplement.

Folic acid deficiency can result in a form of **megaloblastic anemia** that can occur during pregnancy. It is characterized by too few red blood cells and by large immature red blood cells. The body's requirement for folic acid increases dramatically when new red blood cells are being formed. Consequently, the obstetrician might prescribe a folic acid supplement of 400 mcg per day during pregnancy.

Alcohol, Caffeine, Drugs, and Tobacco

Excessive or regular use of alcohol is associated with subnormal physical and mental development of the fetus. This is called **fetal alcohol syndrome (FAS).** When the mother drinks alcohol, it enters the fetal bloodstream in the same concentration as it does the mother's. Unfortunately, the fetus does not have the capacity to metabolize it as quickly as the mother, so it stays longer in the fetal blood than it does in the maternal blood. The effects of moderate alcohol indulgence are not known so abstinence is recommended.

Caffeine is known to cross the placenta, and heavy caffeine use is associated with complications of pregnancy. Birth defects in newborn rats whose mothers were fed very high doses of caffeine during pregnancy have been observed, but there is no data on humans showing that moderate amounts of caffeine are harmful. As a safety measure, however, it is suggested that pregnant women limit their caffeine intake to two cups of caffeine-containing beverages each day.

Drugs vary in their effects, but self-prescribed drugs, including vitamin and mineral supplements and dangerous illegal drugs, can all damage the fetus. Drugs derived from vitamin A can cause **fetal malformations** (physical abnormalities) and **spontaneous abortions** (naturally caused). Illegal drugs can cause the infant to be born addicted to whatever substance the mother used and, possibly, to be born with acquired immunodeficiency syndrome (AIDS).

Tobacco smoking by pregnant women has for some time been associated with babies of reduced birth weight. The baby's birth weight decreases as the number of cigarettes smoked increases. This is thought to be caused because smoking reduces the oxygen and nutrients carried by the blood.

Obviously, because of the indications of toxicity to the fetus, it is advisable that pregnant women limit, if not avoid, the use of these substances.

DIET FOR THE PREGNANT WOMAN WITH DIABETES

Diabetes mellitus is a group of diseases in which one cannot use or store glucose normally because of inadequate production or use of insulin. This impaired metabolism causes fat and glucose to accumulate in the blood where they cause numerous problems if they are not controlled. (See Chapter 19 for additional information on diabetes mellitus.)

Some women have diabetes mellitus when they become pregnant. Others may develop **gestational diabetes** during pregnancy. In most cases, this latter type disappears after the infant is born. Either type increases the risks of physical or mental defects in the infant, stillbirth, and **macrosomia** (birthweight over 9 pounds) unless blood glucose levels are carefully monitored and maintained within normal limits.

Every pregnant woman should be tested for diabetes. Those found to have the disease must learn to monitor their diets to maintain normal blood glucose levels and avoid both **hypoglycemia** (low blood glucose) and **hyperglycemia** (high blood glucose).

In general, nutrient requirements of the pregnant woman with diabetes are the same as for the normal pregnant woman.

The diet should be planned with a diet counselor, as it will depend on the type of insulin and the time and number of injections. Patients with gestational diabetes and diabetic patients who do not normally require insulin to control their diabetes may require insulin during pregnancy to control blood glucose levels. Between-meal feedings help maintain blood glucose at a steady level. Artificial sweeteners are not recommended.

PREGNANCY DURING ADOLESCENCE

Teenage pregnancy is an increasing concern. The nutritional, physical, psychological, social, and economic demands on a pregnant adolescent are tremendous. With the birth of the infant, they increase. Young women who are themselves still in need of nurturing are suddenly responsible for helpless newborns. Without sufficient help, the total effect on mother, child, and society can be devastating.

Prenatal health care, infant care, possibly psychological, nutritional, and economic counseling, as well as help in locating appropriate housing may all be needed. And at this time, the young woman's family may or may not be supportive.

At such a time, nutritional habits can seem to some as being of slight importance. They are, however, of primary importance. An adolescent's eating habits may not be adequate to fulfill the nutritional needs of her own growing body. When she adds the nutritional burden of a developing fetus, both are put at risk. Adolescents are partic-

ularly vulnerable to **pregnancy-induced hypertension** (PIH) and premature delivery. PIH can cause cardiovascular and kidney problems later. Premature delivery is a leading cause of death among newborns. Inadequate nutrition of the mother is related to both mental and physical birth defects.

These young women will need to know their own nutritional needs and the additional nutritional requirements of pregnancy. (See Table 12-3.) They will need much counseling and emotional support from caring, experienced people before nutritional improvements can be suggested.

LACTATION

Lactation is the period during which the mother nurses the infant. At this time, she must maintain her own health while she produces sufficient milk to nourish the infant.

Kcal Requirements During Lactation

The mother's kcal requirement increases during lactation. The kcal requirement depends on the amount of milk produced. Approximately 85 kcal are required to produce 100 ml ($3\frac{1}{3}$ oz) of milk. During the first six months, average daily milk production is 750 ml (25 oz) and for this the mother requires approximately an extra 640 kcal per day. During the second six months, when the baby begins to eat food in addition to breast milk, average daily milk production slows to 600 ml (20 oz) and the kcal requirement is reduced to approximately 510 extra kcal per day.

As noted in Table 12-2, the Food and Nutrition Board suggests that kcal be increased by 500 per day during lactation. This is less than the actual need because it is assumed that some fat has been stored during pregnancy, which can be used for energy in milk production during lacta-

Breakfast	kcal	Lunch	kcal	Dinner	kcal
Grapefruit half	40	½ cup orange juice	50	½ cantaloupe	50
1 poached egg	80	Creamed chicken*	206	3 oz. beef pot roast	250
2 slices bacon	110	*3 ounces white meat—140		1 medium potato	120
2 slices oatmeal toast	150	⅓ cup white sauce—66		½ cup carrots	35
1 tbsp. peanut butter	100	on 1 slice whole wheat toast	75	½ cup gravy	40
1 cup skim milk	85	1 cup mixed green salad	15	1 medium tomato, sliced	25
1 cup black coffee	0	with 2 tbsp. oil & vinegar	140	1 pumpernickel roll	100
		1 small baked apple	125	with 1 tbsp. margarine	100
		with 1 tbsp. brown sugar	45	⅔ cup baked custard	200
		1 cup skim milk	85	1 cup skim milk	85
	565		741		1,005

Table 12-5 Suggested 2600-kcal Menu for Lactating Women

Snacks: 1 cup tomato juice   40 kcal
1 vanilla milkshake   300

tion. The precise amount depends on the size of the infant and its appetite and the size and activities of the mother. Each ounce of human milk contains 20 kcal.

If the mother takes in an insufficient number of kcal, the quantity of milk will be reduced. Thus, lactation is not a good time to go on a strict weight-loss diet. There will be some natural weight loss caused by the burning of the stored fat for milk production.

Nutrient Requirements During Lactation

In general, most nutrient requirements are increased during lactation. The amounts depend on the age of the mother. (See Table 12-3.) Protein is of particular importance because it is estimated that 10 g of protein are secreted in the milk each day.

The Food Guide Pyramid will be helpful in meal planning for the lactating mother (see Table 12-5). She should be sure to include sufficient fruits and vegetables, especially those rich in vi-

tamin C, and extra milk each day. Cheese, ice cream, custards, and puddings can be substituted for milk. Extra milk will provide many of the additional nutrients and kcal required during lactation. It should be noted that potato chips, sodas, candies, and desserts provide little more than kcal.

Vegetarians will need to be especially careful to be sure they have sufficient kcal, iron, zinc, copper, protein, calcium, and vitamin D. A vitamin B_{12} supplement can be prescribed for them.

It is important that the nursing mother have sufficient fluids to replace those lost in the infant's milk. There is no particular beverage that is better than any other.

The mother should be made aware that she must reduce her caloric intake at the end of the nursing period to avoid adding unwanted weight.

Medicines, Caffeine, Alcohol, and Tobacco

Most chemicals enter the mother's milk so it is essential that the mother check with her obstetrician before using any medicines or nutrient supplements. Caffeine can cause the infant to be irritable. Alcohol in excess, tobacco, and illegal drugs can be very harmful.

CONSIDERATIONS FOR THE HEALTH CARE PROFESSIONAL

Good nutrition during pregnancy can make the difference between a healthy, productive life and one shattered by health and economic problems—for both mother and child.

Most pregnant women will want to know what is the best nutritional information for themselves and their children. They also will be concerned about their weight during and after pregnancy. It is essential that they receive advice from a properly trained health care professional. Articles in newspapers and magazines or in pamphlets from health food stores may or may not be correct and should not be taken at face value unless or until approved by a professional in the dietetic field.

Nutrition is currently a popular topic, and people are inclined to believe what is printed. It can be difficult to persuade people that the information they read is incorrect. As always, the health care professional must use great patience in reeducating those patients who may require it.

The pregnant teenager can present the greatest challenge. Her needs are vast but her experience, and thus her perspective, is limited. Teaching pregnant adolescents about good nutrition may be difficult but, if successful, can help not only that particular patient but her child and her friends.

SUMMARY

A pregnant woman is more likely to remain healthy and bear a healthy infant if she follows a well-balanced diet. Research has shown that maternal nutrition can affect the subsequent mental and physical health of the child. Anemia and PIH during pregnancy are two conditions that can be caused by inadequate nutrition. Both kcal and most nutrient requirements increase for pregnant women (especially adolescents) and women who are breastfeeding. The average weight gain during pregnancy is 24 to 30 pounds.

Discussion Topics

1. Discuss the statement, "A pregnant woman must eat for two."
2. Why is it especially important for a pregnant woman to have a highly nutritious diet?
3. Discuss weight gain during pregnancy from the first month through the ninth. Why is an excessive weight gain during pregnancy undesirable? Is pregnancy a good time to reduce? Explain.
4. Of what value are protein-rich foods during pregnancy?
5. It is common for an iron supplement to be prescribed during pregnancy. Why? What may happen if the mother-to-be does not receive an adequate supply of iron? And how might such a condition affect her baby? Discuss the advisability of the pregnant woman's taking a self-prescribed iron or vitamin supplement in addition to that prescribed by the obstetrician.

6. Discuss why the obstetrician regularly checks the pregnant woman's blood pressure, urine, and weight during her pregnancy.
7. Discuss the effects of lactation on the mother's diet.
8. What is morning sickness and how may it be alleviated? If any class member has been pregnant, ask her questions regarding morning sickness. Can this be a truly serious problem? Explain.
9. Why does the infant store iron?
10. Why is it a good idea for a pregnant woman to include a citrus fruit or melon with every meal?
11. Why is the average weight gain 24 to 30 pounds during pregnancy when the infant weighs approximately $7\frac{1}{2}$ pounds?
12. Why does the need for protein increase so dramatically during pregnancy?
13. Describe *pica*. Why is it undesirable?
14. Discuss the dangers to the fetus if the mother uses drugs.
15. How can the mother's diabetes affect the fetus?

Suggested Activities

1. Using Tables A-1 and A-5 in the Appendix, plan a day's menu for a normal 24-year-old pregnant woman. Adapt it to meet the needs of a pregnant 16-year-old. Adapt both menus to suit women who dislike drinking milk.
2. Adapt the first menu in Activity 1 to meet the needs of a 29-year-old pregnant woman.
3. Using Tables A-1 and A-5 in the Appendix, plan a day's menu for a nursing mother who requires 2700 calories.
4. Using Table A-5 in the Appendix, list the nutrients in one quart (500 ml) of skim milk. Do the same for 1 quart of whole milk.
5. Make a list of different ways of including milk in the diet. Compare notes and recipes with other class members.
6. List the foods that you have eaten in the past 24 hours. Adapt these menus to meet your nutritional requirements if you were pregnant.
7. Ask a physician or a dietician to speak to the class on the importance of adequate nutrition before and during pregnancy. Ask the speaker questions regarding the effects of good or poor nutrition on the health of the mother, prenatal development, infant mortality, and the growth and development of the child. Ask the speaker's opinion regarding the use of alcohol; caffeine; and tobacco during pregnancy. During lactation.
8. Invite a physician to speak to the class on the symptoms and dangers of PIH.
9. Invite a nutrition counselor to speak to the class on the possible problems that can occur during the pregnancy of a diabetic mother.

Review

A. Multiple choice. Select the *letter* that precedes the best answer.
  1. The infant developing in the mother's uterus is called the
      a. sperm   c. placenta
      b. fetus   d. ovary
  2. A common form of anemia is caused by
      a. pica   c. a lack of iron
      b. an excess of vitamin A   d. improper cooking of meat
  3. High blood pressure, edema, and albumin in the urine are symptoms of
      a. nausea   c. pica
      b. anemia   d. pregnancy-induced hypertension
  4. A common name given nausea in early pregnancy is
      a. morning sickness   c. pregnancy-induced hypertension
      b. pica   d. mortality
  5. Folic acid and vitamin B_{12} requirements increase during pregnancy because of their roles in
      a. building strong bones and teeth
      b. fighting infections in the placenta
      c. blood building
      d. enzyme action
  6. The average additional daily energy requirement for the pregnant woman is
      a. 100 calories   c. 500 calories
      b. 300 calories   d. 1000 calories
  7. The additional nutrients required during pregnancy can be met by
      a. eating steak each day
      b. drinking a malted milk each day
      c. using an additional pint of skim milk each day
      d. using an iron supplement
  8. Craving for nonfood substances during pregnancy is known as
      a. anemia   c. nausea
      b. megaloblastic anemia   d. pica
  9. During pregnancy, the average weight gain is
      a. 15 to 24 pounds   c. 11 to 24 kilograms
      b. 24 to 30 pounds   d. 15 to 24 kilograms
 10. The period during which a mother nurses her baby is known as
      a. pregnancy   c. lactation
      b. trimester   d. obstetrics

11. Some appropriate substitutes for milk include
   a. orange juice and tomato juice   c. breads and cereals
   b. cheese and custard   d. vegetables and fruit juices
12. The RDA for additional kcal for a nursing mother is
   a. 100 calories   c. 500 calories
   b. 300 calories   d. 1000 calories
13. The daily diet during pregnancy and lactation should:
   a. be based on the Food Guide Pyramid
   b. include at least two quarts of milk
   c. be limited to 1900 kcal
   d. all of the above
14. Appropriate snacks for pregnant and lactating women include
   a. fruits and raw vegetables   c. sodas
   b. potato chips and pretzels   d. hard candies

B. True or False
   The following usually contain milk or cream:

   1. Eggnog
   2. Chocolate pudding
   3. Meat loaf
   4. Strawberry yogurt
   5. Pineapple cottage cheese
   6. Creamed chicken
   7. Caramel custard
   8. New England clam chowder
   9. Hot cocoa
   10. Quiche Lorraine
   11. Chicken gravy
   12. Banana cream pie
   13. Cream of broccoli soup
   14. Sour cream pie
   15. "Light" coffee
   16. Cheesecake
   17. Chipped beef on toast
   18. Macaroni and cheese
   19. Apple pie a la mode
   20. Grilled cheese sandwich
   21. Vanilla shake
   22. Chocolate malt
   23. Pizza
   24. Tuna melt
   25. Rice pudding

Case Study 1

Pregnancy and Weight Gain

When Marcia learned she was pregnant, she decided that since she was 15 pounds overweight, pregnancy would be a good time to lose the weight and save money on food at the same time. The doctor had told her that most women gain about 24 to 30 pounds during pregnancy. She thought if she didn't gain any weight, she should be about 9 to 15 pounds lighter after the baby was born.

Sticking to her "diet" was easy at first as she felt squeamish about food then but, when she was about four months pregnant, her appetite returned. She fought her appetite, however, and ate little. In the morning she had juice, toast, and coffee. At noon, she had a cup of yogurt and a piece of fruit, and at night, she ate vegetables and lots of popcorn—salted, but without butter. She felt tired nearly all the time, but she thought it was related to her pregnancy. She skipped several appointments with her doctor to save money, but in her 20th week when her face and hands became puffy, she saw the doctor.

After her doctor explained PIH and diet to her, she vowed to follow a good diet during the remainder of her pregnancy and to lose weight after the baby was born.

Case Study Questions Based on the Nursing Process

Assess
1. Why is it unwise to gain no weight during pregnancy?
2. What was Marcia probably suffering from? Why?
3. How was Marcia's diet nutritionally deficient?

Plan
4. If Marcia had not become bloated and visited the doctor, what might have happened to her?
5. What probably caused Marcia's fatigue?

Implement
6. If you were the diet counselor, what would you teach Marcia about her dietary needs and ways to meet them?

Evaluate
7. At her next office visit, what will indicate to the doctor that Marcia is following a good diet?

Case Study 2

Effects of Excessive Alcohol Intake During Pregnancy

Mara was a beautiful, vivacious European who had moved to the United States when she was 21. She had an exciting job in an advertising agency and a delightful group of friends with whom she loved to party. Eventually she married Peter, whom everyone expected would one day head the agency.

She was a wonderful hostess, and she and Peter hosted many parties. Perhaps from entertaining, they developed a habit of a predinner cocktail when they were home alone. This soon grew to two or three or more. Often, they skipped dinner. Sometimes, especially after she became pregnant and was home alone all day, she had one or two drinks before lunch. Peter didn't notice. He, too, was indulging in prelunch cocktails.

Their first child was very small but was normally bright. By the time she was pregnant with their second child, she had been in clinics several times to overcome alcoholism. She felt less lonely and bored when she was drinking. Their second child was very small, had wide set eyes—unlike theirs—and was mentally slow.

Following the birth of their second child, Mara stopped drinking. Peter did not, and they eventually divorced.

Case Study Questions Based on the Nursing Process

Assess
1. Is it likely that Mara would have been better off during her pregnancy if she had continued to work? Why?
2. Is this an unusual story? Explain.
3. From what did the second child suffer? Is it likely that the child can overcome this problem? Why?

Plan
4. What may have finally caused Mara to stop drinking?
5. In addition to the excessive alcohol, what else may possibly contribute to the reduced physical and mental development of children born to women who abuse alcohol?

Implement
6. During Mara's second pregnancy, what would the doctor probably have noticed that would have alerted him or her to Mara's alcoholism?
7. What could have been done to help Mara stop drinking during her second pregnancy?

Evaluate
8. If Mara becomes pregnant a third time and does not drink during the pregnancy, is it likely that this child will have FAS?

Diet During Infancy

OBJECTIVES

After studying this chapter, you should be able to
• State the effect inadequate nutrition has on an infant
• Identify the ingredients used in infant formulas
• Describe when and how foods are introduced into the baby's diet
• Describe inborn errors of metabolism and their dietary treatment

Food and its presentation are extremely important during the baby's first year. Physical and mental development are dependent on the food itself, and **psychosocial development** is affected by the time and manner in which the food is offered.

Infants react to their parents' emotions. If food is forced on a child, or withheld until the child is uncomfortable, or if the food is presented in a tense manner, the child reacts with tension and unhappiness. If the parent is relaxed, the infant's mealtime can be a pleasure for both parent and child, figure 13-1.

Although babies have been fed according to prescribed time schedules in the past, it is preferable to feed infants **on demand** (when they are hungry). Feeding on demand prevents the frustrations that hunger can bring, and helps the child develop trust in people. The newborn may require more frequent feedings, but normally the

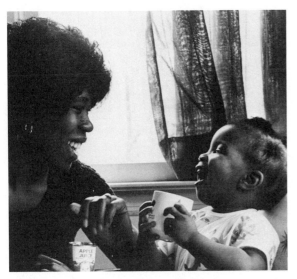

Figure 13-1 Food is better accepted and digested in a happy and relaxed atmosphere.

demand schedule averages approximately every four hours by the time the baby is two or three months old.

NUTRITIONAL REQUIREMENTS OF THE INFANT

The first year of life is a period of the most rapid growth in one's life. A baby doubles its birth weight by six months of age and triples it within the first year. This explains why the infant's energy, vitamin, mineral, and protein requirements are higher per unit of body weight than those of older children or adults. It is important to remember, however, that growth rates vary from child to child. Nutritional needs will depend largely on a child's growth rate.

During this first year, the normal child needs about 100 kcal per kilogram of body weight each day. This is approximately two to three times the adult requirement. Low birth weight infants and infants who have suffered from malnutrition or illness require more than the normal number of kcal per kilogram of body weight. The nutritional status of infants is reflected by many of the same characteristics as those of adults. (See Table 1-2.)

The basis of the infant's diet is milk. It is a highly nutritious, digestible food containing proteins, fats, carbohydrates, vitamins, minerals, and water.

It is recommended that infants up to six months of age have 2.2 g of protein per kilogram of weight each day and from six to twelve months, 1.56 g of protein per kilogram of weight each day. This is satisfactorily supplied by human milk or by infant formulas, figure 13-2.

Infants have more water per pound of body weight than do adults. Thus, they usually need 1.5 ml of water per kcal ingested. This is the same ratio of water to kcal as is found in human milk and in most infant formulas.

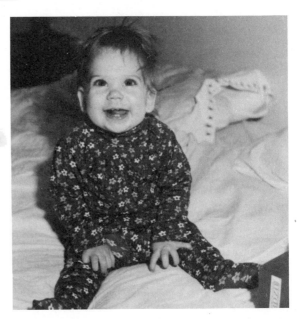

Figure 13-2 A happy, healthy, well-fed six-month-old child.

Table 13-1 Recommended Dietary Requirements for Infants from Birth to One Year of Age

Category	Age (years) or Condition	Weight (kg)	Weight (lb)	Height (cm)	Height (in)	Protein (g)	Fat-Soluble Vitamins Vita-min A (µg RE)	Vita-min D (µg)	Vita-min E (mg α-TE)	Vita-min K (µg)	Water-Soluble Vitamins Vita-min C (mg)	Thia-min (mg)	Ribo-flavin (mg)	Niacin (mg NE)	Vita-min B₆ (mg)	Fo-late (µg)	Vita-min B₁₂ (µg)	Minerals Cal-cium (mg)	Phos-phorus (mg)	Mag-nesium (mg)	Iron (mg)	Zinc (mg)	Iodine (µg)	Sele-nium (µg)
Infants	0.0–0.5	6	13	60	24	13	375	7.5	3	5	30	0.3	0.4	5	0.3	25	0.3	400	300	40	6	5	40	10
	0.5–1.0	9	20	71	28	14	375	10	4	10	35	0.4	0.5	6	0.6	35	0.5	600	500	60	10	5	50	15

Source: Food and Nutrition Board, National Academy of Sciences—National Research Council Recommended Dietary Allowance, Revised 1989

Vitamins and minerals are, of course, essential. (See Table 13-1 for the recommended amounts.)

Milk is, however, a poor source of iron, vitamin C, and usually, vitamin D. An infant is born with a three- to six-month supply of iron. At that age, the pediatrician usually prescribes an iron supplement. Human milk usually does supply the infant with sufficient vitamin C. Babies fed formula that has not had vitamin C added will need supplementary vitamin C. This is usually prescribed within the first ten days of life. Infant formulas contain sufficient vitamin D, but for infants who are nursed and who do not have exposure to sunlight on a regular basis, the pediatrician can prescribe a vitamin D supplement.

Care must be taken that infants do not receive excessive amounts of either vitamin A or D because both can be toxic in excessive amounts. Vitamin A can damage the liver and cause bone abnormalities, and vitamin D can damage the cardiovascular system and kidneys. In addition, some pediatricians prescribe fluoride for breast-fed babies or for formula-fed babies living in areas where the water contains little fluoride.

BREASTFEEDING

While babies will thrive whether nursed or formula fed, there is little doubt that breastfeeding provides advantages that formulas cannot match. Breastfeeding is nature's way of providing a good diet for the baby. It is, in fact, used as the guide by which nutritional requirements of infants are measured.

Mother's milk provides the infant with temporary **immunity** (resistance) to many infectious diseases. It is economical, nutritionally adequate, sanitary, and saves time otherwise spent in shopping for or preparing formula. It is **sterile** (free from microorganisms), easy to digest, and usually does not cause gastrointestinal disturbances or allergic reactions. Breastfed infants grow more rapidly during the first few months of life than formula-fed babies. And because breast milk contains less protein and minerals than cow's milk, it reduces the load on the infant's kidneys.

From the mother's perspective at least, the **bonding** (emotional attachment) that occurs during breastfeeding is unmatched. In addition, breastfeeding helps the mother's uterus return to normal size after delivery.

Breastfeeding had been on the decline for many years, but a growing number of mothers are now nursing their babies. Generally, they tend to be among the better educated. Trends that begin in this group of people are often adopted subsequently by others. If the mother works and cannot be available for every feeding, breast milk can be expressed earlier, refrigerated, and used at the appropriate time or a bottle of formula can be substituted.

BOTTLE FEEDING

Despite the foregoing, some mothers choose to bottle feed their babies. Certain women are unable to produce enough breast milk. Some lack emotional support from their families and some simply find it foreign to their culture. Others who are employed or involved in many activities outside the home find bottle feeding more convenient. Either way is acceptable provided the infant is given love and attention during the feeding. The infant should be cuddled and kept comfortable and warm during the feeding. During and after the feeding, the infant should be **bubbled** (burped) to release gas in the stomach, just as the breast-fed infant should be bubbled,

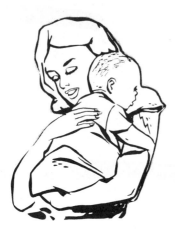

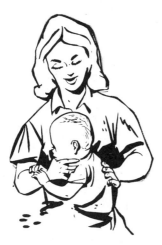

Figure 13-3 To bubble (burp) a baby, hold him or her in one of the two positions shown and gently stroke his or her back.

figure 13-3. Bubbling helps prevent **regurgitation** (spitting up food).

If the baby is bottle-fed, parents receive instructions for feeding from the **pediatrician** (baby and children's doctor). One of the convenient, prepared products may be prescribed. There are many ready-to-use formulas available in disposable bottles and cans. Some of these preparations require the addition of water, but many are complete and ready to serve. Most have vitamins and iron added. The cost of milk formula is directly related to convenience—the most convenient is the most expensive. If parents are more concerned with economy than convenience, the pediatrician can prescribe a homemade formula.

Normally, cow's milk is used in formulas because it is most abundant and easily modified to resemble human milk. It is modified because it has more protein and mineral salts and less milk sugar (lactose) than human milk. Water and sugar are usually added to dilute these nutrients. When an infant is extremely sensitive or allergic to cow's milk, **a synthetic** (manufactured) milk may be given. Synthetic milk is commonly made from soybeans. Goat's milk is sometimes used as a substitute for cow's milk in situations where the baby is allergic to cow's milk, or the baby may be breast fed.

If the infant is given a formula prepared at home, it is essential that it be carefully and accurately prepared. Typically, it is made from water, evaporated cow's milk, and sugar. The pediatrician prescribes a formula that suits the needs of the baby, and adjusts it as the child grows.

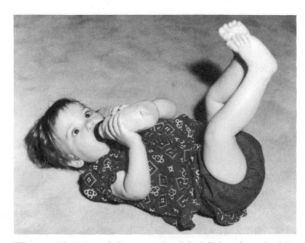

Figure 13-4 An eight-month-old child enjoys holding her bottle.

FOOD Pyramid begins @ 12 mo.

Formula may be given cold, at room temperature, or warmed, but it should be given at the same temperature consistently, figure 13-4. To warm the formula for feeding, bottles should be placed in a saucepan of warm water or a bottlewarmer. The bottles should be shaken occasionally to warm contents evenly. Warming the bottle in the microwave is not advisable because milk can heat unevenly and burn the infant's mouth. The temperature of the milk can be tested by shaking a few drops on one's wrist. The milk should feel lukewarm.

SUPPLEMENTARY FOODS

The age at which infants are introduced to **beikost** (solid and semisolid food) has varied considerably over the years. At the beginning of this century, doctors advocated that children be fed only milk during their first twelve months. By the 1950s, in response to parental demand, some pediatricians advised the introduction of solid food before the age of one month. Now, the general recommendation is that the infant's diet be limited to milk until the age of four to six months, and that milk remain the major food source until the child is one year old. With the appropriate supplements of iron and vitamin D, and possibly vitamin C and fluoride, milk does normally fulfill the nutritional requirements of most children until they reach the age of six months.

The introduction of solid food before the age of four to six months is thought to increase the likelihood of overfeeding and perhaps cause an obesity problem throughout the child's life. Also, the early introduction of solid food may increase the possibility of food allergies, particularly in children whose parents suffer from allergies.

By the age of six months, however, mother's milk or formula alone cannot supply sufficient energy to the growing child. Solid foods are introduced at this stage. These must be introduced gradually and individually. One food is introduced and then no other new food for four or five days. If there is no allergic reaction, another food can be introduced, a waiting period allowed, then another, and so on. The typical order of introduction begins with cereal, usually rice, then wheat, oat, and mixed cereals. Cooked or pureed fruits follow, then cooked or pureed vegetables, egg yolk, and finally, finely ground meats. Between 6 and 12 months, toast, zwieback, teething biscuits, custards, puddings, and ice cream can be added.

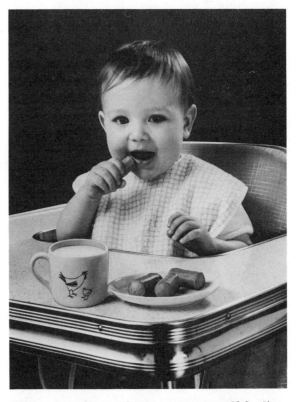

Figure 13-5 Finger foods encourage self-feeding. This baby is enjoying meat sticks specially manufactured for toddlers. *(Courtesy of Gerber Products Company)*

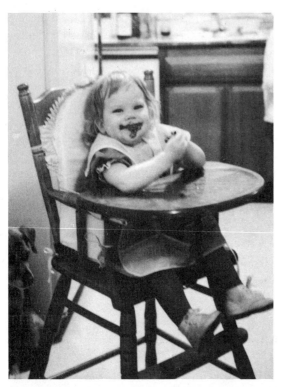

Figure 13-6 Finger foods can be messy but fun.

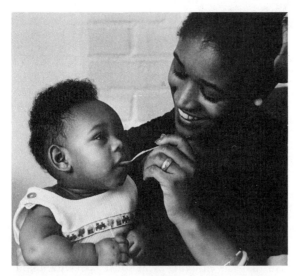

Figure 13-7 Weaning an infant from the bottle actually begins when food is given with a spoon.

By the age of one year, most babies are eating foods from all of the Food Guide Pyramid's groups and may have most any food that is easily chewed and digested, figures 13-5 and 13-6. However, precautions must be taken to avoid offering foods on which the child can choke. Examples include nuts, potato chips, whole peas, grapes, popcorn, small candies, and small pieces of tough meat or raw vegetables. Foods should be selected according to the advice of the pediatrician. It is not necessary to use the commercially prepared "junior" foods. Table foods generally can be used.

The Food Guide Pyramid provides excellent help in determining the baby's menu. Its use will help supply the appropriate nutrients and develop good eating habits. It is particularly important at this time to avoid excess sugar and salt in the infant's diet so the child does not develop a taste for them and, consequently, overuse them throughout life.

Weaning (teaching the infant to drink from a cup instead of the breast or bottle) actually begins when the infant is first given food from a spoon, figure 13-7. It progresses as the child shows an interest in, and ability to drink from a cup. The child will ultimately discard the bottle. If the child shows great reluctance to discard the bottle, the pediatrician's advice should be sought.

It is not advisable for the infant to be given a bottle as a pacifier at bedtime. This increases the difficulty of weaning and, if it contains milk, allows the lactose in the milk to be in contact with the teeth for a long time. This can cause dental caries that in certain cases can be so extreme that the child can lose the upper front baby teeth. This is termed *nursing bottle syndrome*.

METABOLIC DISORDERS

Some infants are born with metabolic disabilities. These congenital disabilities prevent the normal metabolism of specific nutrients. They are called **inborn errors of metabolism.** They are caused by **mutations** (changes) in the genes. There is great variation in the seriousness of the conditions caused by these defects. Some cause death at an early age, and some can be minimized so that life can be supported by adjustments in the normal diet. Among children born with these defects, there is, however, the common danger of damage to the central nervous system because of their abnormal body chemistry. This results in mental retardation and sometimes retarded growth. Early diagnosis of these inborn errors combined with diet therapy increases the chances of preventing retardation. Hospitals test newborns for some of these disorders as a matter of course. Where there is a family history of a certain genetic disorder, genetic screening can be done. In addition, some of these abnormalities can be discovered by **amniocentesis** (testing of the baby in utero).

Galactosemia

Galactosemia is a condition in which there is a lack of the liver enzyme, **transferase.** Transferase normally converts galactose to glucose. Galactose is the simple sugar resulting from the digestion of lactose, the sugar found in milk (see Chapter 3). When transferase is missing, and the infant ingests anything containing galactose, the amount of galactose in the blood becomes so excessive that it is toxic. When this happens to a newborn, she or he suffers diarrhea, vomiting, edema, and the child's liver does not function normally. Cataracts may develop, **galactosuria** (galactose in the urine) occurs, and mental retardation ensues.

Diet Therapy

Diet therapy for galactosemia is the exclusion of anything containing milk from any mam-

mal. During infancy, the treatment is relatively simple because parents can feed the baby lactose-free, commercially-prepared formula and provide supplemental minerals and vitamins. As the child grows, and moves on to adult foods, parents must be extremely careful to avoid any food, beverage, or medicine that contains lactose. Nutritional supplements of calcium, vitamin D, and riboflavin must be given so that the diet is nutritionally adequate. This restricted diet may be necessary throughout life, but some physicians allow a somewhat liberalized diet as the child reaches school age. This may mean only small amounts of baked or processed foods that contain small amounts of milk. Even this must be accompanied by careful and regular monitoring for galactosuria.

Phenylketonuria (PKU)

In **phenylketonuria,** infants lack the liver enzyme, **phenylalanine hydroxylase,** which is necessary for the metabolism of the amino acid, **phenylalanine.** Infants seem to be normal at birth, but if the disease is not treated, most of them become hyperactive, suffer seizures between 6 and 18 months, and become mentally retarded. Most hospitals today test newborns for phenylketonuria. PKU babies typically have light-colored skin and hair.

Diet Therapy

There is a special, nutritionally-adequate, commercial infant formula available for PKU babies. It is called **Lofenalac.** It has had 95 percent of phenylalanine removed from its protein source. This provides just enough phenylalanine for basic needs, but no excess. The specific amount depends on the infant's size and growth rate. Regular blood tests determine the adequacy of the amounts. Diets are carefully monitored for kcal and nutrient intake, and adjusted frequently as needs change. Except for fats and sugars, there is some protein in all foods. Some of that protein is phenylalanine, so diets for the growing child eating normal food must be carefully planned. There are two varieties of synthetic milk available for older children. They are *Phenyl-free* and *PKU-1, -2,* or *-3*. None of these contains any phenylalanine. They can be used as beverages or in puddings and baked products. Diets should be monitored throughout life to avoid mental retardation.

Maple Syrup Urine Disease (MSUD)

Maple syrup urine disease (MSUD) is a congenital defect resulting in the inability to metabolize three amino acids—**leucine, isoleucine,** and **valine.** It is named for the odor of the urine of these patients. When the infant ingests food protein, there are increased blood levels of these amino acids. Hypoglycemia, apathy, and convulsions occur very early. If the disease is not treated promptly, the child will die.

Diet Therapy

The diet must provide sufficient kcal and nutrients, but with extremely restricted amounts of leucine, isoleucine, and valine. A special formula and low-protein foods are used. Diet therapy appears to be necessary throughout life.

CONSIDERATIONS FOR THE HEALTH CARE PROFESSIONAL

Although the physical and mental development of infants depend on the nutrients and kcal they receive, their psychosocial development depends on *how and when* these nutrients and kcal are provided. Some new parents will have a solid knowledge of the nutrition information needed but lack a real understanding of the importance of how and when food should be presented to infants. They may hold the infant during feedings but focus instead on the television or newspaper.

Other parents may know instinctively how important cuddling and attention are to an infant, but they lack accurate knowledge of infant nutrition.

Parents from both "groups" are apt to have opinions based on their parents' knowledge that may or may not be correct.

The health care professional will help these parents most if she or he listens carefully to them. Then, if a *two-way discussion* follows, the parents are more inclined to listen to the advice and suggestions of the health care professional.

SUMMARY

It is particularly important that babies have adequate diets so their physical and mental development is not impaired. Breastfeeding is nature's way of feeding an infant, although formula feeding is quite acceptable. Cow's milk is usually used in formulas because it is most available and is easily modified to resemble human milk. To modify milk, sugar and water are typically added to evaporated milk. The young child's diet is supplemented on the advice of the pediatrician. Added foods should be based on the Food Guide Pyramid.

Inborn errors of metabolism cause various problems, ranging from mental retardation to death, if not properly treated. In these conditions, diet therapy is the primary tool in maintaining the patient's health.

Discussion Topics

1. Do any of the students know a woman who has breast-fed her baby? What were her reactions to the experience?
2. Why is breastfeeding not always possible?
3. Why are some babies not allowed cow's milk? What kind of milk can these children have?
4. Discuss the possible effects of regularly propping the baby's bottle instead of holding the baby during feeding.
5. Why is a rigid time schedule for feeding a baby not advisable?
6. How may weaning be accomplished?
7. What is meant by inborn errors of metabolism? What causes them? How may they affect people?
8. What is galactosemia? How is it acquired? How does it affect the body? Is it serious? How is it treated?
9. Discuss PKU. Include its cause, symptoms, effects, and treatment.
10. Discuss MSUD. Include its cause, reason for its name, symptoms, treatment, and prognosis if it is not treated.

Suggested Activities

1. Have a panel discussion on the advantages and disadvantages of breastfeeding. Invite infant nurses, doctors, and parents as panelists.
2. Observe a demonstration of the actual feeding and bubbling of a baby.
3. Visit a store that carries prepared infant formulas and compare their prices.
4. Organize a panel discussion on metabolic disorders. Assign individual students to individual disorders. Use outside sources.
5. Role-play a situation where the doctor must explain PKU to the parents of a PKU baby. Include cause, symptoms, effects, treatment, and prognosis.
6. Invite a physician to give a talk on inborn errors of metabolism.

Review

A. Complete the following statements.
  1. The mother's milk gives the infant temporary _immun._ to certain diseases.
  2. An infant _does_ (does, does not) react to the emotions of the person feeding her or him.
  3. The doctor who decides what kind of formula to give the baby is the _pediatrician_ .
  4. Cow's milk has more _prot._ and _min salt_ than human milk.
  5. Cow's milk has less _lactose (sugar)_ than human milk.
  6. Usually, the first solid food added to the infant's milk diet is a _____ .

cereal (p. 19)

7. Because milk contains little vitamin _____ , the formula should be supplemented early.
8. When an infant is allergic to cow's milk, _____ may be substituted.
9. Inadequate nutrition during infancy may impair the infant's _____ and _____ development.
10. Phenylketonuria is a congenital condition preventing normal _____ .
11. In galactosemia, the body lacks the enzyme _____ .
12. If untreated, inborn errors of metabolism may cause _____ or _____ .
13. Currently, solid foods are generally not recommended to be given a baby before the age of _____ .
14. Solid foods introduced at an early age are thought to increase the tendency to _____ and _____ in later years.
15. By the age of six months, babies need additional amounts of the mineral _____ .

B. Match the items in column I to the correct statement in column II.

	Column I		Column II
d	1. milk	a.	baby doctor
c	2. supplement	b.	teaching the baby to drink from a cup instead of a nipple
i	3. immunity		
f	4. regurgitation	c.	addition
e	5. bubbling	d.	basis of the infant's diet
a	6. pediatrician	e.	burping
g	7. synthetic	f.	spitting up of food
	8. obstetrician	g.	man-made
h	9. PKU	h.	disease caused by inborn error of metabolism
b	10. weaning	i.	protection from disease
		j.	doctor who delivers the baby

C. Briefly answer the following questions.
1. Why should the mother give her baby special attention during feedings?

2. How is a bottle warmed? Is this always necessary? Explain. Why is a microwave oven not recommended?

3. Why is it not advisable to give an 8-month old child peanuts?

Case Study 1

A PKU Baby

Norma and her husband had looked forward for many years to the time when they would have what they planned as their only child. Norma wanted to nurse her baby, and to stay home and care for it herself. When little Jenny was born, she looked like a dream—beautiful, blond, and fair skinned. She seemed perfect so they were as stunned as they were heartbroken when the doctor told them shortly after the birth that Jenny was a "PKU baby."

Case Study Questions Based on the Nursing Process

Assess
1. What is a "PKU baby?"
2. What did the doctor probably tell them?
3. Will the child's condition allow Norma to nurse her? Why?

Plan
4. What might your reaction be if you were one of Jenny's parents?
5. What will happen to Jenny if she isn't given proper dietary treatment?
6. Will this diet therapy be easy when Jenny is an infant? Why?

Implement
7. At approximately what age will correct diet therapy become difficult for Jenny as well as her parents?
8. If you were Jenny's parent, how might you explain her condition to her? At what age?
9. If you were the diet counselor, what would you teach Norma and her husband about Jenny's dietary needs and how they could fulfill them?

Evaluate
10. Is it necessary for Jenny's parents to read nutritional and ingredient labels for the foods they feed Jenny? Why?
11. If you were Jenny's parents, how and what would you cook for her as she gets older so that she would feel as if she were eating "just like the other kids" in the lunchroom at school?
12. Why will Jenny need to follow a special diet during her entire lifetime?

Case Study 2

Breastfeeding versus Bottle-Feeding

Marion was a busy and successful assistant to a corporate executive. Nevertheless, she decided to take a three-month maternity leave after the birth of Claudia. She nursed the child for a month, but by that time her office was sending her a great deal of paperwork that also needed her attention. She found nursing took too much time and, in consultation with her pediatrician, gradually went from nursing to bottle feeding Claudia. By propping the infant's bottle, Marion could complete more work than if she had been holding the infant. The baby drank the formula and remained healthy but cried more than she had done previously. When Marion returned to work—one month earlier than originally intended—she left the baby with a wonderful older baby nurse named Dolly who had taken care of ten babies during her career. Claudia cried much less after Dolly arrived.

Case Study Questions Based on the Nursing Process

Assess
1. Was nursing the baby for only one month useful? Explain.
2. Is the baby likely to be physically deprived by the change from breast to bottle? Explain.

Plan
3. Why might the pediatrician change the baby's vitamin prescription to exclude vitamin D after she begins receiving formula instead of her mother's milk?

Implement
4. What is one possible reason why this baby cried more when she was fed by bottle than when she was nursed?

Evaluate
5. What might Dolly have done that caused Claudia to cry less?
6. Might both Marion and Claudia have been happier if Dolly had been with them from the time of Claudia's birth? Explain.

CHAPTER 14

DIET DURING CHILDHOOD AND ADOLESCENCE

OBJECTIVES

After studying this chapter, you should be able to
- Identify nutritional needs of children aged 1 to 12 and of adolescents
- State the effects of inadequate nutrition during the growing years
- Describe eating disorders that can occur during adolescence
- Evaluate the nutritive value of the fast-food products available in the U.S. today

CHILDREN AGED ONE TO TWELVE

Although specific nutritional requirements change as children grow, nutrition always affects physical, mental, and emotional growth and development. Studies indicate that the mental ability and size of an individual are directly influenced by diet during the early years. Children who have an inadequate supply of nutrients—especially protein—and calories during their early years may be shorter and less intellectually able than children who receive an adequate diet.

Eating habits develop during childhood. Once developed, poor eating habits will be difficult to change. They can exacerbate emotional and physical problems such as irritability, **depression, anxiety,** fatigue, and illness.

Because children learn partly by imitation, learning good eating habits is easier if the parents have good habits and are calm and relaxed about the child's. Nutritious foods should be available at snack time as well as at mealtime, figure 14-1, and meals should include a wide variety of foods to ensure good nutrient intake.

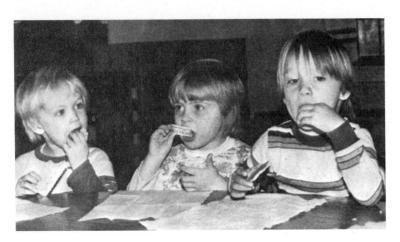

Figure 14-1 Snacks are enjoyed with friends in the playroom. *(From Lesner,* Pediatric Nursing, *Copyright 1983 by Delmar Publishers Inc.)*

Parents should be aware that it is not uncommon for children's appetites to vary. The rate of growth is not constant. As the child ages, the rate of growth actually slows. In addition, children's attention is increasingly focused on their environment rather than their stomachs. Consequently, their appetites and interest in food commonly decrease during the early years. Children between the ages of one and three undergo vast changes. Their legs grow longer; they develop muscles; they lose their baby shape; they begin to walk and talk; and they learn to feed, and generally assert themselves. A two-year-old child's statement "No!" is his or her way of saying: "Let me decide!"

As children continue to grow and develop, they will increasingly and healthfully assert themselves. They want and need to show their growing independence. Parents should respect this need as much as possible. Children's likes and dislikes may change. New foods should be introduced gradually, in small amounts, and as attractively as possible. Allowing the child to assist in marketing and in the preparation of a new food are often good ways of arousing interest in the food and a desire to eat it. Children often prefer foods in small pieces that are simply prepared.

They are wary of foods covered by sauce or gravy. Mealtime should be pleasant, and food should not be forced on the child. When a child is hungry, he or she will eat. Forcing a child to eat can result in life-long weight problems including overweight, **anorexia nervosa,** or **bulimia.** (See pages 203–205 for discussion of these problems.)

Kcal and Nutrient Requirements of Young Children

The *rate* of growth diminishes from the age of one until about ten. This causes a reduction in the kcal requirement per pound of body weight during this period. For example, at six months, a girl needs about 54 kcal per pound of body weight, but by the age of ten, she will require only 35 kcal per pound of body weight (see Table 14-1).

This is not true for nutrient needs, however. From the age of six months to ten years, nutrient needs actually *increase* because of the increase in body size. (See Table 14-2.) Therefore, it is especially important that young children are given nutritious foods *that they will eat.*

Table 14-1 Median Heights and Weights and Recommended Energy Intake

Category	Age (years) or Condition	Weight (kg)	Weight (lb)	Height (cm)	Height (in)	REE (kcal/day)	Multiples of REE	Average Energy Allowance (kcal) Per kg	Average Energy Allowance (kcal) Per day
Infants	0.0–0.5	6	13	60	24	320		108	650
	0.5–1.0	9	20	71	28	500		98	850
Children	1–3	13	29	90	35	740		102	1,300
	4–6	20	44	112	44	950		90	1,800
	7–10	28	62	132	52	1,130		70	2,000
Males	11–14	45	99	157	62	1,440	1.70	55	2,500
	15–18	66	145	176	69	1,760	1.67	45	3,000
Females	11–14	46	101	157	62	1,310	1.67	47	2,200
	15–18	55	120	163	64	1,370	1.60	40	2,200

Source: Food and Nutrition Board, National Academy of Sciences—National Research Council, 1989

The Food Guide Pyramid is a good foundation for developing meal plans that, with possible adjustments, will suit all family members. A variety of foods should be offered and, when possible, the child should be offered some choices of foods. Such a choice at the table helps the child's psychosocial development.

Generally, the young child will need two to three cups of milk each day, or the equivalent in terms of calcium. However, excessive use of milk should be avoided because it can crowd out other, iron-rich foods and possibly cause iron-deficiency anemia. The number of servings of the other food groups is the same as for adults, but the sizes will be smaller. The use of sweets should be minimized as the child is apt to prefer them to nutrient-rich foods.

ADOLESCENCE

Adolescence is a period of rapid growth that causes major changes. It tends to begin between the ages of 10 and 13 in girls, and between 13 and 16 in boys. The growth rate may be three inches a year for girls, and four inches for boys. Bones grow and gain density, muscle and fat tissue develop, and blood volume increases. Sexual maturity occurs. Boys' voices change, girls experience the onset of menses, and both may experience **acne** (pimples).

These changes are obvious and have a tremendous affect on an adolescent's psychosocial development. No two individuals will develop in the same way. One girl may become heavier than she might like; another may be thin; a boy may not develop the muscle or the height he desires; some may develop serious complexion problems. It can be a time of great joy, but also can be a time when counseling is needed.

Adolescent Food Habits

Adolescents typically have enormous appetites. When good eating habits have been established during childhood and there is nutritious food available, the teenager's food habits should present no serious problem.

Table 14-2 Recommended Dietary Allowances

Category or Condition	Age (years)	Weight (kg)	Weight (lb)	Height (cm)	Height (in)	Protein (g)	Vitamin A (µg RE)	Vitamin D (µg)	Vitamin E (mg α-TE)	Vitamin K (µg)	Vitamin C (mg)	Thiamin (mg)	Riboflavin (mg)	Niacin (mg NE)	Vitamin B6 (mg)	Folate (µg)	Vitamin B12 (µg)	Calcium (mg)	Phosphorus (mg)	Magnesium (mg)	Iron (mg)	Zinc (mg)	Iodine (µg)	Selenium (µg)
Infants	0.0–0.5	6	13	60	24	13	375	7.5	3	5	30	0.3	0.4	5	0.3	25	0.3	400	300	40	6	5	40	10
	0.5–1.0	9	20	71	28	14	375	10	4	10	35	0.4	0.5	6	0.6	35	0.5	600	500	60	10	5	50	15
Children	1–3	13	29	90	35	16	400	10	6	15	40	0.7	0.8	9	1.0	50	0.7	800	800	80	10	10	70	20
	4–6	20	44	112	44	24	500	10	7	20	45	0.9	1.1	12	1.1	75	1.0	800	800	120	10	10	90	20
	7–10	28	62	132	52	28	700	10	7	30	45	1.0	1.2	13	1.4	100	1.4	800	800	170	10	10	120	30
Males	11–14	45	99	157	62	45	1,000	10	10	45	50	1.3	1.5	17	1.7	150	2.0	1,200	1,200	270	12	15	150	40
	15–18	66	145	176	69	59	1,000	10	10	65	60	1.5	1.8	20	2.0	200	2.0	1,200	1,200	400	12	15	150	50
Females	11–14	46	101	157	62	46	800	10	8	45	50	1.1	1.3	15	1.4	150	2.0	1,200	1,200	280	15	12	150	45
	15–18	55	120	163	64	44	800	10	8	55	60	1.1	1.3	15	1.5	180	2.0	1,200	1,200	300	15	12	150	50

Source: Food and Nutrition Board, National Academy of Sciences—National Research Council, 1989

Adolescents are imitators, like children, but instead of imitating adults, adolescents prefer to imitate their **peers** (people one's own age) and do what is popular. Unfortunately, the foods that are popular are often empty calorie foods such as potato chips, sodas, and candy. These foods provide mainly carbohydrates and fats, and very few proteins, vitamins, and minerals, except for salt, which is usually provided in excess.

When the adolescent's food habits need improvement, it is wise for the adult to tactfully inform her or him of nutritional needs and of the inferiority of the empty calorie foods. The adolescent has a natural desire for independence and may resent being told what to do.

Before attempting to change an adolescent's food habits, her or his food choices should be carefully checked for nutrient content. It is too easily assumed that because the adolescent chooses the food, the food is automatically a poor choice in regard to nutrient content. This is not always the case. If the adolescent has a problem maintaining an appropriate weight, she or he may need some advice regarding diet.

Kcal and Nutrient Needs of Adolescents

Because of their rapid growth, adolescents' kcal requirements naturally increase. Boys' kcal requirements tend to be greater than girls' because boys are generally bigger in stature, tend to be more physically active, and have more muscle tissue than do girls.

Except for vitamin D, nutrient needs increase dramatically at the onset of adolescence. (See Table 14-2.) Because of menstruation, girls have a greater need for iron than do boys. The RDAs for vitamin D, vitamin C, vitamin B_{12}, calcium, phosphorus, and iodine are the same for both sexes. The RDAs for the remaining nutrients are higher for boys than they are for girls.

♀ ↑ Fe due to menses

ADOLESCENT PROBLEMS RELATING TO NUTRITION

Adolescence is a stressful time for most young people. They are unexpectedly faced with numerous physical changes; an innate need for independence; increased work and extra curricular demands at school; in many cases, jobs; and social and sexual pressures from their peers. For many teens, such stress can cause one or more of the following problems.

Anorexia Nervosa

Generally, adolescent boys in the United States are considered well nourished. This is not always the case with girls who, studies show, are sometimes found to have diets deficient in kilocalories and protein, iron, calcium, vitamin A, or some of the B vitamins.

These deficiencies can be due to poor eating habits caused by concern about weight. A moderate concern about weight is understandable, and possibly even beneficial, provided it does not cause diets to be deficient in essential nutrients or lead to a potentially fatal condition called **anorexia nervosa.**

Anorexia nervosa, commonly called *anorexia,* is a psychological disorder more common to women than men. It begins during the teen years or the early twenties. It causes the patient to drastically reduce the kcal intake so that the reduction disrupts metabolism, and causes hair loss, low blood pressure, weakness, **amenorrhea** (stoppage of monthly menstrual flow), brain damage, and even death.

The causes of anorexia are unclear. Someone with this disorder (an anorexic) has an inordinate fear of being fat. Some anorexics have been overweight and have irrational fears of regaining lost weight. Some young women with demanding parents perceive this as their only means of control. Some may want to resemble slim fashion models. Some fear growing up. Many are perfectionistic overachievers who want to control their bodies. It pleases them to deny themselves food when they are hungry.

These young women usually set a maximum weight for themselves and become expert at "counting calories" to maintain their chosen weight. If the weight declines too far, the anorexic will ultimately die.

Treatment requires

1. development of a strong and trusting relationship between the patient and the health care professionals involved in the case;
2. that the patient learn and accept that weight gain and a change in body contours are normal during adolescence;
3. diet therapy so the patient will understand the need for both nutrients and kcal and how best to obtain them;
4. individual and family counseling so the problem is understood by everyone;
5. close supervision by the health care professional;
6. time and patience from all involved.

Bulimia

Bulimia is a syndrome in which the patient alternately binges and purges by inducing vomiting and using laxatives and diuretics to get rid of ingested food. Bulimics are said to fear that they cannot stop eating. They tend to be high achievers who are perfectionistic, obsessive, and depressed. They generally lack a strong sense of self and have a need to seem special. They know their binge/purge syndrome is abnormal but also fear being overweight. This condition is more common among women than men and can begin any time from the late teens into the thirties.

A bulimic usually binges on high kcal foods such as cookies, ice cream, pastries, and other "forbidden" foods. The binge can take only a few moments or run several hours—until there is no space for more food. This occurs when the person is alone. Bulimia can follow a period of excessive dieting, and stress usually increases the frequency of binges.

Bulimia is not usually life threatening compared with anorexia, but it can cause an upset in electrolytes, irritate the esophagus, and cause malnutrition and dehydration.

Treatment usually includes limiting eating to mealtimes and close supervision after meals to prevent self-induced vomiting. Diet therapy helps teach the patient basic nutritional facts so he or she will be more inclined to treat the body with respect. Psychological counseling will help the patient to understand her fears about food. Group therapy also can be helpful.

Both bulimia and anorexia can be problems that will have to be confronted throughout the patient's life.

Overweight

Overweight during adolescence is particularly unfortunate because it is apt to diminish the individual's **self-esteem** and, consequently, can exclude her or him from the normal social life of the teen years. This further diminishes self-esteem. Also, it tends to make the individual prone to overweight as an adult.

Although numerous studies have been done, the cause of overweight is difficult to determine. Heredity is believed to play a role. Just as one inherits height, color of hair, or artistic talents, it appears that one also inherits the tendency (or lack of it) to overweight. Overfeeding during infancy and childhood also can be a contributing factor. Then, once overweight, the overweight itself contributes further to the problem.

For example, if a teenager becomes the center of his classmates' jokes, he or she may prefer to spend time alone, perhaps watching television, and finding comfort in food. This adds more kcal, reduces activity, and, thus, worsens the condition.

The problem of overweight during adolescence is especially difficult to solve until the individual involved makes the independent decision to lose weight. After making such a decision, the teenager should see a physician to ensure that his or her health is good, to work out the amount of weight that should be lost, the time required for such a loss, and the daily kcal that is advisable.

After a physician's examination, the individual will be helped by discussing the plan with a trained diet counselor. Meals should be planned carefully to include the necessary nutrients but avoid exceeding the kcal allotment. Generally, a plan developed using the Food Guide Pyramid is the easiest for the dieting teen to understand and follow. It's essential that the nutrient and kcal content of fast foods be understood by the teen and that these foods plus other snacks can be built into the weight loss plan. Exercise should also be included in any overweight adolescent's weight loss plan. This helps burn calories and may also inspire the young person to meet new people and to try new activities, such as dancing, baseball, or gymnastics.

Fast Foods

Many Americans have become extremely fond of the **"fast foods"** that are so readily available. Many others are highly critical of their nutrient content. Examples of these foods—most of which are favorites of teenagers—include hamburgers, cheeseburgers, milkshakes, franks, pizza, sodas, hot chocolate, tacos, chili, fried chicken, and onion rings. Because of the criticism they have received, some fast food companies have run tests to determine the nutritional content of their products. These results are usually available in the fast food restaurants.

Generally speaking, fast foods are excessively high in fat and sodium, as well as kcal, and contain only limited amounts of vitamins and minerals (other than sodium), and little fiber. In Table 14-3, the nutrient contents of some varieties of fast foods are shown compared with the RDA for a 16-year-old girl. This shows the potential for problems with a diet that regularly consists of these foods to the exclusion of others.

Nevertheless, these foods are more nutritious than sodas, cakes, and candy. When used with discretion in a balanced diet, they are not harmful.

Alcohol and the Adolescent

In a process called **fermentation,** sugars and starches can be changed to alcohol. Enzyme action causes this change. Alcohol is typically made from fruit, corn, rye, barley, rice, or potatoes. It provides 7 kcal per gram but almost no nutrients.

Alcohol is a drug that can have serious side effects. Initially, it causes the drinker to feel "happy" because it lowers inhibitions. This affects the drinker's judgment and can lead to accidents and crime. Ultimately, alcohol is a depressant as continued drinking leads to sleepiness, loss of consciousness, and, when too much is consumed in a short period, death.

Abuse (overuse) of alcohol is called **alcoholism.** Alcoholism can destroy lives and families and devastate the drinker's nutritional status and thus health. It affects absorption and normal metabolism of glucose, fats, proteins, and vitamins. When thiamin and niacin cannot be absorbed, the cells cannot use glucose for energy. Brain cells, which depend on glucose for energy,

Table 14-3 Some Nutrient and Kcal Contents of Specified Fast Foods Compared With RDA for 16-Year-Old Female

	Wt	kcal	Protein	Fat	Calcium	Iron	Sodium	Vitamin A	Thiamin	Riboflavin	Niacin	Vitamin C
Hamburger	3½ oz	250	12 g	11 g	56 mg	2.2 mg	463 mg	14 RE	0.23 mg	0.24 mg	3.8 mg	1 mg
French Fries	2 oz	160	2 g	8 g	10 mg	0.4 mg	108 mg	0	0.09 mg	0.01 mg	1.6 mg	5 mg
Chocolate Milk Shake	10 oz	335	9 g	8 g	374 mg	0.9 mg	314 mg	59 RE	0.13 mg	0.63 mg	0.4 mg	0
Pizza	4 oz	300	15 g	9 g	220 mg	1.6 mg	700 mg	106 RE	0.34 mg	0.29 mg	4.2 mg	2 mg
Soda	12 oz	160	0	0	11 mg	0.2 mg	18 mg	0	0	0	0	0
Doughnut	2 oz	210	3 g	12 g	22 mg	1.0 mg	192 mg	5 RE	0.12 mg	0.12 mg	1.1 mg	0
Potato Chips	2 oz	315	3 g	21 g	15 mg	0.6 mg	300 mg	0	0.09 mg	0	2.4 mg	24 mg
Chocolate Bar & Peanuts	1½ oz	225	6 g	16 g	75 mg	0.6 mg	30 mg	12 RE	1.0 mg	1.0 mg	2.1 mg	0
RDAs for 16-year-old girl		2,200	44 g	73 g	1200 mg	15 mg	500 mg	800 RE	1.1 mg	1.3 mg	15 mg	60 mg

are particularly affected. Fat may accumulate in the liver, which, if the alcohol abuse continues, can lead to **cirrhosis** of the liver (hardening caused by excessive formation of connective tissue). Alcohol causes the kidneys to excrete larger than normal amounts of water, resulting in an increased loss of minerals. In a poor nutritional state, the body is less able to fight off disease.

Additionally, excessive, long-term drinking can cause high blood pressure and damage the heart muscle. It is associated with cancer of the throat and the esophagus, and can damage the reproductive system.

The risks to the drinker are obvious. When a pregnant or lactating woman drinks, however, she puts the fetus or the nursing infant at risk as well. Alcohol can lower birth weight and cause fetal alcohol syndrome. (See Chapter 12.)

Unfortunately, many teenagers ignore the dangers of alcohol and use it in an effort to appear adult. In addition to the damage to their own health and the accidents and the random acts of violence caused by their drinking, their behavior inspires younger children to emulate them. The health professional is in a good position to spread the message that alcohol is a drug and can cause severe economic and family problems, as well as addiction, disease, and death.

Dental Caries

Dental caries (decayed areas on the outer surface of the teeth) are promoted by the use of sugar in the diet. Sugar aids the development of certain harmful bacteria in the mouth that produce acids that can erode tooth enamel.

To prevent dental caries, sticky sugar foods should be avoided unless the teeth can be brushed or the mouth can be rinsed immediately after eating them.

When fluoride is added to the drinking water, the number of dental caries is reduced. Fluoridated tooth paste also is believed to be helpful. Fluoride is a normal component of bones and teeth but must not be used in excessive amounts, as it can be toxic and affect bone and soft tissues.

Nutrition for the Athlete

Good nutrition during the period of life when one is involved in athletics can prevent unnecessary wear and tear on the body as well as maintain the athlete in top physical form. The specific nutritional needs of the athlete are not numerous, but they are important. The athlete needs additional water, kcal, thiamin, riboflavin, niacin, sodium, potassium, iron, and protein.

The body uses water to rid itself of excess heat through perspiration. This lost water must be regularly replaced during the activity to pre-

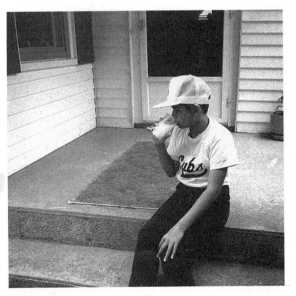

Figure 14-2 All athletes must take time out to rest and replace lost fluids.

vent dehydration, figure 14-2. Plain water is the recommended liquid because the commercial "athletes'" or "electrolyte" drinks contain more sugar, salt, and potassium than is advisable. If these commercial beverages are used, they must be diluted with twice as much water as drink. Salt tablets are not recommended because despite the loss of salt and potassium through perspiration, the loss is not equal to the amount contained in the tablets. If there is an insufficient water intake, these salt tablets can increase the risk of dehydration.

The increase in kcal depends on the activity and the length of time it is performed. The requirement could be double the normal, up to 6,000 kcal per day. Because glucose and fatty acids are used for energy, and not protein, the normal diet proportions of 50 to 55 percent carbohydrate, 30 percent fat, and 10 to 15 percent protein are advised.

There is an increased need for B vitamins because they are necessary for energy metabolism. They are provided in the breads, cereals, fruits, and vegetables needed to bring the kcal count to the total required. Some extra protein is used during training when muscle mass and blood volume are increasing. This amount is included in the RDA for age and is provided in the normal diet. Protein needs are not increased by physical activity. In fact, excess protein can cause increased urine production, which can lead to dehydration.

The minerals sodium and potassium are needed in larger amounts because of loss through perspiration. This amount of sodium can usually be replaced just by salting food to taste, and orange juice can provide the extra potassium.

A sufficient supply of iron is important to the athlete, particularly to the female athlete. Iron-rich foods eaten with vitamin C-rich foods should provide sufficient iron. The onset of menstruation can be delayed by the heavy physical activity of the young female athlete and amenorrhea may occur in those already menstruating.

When weight is a concern of the athlete, such as with wrestlers, care should be taken that the individual does not become dehydrated by refusing liquids in an effort to "make weight" for the class.

When weight must be added, the athlete will need an additional 2500 kcal to develop one pound of muscle mass. The additional foods eaten to reach this amount of kcal should contain the normal proportion of nutrients. A high-fat diet should be avoided because it increases the potential for heart disease. Athletes should reduce kcal intake when training ends. Unused muscles will be converted to fat.

In general, the athlete should select foods using the Food Guide Pyramid. The pregame meal should be eaten three hours before the event, and should consist primarily of carbohydrates, and small amounts of protein and fat. Concentrated sugar foods are not advisable because they may cause extra water to collect in the intestines, creating gas and possibly diarrhea.

Glycogen loading (carboloading) is sometimes used for long activities. This means that muscle stores of glycogen are increased. To accomplish this, the athlete begins six days before the event. For three days the athlete eats a diet consisting of only 10 percent carbohydrate and mostly protein and fat as she or he performs heavy exercise. This depletes the current store of glycogen. The last three days, the diet is 70 percent carbohydrate and the exercise is very light so that the muscles become loaded with glycogen. However, this may cause an abnormal heartbeat and some weight gain. Currently, it is recommended that the athlete exercise heavily and eat carbohydrates as desired. Then, during the week before the competition, exercise should be reduced. On the day before competition, the athlete should eat a high-carbohydrate diet and rest.

After the event, the athlete may prefer to drink fruit juices until relaxed, and then fulfill the appetite with sandwiches or a full meal.

There are no magic potions or diet supplements that will increase an athlete's prowess as may be touted by health food faddists. *Steroid* drugs should not be used to build muscles. They can affect the fat content of the blood, damage the liver, change the reproductive system and even the facial appearance. Good diet, good health habits, and practice combined with innate talent remain the essentials for athletic success.

CONSIDERATIONS FOR THE HEALTH CARE PROFESSIONAL

The health care professional who works with young children will be challenged by the poor eating appetites of her or his patients. Compounding this problem will be the anxiety of the patients' parents. They will be understandably concerned about both their children's appetites and physical conditions. The health care professional can be most helpful to all concerned by exhibiting patience and understanding and by listening to parents and patient.

The problems of adolescent patients, perhaps particularly those with eating disorders, can be especially vexing. For example, telling an anorexic patient to eat could be counterproductive. Health care professionals working with such patients should consult with the patient's psychological counselor.

SUMMARY

Children's nutritional needs vary as they grow and develop. The rate of growth slows between the ages of one and ten, and the child's kcal requirement per pound of body weight slows accordingly. However, nutrient needs gradually increase during these years. During adolescence, growth is rapid, and nutritional and kcal requirements increase substantially. Anorexia nervosa, bulimia, and obesity are problems of weight control that can occur during adolescence. Fast foods are acceptable when used with discretion in a balanced diet. Alcohol can be a serious problem for adolescents, and it is essential that adolescents understand its potential dangers. The nutritional needs of athletes are similar to those of non-athletes except for increased needs for kcal, B vitamins, sodium, potassium, and iron.

Discussion Topics

1. Discuss how parents' anxieties about children's food habits may affect those habits.
2. Discuss the manner in which depression may affect food habits.
3. In what ways does overweight affect an adolescent's self-esteem?
4. Discuss ways of arousing a six-year-old's interest in new foods.
5. Why does an 11-year-old girl require more calcium and vitamin D than her 60-year-old grandmother?
6. Why can it be especially difficult for a parent to influence her or his adolescent's attitudes about food?

7. Discuss the nutrient content of some fast foods. Explain why they can be useful additions to the diet, and also why they should not be used exclusively.

8. What could result if a 30-year-old lawyer continued to eat as he did as a 17-year-old football player?

9. Describe anorexia nervosa. Ask if anyone in the class has suffered from it or knows anyone who has. Ask that individual for descriptions of the patient's attitude, physical condition, possible causes, and case results (if any).

10. Discuss how snack foods can affect one's overall nutrition. Why should they be included in an adolescent's weight-loss plan?

11. Discuss the pros and cons of glycogen loading.

12. What are dental caries? What causes them and how might they be avoided?

Suggested Activities

1. List your favorite snack foods. List nutritious snack foods. Check kcal values of these foods (see Table A-5 in the Appendix) and compare lists for nutrition and taste. Discuss possible improvements in your list of favorite snacks.

2. Role-play a situation where an overweight, patient has been told by her physician that she must lose 25 pounds. Try to convince her to change her food habits. (Remember to consider types of foods as well as amounts, meal hours, and reasons she is overeating.)

3. Plan a talk for fourth grade students on the importance of good food habits. Begin with an outline and develop it into a narrative that nine-year-old children will understand. If possible, ask permission of a fourth-grade teacher to deliver this talk to the class.

4. Role-play a situation where your younger sister, who is considerably overweight, has just asked you how she can lose weight. Ask her why she wants to lose weight; how much weight she wants to lose; how long she is willing to be on a reducing diet; what her favorite foods are; when she eats; the amounts she eats; where she eats; and with whom she eats.

5. Invite a nutritionist to talk to the class on any or all of the following: glycogen loading; fast foods; anorexia nervosa; bulimia; overweight in adolescence.

6. Invite a psychiatrist who specializes in adolescent eating disorders to speak to the class.

7. Hold a panel discussion on alcohol. Assign the following topics to individual class members. They should prepare themselves by doing outside research prior to the panel discussion on:
    What is alcohol?

Why do people use alcohol?

How does alcohol affect the human body?

How can alcohol abuse affect one's nutritional status?

What are the dangers of drinking during pregnancy?

8. Role play a situation where a 15-year-old girl is being coerced by 17-year-old friends at a party to accept an alcoholic drink.

Review

A. Multiple choice. Select the *letter* that precedes the best answer.

1. Anorexia nervosa
   a. is characterized by binges and purges
   b. causes severe acne
   c. is a psychological disorder
   d. typically causes overweight

2. A child's eating habits
   a. can reflect his or her desire to assert self
   b. seldom change after the child reaches the age of one year
   c. usually improve when parents force the child to try new foods
   d. have no relation to the child's growth rate

3. Children's appetites
   a. vary
   b. are static
   c. are irrelevant to their nutritional status
   d. are entirely dependent on the size of the child

4. Of the following foods, children are most apt to prefer
   a. carrot-zucchini casserole   c. raw carrot sticks
   b. creamed carrots with peas   d. carrot and pineapple gelatin
                                          salad

5. Young children's and adults' nutritional requirements are the same for
   a. protein   c. calcium
   b. vitamin D   d. kcal

6. Children's iron requirement is high because it is needed for
   a. healthy bones and teeth   c. prevention of nightblindness
   b. fighting infections   d. blood building

7. As a child grows, his or her kcal requirement per pound of body weight
   a. remains unchanged   c. becomes less
   b. increases   d. doubles each year

8. Meatloaf is a good source of
   a. protein
   b. vitamin C
   c. calcium
   d. all of the above and more

9. Empty calorie foods provide
   a. carbohydrate and fat
   b. proteins, minerals, and vitamins
   c. no calories
   d. fiber

10. Although adolescent boys usually need more kcal than girls, girls usually need more
    a. protein
    b. vitamin C
    c. iron
    d. vitamin D

B. Completion

1. A psychological disorder that causes people to drastically reduce their kcal intake is called _____ .

2. An overweight adolescent who has decided to reduce should plan meals based on _____ .

3. A real criticism of fast foods is their high _____ , _____ , and _____ content, and low _____ , _____ , and _____ content.

4. Allowing a very young child an unlimited amount of milk can crowd out other nutritious foods and possibly cause _____ .

5. Eating habits usually develop during _____ .

6. As children grow, their rate of growth _____ .

7. Excessive amounts of vitamins and minerals can be _____ .

8. The eating disorder in which the patient alternately binges and purges is _____ .

9. The cessation of menstruation is called _____ and can be caused by _____ .

10. The first step in a substantial weight-loss program should be to see a _____ .

C.   Answer the following questions as they relate to this menu.

Breakfast	*Lunch*	*Dinner*
Orange Juice	Macaroni & Cheese	Meat Loaf
Cereal & Milk	Green Beans	Baked Potato
Toast	Bread	Shredded Lettuce
Butter or Margarine	Butter or Margarine	with Tomatoes
Milk	Pineapple Chunks	and Dressing
Coffee	Milk	Roll
		Butter or Margarine
		Custard
		Milk

FAT

Morning Snack
Crackers & Cheese
Apple Juice

Afternoon Snack
Banana

1.   Vitamin C is considered an iron enhancer and should be eaten at each meal. Where is the vitamin C in this menu?

2.   Protein should be included in every meal. Where is the protein in this menu?

3.   List seven sources of iron in this menu.

4.   List the sources of milk in this menu and estimate the approximate amounts included.

Case Study 1

Anorexia Nervosa

Eleanor had noticed recently that her 15-year-old daughter, Millie, was increasingly pale and thin, had one cold after another, and never seemed to have time for snacks after school. In addition, she was always late for meals. When she was at the table, she seemed to "stir" the food on her plate and not eat it. Millie was "always" studying and "always" tired. The family lived only five blocks from the high school. Millie and her brother Joe normally walked to school. When Joe told his mother that Millie was riding the bus to and from school because she felt so weak, Eleanor insisted Millie visit the doctor.

Millie's doctor diagnosed a "mild" case of anorexia nervosa. The doctor explained briefly the dangers of this condition, blamed Millie's frequent colds on it, and discussed food vaguely. In addition, the doctor asked Eleanor if she would prepare milkshakes for Millie once or twice a day, and asked Millie to stop in on Friday afternoons for a while. The doctor subsequently called Eleanor and advised that the situation be treated with deliberate calm and that Millie's favorite foods be casually made available. The Friday visits would be short. They would be devoted largely to talk about school and college as Millie's weight was being checked. The plan worked. Within two months, Millie was looking and feeling better.

Case Study Questions Based on the Nursing Process

Assess
1. Was it wise to advise Millie that she had anorexia nervosa? Why?
2. Should the doctor have been more specific about the dangers of anorexia? Why?

Plan
3. Why did the doctor advise milkshakes "once or twice a day"?
4. Why should favorite foods be "casually" made available? Why not directly offered?

Implement
5. What might have happened to Millie if her mother had not brought her to the doctor? If the doctor had not handled the situation carefully?

Evaluate
6. Is long-term follow-up care advisable for Millie?
7. As time progresses, how might the doctor approach and teach Millie about her need for nutrients and kcal?

Case Study 2   *Bulimia*

Florie was an attractive 17-year-old girl with beautiful, shiny hair. She was 5'7" tall and weighed 135 pounds. She was upset after she and her boyfriend broke up and thought it had happened because she was "too fat." One day on a city bus she overheard a slim and attractive young woman tell her friend that she regularly forced herself to vomit after eating a large dinner. She said it helped her control her weight.

Florie decided this would be her secret way to slimness—that might bring back her boyfriend. She began this new "routine" that evening. Soon, she was using unneeded laxatives and occasionally "borrowing" her grandmother's diuretics. When she was especially hungry, she'd buy two boxes of her favorite cookies and a pint of ice cream and eat them in one hour. Then she'd force herself to vomit.

Within two months, her weight dropped to 110 pounds. She had thought she would be happy about this, but she felt so tired that she didn't care. She noticed, too, that her hair seemed limp and had lost its sheen.

Her mother noticed her weight loss and was concerned. One night she caught Florie gagging herself. They talked; Florie confessed; they cried. They discussed psychological and diet counseling and Florie agreed to try both.

Case Study Questions Based on the Nursing Process

Assess
1. In reviewing the 1983 Metropolitan Height and Weight Table A-2 in the Appendix, would you agree that Florie was overweight before she became bulimic? Explain.
2. Why was Florie tired?
3. What questions might the psychotherapist ask Florie?

Plan
4. What advice might the diet counselor offer Florie?
5. If therapy doesn't help Florie, what problems relating to bulimia can she face in the future?

Implement
6. What might you have said and done if you were Florie's mother?
7. What advice would you offer a friend who admits to being bulimic?

Evaluate
8. If you were Florie's mother, what evidence would you look for to indicate that Florie was getting better?
9. Is it possible that Florie can be cured of bulimia?

DIET DURING YOUNG AND MIDDLE ADULTHOOD

OBJECTIVES

After studying this chapter, you should be able to
- Identify the nutritional needs of young adults and the middle-aged
- Explain sensible, long-range weight control for these people
- Adapt menus to meet their nutritional and kcal requirements

Adulthood can be broadly divided into three periods: young, middle, and late adulthood. The first two periods will be discussed in this chapter. Late adulthood is discussed in Chapter 16.

Young adulthood is a time of excitement and exploration. The age range runs from about 18 to 35 or 40 years of age. Individuals are alive with plans, desires, and energy as they begin searching for and finding their places in the mainstream of adult life. They appear to have boundless energy for both social and professional activities. They are usually interested in exercise for its own sake, and often participate in athletic events as well.

The middle period ranges from about 40 to 65 years of age. This is a time when the physical activities of young adulthood typically begin to decrease, resulting in a lowered kcal requirement for most individuals. During these years, people seldom have young children to supervise, and the strenuous physical labor of some occupations may be delegated to younger people. Middle-aged people may tire more easily than they did when they were younger. Therefore, they may not get as much exercise as they did in earlier years. Because appetite and food intake may not decrease, there is a common tendency toward weight gain during this period.

NUTRIENT REQUIREMENTS

Growth is usually complete by the age of 25. Consequently, except during pregnancy and lactation, the essential nutrients are needed only to maintain and repair body tissue and to produce energy. During these years, the **nutrient requirements** of healthy adults change very little. (See Table 15-1.)

Despite men's generally larger size, only 11 of the given RDAs are greater for men than for women. Six of the RDAs are the same for both sexes. The iron requirement for women remains higher than that for men throughout the childbearing years. Extra iron is needed to replace blood cells lost during menstruation and to help build both the infant's and the extra maternal blood needed during pregnancy. After menopause, this requirement for women matches that of men.

Protein needs for adults are thought to be 0.75 grams per kilogram of body weight. To determine the specific amount, one must divide the weight in pounds by 2.2 to obtain the weight in kilograms and then multiply the weight in kilograms by 0.75.

The current RDA of calcium for adults is 800 mg, and for vitamin D, 200 IU. Both calcium and vitamin D are essential for strong bones, and both are found in milk. Bone loss begins at about the age of 35 to 40 and can lead to osteoporosis later. Therefore, it is wise for young people, especially women who are more prone to osteoporosis than men, to consume foods that provide more than the RDAs of these two nutrients. Two

glasses of milk a day provide the RDA for each of these nutrients. Increasing this amount could prevent osteoporosis later. Skim milk or foods made from skim milk should be used to limit the amount of fat consumed. (See Chapter 4.)

KCAL REQUIREMENTS

The **kcal requirement** begins to diminish after the age of 25, as basal metabolism rates (REE) are reduced by approximately 2 to 3 percent a decade. This is a small amount per year, but, after 25 years, a person will gain weight if the total **kcal intake** is not reduced accordingly. An individual's actual need, of course, will be determined primarily by activity and amount of **lean body mass** (muscle tissue). Those who are more active will require more kcal than those who are sedentary. Those with a high proportion of muscle tissue will require more kcal than those with a high proportion of fat tissue. (See also Chapter 18 on weight control.)

NUTRITION-RELATED CONCERNS

Eating Habits

It is especially important to maintain good eating habits during young and middle adulthood. Women, who may be concerned about weight, cost of food, or time, can easily develop nutritional deficiencies. For example, a woman who settles for a piece of pie at lunchtime while her husband eats a hamburger and salad is being very foolish. If she continues to eat like this, she will jeopardize her health.

A hamburger can have 250 to 400 kcal. The salad will contain less than 50 kcal without dressing, and the dressing could be limited to one tablespoon, or approximately 100 kcal, for a total

Table 15-1 Nutrient Requirements for Adults

Category or Condition	Age (years)	Weight (kg)	Weight (lb)	Height (cm)	Height (in)	Protein (g)	Fat-Soluble Vitamins				Water-Soluble Vitamins							Minerals						
							Vitamin A (µg RE)	Vitamin D (µg)	Vitamin E (mg α-TE)	Vitamin K (µg)	Vitamin C (mg)	Thiamin (mg)	Riboflavin (mg)	Niacin (mg NE)	Vitamin B$_6$ (mg)	Folate (µg)	Vitamin B$_{12}$ (µg)	Calcium (mg)	Phosphorus (mg)	Magnesium (mg)	Iron (mg)	Zinc (mg)	Iodine (µg)	Selenium (µg)
Males	15–18	66	145	176	69	59	1,000	10	10	65	60	1.5	1.8	20	2.0	200	2.0	1,200	1,200	400	12	15	150	50
	19–24	72	160	177	70	58	1,000	10	10	70	60	1.5	1.7	19	2.0	200	2.0	1,200	1,200	350	10	15	150	70
	25–50	79	174	176	70	63	1,000	5	10	80	60	1.5	1.7	19	2.0	200	2.0	800	800	350	10	15	150	70
	51+	77	170	173	68	63	1,000	5	10	80	60	1.2	1.4	15	2.0	200	2.0	800	800	350	10	15	150	70
Females	15–18	55	120	163	64	44	800	10	8	55	60	1.1	1.3	15	1.5	180	2.0	1,200	1,200	300	15	12	150	50
	19–24	58	128	164	65	46	800	10	8	60	60	1.1	1.3	15	1.6	180	2.0	1,200	1,200	280	15	12	150	55
	25–50	63	138	163	64	50	800	5	8	65	60	1.1	1.3	15	1.6	180	2.0	800	800	280	15	12	150	55
	51+	65	143	160	63	50	800	5	8	65	60	1.0	1.2	13	1.6	180	2.0	800	800	280	10	12	150	55

Source: Food and Nutrition Board, National Academy of Sciences—National Research Council, 1989

kcal intake of about 400 to 550. Pies average 100 kcal per one-inch slice. Most slices are about $3\frac{1}{2}$ inches. A scoop of ice cream on the pie would bring the total at least another 100 kcal.

Although the kcal intakes of the husband and wife would be comparable, the nutrient intakes would differ. The wife's would be inadequate. If the woman is of childbearing age and plans to have children, she and her children could suffer from such habits.

Generally, people today are concerned about nutrition and want to limit fats, cholesterol, sugar, salt, and kcal, and increase fiber. Many know the sources of these items; others do not. Unfortunately, both groups tend to select their foods because of convenience and flavor rather than nutritional content. It is easier to heat a prepared frozen dinner in the microwave and complete the meal with ice cream than it is to shop for individual food items, cook them, and wash up after the meal. Consequently, many people ingest more fats, sugar, salt, and kcal, and less fiber and other nutrients than they should.

WEIGHT CONTROL

Weight control is probably one of the top ten concerns of U.S. adults. Whether for reasons of vanity, health, or both, most people are interested in controlling their weight. It is advisable because overweight can introduce health problems. Cases of **diabetes mellitus** and **hypertension** are more numerous among the overweight than among those of normal weight. (See Table 15-2.) Overweight individuals are poor risks for surgery, and their lives are generally shorter. They are prone to social and emotional problems because **obesity** (excess body fat) reduces self-esteem.

The causes of overweight are not always known, but the most common cause appears to be **energy imbalance.** In other words, if one is overweight, chances are that more kcal have been taken in than were needed for energy.

An intake of 3500 kcal more than the body needs for maintenance and activities will result in one extra pound. An individual who overeats by only 200 kcal a day can gain 20 pounds in one year. Obviously, when nutrient requirements remain static but kcal requirements decrease, people must carefully select their foods to fulfill their nutrient requirements. (See Table 15-3.) A hypothyroid condition can also contribute to overweight.

For those individuals who are overweight simply because of energy imbalance, the problem may be solved by eating less, by increasing the amount of exercise (work) performed, or by eating less combined with increased exercise. Exercise will increase the number of kcal burned. However, unless the exercise is sufficient to burn more kcal than are ingested, exercise alone will not solve the problem. See Table 2-2 for the amounts of energy burned by specific types of work. By far the most effective method of weight loss is increased exercise combined with reduced kcal intake. This will help tone the muscles as the excess **adipose tissue** (fatty tissue) is lost.

When weight reduction is to be undertaken, the patient should confirm with his or her physician that he or she is in good health. Then with the help of a trained dietitian, a diet should be developed that will fit the dieter's lifestyle. A diet is easiest to follow when it is based on the Food Guide Pyramid. This will aid the dieter in obtaining needed nutrients, change previously unsatisfactory eating habits, and allow him or her to adapt and, thus, enjoy home, party, or restaurant meals. For additional information about weight loss diets, see Chapter 18.

Table 15-2 Median Heights and Weights and Recommended Energy Intake for Adults

Category	Age (years) or Condition	Weight (kg)	Weight (lb)	Height (cm)	Height (in)	REE (kcal/day)	Average Energy Allowance (kcal) Multiples of REE	Average Energy Allowance (kcal) Per kg	Average Energy Allowance (kcal) Per day
Males	19–24	72	160	177	70	1,780	1.67	40	2,900
	25–50	79	174	176	70	1,800	1.60	37	2,900
	51+	77	170	173	68	1,530	1.50	30	2,300
Females	19–24	58	128	164	65	1,350	1.60	38	2,200
	25–50	63	138	163	64	1,380	1.55	36	2,200
	51+	65	143	160	63	1,280	1.50	30	1,900

Source: Food and Nutrition Board, National Academy of Sciences—National Research Council, 1989

Table 15-3 2000 kcal Daily Menus

Breakfast

½ cup orange juice	50 kcal	
1 cup dry cereal	100	
½ cup skim milk	50	
2 teaspoons sugar	35	
2 slices toast	150	
½ tablespoon margarine	50	
1 cup black coffee	0	435 kcal

Lunch

Roast Beef Sandwich:		
3 oz. roast beef	200	
2 slices bread	150	
2 tablespoons mayonnaise	200	
lettuce	10	
1 cup skim milk	100	
1 orange	75	735

Dinner

3 oz. broiled fish	150	
1 baked potato	100	
1½ tablespoons margarine	150	
½ cup green peas	50	
tossed salad with 1 Tbsp dressing	150	
1 cup skim milk	100	
¾ cup ice cream	200	
1 oatmeal cookie	100	1,000
		2,170 kcal

CONCERNS FOR THE HEALTH CARE PROFESSIONAL

The young and middle years of life are busy. Most people feel they have too many things to do and too little time to accomplish them. Most have families and jobs and, thus, responsibilities. When health problems occur during these years, people can be psychologically devastated. They worry about their children, bills, and jobs.

Some patients this age will require psychological counseling; others will need the assistance of a social service agency; some will need both. Others will simply need reassurance that they will recover and that their lives will continue much as before their accident or illness.

The health care professional can do patients a great service by alerting her or his superiors to serious problems when they exist and, in simpler cases, by helping the patient see that there is a light at the end of the tunnel.

SUMMARY

Although kcal requirements diminish after the age of 25, most nutrient requirements do not. Consequently, food must be selected with increasing care as one ages to ensure that nutrient requirements are met without exceeding the kcal requirement.

Overweight can cause health problems. If it is caused by energy imbalance, a program of weight loss should be undertaken. A sensible weight loss program includes exercise. The diet should be based on the Food Guide Pyramid and eating habits should be improved during the diet so that the lost weight will not be regained later.

Discussion Topics

1. Why do kcal requirements tend to diminish after the age of 25? Why do nutrient requirements not diminish at the same time?
2. How can only an extra 200 kcal a day result in overweight?
3. Why does a 40-year-old carpenter require more kcal than a 40-year-old architect?
4. How would you advise your 30-year-old sister who boasts about eating only an English muffin and coffee at lunch?
5. Why is overweight inadvisable?
6. Why are middle-aged adults more inclined to overweight than young adults?
7. Why is 35-year-old Vera putting on weight even though it's true that she doesn't eat any more than she did as a 17-year-old cheerleader?

Suggested Activities

1. Plan a panel discussion entitled, "How to lose weight at forty!"
2. Role-play a situation where a 50-year-old woman has just been advised by her physician to lose 25 pounds. She does not want to and cannot understand why she should. She insists her eating habits have not changed

in 25 years. Consider kcal requirement, nutrient requirements, activity, age, and psychology.

3. Using Table A-5 in the Appendix, adapt the menus in Table 15-3 to meet the needs of the following people:
   a. a pregnant 18-year-old
   b. a 30-year-old nursing mother
   c. a man of 40 years
   d. a 45-year-old woman who must follow a 1000 kcal diet

Review

A. Multiple choice. Select the *letter* that precedes the best answer.

1. The number of kcal one needs each day is called one's
   a. nutrient requirement   c. kcal requirement
   b. kcal intake   d. nutritional requirement

2. Overweight during middle age is often due to
   a. obesity   c. adipose tissue
   b. hypertension   d. energy imbalance

3. The measure of energy in foods eaten is one's
   a. kcal requirement   c. nutrient requirement
   b. kcal intake   d. energy imbalance

4. Because of menstruation and pregnancy during the young and middle years, women have a greater need than men for
   a. proteins   c. iodine
   b. B vitamins   d. iron

5. Kcal requirements
   a. increase with age   c. remain unchanged throughout
   b. decrease with age   adult life
                                    d. none of the above

6. To lose one pound of weight, kcal intake must be reduced by
   a. 1000 kcal   c. 3500 kcal
   b. 800 kcal   d. none of the above

7. During the childbearing years, women's iron requirement is
   a. higher than men's   c. lower than men's
   b. the same as men's   d. none of the above

8. Exercise
   a. is more important to men than to women
   b. has no effect on muscles after the age of 40
   c. eliminates the need for post-menopausal women to drink milk
   d. helps to burn kcal as it tones the muscles

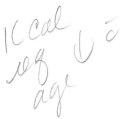

9.   Nutrient requirements during adult life generally
   a. increase with age
   b. decrease with age
   c. remain unchanged throughout adult life
   d. none of the above

10. Women's kcal requirements as compared with men's are generally
   a. higher
   b. lower
   c. the same as
   d. none of the above

Case Study 1

Learning to Maintain a Healthful Weight

Ray was a happy man who had experienced a great deal of success in life. He enjoyed his work and family, and he and his wife were involved in many social events. He loved the cocktail receptions, the dinner parties, the fabulous vacations they took, and having a few neighbors over for a barbecue in their backyard.

His one problem was weight! It seemed he was on a new diet every month, trying to lose the 30 pounds he had added since college. He would lose 5, 10, or even 15 pounds. Then, when the diet was "over," he would inevitably regain the weight and sometimes more than he had lost.

Finally, he visited a diet counselor recommended by his physician. The counselor explained why "miracle weight-loss diets" can only work in the event of a miracle. She provided him with basic nutrition information regarding high- and low-kcal foods, discussed his normal food habits with him, and made some suggestions regarding his weight loss plan. She agreed to counsel him on a weekly basis for a period of three months, during which time he was told to expect to lose 12 pounds if he followed the plan. Three months later, Ray had lost 15 pounds. A year later, he had lost 30 pounds and was delighted to be back in his college shape. He has maintained his "new" weight for over five years.

Case Study Questions Based on the Nursing Process

Assess
1. What probably contributed to Ray's excess weight?

Plan
2. What advice might the diet counselor have offered Ray about cocktails and appetite? Cocktails and calories?

Implement
3. What sort of "basic nutrition information" might the diet counselor have provided Ray?
4. Why would it be advisable for him to meet with the diet counselor each week?

Evaluate
5. Why was Ray finally able to keep the weight off?

Case Study 2

Temporary Depression

Molly was a busy, thin 40-year-old wife and mother. Her two girls were in high school; she had a full-time job that she enjoyed and that provided money for the family; and she had a house that was too big for her to take care of by herself. Her husband was currently unemployed but was spending all his time seeking a new job.

One morning, Molly tripped, fell, and badly fractured her leg. The doctor repaired the leg and told her it would heal well, but that she would be in the hospital for two weeks and would be out of work for at least six months. Molly was devastated. She couldn't eat and could scarcely sleep.

Every morning in the hospital, a young woman came into her room to mop the floor. Every morning this woman was singing. Molly waited for her to come and one day told her what a pleasure it was to see her and asked how she could be so happy. The young woman looked at Molly, leaned on her broom, and said: "Well, you got to make the best of things. Take you, for example, you aren't sick. You're just broken." Molly laughed and her spirits mended after that morning. She never forgot this wonderful young woman.

Case Study Questions Based on the Nursing Process

Assess
1. Why is a sudden physical disability during the young or middle adult years sometimes devastating to a patient?
2. What was Molly probably concerned about as she lay in her hospital bed?
3. Is it likely that Molly's appetite was affected by her worries? If so, how? Is it possible this contributed to her feelings of devastation?

Plan
4. How might her family have helped her to cope with her worries?

Implement
5. Imagine that you are Molly. How would you react to such an accident? What kinds of support might help you?

Evaluate
6. Ultimately, what helped Molly overcome her depression?
7. Is Molly's depression likely to return? How can she help prevent recurrence?

CHAPTER 16

VOCABULARY

arthritis
atherosclerosis
emotional stress
estrogen
food faddists
geriatrics
gerontology
hypertension
nutrient dense foods
occlusions
osteoporosis
periodontal disease
physical stress
physiological
plaque
skeletal system

DIET DURING LATE ADULTHOOD

OBJECTIVES

After studying this chapter, you should be able to
- Explain the nutritional and kcal needs of people 65 and over
- Explain the development of given chronic diseases
- Identify physiological, economic, and psychosocial problems that can affect a senior citizen's nutrition

Currently, the fastest growing age group in the United States is that of people age 65 and older. The average life expectancy in this country has increased to 75 years. It is expected that by the year 2000 there will be 26 million people in the United States 80 years and older. Consequently, **gerontology,** the study of aging, is of increasing importance.

The rate of aging varies. Each person is affected by heredity, **emotional** and **physical** **stress** endured, and nutrition. Experiments continue to teach more about the causes of aging and the role of nutrition in the aging process.

THE EFFECTS OF AGING

As people age, **physiological** (physical), psychosocial, and economic changes occur that affect nutrition.

Physiological

The body's functions slow with age, and its ability to replace worn cells is reduced. The metabolic rate slows; bones become less dense; lean body tissue (muscle) is reduced; eyes do not focus on nearby objects as they once did and some grow cloudy from **cataracts;** the heart and kidneys become less efficient; and hearing, taste, and smell are less acute.

Digestion is affected because the secretion of hydrochloric acid and enzymes is diminished, and the tone of the intestines is reduced, frequently resulting in constipation or in some cases diarrhea.

Psychosocial

Feelings do not decrease with age. In fact, psychosocial problems can increase as one grows older. Age does not diminish the desire to feel useful and appreciated and loved by family and friends. Retirement years may not be "golden" if one suffers a loss of self-esteem from feelings of uselessness. Grief over the loss of a spouse or close friend combined with the resulting loneliness can be devastating. Physical disabilities that develop in the senior years and prevent one from going out independently can destroy a social life. Becoming a fifth wheel in a grown child's home or a sudden resident of a nursing home can lead to severe depression. Problems such as these can diminish a person's appetite and ability to shop and cook.

Economic

Retirement typically results in decreased income. Unless one has carefully prepared for it, this can affect one's quality of life by reducing social activities, add worry about meeting bills, and cause one to select a less than healthy diet by choosing foods on the basis of cost rather than nutrient content.

Sidestepping Potential Problems

Healthy eating habits throughout life, an exercise program suited to one's age, and social activities that please can prevent or delay physical deterioration and psychological depression during the senior years. Their benefits can be said to be circular. The first two contribute largely to one's physical condition, and social activities can prevent or diminish depression. They give purpose to the day, joy to the heart, and zest to the appetite. Whenever there is depression in an elderly person, the patient's nutrition and lifestyle should be carefully reviewed.

NUTRITIONAL REQUIREMENTS OF SENIOR CITIZENS

Although the nutritional needs of growth disappear with age, the normal nutritional needs for maintaining a constant state of good health remain throughout life. Good nutrition can speed recovery from illness, surgery, or broken bones, and generally improve the spirits, quality, and even length of life.

Despite the physical changes the body undergoes after the age of 51, only a few of the RDAs for people in that age category are less than those for younger people.

The protein requirement remains at the average 50 g per day for women and 63 g for men. This is based on the estimated need of 0.8 g per kilogram of body weight. Generally, vitamin requirements do not change after the age of 51, except for a slight decrease in the RDAs for thiamin, riboflavin, and niacin. The need for these three vitamins depends largely on the kcal intake, and kcal requirement is reduced after the age of 51. The need for iron is decreased after age 51 in women because of menopause. (See Table 16-1.)

The kcal requirement decreases with age because metabolism slows and activity is reduced.

Table 16-1 Recommended Dietary Allowances

Category	Age (years) or Condition	Weight (kg)	Weight (lb)	Height (cm)	Height (in)	Protein (g)	Fat-Soluble Vitamins Vita-min A (µg RE)	Vita-min D (µg)	Vita-min E (mg α-TE)	Vita-min K (µg)	Water-Soluble Vitamins Vita-min C (mg)	Thia-min (mg)	Ribo-flavin (mg)	Niacin (mg NE)	Vita-min B$_6$ (mg)	Fo-late (µg)	Vitamin B$_{12}$ (µg)	Minerals Cal-cium (mg)	Phos-phorus (mg)	Mag-nesium (mg)	Iron (mg)	Zinc (mg)	Iodine (µg)	Sele-nium (µg)
Males	25–50	79	174	176	70	63	1,000	5	10	80	60	1.5	1.7	19	2.0	200	2.0	800	800	350	10	15	150	70
	51+	77	170	173	68	63	1,000	5	10	80	60	1.2	1.4	15	2.0	200	2.0	800	800	350	10	15	150	70
Females	25–50	63	138	163	64	50	800	5	8	65	60	1.1	1.3	15	1.6	180	2.0	800	800	280	15	12	150	55
	51+	65	143	160	63	50	800	5	8	65	60	1.0	1.2	13	1.6	180	2.0	800	800	280	10	12	150	55

Source: Food and Nutrition Board, National Academy of Sciences—National Research Council, 1989

Table 16-2 Median Heights and Weights and Recommended Daily Energy Intake

Category	Age (years) or Condition	Weight (kg)	Weight (lb)	Height (cm)	Height (in)	REE (kcal/day)	Average Energy Allowance (kcal)[a] Multiples of REE	Average Energy Allowance (kcal)[a] Per kg	Average Energy Allowance (kcal)[a] Per day[b]
Males	25–50	79	174	176	70	1,800	1.60	37	2,900
	51+	77	170	173	68	1,530	1.50	30	2,300
Females	25–50	63	138	163	64	1,380	1.55	36	2,200
	51+	65	143	160	63	1,280	1.50	30	1,900

[a] In the range of light to moderate activity, the coefficient of variation is ±20%.
[b] Figure is rounded.
Source: Food and Nutrition Board, National Academy of Sciences—National Research Council, 1989

(See Table 16-2.) If the kcal intake is not reduced, weight will increase. This additional weight would increase the work of the heart and put increased stress on the **skeletal system.** It is important that the kcal requirement not be exceeded, and just as important that the nutrient requirements be fulfilled to maintain good nutritional status. An exercise plan appropriate for one's age and health can be helpful in burning excess kcal and toning the muscles.

FOOD HABITS OF SENIOR CITIZENS

If the established food habits of the older person are poor, such habits will undoubtedly have been a long time in the making. These habits will not be easy to change. Poor food habits that begin during old age can also present problems. Decreased income during retirement, physical disability, and inadequate cooking facilities may cause difficulties in food selection and preparation. Anorexia caused by grief, loneliness, boredom, or difficulty in chewing can decrease food consumption.

Studies indicate that many senior citizens consume diets deficient in protein, vitamins C, B_6, and B_{12}, folic acid, calcium, iron, and sometimes kcal.

An elderly patient's diet plan should be based on the Food Guide Pyramid and the nutrients contained compared with the RDA. Older persons' needs can vary considerably, depending on her or his condition, so each should be examined by a physician to determine specific requirements.

Variety and **nutrient dense foods** should be encouraged, as should the use of water. Water is important to help prevent constipation, maintain urinary volume, and prevent dehydration. When there is serious protein and kcal malnutrition (PCM), the reason may be economic or psychosocial. Elderly people who have long hospital stays can develop PCM in the hospital. They may dislike the food, drugs may dull the appetite, they may be lonely and depressed. Sometimes poor or missing teeth can make eating protein foods difficult. In such cases, protein-rich soups can be suggested.

If overweight is a problem, it may be caused by overeating, lack of exercise, drugs, or alcohol.

Any adjustment in food habits will require great tact, and plans for changes must be based on the individual's total situation.

FOOD FADS AND THE ELDERLY

Because!

Some older people are consciously or unconsciously searching for eternal life, if not youth. Consequently, they are frequently susceptible to the claims of **food faddists** who seek to profit from their ignorance. Senior citizens spend money on unnecessary vitamins, minerals, and special honey, molasses, bread, milk, and other foods that may be guaranteed by the salesperson to prevent or cure various diseases. This money could be much more effectively used on ordinary foods from the Food Guide Pyramid that would cost considerably less.

Vit D = ↑ Cal absorb.

NUTRITION AND CHRONIC DISEASES COMMON TO SENIOR CITIZENS

It is estimated that 85 percent of people over 65 have one or more chronic diseases. Examples include osteoporosis, arthritis, cataracts, cancer, diabetes mellitus, hypertension, heart disease, and periodontal disease. The branch of medicine that is involved with diseases of older people is called **geriatrics.**

Osteoporosis

Osteoporosis is a condition in which the amount of calcium in bones is reduced, making them porous. It is estimated that up to 50 percent of elderly people have osteoporosis, and the majority of these are women. It is typically unnoticed at its onset, which is at approximately age 40, and may not be noticed at all until a fracture occurs. One of its symptoms is a gradual reduction in height. Doctors are not certain of its cause. It is thought that years of a sedentary life coupled with a diet deficient in calcium, vitamin D, and fluoride contribute to it, as does **estrogen** (hormone secreted by ovaries) loss, which occurs after menopause. Some doctors are advising patients to consume 1500 mg of calcium, which would require the daily consumption of over one quart of milk or its equivalent. Calcium tablets could be used instead, but the patient would also require supplementary vitamin D. A diet with sufficient calcium and vitamin D plus an appropriate exercise program begun early in the adult years is thought to help prevent this disease.

Another possible cause of osteoporosis may be a diet containing excessive amounts of phosphorus, which can speed bone loss. It is known that Americans are ingesting increasing amounts of phosphorus. Sodas and processed foods contain phosphorus and their consumption is increasing as milk consumption is decreasing in the U.S. Some believe that **periodontal disease** may be a harbinger of osteoporosis. Periodontal disease is characterized by bone loss in the jaw, which can lead to loosened teeth and infection in the gums.

Arthritis

Arthritis is a disease that causes the joints to become painful and stiff. It results in structural changes in the cartilage of the joints. A patient with arthritis should be especially careful to avoid overweight because the extra weight adds stress to joints that are already painful. If the patient is overweight, a weight reduction program should be instituted. The regular use of aspirin by these patients may cause slight bleeding in the stomach lining and subsequent anemia, so their diets may require additional iron. Arthritis can greatly complicate a patient's life because it may partially or completely immobilize the patient to the point where shopping, moving around, and cooking become difficult.

While aspirin and other anti-inflammatory drugs do help relieve the pain of arthritis, there is as yet no cure. Patients should be well informed of this to prevent them from wasting their money on so-called "cures" of tricksters.

Cancer

Research about the role of nutrition in cancer development continues. The American Cancer Society has indicated that diets consistently high in fat, or low in fiber and vitamin A may contribute to cancer. (See Chapter 23.)

Diabetes Mellitus

Diabetes mellitus is a chronic disease. It develops when the body does not produce sufficient amounts of insulin or does not use it effectively for normal carbohydrate metabolism. Diet is very important in the treatment of diabetes. Chapter 19 discusses this treatment in detail.

Hypertension

Hypertension, or high blood pressure, can lead to strokes. It is associated with diets high in salt or possibly low in calcium. Most Americans ingest from two to six times the amount of salt needed each day. It is thought that the earlier a person reduces salt intake, the better that person's chances of avoiding hypertension, particularly if there is a family history of it. Hypertension is discussed in detail in Chapter 20.

Heart Disease

Heart attack and stroke are the major causes of death in the United States. They occur when arteries become blocked (occluded), preventing the normal passage of blood. These **occlusions** (blockages) are caused by blood clots that form and are unable to pass through an unnaturally narrowed artery. Arteries are narrowed by **plaque,** a fatty substance containing cholesterol that accumulates in the walls of the artery. This condition is called **atherosclerosis.** It is believed that excessive cholesterol and saturated fats in the diet over many years contribute to this condition. The therapeutic diet appropriate for atherosclerosis is discussed in Chapter 20.

Current research about the role of nutrition in preventing or relieving these diseases continues. The effects of nutrition are cumulative over many years. The effects of a lifetime of poor eating habits cannot be cured overnight. When diets have been poor for a long time, prevention

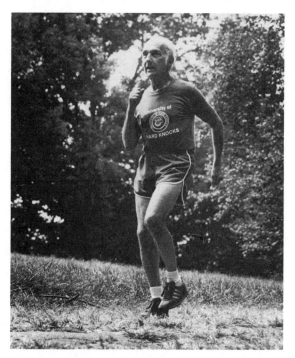

Figure 16-1 Exercising for good health is not limited to the young.

of these chronic diseases may not be possible. It may be possible, however, to use nutrition to help stabilize the condition of a patient with one of these diseases. The prevention of many of the diseases of the elderly should begin in one's youth (see figure 16-1).

APPROPRIATE DIETS FOR SENIOR CITIZENS

The diets of senior citizens should be planned around the Food Guide Pyramid (see Table 16-3). When special health problems exist,

Table 16-3 Suggested Day's Menu Totaling 1995 kcal		
Breakfast		
$\frac{1}{2}$ cup orange juice	50 kcal	
1 cup dry cereal	100	
$\frac{1}{2}$ cup skim milk	42	
2 teaspoons sugar	34	
2 slices whole grain bread, toasted	150	
$\frac{1}{2}$ tablespoon margarine	50	
1 tablespoon jelly	50	
1 cup black coffee	0	475 kcal
Lunch		
$\frac{3}{4}$ cup macaroni and cheese	300	
1 tomato, sliced	25	
$\frac{1}{2}$ cup green beans	25	
1 cup skim milk	85	
$\frac{2}{3}$ cup custard	200	635
Dinner		
$\frac{1}{2}$ cup pineapple juice	75	
3 oz broiled hamburger	240	
$\frac{1}{2}$ cup rice	100	
$\frac{1}{2}$ cup shredded lettuce	10	
1 tablespoon salad dressing	75	
1 cup skim milk	85	
Fresh fruit	100	685
Snacks		
1 banana	100	
5 dried prunes	100	
2 oatmeal cookies	200	400 kcal
		2195 kcal

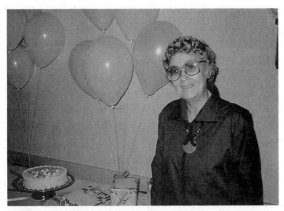

Figure 16-2 Celebrating one's 80th birthday is as much fun as celebrating one's 8th, when health is good.

the normal diet should be adapted to meet individual needs. (See Section 3 on Diet Therapy.)

The federal government provides the states with funds to serve senior citizens hot meals at noon in senior centers across the country. These senior centers become social clubs and are immensely beneficial to the elderly, figure 16-2. They provide companionship in addition to nutritious food. Frequently the noon meal at "the center" becomes the focal point of an older person's day.

The federal government also provides transportation to those who are otherwise unable to reach the senior center for the meal. When individuals are completely homebound, arrangements can be made for the meals to be delivered to their homes. In some communities, there are Meals-on-Wheels projects. Participating people pay according to ability. In addition, food stamps are available, and can sometimes be used for the Meals-on-Wheels programs.

CONSIDERATIONS FOR THE HEALTH CARE PROFESSIONAL

It is essential that the health care professional remember that each patient is an individual with individual needs. It is easy for someone working exclusively with geriatric patients to group them together, but this diminishes the quality of the care they receive and adds to their unhappiness. The 80-year-old patient is just as pleased to see a smile on the face of a nurse as is the 18-year-old patient. The 70-year-old overweight arthritic patient deserves as much help with a weight-loss program as the 45-year-old patient. The 85-year-old patient suffering from senility still enjoys a bright hello and a gentle pat on the back. People's feelings must never be forgotten. The incapacitation that can accompany old age is a terrible indignity, and these patients deserve special care.

SUMMARY

The elderly are becoming an increasingly large segment of the U.S. population and their nutritional needs are of growing concern. It is becoming apparent that many of the chronic diseases of the elderly could be delayed or avoided by maintaining good nutrition throughout life. Most nutrient requirements do not decrease with age, but kcal requirements do. When food habits of senior citizens must be changed, adjustments require great tact and patience on the part of the nutrition counselor. Older people are easily attracted to food fads that promise good health and prolonged life.

Discussion Topics

1. Why are the normal nutrient requirements of people in their seventies the same as those of people in their fifties?
2. Why does the iron requirement usually diminish for women after the age of 50?
3. Why might elderly people suffer from anorexia?
4. How might arthritis affect one's eating habits?
5. In what ways can emotional stress affect eating habits? What kinds of emotional stress do the elderly sometimes suffer?
6. Why are older people inclined to believe food faddists' stories?
7. What is the difference between geriatrics and gerontology?
8. What is periodontal disease and what is its possible significance?
9. What is osteoporosis?
10. Why do kcal requirements diminish as people age?

Suggested Activities

1. Arrange a panel discussion on nutrition for the senior citizen. Consider nutrient requirements, kcal requirements, physical disabilities, food habits, food fads, chronic diseases, appropriate diets, and the means of obtaining them.
2. If possible, visit a nursing home at mealtime. Write your evaluation of the food and a description of patient reaction(s) to it and to you, the visitor.
3. Role-play a situation where a 75-year-old arthritic woman who has just been widowed is depressed and disinterested in food, and is being counseled to eat a nutritious diet.
4. Describe an appropriate response to your 65-year-old aunt who has just become captivated by a salesperson in a local health food store, and has announced that she is buying a six-month supply of vinegar-honey tablets that are guaranteed to prevent arthritis.
5. Plan a talk on nutrition for the Parents' Association of a local high school entitled, "Invest Now for Future Dividends—Eat Well."
6. Adapt the menus in Table 16-3 to meet the kcal requirements of someone who needs 2300 kcal.

Review

A. Multiple choice. Select the *letter* that precedes the best answer.
   1. Gerontology is of increasing interest because it is
      a. the branch of medicine involved with diseases of older people
      b. the study of nutrition

    c. hoped experimentation in this field will explain the causes of aging

    d. the study of heart disease

2. After the age of 51, nutrient requirements generally
   - a. increase
   - b. decrease
   - c. remain unchanged
   - d. none of the above

3. After the age of 51, kcal requirements generally
   - a. increase
   - b. decrease
   - c. remain unchanged
   - d. none of the above

4. The iron requirement for women after the age of approximately 51 generally
   - a. increases
   - b. decreases
   - c. remains unchanged
   - d. none of the above

5. As the metabolic rate slows with age,
   - a. the kcal requirement is increased
   - b. the kcal requirement is decreased
   - c. there is a decreased need for vitamins A, D, and K
   - d. cataracts can develop

6. Osteoporosis is a disease that causes
   - a. poor appetite
   - b. a reduction in the number of red blood cells
   - c. joints to become painful and stiff
   - d. bones to become porous

7. Arthritis is a disease that causes
   - a. poor appetite
   - b. a reduction in the number of red blood cells
   - c. joints to become painful and stiff
   - d. bones to become porous

8. Hypertension is related to diets high in
   - a. cholesterol
   - b. vitamin D
   - c. calcium
   - d. salt

9. Diets high in cholesterol content are thought to contribute to
   - a. diabetes mellitus
   - b. hypertension
   - c. heart disease
   - d. cataracts

B. Completion

1. _Anorexia_ is a condition in which the patient, for psychological reasons, has no appetite or interest in food, and weight loss becomes a concern.

2. _Arthritis_ is a chronic disease in which the joints become painful and stiff.

3. _Diabetes_ is a chronic disease that prevents the normal production of insulin so that carbohydrate metabolism is affected.

4. _Geriatrics_ is the branch of medicine dealing with diseases of the elderly.

5. _Gerentology_ is the study of aging.

6. _Hyp_ is also known as high blood pressure.

7. _Nut.Statis_ is the condition of one's nutrition.

8. _Osteoporo_ is the disease in which bones become porous.

9. _Periodontu_ occurs in the gums and supportive tissue of the teeth.

10. _Skelital_ system is the bone structure of the body.

C. Essay Questions

1. What factors may contribute to the formation of poor food habits during the senior years?

2. Why are the elderly especially susceptible to food fads?

3. Explain how the cumulative effects of diet are thought to be related to the development of osteoporosis and heart disease.

Case Study 1

Diet and Osteoporosis

Evelyn was effortlessly slender as a young woman in the 1920s, and was pleased to be so. However, when her 40th birthday approached, she noticed her clothes seemed tighter than they had previously. And, when she had her annual physical exam, she was shocked to see that she had gained 10 pounds in one year. She decided that she must stop gaining weight despite her busy afternoon social schedule of teas and meetings.

So, while she continued to attend the social events of her day, she indulged less in the sweets that were always offered. And, just to be "safe," she began to skip dinner on the nights she attended a "social." She cooked for her family and sat with them, but ate nothing on those evenings. She also eliminated milk at lunch—saving "room" for the afternoon teas. By the time Evelyn was 65, she had broken ribs and a leg in falls. During a physical exam that year, her doctor noticed that she had a serious case of osteoporosis. The doctor prescribed 1500 mg of calcium, 400 IU of vitamin D, and a two-mile walk each day. She has followed the doctor's instructions to the letter for 15 years. At the age of 80, she is still vigorous, although she has broken a finger, both wrists, more ribs, and some vertebrae. Still, she thinks, it could have been a lot worse!

Case Study Questions Based on the Nursing Process

Assess
1. Is it definite that Evelyn's food habits caused her osteoporosis? Explain. Did they possibly contribute to it?
2. What other factors might have contributed to Evelyn's osteoporosis?
3. If Evelyn had not put a stop to a ten-pound a year weight gain, what other disease(s) might have afflicted her as she aged?

Plan
4. How many kcal does it take to gain 10 pounds in one year?
5. Do you think Evelyn's then middle-aged daughters might have learned anything from the diagnosis of their mother's osteoporosis? Explain.

Implement
6. If you were the diet counselor, what would you teach Evelyn's daughters to help them decrease their risk of developing osteoporosis?

Evaluate
7. What actions did Evelyn take to slow the progression of her osteoporosis?

Case Study 2

Temporary Physical Disability

Maria was a thin 65-year-old widow. She had suffered a severe fracture of her left arm that had required surgery. Her surgeon told her she was healing well and would be released from the hospital on Saturday—exactly two weeks after surgery. Although she did not tell the doctor, she felt weak and feared returning home alone while she was still incapacitated.

On Saturday as she prepared to leave, her favorite nurse, Betsy, said she realized Maria hadn't been eating well during her hospital stay. Betsy said she had asked the local visiting nurse association to have someone call on Maria twice each week. Betsy also urged Maria to eat, reminding her that a good diet would help her arm to heal.

Case Study Questions Based on the Nursing Process

Assess

1. Is it possible that Maria's surgeon had not noticed her weakness? Explain.
2. What may have caused Maria's weakness?

Plan

3. What might Betsy have done in the hospital to improve Maria's appetite?
4. Why might Maria be nervous about returning home?
5. How might a visiting nurse be helpful to Maria?

Implement

6. When Betsy was discussing a "good diet" with Maria, what did she probably suggest Maria eat to aid in the healing process and help her regain her strength?
7. Plan a one-day menu for Maria.

Evaluate

8. What will the visiting nurse look for to confirm that Maria is following the recommended diet plan?

SECTION 3

DIET THERAPY

CHAPTER 17

NUTRITIONAL ASSESSMENT AND THERAPY

OBJECTIVES

After studying this chapter, you should be able to
- List the basic steps in nutritional assessment
- Describe diet therapy
- Name basic hospital diets
- Explain why diet-therapy patients often need nutritional counseling

NUTRITIONAL ASSESSMENT

Patients in health care facilities have different backgrounds, food customs, and problems. Still they share a common goal—the return of good health. Each requires and deserves individualized treatment. Part of this treatment is nutri-tional. Good nutrition is essential for the attainment of good health and for its maintenance.

The varying conditions of the diversified patient population in a health care facility prohibit any generalization of nutritional therapy. Patients require individual **nutritional assessment** (evaluation of nutritional status). Proper nutri-

241

tional assessment includes **anthropometric measurements** (comparative body measurements), **clinical evaluation** (physical signs of good or poor nutrition), **biochemical tests,** and **specific dietary information.**

Anthropometric measurements include height, weight, measurements of the head, chest, arm, and skinfold. The skinfold measurement is done with a **caliper.** It is used to determine the percentage of adipose and muscle tissue in the body.

Clinical evaluation is the physical observation of a patient, in which signs of nutrient deficiencies are noted. While some nutrient deficiencies such as scurvy, rickets, iron-deficiency anemia or kwashiorkor are obvious, others can be far more subtle. Table 17-1 lists some symptoms of nutritional deficiencies and their causes.

Biochemical tests include various blood, urine, and feces tests and, sometimes, liver and bone *biopsies* (microscopic examination of the tissue). These tests are made for nutrients, prod-

ucts of metabolism, or waste materials, depending on the patient's condition. Examples of blood *analyses* (tests) include hemoglobin, red blood cell count, white blood cell count, serum cholesterol, serum triglycerides, and high-density lipoproteins. Examples of urine analyses include creatine (a nitrogen-containing compound in urine; provides information on muscle mass and thus body composition), vitamin C, riboflavin, and thiamin levels.

Dietary assessment (evaluation of food habits) is, or course, very important to the nutritional assessment of any patient, but it cannot be the sole measure. It must be used in conjunction with the laboratory tests, the clinical evaluation, and the anthropometric measurements.

The information provided by the dietary assessment should be evaluated against the patient's personal, social, and economic background.

It can be difficult to obtain an accurate dietary assessment. The most common method is

Table 17-1 Clinical Signs of Nutritional Deficiencies

Clinical Signs	Possible Deficiencies
Pallor; blue half circles beneath eyes	Iron, copper, zinc, B_{12}, B_6, biotin
Edema	Protein
Bumpy "gooseflesh"	Vitamin A
Lesions at corners of mouth	Riboflavin
Glossitis	Folic acid
Numerous "black and blue" spots and tiny, red "pin prick" hemorrhages under skin	Vitamin C
Emaciation	Carbohydrates, proteins; kcal
Poorly shaped bones or teeth or delayed appearance of teeth in children	Vitamin D or calcium
Slow clotting time of blood	Vitamin K
Unusual nervousness, dermatitis, diarrhea in same patient	Niacin
Tetany	Calcium, potassium, sodium
Goiter	Iodine
Eczema	Fat (linoleic acid)

the *24-hour recall.* In this method, the patient is either interviewed by the **dietitian** or completes a lengthy questionnaire. In either case, the patient is asked to give the types, amounts, preparation methods used, and hours of all food eaten in the 24 hours just before hospitalization.

Another common method is the **food diary.** For this, the patient is asked to list all food eaten in a three- or four-day period. Neither method is totally accurate because patients forget and/or are not always totally truthful. They are sometimes inclined to seek approval by saying they have eaten foods because they know they should have done so or vice versa.

When the preceding steps are evaluated together, and in the context of the patient's medical condition, the dietitian has the best opportunity of making an accurate nutritional assessment of the patient. This assessment can then be used by the entire health care team. The doctor will find it helpful in evaluating the patient's condition and treatment. The dietitian can use the information it provides to plan the patient's dietary treatment and counseling, and other health care professionals will be able to use it in terms of assisting and counseling the patient.

DIET THERAPY

Diet therapy is the process by which food is used to build good health. It means *healing with food*—an intriguing idea. Sometimes, in cases such as marasmus or kwashiorkor or anorexia nervosa, it is just that simple. Good food is prescribed and good health is the result. These are times when it is simply a matter of changing a nutritionally inadequate diet to a **nutritionally adequate** one. More often, however, diet therapy means that diets must be changed to fulfill specific nutritional requirements created by disease or injury.

Usually, diet therapy means the addition or subtraction of specific nutrients or kcal in specified amounts to or from a normal diet, or the **modification** (change) of their consistencies. These are called **therapeutic diets.** They are adaptations of the normal diet. Sometimes, the diets themselves can create nutritional deficiencies when their limitations are severe, as in the case of a clear liquid diet. When diets are nutritionally inadequate, they can be used for only a short time and/or dietary supplements of vitamins, minerals, proteins, or fatty acids can be prescribed.

Therapeutic diets are prescribed by the physician. The dietitian or nutritionist plans the meals to fit the physician's prescription, and frequently counsels the patient about the diet. The health professional is usually the individual who is on hand to observe the patient's reaction to the diet, to encourage and assist the patient, and sometimes to counsel.

STANDARD HOSPITAL DIETS

Health facilities such as hospitals and nursing homes usually have **standard diets** that simplify their meal planning. Hospitals typically have liquid, soft, regular, and sometimes light diets.

These basic diets may be modified by changing their consistency, energy value, or nutrient content. For example, a low-kcal diet or a sodium-restricted diet can be prepared as a liquid, soft, light, or regular diet.

The person serving a meal should learn to recognize the types of food allowed in each diet. In some facilities it is the duty of the health professional to double-check the meal tray before it is served.

Liquid Diets

A **liquid diet** consists of foods that will pour or are liquid at body temperature. The nutritive value of liquid diets is low and consequently they are usually used only for very limited periods of time. Liquid diets are subdivided into two types—the **clear liquid** and the **full liquid diet.**

Clear Liquid Diet

The clear liquid diet consists of liquids that do not irritate the gastrointestinal tract, cause **flatulence** (gas in the stomach or intestines), or stimulate peristalsis. A clear liquid diet passes through the body easily and does not create **residue** (indigestible fiber). Therefore, this diet is used when the amount of **fecal matter** (waste material) in the colon must be kept at a minimum. The clear liquid diet can be used after surgery. The diet also can be ordered to replace fluids lost through vomiting or diarrhea.

The clear liquid diet is composed mainly of water and carbohydrates. It does not include milk (see Table 17-2). It is only a temporary diet because it is nutritionally inadequate, and its use is typically limited to 24 to 36 hours. The meals, which are small and frequent, are usually served every two, three, or four hours (see Table 17-3). It is usually followed by the full liquid diet.

Full Liquid Diet

The full liquid diet contains all foods in the clear liquid diet and additional, more nutritious foods as well.

The full liquid diet includes many milk-based foods that make this diet more nutritious

Table 17-2 Foods Allowed in a Clear Liquid Diet
apple and grape juice
fat-free **broths** or **bouillon** (clear soups)
plain gelatin
fruit ice
ginger ale and carbonated water (if permitted by physician)
tea or black coffee with sugar

than the clear liquid diet (see Table 17-4). Compared with a regular diet, however, the nutritive value of a full liquid diet is low. Its nutrient content may be increased by adding commercially prepared liquid supplements. In addition, the physician may prescribe a vitamin supplement. Feedings are usually given every two or three hours.

This diet can be given to patients who have acute infections; to patients who have difficulty chewing; to those who have had heart attacks; and to patients with **gastrointestinal** (relating to the stomach and intestines) disturbances. Table 17-5 shows sample menus for a full liquid diet.

The Soft Diet

The **soft diet** is similar to the regular diet except that the texture of the foods has been modified. The soft diet commonly follows a full liquid diet. It may be ordered for **postoperative** (after surgery) cases, for patients with **acute** (se-

Table 17-3 Sample Menus for a Clear Liquid Diet					
Breakfast	10 A.M.	Dinner	3 P.M.	Lunch or Supper	9 P.M.
Grape Juice Tea with Sugar	Apple Juice	Beef Bouillon Gelatin Tea with Sugar	Grape Juice	Chicken Broth Fruit Ice Tea with Sugar	Beef Bouillon

Table 17-4 Foods Allowed in a Full Liquid Diet

all clear liquids
fruit and vegetable juices
strained soups (cream or water based)
strained, cooked cereals
custard, puddings
ice cream, sherbet, frozen yogurt
plain gelatin
junket (sweetened, flavored, thickened milk dessert)
milk, cream, buttermilk
hot cocoa
eggnog
carbonated beverages

vere) infections, gastrointestinal conditions, or chewing problems.

This diet includes liquids and foods that have a soft texture and are easy to digest (see Table 17-6). The foods allowed are those that contain little fiber and no tough connective tissue. As a result, a soft diet leaves little food residue. Meats in a soft diet are tender. Most fruits must be cooked, but bananas or orange or grapefruit sections (with membranes removed) are sometimes allowed. Usually only young, tender, cooked vegetables are served; frequently these are pureed. Cereals are either refined or cooked.

When patients are unable to chew, the **mechanical soft diet** can be ordered. In this diet, all meats are ground, and fruits and vegetables are pureed. It may be necessary after facial surgery, or when teeth are missing or inadequate.

Generally, foods on the soft diet are mildly flavored, slightly seasoned, or left unseasoned. Although this diet nourishes the body, between-meal feedings are sometimes given to increase the energy value. Table 17-7 shows sample menus for a soft diet.

The Light Diet

The **light diet** is an intermediate diet sometimes used between the soft and the regular diets. It is nutritionally adequate.

The light diet is also called the **convalescent diet** because it is primarily used for **convalescent** (recovering from an injury or illness) patients and for those with minor illnesses. The light diet is considered one of the four standard diets, but some health facilities do not use it because it is similar to the regular diet.

The important fact to remember about the light diet is that the foods must be easy to digest.

Table 17-5 Sample Menus for a Full Liquid Diet

Breakfast	10 A.M.	Dinner	3 P.M.	Lunch or Supper	9 P.M.
Strained Orange Juice	Tomato Juice	Strained Cream of Chicken Soup	Eggnog	Apple Juice	Cocoa
Strained Oatmeal Gruel with Cream and Sugar		Plain Gelatin with Sweetened Whipped Cream		Beef Broth	
Coffee or Tea with Cream and Sugar		Milk		Vanilla Ice Cream	
		Tea with Cream and Sugar		Milk	
				Coffee or Tea with Cream and Sugar	

Table 17-6 Selecting Foods in a Soft Diet

Foods Allowed in Soft Diet	Foods to be Avoided
milk, cream, butter mild cheeses such as cottage or cream cheese eggs, except fried tender chicken, fish, sweetbreads, ground beef and lamb soup broth and strained cream soups tender, cooked vegetables or pureed vegetables fruit juices, cooked fruits, bananas, orange and grapefruit sections with membranes removed refined cereals, cooked cereals, spaghetti, noodles, macaroni, enriched white bread, white crackers tea, coffee, cocoa, carbonated beverages sherbet, ices, plain ice cream, custard, pudding, junket, gelatin, plain cookies, angel and sponge cake salt and some spices in small amounts as allowed by the physician	meat and shellfish with tough connective tissue coarse cereals **condiments** (foods used as seasonings, relishes) rich pastries and desserts foods high in cellulose fried foods raw vegetables and raw fruits (except bananas and citrus fruits with membranes removed) nuts and coconut

Table 17-7 Sample Menus for a Soft Diet

Breakfast	Dinner	Lunch or Supper
Orange juice Cream of Wheat with Milk and Sugar Buttered Toast Tea or Coffee with Milk and Sugar	Cream of Tomato Soup Broiled Ground Beef Patty Mashed Potatoes with Margarine Green Beans Bread and Margarine Stewed Peaches Skim Milk	Apple Juice Creamed Chicken with Peas and Noodles Baked Squash Bread and Margarine Custard Tea with Milk and Sugar

Note: Between meals the patient may have malted milk, milkshakes, eggnog, or cocoa.

Foods are simply cooked, with little seasoning, and served without heavy sauces or spicy seasonings. The diet includes all foods allowed on the soft and liquid diets plus those foods listed in Table 17-8. Table 17-9 shows sample menus for a light diet.

Regular Diet

A **regular diet** is a nearly normal diet based on the Food Guide Pyramid (see Table 17-10).

People on this diet require nutrients for health maintenance only, and not for therapy. A regular diet includes a great variety of foods. However, the kcal value of this diet is somewhat lower than for normal diets because the people on it are not normally active, and consequently require fewer calories than the ordinary person. Except for foods that cause digestive disturbances in some individuals, or are so high-kcal as to cause weight gain, there are seldom limitations on this diet.

Table 17-8 Selecting Foods for a Light Diet

Foods Allowed in Light Diets	Foods to be Avoided
cheddar cheese	rich pastries
tender cuts of beef, lamb, and veal such as steaks, roasts, and chops	heavy salad dressings
	fried foods
bacon, liver	coarse foods such as some very coarse cereals
all soups	fruits and vegetables that are high in cellulose
cooked vegetables and fruits, citrus fruits, bananas, lettuce and tomato salads	foods that cause flatulence
enriched and whole wheat bread and crackers	nuts
plain cakes	

Table 17-9 Sample Menus for a Light Diet

Breakfast	Dinner	Lunch or Supper
Orange Sections	Vegetable Soup	Tomato Juice
Oatmeal with Milk and Sugar	Roast Lamb	Scrambled Eggs with Cottage Cheese
Buttered Toast	Baked Potato	Asparagus Tips
Jelly	Buttered Carrots	Bread and Margarine
Coffee with Milk and Sugar	Lettuce Salad	Orange Sherbet
	Bread and Margarine	Tea with Milk and Sugar
	Frozen Yogurt	
	Tea with Milk and Sugar	

Table 17-10 A Day's Menu with a Regular Diet Can Include a Wide Variety of Foods

Breakfast	Dinner	Lunch or Supper
Orange Juice	Tomato Juice	Apple Juice
Oatmeal	Roast Beef	Poached Egg on Toast
Milk-Sugar	Mashed Potatoes	Cooked Spinach
Toast-Margarine	Steamed Carrots	Fruit Gelatin
Coffee or Tea	Lettuce with French Dressing	Plain Cookie
	Bread-Margarine	Skim Milk or Tea
	Milk Pudding	
	Skim Milk	

NUTRITIONAL COUNSELING

When the physician has diagnosed the patient's condition and the specific form of diet therapy has been prescribed, the work of the diet counselor begins.

It can be difficult to convince a patient to eat meals based on a therapeutic diet. A change in food habits is not an easy or pleasant experience anytime. Sometimes, as in the case of a diabetic patient, the new diet may be needed for a lifetime. People are often reluctant to eat new foods or familiar foods prepared in unfamiliar ways. This is especially true when they are ill. Weakness, exhaustion, illness, pain, fear, loneliness, and self-pity are common among hospitalized patients, and they all discourage appetites. Anorexia and malnutrition in hospitalized patients often result.

The nutritionist typically follows a four-step process.

1. Nutritional assessment
2. Dietary plan
3. Implementation of the plan
4. Evaluation

After making the nutritional assessment, the nutritionist talks with the patient and the patient's family. Sometimes the patient and/or a family member does not understand the need for the diet. Elementary facts of nutrition may need to be explained. A good, but simple, explanation of the reasons for the diet can help improve the patient's attitude and appetite. Food prejudices may need to be overcome.

When the nutritionist feels that the patient understands the need for and basis of the therapy, they work together to form a plan to implement the doctor's dietary prescription. The nutritionist is, of course, the guide, and proceeds on the basis of the patient's dietary habits, likes, needs, and nutritional assessment. It is not just the patient who must adapt when diet therapy is required, however. The new diet must be adapted to satisfy the patient as well, or successful diet therapy is not likely to follow.

Together they discuss the patient's dietary needs, set goals, and discuss means of achieving these goals. When this has been accomplished, they discuss the implementation of this plan. Menus, shopping, recipes, cooking, adapting family meals to conform to the patient's needs, selecting food from restaurant menus, eating at a friend's table—all are discussed. Means of camouflaging disliked foods are noted. Nutritionally acceptable substitutes for prescribed foods are discussed. Milk, for example, can be included in pudding, ice cream, cheese, cream sauce, soup, or custard. In this way, potential problems may be avoided and, if they cannot be avoided, at least the patient is prepared for them when they do occur.

During this process, with the encouragement and help of the diet counselor, the diet becomes less formidable and possibly even a somewhat interesting challenge to the patient.

When the patient has lived for a period with the plans made with the diet counselor, they meet again to reevaluate their plans. Questions are answered. Unexpected problems are brought to light and, hopefully, resolved. Means of coping with disallowed foods that can be expected to be served at upcoming special events such as weddings and holidays are discussed. Plans that were found in the intervening time to be inappropriate, are revised. Plans may be made for a subsequent evaluation. Some patients need repeated encouragement and renewed motivation. Some few do not. Some patients will fail. Many will succeed—with the help of the diet counselor and the health care professional.

CONSIDERATIONS FOR THE HEALTH CARE PROFESSIONAL

If nutritional therapy has been found necessary for the well-being of the patient, it will be helpful to all if the nurse is involved with the nutritionist in instructing the patient about the new diet. The patient will be more familiar with and thus more comfortable asking the nurse rather than the nutritionist questions. The nurse can reinforce the nutritionist's information, if needed, and relay questions to the nutritionist, if necessary.

Most patients will want to learn how to live with their prescribed diets. Some will resist and find ways of having family and friends bring forbidden foods. The first group can try the patience of the nurse with elementary and repetitive questions. The second group can exasperate a busy nurse who does not have time to play detective. It is important that the nurse remember that both types of patients need help.

SUMMARY

The nutritional assessment of hospitalized patients is necessary in determining their nutritional status. The nutritional assessment includes anthropometric measures, clinical evaluation, biochemical tests, and dietary assessment.

Diet therapy means healing with food. It may include the addition or subtraction of specific nutrients, of kcal, or the modification of texture of foods in a normal diet. When specific diet therapy is prescribed, it is essential that the diet counselor work on the basis of the nutritional assessment and with the patient and the patient's family to develop a usable diet plan that fulfills the physician's prescription and fits into the patient's lifestyle.

Health facilities have standard diets. These usually include liquid, soft and regular, and sometimes light diets. The progression moves from clear liquid to full liquid to soft to regular. Each of these can be modified to fulfill specific therapeutic needs.

Discussion Topics

1. Why might the diet counselor need to know the skinfold measurements of patients?
2. Of what value is clinical evaluation of a patient?
3. When might a bone biopsy be helpful?
4. Describe the method of dietary assessment called "24-hour Recall." Compare it to the "Food Diary."
5. Why is malnutrition a problem among hospital patients?
6. What are the usual standard hospital diets? If anyone in the class has eaten or seen any hospital diets, ask that person to describe them.
7. Describe the regular hospital diet. How can it differ from a normal diet?
8. Why is the kcal count sometimes lower on the regular hospital diet than on a normal diet?
9. When is the light diet used? Why is it not included in the diets of all hospitals?
10. What types of foods are included in the light diet?

11. Would the light diet be generally suitable for healthy geriatric patients? For children? Is it nutritionally adequate?

12. Many people have unknowingly been on a self-imposed light diet at home. Under what conditions might this have occurred?

13. Describe a soft diet. Does it nourish the body? When may it be prescribed?

14. Why are between-meal feedings sometimes given to patients on the soft diet?

15. What are condiments and why are they excluded from the soft diet?

16. Name the conditions for which a soft diet may be prescribed.

17. What is indigestible carbohydrate? Why should it be limited in a soft diet? Name several foods that contain a large proportion of indigestible carbohydrate. Name foods containing very little.

18. What are food "membranes"? Why should such membranes be omitted from the soft diet?

19. Why are patients on the clear-liquid diet fed so frequently? Why is it only a temporary diet?

20. How does the full-liquid diet differ from the clear-liquid diet?

21. What is bouillon? How is it prepared?

22. What is junket? If anyone in the class has tasted it, ask that person to describe it.

23. Mr. Brown has recently had a stroke that paralyzed his right side. Why do you think a liquid diet has been prescribed for him?

24. What is diet therapy?

25. Discuss ways in which the health professional may help solve the problem of friends and relatives bringing food to patients on therapeutic diets.

26. What are food prejudices? Name some and discuss how one might attempt to help the patient overcome them.

27. Why is it important to teach the patient about her or his new diet?

28. Why do people who are ill frequently experience a decrease in appetite? How can the nurse encourage patients to eat well?

Suggested Activities

1. Ask a nutritionist to discuss and demonstrate anthropometric measurements.

2. Make a chart of the diets discussed in this chapter and include the foods allowed in each. Compare the charts and correct if necessary. The charts should be kept for reference.

3. Plan a daily menu for each of the diets in this chapter. Compare menus and correct them if necessary.

4. Adapt the menus for the regular diet to suit a 40-year-old woman. How might the diet be changed if the patient were a 16-year-old boy with a broken leg?

5. In some hospitals, regular diets do not include rich, high-kcal foods. Substitute other foods or methods of preparation to make the regular diet that follows more appropriate:

Deep-fried Fish Fillets
French-fried Potatoes
Green Peas
Lettuce with Oil and Vinegar
Bread and Butter
Pecan Pie with Whipped Cream
Whole Milk

6. Make a list of the foods eaten yesterday. Circle those foods that would not be allowed on the light diet.

7. Adapt the following menu to make it appropriate for a patient on a regular hospital diet.

Breakfast	**Dinner**	**Lunch or Supper**
Orange Juice	Roast Beef	Pepper Steak
2 Fried Eggs	Mashed Potato	Cooked Spinach
Danish Pastry	Steamed Carrots	Fruit Gelatin
Coffee or Tea	Lettuce with	Pecan Roll
with	Creamy Garlic Dressing	Milk or Tea
Milk-Sugar	Whole Wheat Bread	
	Milk Pudding	
	Milk	

8. Adapt the following menu to suit the needs of a patient on a soft diet:

Fresh Fruit Cup
Oatmeal with Milk and Sugar
Bran Muffin and Butter
Tea with Sugar

9. Write your dinner menu for last night. Adapt it to suit a patient on the soft diet.

10. Find recipes that are suitable for these standard hospital diets.

11. Begin a Therapeutic Diet Recipe File in which the recipes are coded according to the diet in which they are allowed. Code them by using a special color dot in the upper right-hand corner of each recipe or use the initials of the diet. Many of the recipes may be suitable for several different diets.

12. Observe demonstrations of an electric blender, a food processor, and a microwave oven. Practice using them and cleaning them.

13. Role-play a situation in which the health professional persuades a middle-aged woman who loves sweets that her carbohydrate-controlled diet can be satisfying. The class should evaluate the "nurse's" tact and ingenuity in persuading the "patient" to accept her new diet.

14. Plan a visit to a hospital kitchen. If possible, ask the dietitian to explain the various procedures to the class. Discuss this visit in class.

Review

A. Multiple choice. Select the *letter* that precedes the best answer.

1. The use of diet to build health during and after illness is called
   a. diet therapy   c. dietitian
   b. dietetics   d. physical therapy

2. Special diets are prescribed by the
   a. nurse   c. physician
   b. dietitian   d. physical therapist

3. Basic diets may be modified by changing their
   a. color, flavor, or satiety value
   b. consistency, energy value, or nutrient content
   c. temperatures and serving times
   d. cost and efficiency of preparation

4. A therapeutic diet
   a. is used only in hospitals
   b. may add or subtract certain nutrients and foods in specified amounts
   c. is always nutritious
   d. never affects the kcal content of a diet

5. A modification in consistency means a change in
   a. texture   c. color
   b. flavor   d. satiety value

6. A modification in energy value means a change in
   a. nutrient content   c. kcal content
   b. vitamin content   d. all of the above

7. The standard hospital diets are usually
   a. liquid, soft, regular, and light
   b. soft, light, and salt-free
   c. low fat, regular, soft, and normal
   d. liquid, soft, and diabetic

8. Regular hospital diets usually limit
   a. pastries and fried foods   c. broiled and boiled foods
   b. all fats   d. meats and meat products

9. Regular diets are based on
   a. individual doctors' prescriptions
   b. low-kcal foods only
   c. all-vegetable diets
   d. the Food Guide Pyramid

10. The light diet is
    a. always one of the standard hospital diets
    b. more restrictive than the soft diet
    c. similar to a regular diet
    d. rarely used for obese patients

11. The light diet, if used, is typically given
    a. after the full liquid diet and before the soft diet
    b. after the regular diet and before the soft diet
    c. after the soft diet and before the regular diet
    d. immediately after surgery

12. The light diet is given to
    a. newborns
    b. patients recovering from an illness
    c. patients preparing for surgery
    d. all patients over 60

13. A major difference between the regular and soft diet is the
    a. nutrient content
    b. texture of the foods
    c. energy values
    d. satiety value of the foods

14. It is not unusual for the soft diet to be
    a. ordered to precede the clear liquid diet
    b. ordered to precede the full liquid diet
    c. ordered to follow the full liquid diet
    d. used in place of the clear liquid diet

15. The soft diet is sometimes ordered for
    a. preoperative patients
    b. postoperative patients
    c. comatose patients
    d. all of these

16. The following would not be included in a soft diet:
    a. ground beef
    b. leg of lamb
    c. roast chicken
    d. baked pork chops

17. Fiber is
    a. a complete protein
    b. an indigestible carbohydrate
    c. a saturated fat
    d. an essential mineral

18. The clear liquid diet consists of liquids that
    a. prevent constipation
    b. prevent infections
    c. do not stimulate peristalis
    d. do not stimulate the pancreas glands to produce insulin

19. The clear liquid diet
    a. replaces lost body fluids
    b. provides a nutritionally adequate diet
    c. includes any food that pours
    d. is never used after surgery

20. The following group of foods would be allowed on a clear liquid diet:
    a. cream of chicken soup, coffee, and tea
    b. tomato juice, sherbet, and strained cooked cereal
    c. raspberry ice, beef bouillon, and apple juice
    d. tea, coffee, and eggnog

21. The full liquid diet
    a. is always nutritionally adequate
    b. is followed by a clear liquid diet
    c. does not include milk in any form
    d. is sometimes given to patients with acute infections

22. The clear liquid diet
    a. is given all patients with chewing difficulties
    b. may be used after surgery
    c. includes milk foods
    d. is nutritionally adequate

23. One of the reasons for giving the clear liquid diet is to
    a. rest the teeth and gums
    b. cause weight reduction
    c. activate the colon
    d. reduce peristalsis

24. Eggnog and beef bouillon are
    a. allowed on both liquid diets
    b. not allowed on either liquid diet
    c. allowed only on the clear liquid diet
    d. allowed on the full liquid diet

25. Calipers are used to measure
    a. kcal content of a diet
    b. nutrient content of a diet
    c. percentage of fat and muscle tissue
    d. serum cholesterol

B. Completion
    1. Nutritional assessment is the _____ of nutritional status.
    2. Anthropometric measurements are measurements of _____ .
    3. An example of a biochemical test might be

    _____ .

4. Clinical evaluation is the physical _____ of a patient.
5. Diet therapy means _____ with food.
6. Among hospitalized patients, loneliness, disease, and self-pity often contribute to _____ .
7. The instrument used to measure skinfold is the _____ .
8. The 24-Hour Recall or the _____ can be used to inform the diet counselor of foods the patient has recently eaten.
9. Generally, therapeutic diets have had _____ and/or _____ content increased or decreased, or the _____ modified.
10. A blood analysis is an example of a _____ .

Case Study 1

An Elderly Woman With a Bone Fracture

Mrs. J., age 75, was hospitalized after a fall at home. Initial assessment revealed a thin, pale, frail, but alert, female. X-ray results determined she had a fractured right hip and osteoporosis. Surgery was performed, and Mrs. J. had an uneventful recovery. During her two-week hospitalization, her incision was healing normally and she was increasing her ambulation progressively. She had many visitors, including her husband, grandchildren, and many friends.

However, as she approached discharge, Mrs. J. became increasingly depressed and wept often. She was listless and resisted increasing her activity level. The physician ordered a complete blood count that revealed her hemoglobin was low at 10 g/dl. As a result, she was started on an iron tablet daily.

The dietitian was asked to interview her because the nurses had identified a continual poor intake of food at meals. The dietitian obtained a diet history and noted that Mrs. J. had a limited amount of dairy products and meat in her diet. Mrs. J. stated her favorite meal consisted of toast, tea, and bananas. Further evaluation indicated that Mrs. J. had been suffering from periodontal disease for years and had not kept her dental appointments. As the disease progressed, Mrs. J. had been increasingly unable to chew meats and fresh vegetables. During her hospitalization, she was too embarrassed to discuss her needs with the nurses and simply did not eat the foods on her trays that required chewing.

Case Study Questions Based on the Nursing Process

Assess

1. What may have contributed to Mrs. J.'s developing osteoporosis?
2. What is missing from Mrs. J.'s diet that would predispose her to anemia?
3. Is Mrs. J.'s diet at home likely to be nutritionally adequate?
4. What nutrients must be increased to help Mrs. J.'s fracture heal properly?

Plan

5. What will the dietitian include in the diet plan for Mrs. J. to improve her overall nutrition?
6. What would you include in her diet plan to increase kcal while maintaining a soft, easily-chewed texture?

Implement

7. How will you teach Mrs. J. about her current nutritional needs?
8. As you work with Mrs. J. to improve her diet, how will you ensure she seeks dental follow-up?

Evaluate

9. When Mrs. J. returns to the physician for follow-up, what clinical signs will indicate that Mrs. J. is following her recommended diet?
10. If Mrs. J.'s nutritional status improves, what effect would you expect to see on her emotional well-being and general physical status?

Case Study 2

The Untruthful Patient

Dennis was a 55-year-old unemployed accountant, hospitalized with a fractured leg suffered in a fall down the basement stairs. He had had a series of jobs during his life, most of which he'd lost because of a drinking problem.

He was seriously underweight, anemic, and his potassium and thiamin levels were low. During his dietary assessment in the presence of his wife, he told the nutritionist that he regularly ate three well-balanced meals a day and drank only "in company."

His wife interrupted and said: "One meal of gin, one of rye, and one of Scotch. All in the company of yourself," and began to cry.

The nutritionist left them alone while she went to get some tea and crackers for them. She asked the nurse to join them as she discussed the need to improve

Dennis's diet and to reduce his alcohol intake. He agreed to the recommended high-kcal/high-vitamin diet and said he would be "dry from now on."

When his wife came to visit him the next day, he was intoxicated.

Case Study Questions Based on the Nursing Process

Assess
1. What probably caused Dennis's fall?
2. Was it appropriate for the nutritionist to leave them alone as she did?

Plan
3. Why was it appropriate for the nutritionist to bring the nurse into the private conversation?
4. How might Dennis have obtained the liquor he drank in the hospital?
5. What can be done to ensure that Dennis does not obtain more liquor while in the hospital?
6. How can the nurse help Dennis and his wife learn about the management of alcoholism?

Implement
7. What organizations will the nurse recommend Dennis contact?
8. How will the nurse's attitude about alcoholism affect his or her ability to help Dennis?

Evaluate
9. After contacting Alcoholics Anonymous, Dennis and his wife agreed to attend meetings. How can the nurse ensure they will go?
10. What factors will influence Dennis's recovery from drinking?

DIET AND WEIGHT CONTROL

OBJECTIVES

After studying this chapter, you should be able to
- Discuss the causes and dangers of overweight
- Discuss the causes and dangers of underweight
- Identify foods suitable for high-kcal diets and those suitable for low-kcal diets
- Adapt family menus to meet the needs of people on low-kcal or high-kcal diets

One must understand some commonly used terms before discussing weight control. Normal weight can be translated to read **average, desired,** or **standard. Normal weight** is that which is appropriate for the maintenance of good health for a particular individual at a particular time. **Overweight** is defined as weight 10 to 20 percent above average. **Obesity** is defined as excessive body fat, with weight 20 percent above average. **Underweight** is weight 10 to 15 percent below average.

Body weight is composed of fluids, organs, fat, muscle, and bones so large variation exists

among people. In addition to height, age, physical condition, heredity, sex, and general frame size (small, medium, or large) are all critical factors in determining desired weight. For example, a 6'2" man with a 44" chest, 36" long arms, and 8½" wrists will weigh more than a 6'2" man with a 40" chest, 35" long arms, and 7½" wrists because he has more body tissue. Table 18-1 gives lists of median (midpoint) weights according to age, sex, and height.

Some people can weigh more than is indicated on Table 18-1 and still be in good physical condition. Professional football players, because

Table 18-1 Median Weights for Heights and Ranges for Males and Females

Category	Age (years) or Condition	Weight (kg)	Weight (lb)	Height (cm)	Height (in)
Infants	0.0–0.5	6	13	60	24
	0.5–1.0	9	20	71	28
Children	1–3	13	29	90	35
	4–6	20	44	112	44
	7–10	28	62	132	52
Males	11–14	45	99	157	62
	15–18	66	145	176	69
	19–24	72	160	177	70
	25–50	79	174	176	70
	51+	77	170	173	68
Females	11–14	46	101	157	62
	15–18	55	120	163	64
	19–24	58	128	164	65
	25–50	63	138	163	64
	51+	65	143	160	63

Recommended Dietary Allowances 10th Edition National Academy Press, Washington, DC. 1989

of the amount of muscle they develop, are examples of this. However, when they retire and reduce their physical activity, that same muscle can change to fat. If their weights remain the same, they then will be considered overfat because the proportion of fat will have become too high. Some can weigh what Table 18-1 indicates they should weigh and yet be overfat because too great a percentage of the weight is made up of fat.

To measure body fat, a **caliper** is used. Because the fat under the skin on the stomach and the upper arm is representative of the percentage of overall body fat, it is usually measured when knowledge of the percentage of body fat is required. If it is more than 1½ inches, one is considered overweight. If it is under ½ inch, one is considered underweight.

A moderate amount of fat is a necessary component of the body. It provides stored energy, protects organs from injury, and acts as insulation. The final determination of desirable weight depends on common sense. One can usually see when one is overweight.

OVERWEIGHT AND OBESITY

Overweight is a serious health hazard. It puts extra strain on the heart, lungs, muscles, bones, and joints, and increases the susceptibility to **diabetes mellitus** and **hypertension.** It increases surgical risks, shortens the life span, causes psychosocial problems, and is associated with heart disease and some forms of cancer.

Causes

The most common cause of overweight is **energy imbalance.** People eat more than they need. Excess weight can accumulate during and after middle age because people reduce their activity and metabolism slows with age. Consequently, weight accumulates unless kcal intake is reduced. **Hypothyroidism** is a possible, but rare, cause of obesity. In this condition, the basal metabolism rate is lowered, thereby reducing the number of kcal needed for energy. Unless corrected, this can result in excess weight.

Although neither has been proven, there are two popular theories about weight loss: the **fat cell theory** and the **set point theory.**

According to the fat cell theory, obesity develops when the size of fat cells increases. When their size decreases as during a reducing diet, the individual is driven to eat in order for the fat cells to regain their former size. Therefore, it is difficult to lose weight and keep it off.

According to the set point theory, everyone has a set point or natural weight at which the body is so comfortable that it does not allow for deviation. This is said to be the reason why some people cannot lose weight below a "set point" or why, if they do, they quickly regain to that "set point."

DIETARY TREATMENT OF OVERWEIGHT AND OBESITY

Obviously, if the most common cause of overweight is overeating, the solution is to reduce one's food intake. This is seldom easy. To accomplish it, a weight-reduction (low-kcal) diet must be undertaken. For the diet to be effective, one must have a genuine desire to lose weight.

The simplest and, therefore, perhaps the best weight-reduction diet is the normal diet based on the Food Guide Pyramid, but with the kcal content controlled. If necessary, its consistency can also be adapted to meet individual needs by using a food processor or a blender.

The exchange lists provide another excellent method frequently used to healthfully control the kcal content of the diet. These lists were originally developed by the American Diabetes Association and the American Dietetic Association for the use of diabetic patients. They are organized to provide specific numbers of kcal and nutrients according to six lists and are discussed in detail in Chapter 19.

A reduction of 3500 kcal will result in a weight loss of one pound. Physicians frequently recommend that no more than two pounds of weight be lost in one week. To accomplish this, one must reduce one's weekly kcal intake by 7,000, or daily intake by 1,000. Diets should not be reduced below 1000 kcal per day or the dieter will not receive the necessary nutrients. The diet should consist of 15–20 percent protein, 45–55 percent carbohydrate, and 30 percent fat, in other words, normal proportions of nutrients, but in reduced amounts. The number of meals and snacks each day should be determined by the dieter's needs and desires, but the total number of kcal must not be exceeded.

There is no magic way of losing weight and maintaining the reduced weight, but there is a key to it. That *key is revised eating habits.* In fact, unless eating habits are truly revised, it is likely that the lost weight will be regained once the weight reduction has been accomplished because at that point the dieter may be euphoric about the weight loss and forget its cost. The cost of slimness is eating less than one might prefer.

Food Selection

The dieter must learn to "eat lean." It is useful to learn the kcal values of favorite foods, and to consider them before indulging. Kcal counting is not necessary, however, if one learns a basic list of foods that are allowed on low-kcal diets because of their low-kcal values, and anoth-

Table 18-2 Foods to Allow/Avoid on a Low-kcal Diet

Foods Allowed on a Low-kcal Diet	Foods to Avoid on a Low-kcal Diet	
skim milk, buttermilk, low-fat yogurt	cream soups	nuts
cottage cheese and other skim milk cheeses	cream sauces	jellies/jams
eggs, except prepared with fat	cream in any form	fatty meats
lean beef, lamb, veal, pork, chicken, turkey, fish	gravies	salad dressing
clear soups	rich desserts	cakes
whole grain or enriched bread as allowed by doctor	sweet drinks/sodas	cookies
vegetables should be low in carbohydrate	alcoholic beverages	pastries
fresh fruits and those canned without sugar	candy	oily fish
coffee or tea, without milk and sugar	fried foods	whole milk
salt, pepper, herbs, garlic, and onions		

er list of foods that should be avoided because of their high-kcal values (see Table 18-2). The high-kcal foods should be avoided during the diet, and except for special occasions, after the diet.

In addition, one should remember that the following foods must be used judiciously:

- cheese—1 oz natural cheese contains 80 to 100 kcal
- butter or margarine—one tablespoon contains 100 kcal
- sugar—one teaspoon contains 16 kcal
- crackers—kcal contents vary, but may run from 15 for a soda cracker to 50 for a graham cracker

Substitutions of foods with very low kcal contents should be made for those with high kcal contents whenever possible. The following are examples:

- skim milk for whole milk
- yogurt for sour cream
- lemon juice and herbs for heavy salad dressings
- fruit for rich appetizers or desserts
- consomme or bouillon instead of cream soups

- water-pack canned foods rather than those packed in oil or syrup

Generally, "diet" or "dietetic" foods are not advisable. Although these foods are more expensive than the same foods in normal packs, frequently their kcal contents are only slightly lower if at all. Diet sodas may pacify the appetite for some dieters but many cause diarrhea. Until there is certainty that artificial sweeteners are not dangerous to health, their use seems unwise. Fresh ice water or seltzer water make pleasant kcal-free drinks, and they help prevent an addiction to sodas.

Table 18-3 Low-kcal Foods That May Be Used Freely on a Weight-Loss Diet

black coffee	zucchini
plain tea or tea with lemon	cauliflower
	broccoli
cantaloupe	celery
strawberries	cucumbers
lettuce	red and green peppers
cabbage	bean sprouts
asparagus	mushrooms
tomatoes	spinach

Some foods that can be eaten with relative disregard for kcal content (provided they are served without additional kcal-rich ingredients) are listed in Table 18-3.

Cooking Methods

Cooking methods should be considered. Broiling, baking, roasting, poaching, or boiling are the preferred methods because they do not require the addition of fat, as frying does. Skimming of fat from the tops of soups, meat dishes, and vegetables reduces their fat content as does trimming fat from meats before cooking. The addition of extra butter or margarine to foods should be avoided.

Patience and encouragement are needed throughout the ordeal of the diet. Temptation is everywhere, and the dieter should be forewarned.

Just one piece of chocolate cake could set the diet back for half a day (400 to 500 kcal) and lower resistance to future temptation. Breaking the diet one day will make it seem easy to break it a second day, and so on. Fresh vegetables and drinks of water may be used to harmlessly prevent or assuage the hunger pains that are bound to appear. A short walk or a few minutes of exercise may help to turn the dieter's thoughts from food. Sample menus for a low-kcal diet are shown in Table 18-4.

Exercise

Exercise, particularly aerobic exercise, is an excellent adjunct to any weight-loss program. Aerobic exercise uses energy from the body's fat reserves as it increases the amount of oxygen the body takes in. Examples are dancing, jogging,

Table 18-4 Sample Menus for a Low-kcal Diet—1200 Calories

Breakfast	Dinner	Lunch or Supper
Orange Juice ($\frac{1}{2}$ cup = 50 kcal)	Half Grapefruit (40 kcal)	Sliced Chicken
Poached Egg (80 kcal)	Lean Roast Beef	($\frac{1}{2}$ breast = 3 oz at 140 kcal)
Whole Wheat Toast	(3 oz = 200 kcal)	Asparagus on Lettuce
(1 sl = 75 kcal)	Baked Potato (100 kcal)	(4 spears = 10 kcal
Margarine (1 tsp = 33 kcal)	Cooked Carrots	+ lettuce leaves at 5 kcal) with
Skim Milk ($\frac{1}{2}$ cup = 45 kcal)	($\frac{1}{2}$ cup = 35 kcal)	Cottage Cheese (2 oz = 50 kcal)
Black Coffee	Lettuce and Tomato Salad	Bread (1 sl = 75 kcal)
	($\frac{1}{8}$ head lettuce = 8 kcal	Margarine (1 tsp. = 33 kcal)
	$\frac{1}{2}$ tomato = 15 kcal)	Cantaloupe ($\frac{1}{2}$ melon = 50 kcal)
	Bread	Black Coffee or Tea
	($\frac{1}{2}$ sl = 35 kcal)	
	Margarine	
	(1 tsp = 33 kcal)	
	Strawberries	
	(1 cup fresh = 55 kcal)	
	Skim Milk	
	($\frac{1}{2}$ cup = 45 kcal)	
	Black Coffee or Tea	

bicycling, skiing, rowing, and power walking. Such exercise helps tone the muscles, burns kcal, increases the BMR so food is burned faster, and is fun for the participant. Any exercise program must begin slowly and increase over time so no physical damage occurs.

Exercise alone can only rarely replace the actual diet, however. The dieter should be made aware of the number of kcal burned by specific exercises so as to avoid overeating after the workout. See Table 2-2, giving numbers of kcal required for specific activities.

Helpful Tips for Those on Weight Loss Diets

1. Record food for two weeks before diet. Figure kcal and circle those items that could easily have been avoided.
2. Plan your weight-loss diet to include some favorite foods.
3. Weigh regularly (for example, once a week) but do not weigh yourself daily.
4. Don't wait too long between meals. Allow kcal for snacks.
5. Watch size of portions.
6. Join a support group and go to meetings, if necessary, during and after the weight loss.
7. Eat slowly.
8. Use small plates.
9. Use low-kcal garnishes.
10. Eat whole, fresh foods. Avoid processed foods.
11. Treat yourself with something other than food.
12. Anticipate problems (e.g., banquets and holidays). "Undereat" slightly before and after.
13. "Save" some kcal for treats later.
14. If something goes wrong, don't punish yourself by eating.
15. If there is no weight loss for one week, begin a new food diary and evaluate your diet honestly.
16. As you near your goal, keep a diary and indicate adjustments for your new regimen of no further loss, but no gain either.
17. Write a lifetime diet plan to use after the weight loss. Allow for special occasions and treats.
18. If a binge does occur, don't punish yourself by continuing the binge. Stop it! Go for a walk, to a movie, to a museum. Call a friend.
19. Adapt family meals to suit your needs. Don't make a production of your diet. Avoid the heavy kcal items. Limit yourself to a spoonful of something too rich for a weight-loss diet. Substitute something you like that is low in kcal.

Fad Diets

Many of the countless fad reducing diets regularly published in magazines and books are **crash-reducing diets.** This means they are intended to cause a very rapid rate of weight reduction. Often **fad diets** require the purchase of expensive foods. Others are part of a weight-loss plan including exercise with special equipment. Expensive food items and equipment can add to the burden of dieting.

A crash diet usually does result in an initial rapid weight loss. However, the weight loss is thought to be caused by a loss of body water rather than body fat. Sudden weight loss of this type is followed by a **plateau period,** that is, a period in which weight does not decrease. Disillusionment is apt to occur during this period and may cause the dieter to go on an "eating binge." This can result in regaining the weight that was lost and sometimes more. This in turn causes the dieter to try another weight loss diet, creating a **yo-yo effect.**

Some popular reducing diets severely limit the foods allowed, providing a real danger of nutrient deficiencies over time, and their restricted nature makes them boring. Some provide too much cholesterol and fat, contributing to atherosclerosis. Some contain an excess of protein, which puts too great a demand on the kidneys. The powdered varieties of weight-loss diets available are not only expensive and inconvenient (if one is not at home to prepare them), they can be life threatening if they fail to supply sufficient potassium for the heart.

These diets ultimately fail because they defeat the dual purpose of the dieter, which is to lose weight and prevent its returning. To accomplish both, eating habits must be changed and crash diets do not do this.

Surgical Treatment of Obesity

When obesity becomes **morbid** (damaging health), and the individual lacks the self-control to reduce weight by dieting, surgery could be indicated. Two of the surgical procedures used for this include the **jejunoileal bypass** and the **gastric bypass.** In the former, the **jejunum** (the middle section of the small intestine) is surgically attached to a small section of the **ileum** (the last part of the small intestine). This results in fewer nutrients being absorbed and consequent loss of weight.

Some obese people think that such a procedure would be their salvation, believing that following it, they could eat as much as they wanted and still lose weight. It may not be salvation. Common complications of this type of surgery include diarrhea and consequent electrolyte and fluid imbalances, liver problems, kidney stones, and bone disease—the last probably caused by reduced absorption of minerals and vitamins.

Gastric bypass is a procedure in which the stomach is stapled so that it is reduced in size. This reduced stomach capacity reduces the amounts of food that can be eaten. Post-surgery complications (nausea and vomiting) are fewer than with jejunoileal bypass surgery, but there is comparatively less weight lost.

Pharmaceutical Treatment of Obesity

Amphetamines (pep pills) have been prescribed for the treatment of obesity because they depress the appetite. However, it has been learned that their effectiveness is reduced within a relatively short time. The dosage must be regularly increased; they cause nervousness and insomnia; and they can become habit-forming. Consequently, they are rarely prescribed now. Over-the-counter diet pills are available. They are intended to reduce appetite but are not thought to be effective. In addition to caffeine and artificial sweeteners, they contain **phenylpropanolamine** that can damage blood vessels and should be avoided.

Some people believe that **diuretics** (medications that cause frequent urination) and laxatives promote weight loss. They do, but only of water. They do not cause a reduction of body fat, which is what the dieter is seeking. An excess of either could be dangerous because of possible upsets in fluid and electrolyte balance. In addition, laxatives can become habit-forming. They should not be used on any frequent or regular basis without the supervision of a physician.

UNDERWEIGHT

Dangers

Underweight can cause complications of pregnancy and various nutritional deficiencies. It may lower one's resistance to infections and, if carried to the extreme, can cause death.

Causes

Underweight can be caused by inadequate consumption of nutritious food because of depression, disease, anorexia nervosa, bulimia, or poverty. It also can be caused by excessive activity, the tissue wasting of certain diseases, poor absorption of nutrients, infection, or **hyperthyroidism** (a condition in which the basal metabolism rate is increased and consequently the number of kcal needed for energy is increased; unless corrected, it usually results in weight loss). For further discussion of anorexia nervosa and bulimia, see Chapter 14.

Treatment

Underweight is treated by a high-kcal diet, or by a high-kcal diet combined with psychological counseling if the condition is psychological in origin as, for example, in depression or anorexia nervosa. In many cases, a high-kcal diet will be met with resistance. It can be as difficult for an underweight person to gain weight as it is for an overweight person to lose it.

The diet should be based on the Food Guide Pyramid so it can be easily adapted from the

---

Table 18-5 Sample Menus for a High-kcal Diet—3000 Calories

Breakfast	Dinner	Lunch or Supper
Orange Juice (1 cup = 100 kcal)	Sirloin Steak (4 oz = 320 kcal)	Grapefruit Juice ($\frac{1}{2}$ cup = 50 kcal)
Oatmeal (1 cup = 130 kcal) with Milk and Sugar ($\frac{1}{2}$ cup whole milk = 80 kcal + 2 tbsp sugar = 90 kcal)	Baked Potato (100 kcal) with Margarine* (1 tbsp = 100 kcal)	Lamb Chop (150 kcal)
Soft Cooked Egg (80 kcal)	Lima beans ($\frac{1}{2}$ cup = 90 kcal)	Mashed Potatoes ($\frac{3}{4}$ cup = 145 kcal)
Bacon (2 sl = 65 kcal)	Lettuce and Tomato Salad ($\frac{1}{8}$ head lettuce = 8 kcal + $\frac{1}{2}$ tomato at 20 kcal)	Cooked Carrots ($\frac{1}{2}$ cup = 35 kcal)
Whole Wheat Toast (1 sl = 75 kcal) with Margarine* (2 tsp = 66 kcal)	Salad Dressing* (1 tbsp commercial "French" type = 65 kcal)	Celery-Apple Salad (1 stalk celery = 5 kcal + $\frac{1}{2}$ apple at 35 kcal + 1 tbsp mayonnaise at 100 kcal)
Coffee with Milk and Sugar (2 tbsp milk = 20 kcal + 1 tbsp sugar = 45 kcal)	Roll and Margarine* (200 kcal)	Bread and Margarine (125 kcal)
	Chocolate Ice Cream ($\frac{1}{2}$ cup = 160 kcal)	Baked Apple (small apple = 80 kcal + 2 tbsp sugar at 90 kcal)
	Coffee	Milk (160 kcal)
		Coffee or Tea
Snack		**Snack**
$\frac{1}{2}$ cup Milk (80 kcal) 1 Cookie (100 kcal)		$\frac{1}{2}$ cup Milk (80 kcal) 2 Graham Crackers (55 kcal)

*If patient tolerates the fat.

regular, family menus, or to a soft textured diet. The total number of kcal prescribed per day will vary from person to person, depending on the person's activity, age, size, sex, and physical condition.

If the individual is to gain one pound a week, 3500 kcal in addition to the individual's basic normal weekly kcal requirement are prescribed. This means an extra 500 kcal must be taken in each day. If two pounds of weight gain per week are required, an additional 7000 kcal each week, or an addition of 1000 kcal each day are necessary. This diet cannot be immediately accepted at full kcal value. Time will be needed to gradually increase the daily kcal value. In this diet, there is an increased intake of foods rich in carbohydrates, some fats, and proteins. Vitamins and minerals are supplied in adequate amounts. If there are deficiencies of some vitamins and minerals, supplements are prescribed.

Nearly all nutritious foods are allowed in the high-kcal diet, but easily digested foods (carbohydrates) are recommended (see Table 18-5). Because an excess of fat can be distasteful and spoil the appetite, fatty foods must be used with discretion. Fried foods are not recommended. Bulky foods should be used sparingly. Bulk takes up stomach space that could be better used for more concentrated, higher kcal foods.

Those requiring this diet frequently have poor appetites so meals should be made especially appetizing. Favorite foods should be served, and portions of all foods should be small to avoid discouraging the patients. Many of the extra kcal needed may be consumed as snacks between meals, unless these snacks reduce the patient's appetite for meals and consequently reduce the total kcal intake. In some cases, the patient may consume more kcal each day if the number of meals is reduced, thereby increasing the appetite for each meal served. When the causes of underweight are psychological, therapy is required before the diet is begun, and the diet counselor and therapist may well need to consult one another before and during treatment. Foods to be avoided in a high-kcal diet are foods the patient dislikes, fatty foods, and bulky, low-kcal foods.

CONSIDERATIONS FOR THE HEALTH CARE PROFESSIONAL

Even for the most determined patients, a successful weight-loss program will be charged with anxiety. There will be days of disappointment. It will take a long time to reach the ultimate goal. The health care professional will need to supply psychological support and nutritional advice. There may be times when sympathy over disappointing results will be the most important thing the health care professional could offer the dieter. It is essential that the health care professional see the problems, sympathize with the patient, and then effectively lead her or him back to the diet. The key word for the health care professional is *support*.

SUMMARY

Excessive weight endangers health and should be lost by the use of a restricted-kcal diet based on the Food Guide Pyramid. Such a diet helps the dieter revise eating habits and avoid regaining the lost weight. Excess weight is usually caused by energy imbalance. Exercise is beneficial to weight-loss regimens but rarely can replace the restricted-kcal diet. Fad diets are expensive, boring, and conducive to nutritional deficiencies. They ultimately fail because they do not revise eating habits. Underweight is also dangerous to health, psychological counseling as well as a high-kcal diet may be required for proper treatment.

Discussion Topics

1. Discuss *overweight, obesity,* and *underweight.* Tell how someone may be overweight according to the height/weight charts and still be considered to be in good physical condition. What factors contribute to the determination of one's correct weight?
2. What are some causes of overweight? Discuss why some people eat more than they need. Discuss how this can be prevented or changed.
3. Explain why revised eating habits are essential to an effective weight-loss program.
4. Describe three cooking methods that are preferred for people on low-kcal diets, and explain why they are preferred.
5. Name ten foods that should be avoided during a weight-loss program. Tell why.
6. Name ten foods that may be used without concern as to kcal during a weight-loss program. Explain why.
7. In addition to its high kcal content, how could a slice of chocolate cake be detrimental to a weight-loss diet?
8. Describe the use of exercise during a weight-loss program. Could it be used in lieu of the diet? Why?
9. Describe one or two popular reducing diets. Could such a diet have any effect on the nutrition of those people who subscribe to it? If so, what? Ask if anyone in the class has used such a diet. If so, ask that person to describe the diet, the physical effects felt during the diet, and the ultimate result.
10. Explain why a high-kcal diet could be unpleasant for a patient.
11. Discuss the causes and dangers of underweight.

Suggested Activities

1. Using Table A-5 in the Appendix, look for kcal values of ten favorite foods. Make two lists. On the left, list which of the ten foods would be suitable for a high-kcal diet. On the right, list those foods suitable for a low-kcal diet.
2. Make a list of foods eaten yesterday. Circle those foods that would not be suitable for a low-kcal diet. Explain why.
3. Find recipes that are suitable for the high-kcal diet and others that are suitable for the low-kcal diet. Add these to the special diet recipe file.
4. Adapt a sample menu for the 1200-kcal diet in this chapter to make it suitable for a regular 2400-kcal diet. Adapt it for a high-kcal diet (3000 kcal). Use Table A-5 in the Appendix for kcal values of foods.
5. Plan a day's menu for a 1200-kcal diet. Compare menus with other class members and correct them if necessary. Adapt them for a 3000-kcal diet.

6. Prepare at least one of the meals on the planned menu and evaluate it in terms of nutritive content, flavor, aroma, color, shape, appearance, texture, and satiety value, as well as kcal value.

A. Multiple choice. Select the *letter* that precedes the best answer.

1. The general type of foods that should be avoided in the high-kcal diet are
   a. fatty foods
   b. foods the patient likes
   c. breads and cereals
   d. coffee and tea

2. In the high-kcal diet, the energy value
   a. is increased
   b. is decreased
   c. is reduced to minimal levels
   d. remains the same as on the regular diet

3. The low-kcal diet may be prescribed for
   a. obesity
   b. anorexia nervosa
   c. hyperthyroidism
   d. severe allergies

4. In the low-kcal diet, the energy value
   a. remains the same as for the regular diet
   b. is decreased
   c. is increased
   d. should equal that of the clear liquid diet

5. A proper weight reduction plan allows for loss of
   a. 1 to 2 pounds per day
   b. 1 to 2 pounds per week
   c. 3 to 5 pounds per week
   d. 15 to 20 pounds per month

6. Popular crash-reducing diets
   a. are always effective and totally harmless
   b. are useful for teenagers
   c. result in a slow, even loss of weight
   d. are potentially hazardous

7. Normal weight
   a. is always the same for two people of the same sex and height
   b. does not change during one's lifetime
   c. may be greater than the amounts indicated on the height/weight charts in some cases
   d. all of the above

8. A caliper is used
   a. to measure the amount of weight to be lost
   b. to determine the percentage of body fat
   c. to determine the percentage of bone tissue
   d. only in cases of gross obesity

9. The most common cause of overweight is
   a. hypothyroidism
   b. hyperthyroidism
   c. energy imbalance
   d. all of the above

10. The dysfunction of the thyroid gland in which the basal metabolism rate is lowered and the need for kcal is reduced is called
   a. hypothyroidism
   b. hyperthyroidism
   c. energy imbalance
   d. none of the above

11. The dysfunction of the thyroid gland in which the basal metabolism rate is raised and the need for kcal is increased is called
   a. hypothyroidism
   b. hyperthyroidism
   c. energy imbalance
   d. either a or b

12. To lose two pounds per week, one's weekly kcal intake must be reduced by
   a. 500
   b. 1000
   c. 3500
   d. 7000

13. To lose one pound per week, one's weekly kcal intake must be reduced by
   a. 500
   b. 1000
   c. 3500
   d. 7000

14. The "key" to losing weight and maintaining the reduced weight is
   a. skipping lunch
   b. fasting one day each week
   c. revising eating habits
   d. assiduously counting kcal each meal

15. Strawberries, yogurt, poached egg, and whole wheat toast would
   a. be allowed on a kcal-restricted diet
   b. not be allowed on a low-kcal diet
   c. constitute a poor breakfast for someone on a high-kcal diet
   d. not be a nutritious breakfast for someone on a weight-controlled diet

16. Baking, roasting, broiling, boiling, and poaching are recommended for
   a. low-kcal diets only
   b. high-kcal diets only
   c. both high- and low-kcal diets
   d. none of the above

17. Large green salads with creamy dressings are
   a. recommended for low-kcal diets
   b. recommended for high-kcal diets
   c. recommended for either low- or high-kcal diets
   d. not recommended for either low- or high-kcal diets

18. Fad diets are not recommended as reducing diets because they
    a. usually cause illness
    b. alter eating habits excessively
    c. do not alter eating habits
    d. require an excessive amount of time before weight loss occurs
19. The jejunoileal bypass
    a. prevents food from reaching the large intestine
    b. reduces the stomach capacity
    c. reduces the absorption capacity of the small intestine
    d. is highly recommended for obese patients
20. Amphetamines are
    a. an excellent method of maintaining a depressed appetite
    b. interchangeable with diuretics
    c. frequently used today
    d. dangerously habit forming

B. Complete the following statements.
    1. The high-kcal diet is one in which the energy value is _____ .
    2. The patient requiring a _____ -kcal diet usually has a poor appetite; therefore, serving sizes should be _____ .
    3. When the thyroid gland is overactive and raises the metabolism rate, the condition is called _____ .
    4. The diet ordered for a patient with an overactive thyroid gland is the _____ .
    5. Bulky foods such as fresh fruits and vegetables are usually advisable for _____ -kcal diets.
    6. A type of milk recommended for patients on the low-kcal diet is _____ or _____ .
    7. Steak, lima beans, and ice cream are examples of food allowed on the _____ -kcal diet.
    8. Lean meat, strawberries, and skim milk are examples of foods recommended for the _____ -kcal diet.
    9. Underweight caused by anorexia nervosa will probably require _____ in addition to a high-kcal diet.
    10. The surgical procedure used to reduce stomach capacity is called the _____ .

Case Study 1

Marilyn E. was finding it increasingly difficult to breathe after any sort of exertion. Her knees were giving her a great deal of pain and she was ashamed of her shape. She was 5′6″, of medium build, and weighed 180 pounds. Her friend convinced her to see a doctor. The doctor examined her and advised her to lose 60 pounds. He told her that her breathing would be easier and her knees should give her no trouble if she were lighter. The doctor put her on a low-kcal diet.

Marilyn could not understand why she was heavy. She never ate breakfast—"just coffee and Danish after I get to the office." Furthermore, she did not always eat lunch, but usually had coffee and doughnuts with the people in her office around 4 P.M. Dinner was usually a sandwich at the local coffee shop where they baked delicious pies. She admitted to sometimes having more than one slice. She said she seldom snacked on anything except cookies and soda. Marilyn's favorite activity was watching TV.

Case Study Questions Based on the Nursing Process

Assess

1. How many pounds a week has Marilyn probably been told to lose?
2. How long should she expect this to take?
3. How many kcal each day will she have to omit from her diet?
4. Approximately how many kcal did Marilyn probably ingest each day on her pre-diet regimen?
5. What should Marilyn's first step be in beginning her diet?

Plan

6. When Marilyn visits her parents, they always have her favorite meal— leg of lamb with gravy, mashed potatoes, lima beans, coleslaw, and apple pie with whipped cream and pecans. How many kcal would an average-sized meal of these foods total? What can Marilyn say to her parents?

Implement

7. How can Marilyn improve her breakfast habits?
8. How can Marilyn improve her lunch habits? She does not feel she has a great deal of money.
9. What should Marilyn be told about her evening meal? Her snacks?
10. What snacks could Marilyn have on her low-kcal diet? Why?
11. Will Marilyn ever be able to eat her favorite apple pie again?
12. Marilyn admits that while she likes meats and vegetables, she does not know how to cook. What advice can she be given?
13. Plan a week's menu for Marilyn who is on a 1200-kcal diet. What questions should Marilyn be asked before the menus are planned? Why?

Evaluate

14. When Marilyn returns for a one-month checkup, how many pounds should she have lost?
15. As Marilyn discusses her new diet, what will indicate that she has accepted the changes?

Case Study 2   *Overweight*

Charles was a 6-foot tall, 40-year-old lawyer with a medium frame who weighed 250 pounds. He visited his physician because he needed a statement of good health to purchase a life insurance policy.

After examining him and discussing his lifestyle and eating habits, his doctor told him he was lucky. His cholesterol was 250 mg, and he was 75 pounds overweight.

Case Study Questions Based on the Nursing Process

Assess
1. Why did the doctor say Charles was lucky?
2. What should Charles weigh, and what would his normal cholesterol range be?

Plan
3. What type of diet(s) is the doctor likely to recommend?
4. How might Charles' lifestyle have to be adapted for him to lose the weight the doctor recommended?

Implement
5. How long should Charles expect it will take him to lose 75 pounds?
6. How might an exercise program help Charles' weight-loss program?

Evaluate
7. How might this weight loss affect Charles' cholesterol count?
8. After one year, Charles had lost 50 pounds and his cholesterol was 212 mg. Is this an appropriate and healthy rate of weight loss? Explain.

DIET AND DIABETES MELLITUS

OBJECTIVES

After studying this chapter, you should be able to
- Describe diabetes mellitus and identify the types
- Describe the symptoms of diabetes mellitus
- Explain the relationship of insulin to diabetes mellitus
- Discuss appropriate nutritional management of diabetes mellitus

Diabetes mellitus is the name for a group of serious and **chronic** (long standing) disorders affecting the metabolism of energy nutrients. These disorders are characterized by **hyperglycemia** (abnormally large amounts of sugar in the blood). Diabetes mellitus afflicts between 10 and 12 million people in the United States. It is a major cause of death; blindness; heart and kidney disease; amputations of toes, feet, and legs; and infections.

Hundreds of years ago a Greek physician named it "diabetes," which meant "to flow through," because of the large amounts of urine generated by victims. Later, the Latin word, "mellitus," which means "honeyed," was added because of the amount of sugar in the urine.

Diabetes insipidus is a different disorder. It also generates large amounts of urine, but it is "insipid," not sweet. This is a rare condition, caused by a damaged pituitary gland. It is not discussed in this chapter.

The body needs a constant supply of energy, and glucose is its primary source. Carbohydrates provide most of the glucose, but about 10 percent of fats and up to nearly 60 percent of proteins can be converted to glucose if necessary.

For the maintenance of good health, the distribution of glucose must be carefully managed. It is transported by the blood, and its entry into the cells is controlled by **hormones.** The primary hormone in this work is **insulin.**

Insulin is secreted by the beta cells of the islets of Langerhans in the pancreas gland. When there is inadequate production of insulin or the body is unable to use the insulin it produces, glucose cannot enter the cells. This causes glucose to accumulate in the blood creating hyperglycemia.

Another hormone, **glucagon,** which is secreted by the alpha cells of the islets of Langerhans, helps release energy when needed by converting glycogen to glucose. **Somatostatin** is a hormone produced by the delta cells of the islets of Langerhans and the hypothalamus. It is thought to participate in the regulation of insulin secretion.

The amount of glucose in the blood normally rises after a meal. The **pancreas** reacts by providing insulin. As the insulin circulates in the blood, it binds to special insulin receptors on cell surfaces. This causes the cells to accept the glucose and amino acids and fats so they can be converted to energy. This results in a reduced amount of glucose in the blood that in turn signals the pancreas to stop sending insulin.

When the cells are unable to accept and use glucose, fats, and amino acids, their concentration increases in the blood. These accumulations can cause serious complications.

SYMPTOMS OF DIABETES MELLITUS

The abnormal concentration of nutrients in the blood of diabetic patients draws water from the cells to the blood. When hyperglycemia exceeds the **renal threshold** (kidneys' capacity to reabsorb the glucose), the glucose is excreted in the urine (**glycosuria**). With the loss of the cellular fluid, the patient experiences **polyuria** (excessive urination), and **polydipsia** (unusual thirst) typically results.

This inability to metabolize energy nutrients causes the body to break down its own tissue for protein and fat. This causes **polyphagia** (excessive appetite) but at the same time a loss of weight, weakness, and fatigue occur. The body's use of protein from its own tissue causes it to excrete nitrogen.

Because the diabetic patient cannot use carbohydrates for energy, excessive amounts of fats are broken down. This causes the liver to produce **ketones** from the fatty acids. In healthy people, ketones are subsequently broken down to carbon dioxide and water, yielding energy. In diabetic patients, fats break down faster than the body can handle them. Ketones collect in the blood (**ketonemia**) and must be excreted in the urine (**ketonuria**). Ketones are acids that lower blood pH, causing **acidosis.** Acidosis can lead to **diabetic coma,** which can result in death if the patient is not treated quickly with fluids and insulin.

In addition to the symptoms previously mentioned, diabetic patients also suffer from diseases of the **vascular system. Atherosclerosis** (condition in which there is a heavy buildup of fatty substances inside artery walls, reducing blood flow) is a major cause of death among diabetic patients. Nerve damage (**neuropathy**) is not uncommon, and infections, particularly of the urinary tract, are frequent problems.

ETIOLOGY

The **etiology** (cause) of diabetes mellitus is not confirmed. Although it appears that diabetes mellitus is hereditary, environmental factors also may contribute to its occurrence. For example, viruses or obesity may precipitate the disease in people who have a **genetic predisposition.**

The World Health Organization indicates that the prevalence of the disease is increasing worldwide, especially in areas showing improvement in living standards.

CLASSIFICATION

The two major types of diabetes mellitus are **Type I,** which is also known as **insulin dependent diabetes mellitus (IDDM),** and **Type II,** also known as **non-insulin dependent diabetes mellitus (NIDDM).**

Type I was formerly classified as juvenile-onset diabetes mellitus. It occurs between the ages of 1 and 40, and includes from 10 to 20 percent of all diabetes cases. These patients secrete little, if any insulin and thus become insulin dependent, requiring both insulin injections and a carefully controlled diet. This type of diabetes occurs suddenly, exhibiting many of the symptoms described in the preceding section. It can be difficult to control.

Type II was previously called adult-onset diabetes. It is less severe than Type I. It usually occurs after the age of 40. Its onset is gradual as the amount of insulin produced each day gradually diminishes. It is not uncommon for the patient to have no symptoms and to be totally ignorant of her or his condition until it is discovered accidentally during a routine urine or blood test. This type of diabetes can usually be controlled by diet, or diet and oral **hypoglycemic agents.** Hypoglycemic agents stimulate the pancreas to produce insulin. Approximately 80 percent of Type II patients are overweight. Consequently, these patients are typically placed on weight-reduction diets until their weights reach an acceptable level.

Gestational diabetes is the form of Type II diabetes mellitus that can occur in obese patients during the last trimester of pregnancy. Concentrated sugars should be avoided. Weight gain should continue but not in excessive amounts. Usually, it disappears after the infant is born. However, diabetes mellitus can develop five to ten years after the pregnancy. (See Chapter 12.)

Secondary diabetes mellitus occurs infrequently and is caused by certain drugs or by a disease of the pancreas.

TREATMENT OF DIABETES MELLITUS

The treatment of diabetes mellitus is intended to:

1. Control blood glucose levels
2. Provide optimal nourishment for the patient
3. Prevent symptoms and thus delay the complications of the disease

Treatment is typically begun when blood tests indicate hyperglycemia or when other previously discussed symptoms occur. Normal blood glucose levels are from about 70 to 120 mg per dl.

Treatment can be by diet alone or by a diet combined with insulin or a hypoglycemic agent plus regulated exercise and the regular monitoring of the patient's blood glucose levels.

The physician and diet counselor can provide essential testing, information, and counseling, and help the patient delay potential damage. The ultimate responsibility, however, rests with the patient. If he or she eats carelessly, forgets insulin, ignores symptoms, and neglects appropriate blood tests, the health care professionals cannot repair the damage.

NUTRITIONAL MANAGEMENT OF DIABETES MELLITUS

The counselor will need to know the patient's diet history, food likes and dislikes, and lifestyle at the onset. The patient's kcal needs will depend on age, activities, lean body mass, size, REE, and, if prescribed, amount of insulin.

It is recommended that carbohydrates provide 50 to 55 percent of the kcal. Approximately 40 to 50 percent of this should be from complex carbohydrates (starches). This is important because complex carbohydrates break down more slowly than do simple sugars so the glucose they provide is released over time. The remaining 5 to 15 percent of carbohydrates can be from simple sugars.

Fats should be limited to 30 percent of total kcal and proteins should provide from 15 to 20 percent of total kcal. Lean protein foods are advisable because they contain limited amounts of fats.

Regardless of the percentages of energy nutrients prescribed, the foods ultimately eaten should provide sufficient vitamins and minerals as well as energy nutrients.

The patient with *IDDM* needs a nutritional plan that balances kcal and nutrient needs with insulin therapy and exercise. It is important that meals and snacks are composed of similar nutri-

ents and kcal and eaten at regular times each day. Smaller meals plus two to three snacks may be more helpful in maintaining steady blood glucose levels for these patients than three large meals each day.

The IDDM patient should anticipate the possibility of missing meals occasionally and carry a few crackers to provide sufficient carbohydrate to prevent **hypoglycemia** (low blood sugar), which can occur in such a circumstance.

The patient with *NIDDM* may be overweight. The nutritional goal for this patient is not only to keep blood glucose levels in the normal range but to lose weight as well. Exercise can help attain both goals.

Diets Based on Exchange Lists

The method of diet therapy most commonly used for diabetic patients is that based on the **exchange lists.** These lists were developed by the American Diabetes Association in conjunction with the American Dietetic Association and are summarized in Table 19-1 and included completely in Table 19-2.

Table 19-1 Summary of Exchange Lists

Food Group		kcal	Carbohydrates	Proteins	Fats
Starch/ Bread Exchanges		80	15 g	3 g	trace
Meats					
Lean	1 oz	55		7	3 g
Medium Fat	1 oz	75		7	5 g
High Fat	1 oz	100		7	8 g
Vegetables		25	5 g	2	
Fruits		60	15 g		
Milk					
Skim	1 cup	90	12 g	8	trace
Low Fat	1 cup	120	12 g	8	5 g
Whole	1 cup	150	12 g	8	8 g
Fat		45			5 g

Table 19-2 Exchange Lists for Meal Planning

STARCH/BREAD EXCHANGES: Each item on this list contains 15 grams of carbohydrate, 3 grams of protein, a trace of fat, and 80 calories. One exchange is equal to any of the following items:

Cereals/Grains/Pasta:

Bran cereals, concentrated	$\frac{1}{3}$ cup
Bran cereals, flaked	$\frac{1}{2}$ cup
(such as Bran Buds, All Bran)	
Bulgar (cooked)	$\frac{1}{2}$ cup
Cooked cereals	$\frac{1}{2}$ cup
Cornmeal (dry)	$2\frac{1}{2}$ tbsp
Grapenuts	3 tbsp
Grits (cooked)	$\frac{1}{2}$ cup
Other ready-to-eat	$\frac{3}{4}$ cup
unsweetened cereals	
Pasta (cooked)	$\frac{1}{2}$ cup
Puffed cereal	$1\frac{1}{2}$ cup
Rice, white or brown	$\frac{1}{3}$ cup
(cooked)	
Shredded wheat	$\frac{1}{2}$ cup
Wheat germ	3 tbsp

Dried Beans/Peas/Lentils:

Beans and peas (cooked)	$\frac{1}{3}$ cup
(such as kidney, white,	
split, blackeye)	
Lentils	$\frac{1}{3}$ cup
Baked beans	$\frac{1}{4}$ cup

Starchy Vegetables:

Corn	$\frac{1}{2}$ cup
Corn on cob, 6 in. long	1
Lima beans	$\frac{1}{2}$ cup
Peas, green (canned or	$\frac{1}{2}$ cup
frozen)	
Plantain	$\frac{1}{2}$ cup
Potato, baked	1 small (3 oz)
Potato, mashed	$\frac{1}{2}$ cup
Squash, winter (acorn,	$\frac{3}{4}$ cup
butternut)	
Yam, sweet potato, plain	$\frac{1}{3}$ cup

Bread:

Bagel	$\frac{1}{2}$ (1 oz)
Bread sticks, crisp,	2 ($\frac{2}{3}$ oz)
4 in. long $\times$ $\frac{1}{2}$ in.	
Croutons, low fat	1 cup
English muffin	$\frac{1}{2}$
Frankfurter or hamburger bun	$\frac{1}{2}$ (1 oz)
Pita, 6 in. across	$\frac{1}{2}$
Plain roll, small	1 (1 oz)
Raisin, unfrosted	1 slice (1 oz)
Rye, pumpernickel	1 slice (1 oz)
Tortilla, 6 in. across	1
White (including French	1 slice (1 oz)
Italian)	
Whole wheat	1 slice (1 oz)

Crackers/Snacks:

Animal crackers	8
Graham crackers, $2\frac{1}{2}$ in.	3
square	
Matzoth	$\frac{3}{4}$ oz
Melba toast	5 slices
Oyster crackers	24
Popcorn (popped, no fat	3 cups
added)	
Pretzels	$\frac{3}{4}$ oz
Rye crisp, 2 in $\times$ $3\frac{1}{2}$ in.	4
Saltine-type crackers	6
Whole wheat crackers	2–4 slices
no fat added (crisp	($\frac{3}{4}$ oz)
breads, such as Finn,	
Kavli, Wasa)	

Starch Foods Prepared With Fat:
(Count as 1 starch/bread serving, plus 1 fat serving.)

Biscuit, $2\frac{1}{2}$ in. across	1
Chow mein noodles	$\frac{1}{2}$ cup
Corn bread, 2 in. cube	1 (2 oz)
Cracker, round butter type	6
French fried potatoes,	10
2 in. to $3\frac{1}{2}$ in. long	($1\frac{1}{2}$ oz)
Muffin, plain, small	1
Pancake, 4 in. across	2
Stuffing, bread (prepared)	$\frac{1}{4}$ cup
Taco shell, 6 in. across	2
Waffle, $4\frac{1}{2}$ in. square	1
Whole wheat crackers,	4–6 (1 oz)
fat added (such as Triscuits)	

Table 19-2 (*Continued*)

MEAT LIST

Lean Meat and Substitutes:

Each item on this list contains 7 grams of protein, 3 grams of fat, and 55 calories. One exchange is equal to any one of the following items:

Beef:	USDA Good or Choice grades of lean beef, such as round, sirloin, and flank steak; tenderloin; chipped beef	1 oz
Pork:	Lean pork, such as fresh ham; canned, cured, or boiled ham; Canadian bacon; tenderloin	1 oz
Veal:	All cuts are lean except for veal cutlets (ground or cubed). Examples of lean are chops and roasts.	1 oz
Poultry:	Chicken, turkey, cornish hen (without skin)	1 oz
Fish:	All fresh and frozen fish	1 oz
	Crab, lobster, scallops, shrimp, clams (fresh or canned in water)	2 oz
	Oysters	6 medium
	Tuna (canned in water)	$\frac{1}{4}$ cup
	Herring (uncreamed or smoked)	1 oz
	Sardines (canned)	2 medium
Wild Game:	Venison, rabbit, squirrel	1 oz
	Pheasant, duck, goose (without skin)	1 oz
Cheese:	Any cottage cheese	$\frac{1}{4}$ cup
	Grated parmesan	2 tbsp
	Diet cheeses (with less than 55 calories per ounce)	1 oz
Other:	95% fat-free luncheon meat	1 oz
	Egg whites	3 whites
	Egg substitutes with less than 55 calories per $\frac{1}{4}$ cup	$\frac{1}{4}$ cup

Medium-Fat Meat and Substitutes: Each item on this list contains 7 grams of protein, 5 grams of fat, and 75 calories. One exchange is equal to any one of the following items:

Beef:	Most beef products fall into this category. Examples are all ground beef, roast (rib, chuck, rump), steak (cubed, Porterhouse, T-bone), and meatloaf.	1 oz
Pork:	Most pork products fall into this category. Examples are chops, loin roast, Boston butt, cutlets.	1 oz
Lamb:	Most lamb products fall into this category. Examples are chops, leg, and roast.	1 oz
Veal:	Cutlet (ground or cubed, unbreaded)	1 oz
Poultry:	Chicken (with skin), domestic duck or (well-drained of fat) ground turkey	1 oz
Fish:	Tuna (canned in oil and drained)	$\frac{1}{4}$ cup
	Salmon (canned)	$\frac{1}{4}$ cup
Cheese:	Skim or part-skim milk cheeses, such as Ricotta	1 oz
	Mozzarella, diet cheeses (with 56–80 calories per ounce)	
Other:	86% fat-free luncheon meat	1 oz
	Egg (high in cholesterol, limit to 3 per week)	1
	Egg substitutes with 56–80 calories per $\frac{1}{4}$ cup	$\frac{1}{4}$ cup
	Tofu ($2\frac{1}{2}$ in. × $2\frac{3}{4}$ in. × 1 in.)	4 oz
	Liver, heart, kidney, sweetbreads (high in cholesterol)	1 oz

Table 19-2 (Continued)

High-Fat Meats and Substitutes: Each item on this list contains 7 grams protein, 8 grams of fat, and 100 calories. *Remember: these items are high in saturated fat, cholesterol, and calories and should be used only three times per week.* One exchange is equal to any one of the following items:

Beef:	Most USDA Prime cuts of beef, such as ribs, corned beef	1 oz
Pork:	Spareribs, ground pork, pork sausage (patty or link)	1 oz
Lamb:	Patties (ground lamb)	1 oz
Fish:	Any fried fish product	1 oz
Cheese:	All regular cheeses, such as American, Blue, Cheddar, Monterey, Swiss	1 oz
Other:	Luncheon meat, such as bologna, salami, pimento loaf	1 oz
	Sausage, such as Polish, Italian	1 oz
	Knockwurst, smoked	1 oz
	Bratwurst	1 oz
	Frankfurter (turkey or chicken)	1 frank (10/lb)
	Peanut butter (contains unsaturated fat)	1 tbsp
	Count as one high-fat meat plus one fat exchange:	
	Frankfurter (beef, pork or combination)	1 frank (10/lb)

VEGETABLE LIST: Each vegetable serving on this list contains 5 grams of carbohydrate, 2 grams of protein, and 25 calories. One exchange is ½ cup of cooked vegetables or ½ cup of vegetable juice or 1 cup of raw vegetables.

Artichoke (½ medium)	Cauliflower	Peppers (green)
Asparagus	Eggplant	Rutabaga
Beans (green, wax, Italian)	Greens (collard, mustard, turnip)	Sauerkraut (cooked)
Bean sprouts	Kohlrabi	Summer squash (crookneck)
Beets	Leeks	Tomato (one large)
Broccoli	Mushrooms (cooked)	Tomato/vegetable juice
Brussels sprouts	Okra	Turnips
Cabbage (cooked)	Onions	Water chestnuts
Carrots	Pea pods	Zucchini (cooked)

Under this plan, foods are categorized by type and included in six major lists.

The foods within each list contain approximately equal amounts of kcal, carbohydrates, proteins, and fats. This means that any one food on a particular list can be substituted for any other food on that *particular list* and still provide the patient with the prescribed types and amounts of nutrients and kcal.

The amounts of nutrients and kcal on one list are not the same as those on any other list. Each list includes serving size by volume or weight and the number of kcal per food item, in addition to the grams of carbohydrates, and, when appropriate, proteins and fats are provided. The number of kcal needed will determine the number of items prescribed from any particular list. These lists also can be used to control kcal content of diets and are thus appropriate for low-kcal diets.

The total energy requirements for adult diabetic patients who are not overweight will be the same as for nondiabetic individuals. When patients are overweight, a reduction in kcal will be

Table 19-2 (*Continued*)

FRUIT LIST: Each item on this list contains 15 grams of carbohydrate and 60 calories. One exchange is equal to any one of the following items:

Fresh, Frozen, and Unsweetened Canned Fruit

Apple (raw, 2 in. across)	1	Mango (small)	½
Applesauce (unsweetened)	½ cup	Nectarine (1½ in. across)	1
Apricots (medium, raw) or	4	Orange (2½ in. across)	1
Apricots (canned)	½ cup or 4 halves	Papaya	1 cup
	½	Peach (2¾ in. across)	1 or ¾ cup
Banana (9 in. long)	¾ cup		
Blackberries (raw)	⅓ melon	Peaches (canned)	½ cup or
Cantaloupe (5 in. across)	1 cup		2 halves
(cubes)	12		or 1 small
Cherries (large, raw)	½ cup	Pears (canned)	½ cup or
Cherries (canned)	2		2 halves
Figs (raw, 2 in. across)	½ cup	Persimmon (medium, native)	2
Fruit cocktail (canned)	½	Pineapple (raw)	¾ cup
Grapefruit (medium)	¾ cup	Pineapple (canned)	⅓ cup
Grapefruit (segments)	15	Plum (raw, 2 in. across)	2
Grapes (small)	⅛ melon	Pomegranate	½
Honeydew Melon (medium)	1 cup	Raspberries (raw)	1 cup
(cubes)	1	Strawberries (raw, whole)	1¼ cup
Kiwi (large)	¾ cup	Tangerine (2½ in. across)	2
Mandarin oranges		Watermelon (cubes)	1¼ cup

Dried Fruit

Apples	4 rings	Figs	1½
Apricots	7 halves	Prunes	3 medium
Dates (medium)	2½	Raisins	2 tbsp

Fruit Juice

Apple juice/cider	½ cup	Orange juice	½ cup
Cranberry juice cocktail	⅓ cup	Pineapple juice	½ cup
Grapefruit juice	½ cup	Prune juice	⅓ cup
Grape juice	⅓ cup		

built into the diet plans, typically allowing for a weight loss of one pound a week.

The diet is given in terms of exchanges rather than as particular foods. For example, the menu pattern for breakfast may include 1 fruit exchange, 1 meat exchange, 2 bread exchanges, and 2 fat exchanges. The patient may choose the desired foods from the exchange lists for each meal but must adhere to the specific exchange lists named and the specific number of exchanges on each list. Snacks are built into the plan. In this way, the patient has variety in a simple yet controlled way.

When there are changes in one's physical condition such as pregnancy or lactation or in one's lifestyle, the diet will need to be modified. A change in job or in working hours can affect nutrient and kcal requirements. When such

Table 19-2 (*Continued*)

MILK LIST

Skim and Very Lowfat Milk: Each item on this list contains 12 grams of carbohydrate, 8 grams of protein, a trace of fat, and 90 calories. One exchange is equal to any one of the following items:

Skim milk	1 cup
$\frac{1}{2}$% milk	1 cup
1% milk	1 cup
Lowfat buttermilk	1 cup
Evaporated skim milk	$\frac{1}{2}$ cup
Dry nonfat milk	$\frac{1}{3}$ cup
Plain nonfat yogurt	8 oz

Lowfat Milk: Each item on this list contains 12 grams of carbohydrate, 8 grams of protein, 5 grams of fat, and 120 calories. One exchange is equal to any one of the following items:

2% milk	1 cup
Plain lowfat yogurt (with added nonfat milk solids)	8 oz

Whole Milk: Each item on this list contains 12 grams of carbohydrate, 8 grams of protein, 8 grams of fat, and 150 calories. One exchange is equal to any one of the following items:

Whole milk	1 cup
Evaporated whole milk	$\frac{1}{2}$ cup
Whole plain yogurt	8 oz

changes occur, the patient should be advised to consult her or his physician or diet counselor so that kcal and insulin needs can be promptly adjusted.

MISCELLANEOUS CONCERNS OF THE DIABETIC PATIENT

Fiber

The therapeutic value of fiber in the diabetic diet has become increasingly evident. High fiber intake appears to reduce the amount of insulin needed because it lowers blood glucose. It also appears to lower the blood cholesterol and the triglyceride levels. High fiber may mean 25 or 30 grams of dietary fiber a day. Such high amounts can be difficult to include. Its use should be increased very gradually, as an abrupt increase can create intestinal gas and discomfort. In addition, it can affect mineral absorption. (See Chapter 7.)

Artificial Sweeteners

Saccharin has been shown to produce bladder cancer in rats. **Aspartame** is the generic name for an artificial sweetener composed of two amino acids, phenylalanine and aspartic acid. It does not require insulin for metabolism. Both have been approved by the FDA, and the American Diabetes Association has given its approval for their use.

Table 19-2 (Continued)

FAT LIST: Each item on this list contains 5 grams of fat and 45 calories. One exchange is equal to any one of the following items:

Unsaturated		Saturated	
Avocado	$\frac{1}{8}$ medium	Butter	1 tsp
Margarine	1 tbsp	Bacon	1 slice
Margarine, diet	1 tbsp	Chitterlings	$\frac{1}{2}$ oz
Mayonnaise	1 tsp	Coconut, shredded	2 tbsp
Mayonnaise, reduced-calorie	1 tsp	Coffee whitener, liquid	2 tbsp
Nuts and Seeds:		Coffee whitener, powder	4 tbsp
Almonds, dry roasted	6 whole	Cream (light, coffee, table)	2 tbsp
Cashews, dry roasted	1 tbsp	Cream, sour	2 tbsp
Pecans	2 whole	Cream (heavy, whipping)	1 tbsp
Peanuts	20 small or 10 large	Cream cheese	1 tbsp
		Salt pork	$\frac{1}{4}$ oz
Walnuts	2 whole		
Other nuts	1 tbsp		
Seeds, pine nuts, sun- flower (without shells)	1 tbsp 2 tsp		
Pumpkin seeds	1 tsp		
Oil (corn, cottonseed, safflower, soybean, sun- flower, olive, peanut)	10 small or 5 large		
Olives	2 tsp		
Salad dressing, mayonnaise-type	1 tbsp		
Salad dressing, mayonnaise type, reduced-calorie	1 tbsp		
Salad dressing (all varieties)	2 tbsp		
Salad dressing, reduced-calorie			

Credit: The American Diabetes Association and the American Dietetic Association

Dietetic Foods

The use of diabetic or dietetic foods is generally a waste of money and can be injurious to the patient. Often the containers of foods will contain the same ingredients as containers of foods prepared for the general public, but the cost is typically higher for the dietetic foods. The inherent danger for diabetic patients is that some may not read the labels on the food containers, assuming that because they are labeled "dietetic" foods, they can be used with abandon. In reality, their use should be in specified amounts only as these foods will contain carbohydrates, fats, and/or proteins that must be calculated in the total day's diet.

It is advisable for the diabetic patient to use foods prepared for the general public, but to avoid those packed in syrup or oil. The important thing is for the diabetic patient to *read the label* on all food containers purchased.

Alcohol

While alcohol is not recommended for diabetic patients, its limited use is sometimes allowed if approved by the physician. However, some diabetic patients who use hypoglycemic agents cannot tolerate alcohol. When used, its kcal must be included in the diet plan.

Exercise

Exercise helps the body use glucose by increasing insulin receptor sites and stimulating the creation of glucagon. It lowers cholesterol and blood pressure and reduces stress and body fat as it tones the muscles. For patients with NIDDM, exercise helps improve weight control, glucose levels, and the cardiovascular system.

However, for patients with IDDM exercise can complicate glucose control. As it lowers glucose levels, hypoglycemia can develop. It must be carefully discussed with the patient's physician. If done, it should be on a regular basis and it must be considered carefully as the meal plans are developed so sufficient kcal and insulin are prescribed.

Insulin Therapy

Patients with IDDM must have injections of insulin every day to control their blood glucose levels, figure 19-1. This insulin is called **exogenous insulin** because it is produced outside the body. **Endogenous insulin** is produced by the body.

Exogenous insulin must be injected because it is a protein and, if swallowed, it would be digested and would not reach the bloodstream as

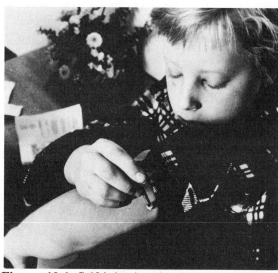

Figure 19-1 Self-injection into the upper arm. *(From Reiss and Melick,* Pharmacological Aspects of Nursing Care, *Second Edition, Copyright 1987 by Delmar Publishers Inc.)*

the complete hormone. After insulin treatment is begun, it is usually necessary to continue it throughout the life of the patient.

The insulin given to diabetic patients is made from the pancreas glands of cattle or pigs, a combination of both, or from a laboratory process in which bacteria duplicate human insulin.

There are various types of insulin available. They differ in the length of time required before they are effective and in the length of time they continue to act. Consequently, they are classified as rapid, intermediate, and long-acting. Those most commonly used are intermediate-acting types that work within 2 to 8 hours and are effective for 24 to 28 hours. For Type I diabetes, insulin is often given in two injections daily, at prescribed times.

Insulin Reactions

When patients do not eat the prescribed diet but continue to take the prescribed insulin, **hypo-**

glycemia (subnormal level of blood sugar) can result. This is called an **insulin reaction** or *hypoglycemic episode,* and may lead to **insulin coma.** Symptoms include headache, blurred vision, tremors, confusion, poor coordination, and eventual unconsciousness. Insulin reaction is dangerous because if frequent or prolonged, brain damage can occur. (The brain must have sufficient amounts of glucose in order to function.) The physician should be consulted if an insulin reaction occurs or seems imminent.

Conscious patients may be treated by giving them hard candy, a glucose tablet, a sugar cube, or a beverage containing sugar. If the patient is unconscious, intravenous treatment of dextrose and water is given. It is advisable for the diabetic patient to carry identification explaining the condition so people do not think she or he is drunk when in reality the person is experiencing an insulin reaction.

CONSIDERATIONS FOR THE HEALTH CARE PROFESSIONAL

It is important to point out to the diabetic patient that one can live a near-normal life if the diet is followed, medication is taken as prescribed, and time is allowed for sufficient exercise and rest. The importance of eating all of the prescribed food must be emphasized. It is important for meals to be eaten at regular times so the insulin-glucose balance can be maintained. It is imperative that the patient learn to read carefully all labels on commercially prepared foods. This is necessary to avoid eating or drinking anything that might contain an unknown amount of sugar. It must be explained that prepared foods with unknown amounts of sugar added are not allowed because they upset the insulin-glucose balance.

Table 19-3 Foods to Avoid	
sugar	honey
cookies, pastries	condensed milk
pies	jam, jelly
candy	chewing gum
syrup	marmalade
cakes	soft drinks
fried, scalloped, or creamed foods	

Adjustments must be made in the shopping, cooking, and eating habits so the diet plan can be followed. Family meals can be simply adapted for the diabetic diet. For example, sugar and flour can be omitted from the patient's portions, and lemon juice, herbs, and spices can be substituted for rich sauces on salads, vegetables, and meats. The diabetic patient soon learns which exchange lists are to be included at each meal and at snack times, and the foods within each exchange list. (See Tables 19-3 and 19-4 for foods omitted and allowed in diabetic diets. Table 19-5 gives samples of useful food seasonings.)

SUMMARY

The diabetic diet is used in treating diabetes mellitus, a metabolic disease caused by the improper functioning of the pancreas that results in inadequate production or utilization of insulin. If the condition is left untreated, the body cannot use glucose properly and serious complications leading to death can occur. Treatment includes diet, medication, and exercise. Diabetic diets are prescribed by the physician or diet counselor in consultation with the patient.

Table 19-4 Free Foods Allowed on the Exchange List

A free food is any food or drink that contains less than 20 calories per serving. You can eat as much as you want of those items that have no serving size specified. You can eat two or three servings per day of those items that have a specific serving size. Be sure to spread them out through the day.

Drinks
Bouillon or broth
   without fat
Bouillon, low sodium
Carbonated drinks,
   sugar-free
Carbonated water
Club soda
Cocoa powder,
   unsweetened (1 tbsp)
Coffee/tea
Drink mixes, sugar-free
Tonic water, sugar-free

Fruit
Cranberries,
   unsweetened ($\frac{1}{2}$ cup)
Rhubarb
   unsweetened ($\frac{1}{2}$ cup)

Vegetables
   (raw, 1 cup)
Cabbage
Celery
Chinese cabbage
Cucumber
Green onion
Hot peppers
Mushrooms
Radishes
Zucchini

Salad Greens
Endive
Escarole
Lettuce
Romaine
Spinach

Nonstick pan spray

Sweet Substitutes
Candy, hard, sugar-free
Gelatin, sugar-free
Gum, sugar-free
Jam/jelly, sugar-free
   (2 tsp)
Pancake syrup, sugar-free
   (1–2 tbsps)
Sugar substitutes
   (saccharin, aspartame)
Whipped topping (2 tbsp)

Condiments
Catsup (1 tbsp)
Horseradish
Mustard
Pickles, dill, unsweet.
Salad dressing,
   low-calorie (2 tbsp)
Taco sauce (1 tbsp)
Vinegar

Source: American Diabetes Association

Table 19-5 Useful Seasonings

Read the label, and choose those seasonings that do not contain sodium or salt.

Basil (fresh)
Celery seeds
Cinnamon
Chili powder
Chives
Curry
Dill
Flavoring extracts
   (vanilla, almond, walnut, pepper-
   mint, lemon, butter, etc.)

Garlic
Garlic powder
Herbs
Hot pepper sauce
Lemon
Lemon juice
Lemon pepper
Lime
Lime juice
Mint
Onion powder

Oregano
Paprika
Pepper
Pimento
Spices
Soy sauce
Soy sauce, low sodium
   ("lite")
Wine, used in cooking
   ($\frac{1}{4}$ cup)
Worcestershire sauce

Source: American Diabetes Association and the American Dietetic Association

Discussion
Topics

1. Describe diabetes mellitus. Explain why it is a serious disease.
2. What is insulin? What is its use? Why can it not be taken orally?
3. What is the function of oral hypoglycemic agents? For which type of diabetes are they usually prescribed?
4. Explain the differences between Type I and Type II diabetes mellitus.
5. Describe the symptoms of Type I diabetes mellitus. Include the following terms: hyperglycemia, renal threshold, glycosuria, polydipsia, polyuria, polyphagia, ketones, ketonuria, acidosis.
6. Name the six exchange lists and explain how they are used.
7. Explain why it is essential that diabetic patients read labels on foods.
8. Why should a diabetic patient avoid adding flour to foods during the cooking process?
9. Why are "dietetic" foods not recommended for diabetic patients?
10. Discuss how an insulin reaction might occur.
11. Why must a diabetic patient's tray be checked carefully after meals?
12. Why is the use of exchange lists the most commonly used method of dietary treatment of diabetes mellitus?
13. How would pregnancy affect one's diet? Lactation?
14. Discuss the effects of exercise on glucose utilization.

Suggested
Activities

1. Ask a physician or registered nurse to speak to the class on diabetes mellitus and its treatment.
2. Ask a diet counselor to explain and demonstrate the planning of diabetic diets using the exchange lists.
    a. Observe the diet counselor planning a 1300-kcal and a 1500-kcal diabetic diet using the exchange lists.
    b. Observe the diet counselor adapting a normal, 2400-kcal daily menu to suit the needs of the diabetic patient on a 1500-kcal diet.
3. After observing the diet counselor, use the information in Table 19-2 to plan an 1800-kcal diet in which 55 percent of kcal is from carbohydrates, 15 percent is from proteins, and 30 percent is from fats. Compare your diets with those of other students. Discuss methods used and correct if necessary.
4. Find recipes suitable for the diabetic diet and add them to the diet recipe file.
5. Prepare and serve a meal planned in activity 2. Evaluate it in terms of nutritive content, flavor, aroma, color, shape, appearance, texture, and satiety value.

6. Visit a local supermarket and compare regular and "dietetic" containers of food in terms of cost, kcal, and nutrient content.
7. Invite someone with IDDM to talk to the class about his or her condition.
8. Invite someone with NIDDM to talk to the class about his or her condition.

Review

A.   Multiple choice. Select the *letter* that precedes the best answer.

1. Diabetes mellitus is a metabolic disorder
   1. caused by malfunction of the pancreas gland
   2. for which a diabetic diet may be ordered
   3. in which sugar accumulates in the blood
   4. for which a regular diet is adequate
   5. that is contagious
      a) all   b) 1,2,3   c) 4,5   d) 1,2,4,5

2. The metabolism of glucose
   1. depends on insulin secreted by the islets of Langerhans
   2. depends on enzymes present in pancreatic juice
   3. is inefficient if diabetes is left untreated
   4. is directly related to secretions from the thyroid gland
      a) 1,3,4   b) all   c) 2,3   d) 1,3

3. Type I diabetes mellitus is treated by
   1. administration of insulin
   2. exclusion of foods that contain glucose
   3. administration of thyroxine
   4. use of a diabetic diet
      a) 1,3,4   b) 1,4   c) all   d) 1,2,3

4. As part of the nutritional management of diabetes mellitus, the physician may recommend that the diet
   1. consist of 40 to 50 percent complex carbohydrates
   2. consist of no more than 30 percent fats
   3. contain 15 to 20 percent proteins
   4. exclude all simple sugars
      a) all   b) 1,2   c) 1,2,3   d) 1,2,4

5. Diets based on the exchange lists
   1. are appropriate only for patients with IDDM
   2. can be used by all diabetic patients
   3. eliminate all carbohydrates
   4. are sometimes used by nondiabetic persons who want to control their kcal
      a) all   b) 1,2   c) 1,2,3   d) 2,4

6. When an excessive amount of glucose accumulates in the blood, the condition
   1. is called hyperglycemia
   2. leads to glycosuria
   3. contributes to polydipsia
   4. is known as acidosis
   5. leads to insulin coma
      a) all   b) 1,2,4   c) 1,3,4,5   d) 1,2,3
7. Diabetic coma
   1. is called acidosis
   2. is caused by excessive insulin
   3. is preceded by ketonuria
   4. causes polyuria
   5. is caused by insufficient insulin
      a) 1,2   b) 2,3,4   c) 1,3,5   d) 1,2,4
8. Type II (NIDDM) diabetes mellitus
   1. usually occurs before the age of 40
   2. usually occurs after the age of 40
   3. usually requires insulin
   4. can usually be controlled by diet and hypoglycemic agent
   5. occurs more often than Type I IDDM
      a) 2,4,5   b) 1,2,3   c) 2,3,4   d) 1,4,5
9. Hypoglycemic agents
   1. have exactly the same effect as insulin
   2. cannot be used for patients over 40
   3. stimulate the pancreas to produce insulin
   4. are used for NIDDM patients
   5. must be injected into the vascular system
      a) 1,2,3   b) 1,2,5   c) 3,4   d) 4,5
10. Diabetic diets based on the Exchange Lists regulate amounts of
    1. carbohydrate
    2. kcal
    3. protein
    4. fat
    5. fiber
       a) 1,2,3,5   b) 1,2,3,4   c) 1,3,4,5   d) all

B. Match the items in column I with the definition in column II.

	Column I		Column II
_____	1. acidosis	a.	long standing
_____	2. aspartame	b.	subnormal level of glucose in blood
_____	3. chronic		
_____	4. endogenous insulin	c.	artificial sweetener
_____	5. glycosuria	d.	insulin injected into the body
_____	6. hyperglycemia	e.	diabetic coma
_____	7. ketonuria	f.	relating to the kidneys
_____	8. polydipsia	g.	hormone essential for metabolism of glucose
_____	9. renal		
_____	10. polyuria	h.	excessive thirst
_____	11. exogenous insulin	i.	excessive hunger
_____	12. hypoglycemia	j.	excessive production of urine
_____	13. insulin	k.	excessive glucose in the blood
_____	14. ketones	l.	relating to the vascular system
_____	15. polyphagia	m.	insulin produced in the body
		n.	excessive sugar in the urine
		o.	ketones in the urine
		p.	dismantled parts of fatty acids

Case Study 1

Diabetes Mellitus

Karen W. is a 20-year-old college student who, early in her fall term, began to experience polyuria, combined with polydipsia and polyphagia. She felt weak and tired most of the time. She expressed a slight concern about this to her friend one day, but her friend only laughed, saying, "How can you possibly worry about being sick? You're tired because you study when you should be sleeping. And you have the best appetite I have ever seen." This was all true. Karen did study a great deal, and she was usually hungry.

However, when Karen's parents arrived for a weekend visit early in October, they were shocked to see how thin she had become. Karen agreed to see a doctor on Monday. The doctor took her history and tested her blood and urine.

Case Study Questions Based on the Nursing Process

Assess

1. What type of diabetes mellitus do Karen's symptoms suggest?
2. What did the blood and urine tests show that caused the doctor to hospitalize Karen immediately?

Plan

3. Will the doctor prescribe insulin or hypoglycemic agents for Karen? What will she need to be taught about the medication?
4. The doctor put Karen on 2400-kcal diet and ordered a nutritional consultation to help her learn to plan her meals, using the exchange lists. Determine the number of grams of protein, carbohydrate, and fat Karen should have each day.
5. Using the exchange lists, plan a day's menu for Karen.

Implement

6. What questions should the nutrition counselor ask Karen before beginning to develop her meal plans?
7. What food items should Karen be careful to avoid?
8. What food items can Karen eat without concern?

Evaluate

9. When Karen's diabetes mellitus is under control, what will be the range of her blood glucose levels? Will she still spill glucose and have ketones in her urine? Explain.
10. Why will Karen's doctor want to see her again soon after discharge when she has followed her diet and participated in her normal activities for a few days?
11. Karen's dormitory is having an International Food Festival running for the next six weeks, featuring typical meals of various countries on Friday nights. This Friday there will be a Swedish dinner including the following foods. Karen is not familiar with some of these foods. Which should she avoid? Why? Which should she eat? Why?

Mixed, Fresh Vegetables with Sourcream Horseradish Dip	Flatbread
	Rye bread
Pickled Herring	Boiled Potatoes
Boiled Shrimp with Lemon Wedges	Beet Salad
	Pound-type Cake with Whipped Cream
Swedish Meat Balls	
Baked Ham	Cookies
Roast Pork with Prunes	Lingonberry Sauce

Case Study 2

NIDDM

Arnie was a big, strapping, "self-made" man who had sold his business and was about to retire at the age of 65. He was proud of the money he had made and of his investments that would now provide him with a comfortable retirement income. At the request of his wife, Eva, he went for a physical examination the week after he sold his business.

The doctor told him he was 30 pounds overweight and that he had NIDDM. Arnie was shocked and angry, but listened to the doctor and agreed to see the diet counselor the doctor recommended.

Case Study Questions Based on the Nursing Process

Assess
1. Why was Arnie angry? Is he likely to be angry at Eva? Explain
2. Is it probable that Arnie will require insulin? Why?

Plan
3. Will Arnie be able to play golf as he'd planned to do in retirement? Explain.
4. Arnie has always liked sweets. How will his new diet affect his sweet tooth?
5. Eva has always enjoyed baking and prides herself on her desserts. How will Arnie's NIDDM affect her life?

Implement
6. What should Arnie and his wife be taught about diet changes?
7. Can Eva adjust her baking recipes so Arnie could have an occasional dessert?

Evaluate
8. Is it possible that Arnie and Eva might require some psychological counseling as a result of Arnie's condition? Explain.
9. What will indicate to the doctor that Arnie is following his new diet?

CHAPTER 20

DIET AND CARDIOVASCULAR DISEASE

OBJECTIVES

After studying this chapter, you should be able to

- Identify factors that contribute to heart disease
- Explain why cholesterol and saturated fats are limited in some cardiovascular conditions
- Identify foods to avoid or limit in a cholesterol-controlled diet
- Explain why sodium is limited in some cardiovascular conditions
- Identify foods that are limited or prohibited in sodium-controlled diets
- Adapt family meals to meet the requirements of heart patients on low-cholesterol or sodium-restricted diets

Cardiovascular disease (CVD) affects the heart and blood vessels. It is the leading cause of death and permanent disability in the United States today. The grief and economic distress it causes are staggering. Organizations, especially the American Heart Association, are promoting programs designed to alert people to the risk factors for cardiovascular disease and thereby reduce its frequency.

Cardiovascular disease can be **acute** (sudden) or chronic. **Myocardial infarction** or **MI** (heart attack) is an example of the acute form. Chronic heart disease develops over time and causes the loss of heart function. If the heart can maintain blood circulation, the disease is classified as **compensated heart disease.** Compensation usually requires that the heart beat unusually fast. Consequently, the heart enlarges. If the heart cannot maintain circulation, the condition is classified as **decompensated heart disease,** and congestive heart failure (CHF) occurs. The heart muscle (**myocardium**), the valves, the lining (**endocardium**), the outer covering (**pericardium**), or the blood vessels may be affected by heart disease.

ATHEROSCLEROSIS

Arteriosclerosis is the general term for **vascular disease** (of the blood vessels) in which arteries harden (become thickened), making the passage of blood difficult and sometimes impossible. **Atherosclerosis** is the form of arteriosclerosis that most frequently occurs in developed countries. It is believed to begin in childhood and is considered one of the major causes of heart attack.

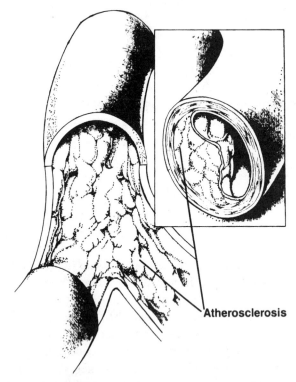

Atherosclerosis

Figure 20-1 Internal views of artery, showing the formation of plaque. *(Reproduced with permission from* About Your Heart and Diet, *American Heart Association.)*

Atherosclerosis affects the inner lining of arteries (the **intima**) where deposits of **cholesterol** (fat-like substance found in animal foods and body tissues), fats, and other substances accumulate over time, thickening and weakening artery walls. These deposits are called **plaque.** (See figure 20-1.) Plaque deposits gradually reduce the size of the **lumen** (tube area) of the artery and, consequently, the amount of blood flow. The reduced blood flow causes an inadequate supply of nutrients and oxygen delivery to and waste removal from the tissues. This condition is called **ischemia.**

The reduced oxygen supply causes pain. When the pain occurs in the heart, it is called **angina pectoris** and should be considered a warning. When the lumen narrows so that a blood clot (**embolus**) occurs in a coronary artery and blood flow is cut off, a heart attack occurs. The dead tissue that results is called an **infarct.** The heart muscle that should have received the blood is the myocardium. Thus, such an attack is commonly called an acute myocardial infarction.

When this occurs in the brain, a stroke or **cerebral hemorrhage** results. When it occurs in tissue some distance from the heart, it is called **peripheral vascular disease.**

Risk Factors

Hyperlipidemia (increased concentration of blood lipids), hypertension (high blood pressure), and smoking are major risk factors for the development of atherosclerosis. Other contributory factors are believed to include obesity, diabetes mellitus, male sex, heredity, personality type (ability to handle stress), age (risk increases with years), and sedentary lifestyle. Although some of these factors are beyond one's control, some factors are not.

It is known that dietary cholesterol and **triglycerides** (fats in foods and in adipose tissue) contribute to hyperlipidemia. Foods containing **saturated fats** increase **serum cholesterol,** whereas **polyunsaturated fats** tend to reduce it.

Lipoproteins carry cholesterol and fats in the blood to body tissues. **Low-density lipoproteins** (**LDL**) carry most of the cholesterol to the cells, and elevated blood levels of LDL are believed to contribute to atherosclerosis. **High-density lipoproteins** (**HDL**) carry cholesterol from the tissues to the liver for eventual excretion. It is believed that low serum levels of HDL can contribute to atherosclerosis.

Diet can alleviate hypertension (discussed later in this chapter), reduce obesity, and help control diabetes mellitus. A sedentary lifestyle can be changed. Exercise can help the patient lose weight, lower blood pressure, and increase the HDL ("good") cholesterol level. It must be done in consultation with the physician and be increased gradually. Also, one can stop smoking. In sum, a person can considerably reduce the risk of atherosclerosis and thus heart attack and stroke.

NUTRITIONAL THERAPY FOR HYPERLIPIDEMIA

Nutritional therapy is the primary treatment for hyperlipidemia. It involves reducing the quantity and types of fats and often kcal in the diet. When the amount of dietary fat is reduced, there is typically a corresponding reduction in the amount of cholesterol and saturated fats ingested and a loss of weight. In overweight persons, weight loss alone will help reduce serum cholesterol levels. (See Table 20-1.)

The American Heart Association categorizes blood cholesterol levels of less than 200 mg/dl to be desirable; 200–239 mg/dl to be borderline high, and 240 mg/dl and greater to be high.

In an effort to prevent heart disease, the American Heart Association has developed guidelines in which it is recommended that adult diets contain less than 300 mg of cholesterol per day and that fats provide no more than 30% of kcal, with a maximum of 10% from saturated fats and a maximum of 10% from polyunsaturated fats. Carbohydrates should make up 50 to 55 percent of the kcal, and proteins from 12 to 20 percent of them. Currently, it is believed that nearly 50 percent of the kcal in the average American diet come from fats. (See Table 20-2.)

A fat-restricted diet can be difficult for the patient to accept. A diet very low in fat will seem unusual and highly **unpalatable** (unpleasant tasting) to most patients. If the physician will allow it, the change in the nutrient makeup of the diet should be made gradually. (See Table 20-1.)

Information about the fat content of foods and methods of preparation that minimize the amount of fat in the diet are essential to the patient. The patient must be taught to select whole, fresh foods and to prepare them without the addition of any fat. Only lean meat should be selected, and all visible fat must be removed. Skim milk and skim milk cheeses should be used instead of whole milk and natural cheeses. Desserts containing whole milk, eggs, and cream are avoided.

In a fat-controlled diet, one must be particularly careful when using animal foods. Cholesterol is found only in animal tissue. Organ meats, egg yolks, and some shellfish are especially rich in cholesterol and should be used in limited quantities, if at all. Saturated fats are found in all animal foods and in coconut, chocolate, and palm oil. They tend to be solid at room temperature. Polyunsaturated fats are derived from plants and some fish and are usually soft or liquid at room temperature. Soft margarine containing mostly liquid vegetable oil is substituted for butter, and liquid vegetable oils are used in cooking.

Table 20-1 Foods to Allow/Avoid on Fat-restricted Diets

Foods to Include	Foods to Avoid
Breads and Cereals	
Whole grain breads and rolls	Breads made with egg or cheese, croissants
Plain buns, bagels, pita bread	Bakery products
Cereals without coconut	Butter crackers
Saltines, matzos, rusks	
Rice, pasta	
Vegetables and Fruits	
Any fresh fruit or vegetable, except those on the "Avoid" list	Coconut, palm oil
	Avocados, olives
Meats, Poultry, and Fish	
After trimming fat and removing skin before eating:	Fatty or prime grade meats; pastrami; spareribs; sausage; bacon; luncheon meats; domestic ducks and geese; organ meats
Fish, but limited shrimp or lobster	
Lean beef, pork, lamb, veal, egg whites; yolks should be limited to 3 a week	
Dairy	
Skim milk or 1% milk	Milk c/ more than 1% fat, cream, non-dairy creamers
Dry curd or lowfat cottage cheese	
Buttermilk	Most cheeses, especially process or blue
Puddings made with skim milk	
Other Foods	
Limited vegetable oils	Butter
Syrup	Lard
Gelatin	Bakery desserts
Jelly	Ice creams
Honey	Fried foods
Fat-free broths	Commercially prepared meals; salad dressings
Margarine made from liquid corn, sesame, olive, or sunflower oil (in limited amounts)	Cream soups
	Cream sauces; gravies
Limited nuts	
Limited home-made salad dressings	
Sherbet	
Hard candy	

Studies indicate that water-soluble fiber, such as that found in oat bran, legumes, and fruits, bind with cholesterol-containing substances and prevent their reabsorption by the blood. Twenty-five grams of soluble fiber per day is thought to effectively reduce serum cholesterol by as much as 15 percent. This is a large amount of fiber and must be introduced gradually to the diet or the patient will suffer from flatulence.

Table 20-2 Foods to Avoid on a Low-cholesterol Diet

Fats on meats and fish
Lard
Organ meats
Bacon
Luncheon meats
Prime grade meats marbled with fat
Duck
Skin on chicken and turkey
Crab meat
Shrimp
Lobster
Egg yolks
Butter
Cream
Whole milk
Natural cheeses
Commercially fried foods
Commercially prepared baked goods
Commercially prepared meat loaf
Commercially prepared mayonnaise
Quiche Lorraine
Chicken a la king
Cheeseburgers
Chicken livers
Custard
Soufflé
Lemon meringue pie
Cheesecake
Ice cream
Eggnog

Some patients will find the use of the diabetic exchange lists useful for controlling the fat content of their diets.

When fat-controlled diets are severely restricted, limiting kcal intake to 1200, they may be deficient in fat-soluble vitamins. Consequently, a vitamin supplement may be prescribed.

If appropriate blood lipid levels cannot be attained within three to six months by the use of fat-restricted diet alone (see Table 20-3 for menus), the physician can prescribe a cholesterol-lowering drug.

MYOCARDIAL INFARCTION

Myocardial infarction (MI) is caused by the blockage of a coronary artery supplying blood to the heart. The heart tissue denied blood because of this blockage dies. Atherosclerosis is a primary cause, but hypertension, abnormal blood clotting, and infection such as that caused by rheumatic fever (which damages heart valves) are also contributory factors.

Following the attack, the patient is in shock. This causes a fluid shift and the patient may feel thirsty. The patient should be given nothing by mouth (NPO), however, until the physician evaluates the condition. If the patient remains nauseated after the period of shock, IV infusions are given to prevent dehydration.

After several hours, the patient may begin to eat. A liquid diet may be recommended for the first 24 hours. Following that, meals may be gradually changed to soft, bland foods offered frequently in small amounts. The daily kcal total for the first five to ten days should be 1000 to 1200. If the patient is obese, the kcal level may be kept at a reduced number.

Foods should not be extremely hot or extremely cold. They should be easy to chew and digest and contain little roughage so the work of the heart is minimal. Both chewing and the increased activity of the gastrointestinal tract that follow ingestion of high-fiber foods cause extra work for the heart. The percentage of energy nutrients will be based on the particular needs of the patient but, in most cases, the types and amounts of fats will be limited. Sodium may be limited, depending on the patient's condition. The intention is to prevent fluid accumulation. Some physicians will order a restriction on the amount of

Table 20-3 Sample Menus for a Fat-controlled Diet

Breakfast	Dinner	Lunch or Supper

Orange Juice
Cream of Wheat with 1 Tbsp
  Sugar and 1 Cup Skim Milk
1 Slice Toast
1 Tbsp Jelly
Coffee
	3 oz Chicken
	Baked Potato
	Baked Acorn Squash with
	  1 Tbsp Honey
	Lettuce Salad
	1 Slice Bread
	1 Tbsp Jelly
	Canned Peaches
	1 Cup Skim Milk
	Tea
		Tomato Juice
		Uncreamed Cottage Cheese
		  on Fruit Salad*
		2 Slices Toast with
		  2 Tbsp Honey
		Angel Cake
		1 Cup Skim Milk
		Tea

*No Avocado

caffeine for the first few days after an MI. The dual goal is to allow the heart to rest and its tissue to heal.

CONGESTIVE HEART FAILURE

Congestive heart failure (CHF) is an example of decompensation, or severe heart disease. It can result from injury to the heart muscle due to atherosclerosis, hypertension, or rheumatic fever. In this situation, when damage is extreme and the heart cannot provide adequate circulation, the amount of oxygen taken in is insufficient for body needs. Shortness of breath is common and chest pain can occur on exertion.

Because of the reduced circulation, tissues retain fluid that would normally be carried off by the blood. Sodium builds up and more fluid is retained, resulting in **edema.** In an attempt to compensate for this pumping deficit, the heart beats faster and enlarges. This adds to the heart's burden. In advanced cases when edema affects the lungs, death can occur.

With the inadequate circulation, body tissues do not receive sufficient amounts of nutrients. This can cause malnutrition and under-

Table 20-4 Potassium-rich Foods

Fruits
apricots
oranges
bananas
avocados
cantaloupe
dates
figs
raisins
honeydew melon
grapefruit
kiwi fruit
peaches
pineapple
prunes
strawberries

Vegetables
asparagus
broccoli
cabbage
green beans
potatoes, sweet potatoes, yams
pumpkin
squash
tomatoes
spinach

Table 20-5 Sodium-restricted; Fat-controlled; High-Potassium Diet of 1800 kcal

Breakfast

½ cup orange juice
1 cup puffed wheat with ½ cup skim milk
1 slice whole wheat toast
½ tablespoon whipped margarine
Coffee
Snack: 6 dried apricots

Lunch or Supper

3 oz sliced chicken, white meat on lettuce with fresh tomato
1 serving bread
½ tablespoon whipped margarine
1 cup skim milk
1 cup fresh pineapple chunks
Snack: 1 banana

Dinner

½ cantalope
3 oz broiled fish
1 medium baked potato
½ tablespoon whipped margarine
⅓ cup coleslaw
1 serving bread
½ tablespoon whipped margarine
1 cup skim milk
1 cup fresh strawberries
Snack: orange

weight, although the edema can mask the problems.

   Diuretics to aid in the excretion of water and sodium and a sodium-restricted diet are typically prescribed. Because diuretics can cause an excessive loss of potassium, the patient's blood potassium should be carefully watched to prevent **hypokalemia** (low blood potassium), which can upset the heartbeat. (See Table 20-4.) Fruits, especially oranges, bananas, and prunes, can be useful in such a situation because they are excellent sources of potassium and contain only negligible amounts of sodium. When necessary, the physician will prescribe supplementary potassium. (See Table 20-5.)

HYPERTENSION

   When blood pressure is chronically high, the condition is called **hypertension.** In 90 percent of hypertension cases, the cause is unknown and the condition is called **essential** or **primary hypertension.** Ten percent of the cases are called

secondary hypertension because the condition is caused by another problem. Some causes of secondary hypertension include kidney disease, problems of the adrenal glands, and use of oral contraceptives.

The blood pressure commonly measured is that of the artery in the upper arm. This is done with an instrument called the **sphygmomanometer.** The top number is the **systolic pressure,** taken as the heart contracts. The lower number is the **diastolic pressure,** taken when the heart is resting. The pressure is measured in millimeters of mercury (mm Hg). Hypertension can be diagnosed when, on several occasions, the systolic pressure is 140 mm Hg or more and the diastolic pressure is 90 mm Hg or more.

Hypertension contributes to heart attack, stroke, heart failure, and kidney failure. It is sometimes called the *silent disease* because sufferers can be **asymptomatic** (without symptoms). Its frequency increases with age, and it is more prevalent among African-Americans than others.

Heredity and obesity are predisposing factors in hypertension. Weight loss usually lowers the blood pressure and, consequently, patients are often placed on weight reduction diets. Smoking and stress also contribute to hypertension.

Excessive use of ordinary table salt also is considered a contributory factor in hypertension. Table salt consists of over 40 percent sodium plus chloride. Both are essential in maintaining fluid balance and thus blood pressure. When consumed in normal quantities by healthy people, they are beneficial.

When the fluid balance is upset and sodium and fluid collect in body tissue causing edema, extra pressure is placed on the blood vessels. To alleviate this condition, a sodium-restricted diet, often accompanied by diuretics, can be prescribed. When the sodium content in the diet is reduced, the water and salts in the tissues flow back into the blood to be excreted by the kidneys.

In this way, the edema is relieved. The amount of sodium restricted is determined by the physician, based on the patient's condition.

Previous research focused primarily on sodium as a primary factor in the development of hypertension but, as research continues, the effects of chloride also are receiving increasing scrutiny. Additionally, the particular roles of calcium and magnesium in relation to hypertension also are being studied.

DIETARY TREATMENT FOR HYPERTENSION

As indicated above, weight loss for the obese patient with hypertension usually lowers blood pressure and, thus, a kcal-restricted diet (see Chapter 18) might be prescribed. A sodium-restricted diet frequently is prescribed for patients with hypertension. A discussion of this follows. When diuretics are prescribed together with a sodium-restricted diet, the patient may lose potassium via the urine and, thus, be advised to increase the amount of potassium-rich foods in the diet. (See Table 20-4.)

Sodium-Restricted Diets

A sodium-restricted diet is a regular diet in which the amount of sodium is limited. Such a diet is used to alleviate edema and hypertension. Most people obtain far too much sodium from their diets. It is estimated that the average adult consumes 10 g of salt a day, providing 4 g of sodium. A committee of the Food and Nutrition Board recently recommended that the daily intake of sodium chloride be limited to no more than 6 g (2.4 g sodium), and the Board itself set a safe minimum at 500 mg/day for adults. (See Table 7-4.) Sodium is found in food, water, and medicine.

It is impossible to have a diet totally free of sodium. Meats, fish, poultry, dairy products, and eggs all contain substantial amounts of sodium naturally. Cereals, vegetables, fruits, and fats contain small amounts of sodium naturally. Water contains varying amounts of sodium. However, sodium often is added to foods during processing, cooking, and at the table. The food label should indicate the addition of sodium to commercial food products. In some of these foods, the addition of sodium is obvious because one can taste it, as in prepared dinners, potato chips, and canned soups. In others, it is not. The following are examples of sodium-containing products frequently added to foods that the consumer may not notice.

- Salt (sodium chloride)—used in cooking or at the table, and in canning and processing.
- **Monosodium glutamate** (called **MSG,** and sold under several brand names)—a seasoning used in home, restaurant, and hotel cooking, and in many packaged, canned, and frozen foods.
- Baking powder—used to leaven quick breads and cakes.
- Baking soda (sodium bicarbonate)—used to leaven breads and cakes; sometimes added to vegetables in cooking or used as an "alkalizer" for indigestion.
- **Brine** (table salt and water)—used in processing foods to inhibit growth of bacteria; in cleaning or blanching vegetables and fruits; in freezing and canning certain foods; and for flavor, as in corned beef, pickles, and sauerkraut.
- Di-sodium phosphate—present in some quick-cooking cereals and processed cheeses.
- Sodium alginate—used in many chocolate milks and ice creams for smooth texture.
- Sodium benzoate—used as a preservative in many condiments such as relishes, sauces, and salad dressings.

- Sodium hydroxide—used in food processing to soften and loosen skins of ripe olives, hominy, and certain fruits and vegetables.
- Sodium propionate—used in pasteurized cheeses and in some breads and cakes to inhibit growth of mold.
- Sodium sulfite—used to bleach certain fruits in which an artificial color is desired, such as maraschino cherries and glazed or crystallized fruit; also used as a preservative in some dried fruit, such as prunes.

Because the amount of sodium in tap water varies from one area to another, the local Department of Health or the American Heart Association affiliate should be consulted if this information is needed. Softened water always has additional sodium. If the sodium content of the water is high, the patient may have to use **distilled water** (minerals have been removed).

Some medicines contain sodium. A patient on a sodium-restricted diet should obtain the physician's permission before using any medication or salt substitute. Many salt substitutes contain potassium, which affects the heartbeat.

The amount of sodium allowed depends on the patient's condition and is prescribed by the physician. In extraordinary cases of fluid retention, a diet with 0.5 g or even 0.25 g a day can be ordered, but this is rare. A moderate restriction limits sodium to 1 g a day. A mild restriction limits sodium to 2 to 3 g a day.

Adjustment to Sodium Restriction

Sodium-restricted diets range from "different" to "tasteless" because most people are accustomed to salt in their food. It can be difficult for the patient to understand the necessity for following such a diet, particularly if it must be followed for the remainder of his or her lifetime. If the physician allows, it will be helpful to the

Table 20-6 Foods to Allow/Avoid on Sodium-restricted Diets

Foods Permitted on Most Sodium-restricted Diets	Foods to Limit or Avoid
Fruit juices without additives	Tomato juice and vegetable cocktail
Fresh fruits	Canned vegetables
Fresh vegetables (except for those on List B)	Sauerkraut
Dried peas or beans	Frozen vegetables if prepared with salt
Skim milk	Artichokes, beets, carrots, celery, chard, dandelion
Puffed-type cereals	greens, kale, spinach, white turnips
Shredded wheat	Dried, breaded, smoked, or canned fish or meats
Regular, cooked cereals without added salt, sugar, or flavorings	Cheeses; salted butter or margarine
Plain pasta	Salt-topped crackers or breads
Rice	Salty foods such as potato chips, salted nuts,
Unsalted, uncoated popcorn	peanut butter, pretzels
Fresh fish	Canned fish, meats, or soups
Fresh unsalted meats	Ham, salt pork, corned beef, luncheon meats,
Unsalted margarine	smoked or canned fish
Oil	Prepared relishes, salad dressings, catsup, soy
Vinegar	sauce
Spices containing no salt, herbs, lemon juice	Bouillon, baking soda, baking powder, MSG
Unsalted nuts	Commercially prepared meals
Hard candy	
Jams, jellies, honey	
Coffee, tea	

patient's adjustment if the sodium content of the diet can be reduced gradually.

It is helpful, too, to remind the patient of the numerous herbs, spices, and flavorings allowed on sodium-restricted diets. (See Table 20-6.) Patients will also find it useful to practice ordering from a menu so as to learn to choose those foods lowest in sodium content.

CONSIDERATIONS FOR THE HEALTH CARE PROFESSIONAL

Patients with heart conditions serious enough to require hospitalization can be frightened, depressed, or angry. The added indignity of being told they must reduce the fats, sodium and, sometimes, the amount of kcal in their diets is not helpful to their psychological well-being. The health care professional will find various moods among these patients. Most will need nutritional advice. Some will want it. Some will be against the new diets. The most important thing the health care professional can do is help the cardiac patient want to learn how to help himself or herself via nutrition.

SUMMARY

Cardiovascular disease represents the leading cause of death in the United States. It may be acute as in myocardial infarction, or chronic as in hypertension and atherosclerosis. Hypertension may be a symptom of other disease. Weight loss, if the patient is overweight, and a salt-restricted diet are typically prescribed.

Atherosclerosis is a vascular disease in which the arteries are narrowed by fatty deposits, reducing blood flow. Angina pectoris, myocar-

dial infarction, or stroke can result. Because cholesterol is associated with atherosclerosis, a low-cholesterol diet, or a fat-restricted diet might be prescribed.

By maintaining one's weight and activities at a healthy level, limiting salt and fat intake, and avoiding smoking, one reduces the risks of heart disease.

Discussion Topics

1. Why are sodium-restricted diets prescribed for patients with hypertension or heart failure?
2. What precautions might one take to prevent hypertension? Atherosclerosis? Explain your answers.
3. What may occur in severe myocardial infarction? What causes myocardial infarction?
4. Describe the dietary progression following a myocardial infarction.
5. What are diuretics? How could they be harmful? How could this danger be avoided?
6. What is edema? How is it related to cardiovascular disease?
7. Are sodium-restricted diets nutritious? Why?
8. If a class member knows anyone who must follow a sodium-restricted diet, discuss that person's initial reaction to this diet. Has this person become accustomed to it?
9. Why is it impossible to prepare a diet absolutely free of salt?
10. Why may a sodium-restricted diet be unpleasant for a patient?
11. Why are potato chips and peanuts not allowed on sodium-restricted diets?
12. Why is table salt restricted in sodium-restricted diets?
13. For what heart condition might fat-controlled diets be ordered? What foods should be avoided? What foods are allowed?
14. In what respects are fat-controlled diets modified? Is the patient apt to notice these modifications?
15. Are fat-controlled diets always nutritious? If not, explain and tell which nutrient(s) may be lacking. Why?
16. What is cholesterol? How is it associated with atherosclerosis? What has been published recently in newspapers and magazines concerning cholesterol and heart problems?
17. Why is skim milk allowed on low-fat diets when whole milk is not?
18. Discuss the differences between saturated and polyunsaturated fats. In what foods is each of these fats predominantly found?
19. What is hyperlipidemia? How is it related to atherosclerosis?

20. Discuss known risk factors for the development of atherosclerosis. Which could be avoided? Explain.

Suggested Activities

1. Find recipes suitable for fat-controlled diets and for a low-cholesterol diet. Compare recipes and check one another's for correctness. Suggest alternate ingredients for any that are not suitable for these diets.

2. Make a list of the foods eaten yesterday. Circle those foods that would not be allowed on a low-cholesterol diet and suggest satisfactory substitutions. Underline those not allowed on mild sodium-restricted diets. Are any both circled and underlined?

3. Plan a day's menu for a very low-fat diet, using Tables 20-1 and A-5 in the Appendix.

4. Plan a day's menu for a low-cholesterol diet. Use Table A-5 in the Appendix. Compare them with the low-fat menus in Number 3 above. Explain the differences.

5. Prepare at least one of these meals and evaluate it in terms of nutritive content, flavor, aroma, color, shape, appearance, texture, satiety value, and kcal.

6. Visit a local supermarket. List the foods containing sodium compounds. Suggest substitutes for these foods for patients on sodium-restricted diets.

7. Find recipes suitable for sodium-restricted diets. Compare them with other students' recipes and discuss their appropriateness.

8. Plan a day's menu for a patient on a mild sodium-restricted diet. Use Tables 20-5 and A-5.

9. Prepare and evaluate at least one of the meals on the menu and evaluate it in terms of nutritive content, flavor, aroma, color, shape, appearance, and satiety value.

10. Mary Jones was placed on a fat-restricted diet containing no more than 70 grams fat. She wants to order the following breakfast. Would this be acceptable? Explain your answer and, if necessary, suggest alternate foods that would be acceptable.

Sliced Avocado
Poached Egg with Ham in Cheese Sauce
on English Muffin
Coffee with Cream

11. John Brown has been told that he has atherosclerosis and must follow a low-cholesterol diet. He is visiting his aunt who is serving the following meal. Which of the foods can John eat and which must he avoid? Why? Can he eat certain parts of any of the foods? If so, which? Why?

Cream of Broccoli Soup
Roast Chicken
Mashed Potatoes with Gravy
Lima Beans with Butter
Green Salad with Vinegar and Oil Dressing
Rolls and Butter
Milk
Angel Food Cake with Whipped Cream
and Strawberries

12. Susan Smith has developed hypertension and has been placed on a mild sodium-restricted diet. She has planned the following dinner for her daughter's graduation party. Which of the foods can she eat and which must she avoid? Explain.

Fresh Fruit Cup
Baked Ham
Potato Chips
Fresh Frozen Broccoli Chunks Baked in
Canned Cream of Chicken Soup
Homemade Coleslaw
Rolls and Butter
Pickles and Olives
Chocolate Cake with Peppermint Ice Cream

Review

A. Multiple choice. Select the *letter* that precedes the best answer.
1. Sodium
   1. is an essential vitamin
   2. regulates the water balance in the body
   3. adds flavor to foods
   4. is found in table salt
      a) 1,2,3   b) 1,3,4   c) 2,3,4   d) all
2. Sodium is found in
   1. most foods
   2. water
   3. baking soda and baking powder
   4. brine
      a) 1,2,3   b) 2,3,4   c) 1,3,4   d) all
3. A patient with angina pectoris might be advised to follow a diet
   1. that contains limited sodium

    2. in which the kcal are reduced

    3. containing minimum amounts of cholesterol

    4. in which saturated fats are limited

        a) only 4   b) 1,2,4   c) 2,3,4   d) all

4.   Herbs, spices, and flavorings may

    1. be used in sodium-restricted diets

    2. never be used in sodium-restricted diets

    3. detract from the blandness of sodium-restricted diets

    4. be used only in the mild sodium-restricted diet

        a) 1,3   b) 2   c) 4   d) 3,4

5.   Lipoproteins

    1. carry proteins to the cells

    2. carry cholesterol to the liver

    3. always contribute to myocardial infarction

    4. are related to the amount of fats in the blood

        a) 1,2   b) 2,3,4   c) 1,3,4   d) 2,4

6.   A sodium-restricted diet may be ordered for patients with

    1. edema

    2. hypertension

    3. congestive heart failure

    4. atherosclerosis

        a) 1,2,3   b) 2,4   c) 1,4   d) all

7.   When water accumulates in body tissues,

    1. the condition is called edema

    2. a sodium-restricted diet may be prescribed

    3. it is a definite symptom of myocardial infarction

    4. salt is completely eliminated from the diet

        a) 1,3   b) 2,3,4   c) 1,2   d) all

8.   It is thought that excessive fats in the blood over time contribute to

    1. atherosclerosis

    2. myocardial infarction

    3. plaque

    4. peripheral vascular disease

        a) 1,3   b) 1,2,3   c) 2,3   d) all

9.   Table salt

    1. is 100 percent sodium

    2. is over 40 percent sodium

    3. contains only negligible amounts of sodium

    4. must be restricted in sodium-restricted diets

        a) 1,3,4   b) 2,3,4   c) 2,4   d) 2,3

10.   In a low-cholesterol diet

    1. eggs are used freely

    2. skim milk is used instead of whole milk

    3. lean muscle meats and fish are permitted

    4. vegetable oils are permitted

       a) 1,2,3   b) 2,3,4   c) 1,3,4   d) all

11. Triglycerides

    1. are interchangeable with lipoproteins

    2. are fats in food and adipose tissue

    3. usually cause congestive heart failure

    4. can contribute to atherosclerosis

       a) 1,2   b) 2,3   c) 2,4   d) all

12. Persons on a low-fat diet will

    1. need information about the fat content of foods

    2. need information about cooking methods for their diets

    3. never be allowed butter or margarine

    4. probably find the diet somewhat unpalatable

       a) 1,3,4   b) 1,2,3   c) 1,2,4   d) all

13. Foods allowed in a low-fat diet include

    1. all cheeses

    2. cooked vegetables

    3. cereals

    4. limited amounts of lean meats

       a) 1,3,4   b) 2,3,4   c) 1,3,4   d) all

14. When preparing foods for the low-fat diet,

    1. small amounts of fat can be added

    2. visible fats must be removed from meats

    3. skim milk is never used

    4. no frying is permitted

       a) 1,4   b) 2,3,4   c) 2,4   d) all

15. On the low-cholesterol diet, saturated fats are

    1. reduced

    2. eliminated

    3. increased

    4. unchanged from that of the regular diet

       a) 1,2   b) 2 only   c) 1 only   d) all

16. Saturated fats are usually

    1. solid at room temperature

    2. liquid at room temperature

    3. found in animal foods

    4. derived from plants

       a) 1,3   b) 2,3   c) 1,4   d) all

17. Polyunsaturated fats are usually

    1. solid at room temperature

    2. liquid at room temperature

    3. found in animal foods

    4. derived from plants

       a) 1,3   b) 2,4   c) 1,4   d) all

18. When the heart muscle reacts with pain because of inadequate blood supply after activity, the condition is called

    1. cerebral accident

    2. edema

    3. hypertension

    4. angina pectoris

       a) 1,3   b) 2,3   c) 3   d) 4

19. Some examples of blood lipids are

    1. triglycerides

    2. lumens

    3. cholesterol

    4. plaques

       a) 2,3   b) 1,3   c) 1,2   d) 3,4

20. Examples of foods particularly rich in potassium are

    1. milk and ice cream

    2. beef and lamb

    3. whole grain breads and cereals

    4. bananas and oranges

       a) 1,2   b) 2,3   c) 4   d) 1

Case Study 1

Heart Conditions

Joe G., a 45-year-old married lawyer with two teen-aged children, suffered an acute myocardial infarction. It was noted that Joe was 20 pounds overweight and had atherosclerosis. Immediately after admission, Joe was placed on a clear liquid diet, then progressed to a soft diet. Within a week, he was allowed a regular diet, with kcal and cholesterol controlled.

After ten days in the hospital, Joe was ready for discharge. As the doctor discussed Joe's future, he was encouraging, telling him that with rest for six to eight weeks, diet and weight control, and a planned cardiovascular rehabilitation program, he should be able to return to a normal life.

The doctor prescribed a low-cholesterol, low-kcal diet and described it. The doctor told Joe he should follow the low-cholesterol diet for the rest of his life. He explained the dangers of the excess weight, and said that after losing 20 pounds, Joe should not have to continue the low-kcal diet. The rehabilitation program was discussed as a way to improve Joe's circulation and help prevent complications.

Joe was surprised by all the information. He weighed exactly the same as when he was a quarterback at the university, 20 years ago. He and his wife had considered themselves "health freaks" in regard to diet. They always ate a balanced breakfast of bacon or ham, eggs, and toast. They never sent their children to school having eaten only cereal. They all carry their lunches, which include meat sandwiches, fruit, and whole milk. At dinner they enjoy steaks, chops, and fish—especially shrimp and lobster—with vegetables.

They use real butter and whole milk purchased at the local health food store so they know it's healthy. They do not indulge in sweets, except for a bedtime snack of ice cream.

Case Study Questions Based on the Nursing Process

Assess
1. Why was Joe started on a clear liquid diet during the acute phase of his illness and then progressed to a soft diet?
2. Why was Joe put on a low-cholesterol diet? Would it harm his wife and children to eat the same foods as Joe? Explain.
3. What foods regularly eaten by Joe in the past will have to be avoided in the future?

Plan
4. Joe's diet had averaged 3500 kcal each day. The doctor put him on a 2500-kcal diet. How much weight will Joe lose each week? How many weeks will be required for Joe to lose 20 pounds?
5. What foods could Joe substitute for some of those he must avoid in his low-kcal, low-cholesterol diet?
6. Joe likes shrimp cooked in garlic butter. Is this advisable for him now? Why?

Implement
7. What problems might Joe encounter as he adjusts to his new diet? How might he cope with them?
8. Plan a day's menu for Joe when he gets home from the hospital. Adapt it for his family.
9. Why is it important for Joe to add exercise to his daily regimen as prescribed by the cardiac rehabilitation program coordinator?

Evaluate
10. What may happen if Joe disregards his doctor's advice?
11. When Joe returns to the doctor's office one month later, what will the doctor look for to confirm that Joe is following the recommendations?

Case Study 2

Despite being 30 pounds overweight, Margaret recovered well from her mitral valve replacement. Following surgery, her chief complaints related to food. She disliked the sodium- and kcal-restricted diet her physician had prescribed. She complained about the dry, white meat of the chicken; the tastelessness of the vegetables; the lack of ice cream and butter; not being able to eat her favorite canned soup; and not having any potato chips.

Case Study Questions Based on the Nursing Process

Assess
1. Why is Margaret's reaction to her new diet not surprising?

Plan
2. What might be done to improve the taste of the "dry, white meat of the chicken" and still keep it within the physician's dietary guidelines?
3. Why can't Margaret have canned bouillon? (It contains only a few kcal.)
4. Explain why Margaret should not have ice cream.

Implement
5. What might Margaret substitute for butter on her fresh asparagus?
6. Margaret's favorite meal is the following. Adapt it to fit her new dietary requirements:

Clam chowder
Roast lamb
Mashed potatoes with gravy
Green beans with cheese sauce
Coleslaw made with mayonnaise
Salt-topped dinner rolls
Canned peaches with whipped cream

Evaluate
7. At her next visit to her physician, Margaret will be asked what foods she eats for breakfast, lunch, dinner, and snacks. Which foods should she be avoiding on a sodium- and kcal-restricted diet?
8. What will the doctor note during the physical exam that may indicate Margaret is not following her diet?

DIET AND RENAL DISEASE

OBJECTIVES

After studying this chapter, you should be able to
- Describe, in general terms, the work of the kidneys
- Explain why protein is sometimes increased or decreased for renal patients
- Explain why sodium and water are sometimes restricted for renal patients
- Explain why potassium and phosphorus are sometimes restricted for renal patients

The kidneys are intricate and efficient processing systems that excrete wastes, maintain volume and composition of body fluids, and secrete certain hormones. To accomplish these tasks, they filter the blood, cleansing it of waste products, and recycle other usable substances so that the necessary constituents of body fluids are constantly available.

Each kidney contains approximately one million working parts called **nephrons.** Each nephron contains a filtering unit called a **glomer-ulus** in which there is a cluster of specialized capillaries (tiny blood vessels connecting veins and arteries). Approximately 180 liters of **filtrate** (substance to be filtered) are processed each day. As the filtrate passes through the nephrons, the kidneys are able to concentrate or dilute it to meet the body's needs. This enables the kidneys to help maintain both the composition and the volume of body fluids and, consequently, fluid balance, acid-base balance, and electrolyte balance. The waste materials are sent via two tubes called **ureters** from the kidneys to the bladder from which they are excreted in urine. These include end products of protein metabolism (**urea, uric acid, creatinine,** ammonia, and sulfates), excess water, dead renal cells, and toxic substances. The recycled materials are **resorbed** (taken back) by the blood. They include amino acids, glucose, minerals, vitamins, and water.

The kidneys synthesize and secrete certain hormones as needed. For example, it is the kidneys that make the final conversion of vitamin D so it can play its role in the absorption of calcium. The kidneys indirectly stimulate the bone marrow to produce red blood cells.

TYPES OF RENAL DISORDERS

Kidney disorders can be initially caused by infection, degenerative changes, cardiovascular disorders, **cysts** (growths), **renal calculi** (stones), or **trauma** (surgery, burns, poisons). When they are severe, renal failure may develop. It may be acute or chronic. **Acute renal failure** occurs suddenly and may last a few days or a few weeks. It is caused by another medical problem such as a serious burn, a crushing injury, or cardiac arrest. It can be expected in some of these situations so preventive steps may be taken.

Chronic renal failure develops slowly with the number of functioning nephrons constantly diminishing. When renal tissue has been destroyed to the point that the kidneys are no longer able to filter the blood, excrete wastes, or recycle nutrients as needed, uremia occurs. **Uremia** is a condition in which protein wastes that should normally have been excreted are instead circulating in the blood. Symptoms include nausea, headache, coma, and convulsions. Severe renal failure will result in death unless **dialysis** (filtration to remove toxic substances) is begun or a kidney transplant is performed.

Nephritis is a general term referring to the inflammatory diseases of the kidneys. Nephritis can be caused by infection, degenerative processes, or vascular disease.

Glomerulonephritis is a nephritis affecting the **capillaries** in the glomeruli. It may occur acutely in conjunction with another infection and be self-limiting, or it may lead to serious renal deterioration.

Nephrosclerosis is the hardening of renal arteries. It is caused by arteriosclerosis and hypertension. Although it usually occurs in older people, it sometimes develops in young diabetics.

Polycystic kidney disease is a relatively rare, hereditary disease. Cysts form and press on the kidneys. The kidneys enlarge and lose function. Although people with this condition have normal kidney function for many years, renal failure may develop near the age of 50.

Renal calculi or **nephrolithiasis** is a condition in which stones develop in the kidneys, the ureters, or the bladder. The size varies from that of a grain of sand to much larger. Some remain at their point of origin and others move. While the condition is sometimes asymptomatic, symptoms include **hematuria** (blood in the urine), infection, obstruction and, if the stones move, intense pain. The stones are classified according to their composition—calcium, uric acid, **cystine** (amino acid), and oxalic acid. They are associated with metabolic disturbances and immobilization of the patient.

NUTRITIONAL TREATMENT OF RENAL DISORDERS

Dietary Treatment of Renal Disease

The dietary treatment of renal disease can be extremely complicated. It is intended to reduce the amount of excretory work demanded of the kidneys while assisting them in maintaining fluid, acid-base, and electrolyte balance. Patients require sufficient protein to prevent malnutrition and muscle wasting. Too much, however, can contribute to uremia. Typically, the patient with chronic renal failure will have protein and sodium, and possibly potassium and phosphorus, restricted.

It is essential that renal patients receive sufficient kcal—35 to 40 kcal per kilogram of body weight—unless they are overweight. Energy requirements should be fulfilled by carbohydrates and fat. The fats must be polyunsaturated to prevent or check hyperlipidemia. If the energy requirement is not met by carbohydrates and fat, ingested protein or body tissue will be metabolized for energy. Either would increase the work of the kidneys because protein increases the amount of nitrogen waste the kidneys must handle. The diet may limit protein to 20 grams. The specific amount of protein allowed is calculated according to the patient's **glomerular filtration rate (GFR)** and weight. Rarely, protein may be increased in an effort to increase blood protein, and the requirement can go as high as 125 grams.

Sodium may be limited if the patient tends to retain it. Retained sodium and water could contribute to edema, hypertension, and congestive heart failure. Fluids are typically restricted for renal patients.

Calcium supplements may be prescribed. In addition, vitamin D may be added and phosphorus limited, to prevent **osteomalacia** (softening of the bones due to excessive loss of calcium). Phosphorus appears to be retained in patients with kidney disorders, and a disproportionately high ratio of phosphorus to calcium tends to increase calcium loss from bones.

Potassium may be restricted in some patients because **hyperkalemia** (high blood potassium) tends to occur in renal failure. Excess potassium can cause cardiac arrest. Because of this danger, renal patients should not use salt sub-

stitutes or low-sodium milk because the sodium in these products is replaced with potassium. Potassium restriction can be especially difficult for a renal patient who probably must limit sodium intake. Potassium is particularly high in fruits—one of the few foods a patient on a sodium-restricted diet may eat without concern.

Renal patients often have an increased need for vitamins B, C, and D, and supplements are often given. Vitamin A should not be given because the blood level of vitamin A tends to be elevated in uremia. If a patient is receiving antibiotics, a vitamin K supplement may be given. Otherwise, supplements of vitamins E and K are not necessary. Iron is commonly prescribed because anemia frequently develops in renal patients. To ensure sufficient kcal, it is sometimes necessary to increase the amount of simple carbohydrates and fats.

Diet During Dialysis

Dialysis patients may need additional protein, but the amount must be carefully controlled to prevent the accumulation of protein waste between treatments.

Potassium levels will vary and must be carefully monitored. Some patients will require supplements, whereas other patients will have potassium restricted. Fluids and sodium are usually restricted to prevent fluid retention. There is often a need for supplements of water-soluble vitamins, vitamin D, calcium, and iron.

Diet After Kidney Transplant

After kidney transplant, there may be a need for extra protein or for the restriction of protein. Carbohydrates and sodium may be restricted. The appropriate amounts of these nutrients will depend largely on the medications given at that time.

Additional calcium and phosphorus may be necessary if there has been substantial bone loss before the transplant. There may be an increase in appetite after transplants. To prevent excessive weight gain, fats and simple carbohydrates may be limited.

Dietary Treatment of Renal Calculi

Because the causes of renal calculi have not been confirmed, treatment of them may vary. Generally, however, large amounts of fluid—at least half of it water—are helpful in diluting the urine, as is a well-balanced diet. Once the stones have been analyzed, specific diet modifications may be indicated.

Alkaline-ash and acid-ash diets are sometimes used in an effort to change the pH of the urine and consequently, the incidence of stones. In these diets, foods are labeled by the ash they leave after oxidation. If the ash is acid, the food is labeled *acid-ash;* if alkaline, it is labeled *alkaline-ash*. Foods that cause the urine to become acidic (a pH below 7) are called acid-ash and those that cause the urine to become alkaline (a pH above 7), alkaline-ash. (See Chapter 8.) Both diets become tedious and difficult to follow.

Calcium Stones

About two-thirds of the kidney stones formed contain calcium. If the patient has a history of calcium stones, this mineral is restricted in the diet, but not usually to less than 600 mg

Table 21-1 Calcium Content of Common Dairy Products

1 cup whole milk	291 mg Calcium
1 cup skim milk	302 mg Calcium
$\frac{1}{2}$ cup ice cream	90 mg Calcium
1 oz. wedge cheddar cheese	204 mg Calcium
$\frac{1}{2}$ cup cottage cheese	70 mg Calcium
1 oz. process cheese	174 mg Calcium
1 cup eggnog	330 mg Calcium

Table 21-2 Purine-rich Foods

Avoid	Limit
liver	meats
kidneys	fish
sweetbreads	poultry
brains	meat soups
heart	
anchovies	
sardines	
meat extracts	
bouillon	
broth	

per day. Obviously, foods rich in calcium will have to be limited (see Table 21-1).

Uric Acid Stones

When the stones contain uric acid, purine-rich foods may be restricted (see Table 21-2). **Purines** are the end products of nucleoprotein metabolism and are found in all meats, fish, and poultry. Organ meats, anchovies, sardines, meat extracts, and broths are especially rich sources of them.

Oxalic Acid Stones

Stones containing oxalic acid are thought to be partially caused by a diet especially rich in oxalic acid, which is found in broccoli, asparagus, chocolate, tea, rhubarb, and spinach. Evidence also indicates that deficiencies of pyridoxine, thiamin, and magnesium may contribute to the formation of oxalic acid kidney stones.

Cystine Stones

Cystine is an amino acid. Cystine stones may form when the cystine concentration in the urine becomes excessive due to a hereditary metabolic disorder. The usual practice is to increase fluids and recommend an alkaline-ash diet.

The High-Protein Diet

The high-protein diet is a regular diet with increased protein content. The protein is provided by normal protein-rich foods (see Table 21-3) and may be further increased by the addition of skim milk powder to soups, cream sauces, gravies, and baked products. It is highly nutritious. It may be used for patients following surgery or during convalescence from burns. Table 21-4 shows sample menus for a high-protein diet.

The Low-Protein Diet

When a low-protein diet is prescribed, it is important that the protein be equally distributed among the three meals (see Table 21-5). This diet contains insufficient protein, minerals, vitamins, and in some cases, kcal.

Table 21-3 Foods Included in a High-Protein Diet

milk: 3 to 4 cups
cheeses
eggs
lean meats, fish, and poultry
vegetables
fruits
cereals (whole grain or enriched) and breads as desired

CONSIDERATIONS FOR THE HEALTH CARE PROFESSIONAL

The patient with renal disease has a severe burden. Anger and depression are common among these patients. These feelings complicate

Table 21-4 Sample Menus for a High-Protein Diet

Breakfast	Dinner	Lunch or Supper
Orange Juice	Roast Chicken	Ground Round Steak
Scrambled Eggs	Baked Potato	Corn
Bacon	Green Peas	Tomatoes and Lettuce
Toast with Butter and Jelly	Lettuce Salad	Bread and Butter
Skim Milk	Bread and Butter	Frozen Yogurt with Strawberries
Coffee with Skim Milk	Custard made from Skim Milk	Skim Milk
	Skim Milk	Tea with Milk

Table 21-5 Sample Menus for a Low-Protein (30 Gram) Diet

Breakfast	Dinner	Lunch or Supper
Orange Juice	1 Cup Pineapple Juice	1 Cup Apple Juice
1 Cup Rice Cereal with $\frac{1}{2}$ Cup Milk and Sugar	1 oz. Roast Beef	1 oz. Roast Chicken
Coffee	$\frac{1}{2}$ Cup Baked Squash with Butter	1 Boiled Potato
	Baked Apple with Sugar	Sliced Cucumber
	Tea	1 Cup Strawberries with Sugar and Cream
		Tea with Sugar

management of the disease if they contribute to the patient's unwillingness to learn about his or her nutritional needs. These complications then add to the patient's problems.

The health care professional can be extremely helpful if he or she can develop a trusting relationship with the patient. Such a relationship can be established by listening to the patient's complaints, needs, and concerns and responding with sincere understanding and sympathy. This can ultimately help motivate the patient to want to learn how to manage his or her nutritional requirements and help the nutrition counselor assist the patient.

SUMMARY

The kidneys rid the body of wastes, maintain fluid, electrolyte, and acid-base balance, and secrete hormones. When they are damaged by disease or injury, the entire body is affected. Diet therapy for renal disorders can be extremely complex because of the multifaceted nature of the kidneys' functions. Untreated severe kidney disease can result in death unless dialysis or kidney transplant is undertaken.

Discussion Topics

1. Discuss the three main tasks of the kidneys.
2. Define nephrons and explain what they do.
3. Discuss some causes of kidney disease.
4. What is nephritis? glomerulonephritis? nephrosclerosis?
5. Why is diet therapy of renal disease so complex?
6. Discuss why protein is typically decreased for patients with renal disease.
7. Why are sodium and water sometimes restricted in renal disease?
8. Why is potassium sometimes restricted in renal disease? What is hyperkalemia?
9. Why is phosphorus sometimes restricted in renal disease?
10. Why might kcal be restricted in renal disease?
11. What is nephrolithiasis? How is it treated?

Suggested Activities

1. Using outside sources, prepare a short report on the functions of the circulatory system, the liver, and the kidneys in eliminating nitrogenous waste products from the body.
2. Find recipes that are suitable for high-protein and low-protein diets.
3. List the foods you ate yesterday. Compute the amount of protein by using Table A-5 in the Appendix. Compare the total protein with the RDA of protein for someone your age and sex as listed on Table A-1 in the Appendix. Would such a diet meet the limitations of someone on a 30-g low-protein diet? Does it contain adequate protein for you? If not, how could you improve it?

4. Plan a day's menu for a 100 g high-protein diet. Plan a day's menu for a 30 g low-protein diet by adapting the high-protein menus and correct if necessary. Adapt them to suit the needs of your family.
5. Prepare at least one meal on each of the menus. Evaluate each in terms of nutritive content, flavor, aroma, color, shape, appearance, texture, and satiety value.
6. Using Table A-5 in the Appendix, compute the protein in the sample high-protein diet menu in this chapter.
7. Plan a day's menus for a patient on a calcium-restricted (600 mg) diet. Adapt the menus to suit your family's needs. Use Table A-5 in the Appendix.
8. Plan a day's menus for a patient who must limit her or his intake of oxalic acid. Adapt it to suit your needs.
9. Invite a registered nurse to discuss renal disease with your class.

Review

Multiple choice. Select the *letter* that precedes the best answer.
1. The kidneys maintain the body's
   a. acid-base balance
   b. electrolyte balance
   c. fluid balance
   d. all of these
2. The specialized part within each nephron that actually filters the blood is called the
   a. ureter
   b. filter
   c. glomerulus
   d. capillary bunch
3. Kidney disorders may be caused by
   a. cysts
   b. infections
   c. burns
   d. all of these
4. When renal tissue has been destroyed to the point that it can no longer filter the blood, the following occurs:
   a. nephritis
   b. nephrosclerosis
   c. uremia
   d. nephrolithiasis
5. The general term referring to the inflammatory diseases of the kidneys is
   a. nephritis
   b. nephrosclerosis
   c. uremia
   d. nephrolithiasis
6. The term referring to the hardening of renal arteries is
   a. nephritis
   b. nephrosclerosis
   c. uremia
   d. nephrolithiasis
7. The rare hereditary disease causing cysts to develop on the kidneys is called
   a. nephritis
   b. glomerulonephritis
   c. renal calculi
   d. polycystic kidney disease

8. The condition in which stones develop in the kidneys, ureters, or bladder is called
    a. nephritis   c. polycystic kidney disease
    b. nephrolithiasis   d. glomerulonephritis
9. Because its nitrogenous wastes contribute to uremia, the following nutrient may be restricted in diets of renal patients
    a. carbohydrate   c. protein
    b. saturated fat   d. vitamin A
10. Kidney dialysis
    a. is a means of filtering all protein from the blood
    b. is a means of removing toxic substances from the blood
    c. always requires the patient be on a low-protein diet
    d. requires the patient to increase his or her sodium intake
11. Sodium and water may be restricted in the diets of renal patients because they
    a. contribute to uremia   c. contribute to hyperlipidemia
    b. increase hypercalcemia   d. contribute to hypertension
12. If osteomalacia occurs in renal patients, the following nutrient may be prescribed
    a. potassium   c. calcium
    b. protein   d. phosphorus
13. In a case of hyperkalemia, the following nutrient may be restricted
    a. potassium   c. calcium
    b. protein   d. phosphorus
14. Fruits are an especially rich source of
    a. potassium   c. calcium
    b. protein   d. phosphorus
15. Because anemia may be present in renal patients, the following nutrient may be prescribed
    a. phosphorus   c. calcium
    b. carbohydrate   d. iron
16. The vitamins renal patients may have an increased need for are
    a. the water-soluble vitamins   c. only the B vitamins
    b. the fat-soluble vitamins   d. vitamins E and A
17. An excess of the following nutrient can compound bone loss in renal patients
    a. phosphorus   c. calcium
    b. carbohydrate   d. iron

18. Acid-ash foods include
    a. meats
    b. dairy foods
    c. vegetables, except corn and lentils
    d. fruits, except cranberries, plums, and prunes
19. Purine-rich foods include
    a. meats
    b. dairy foods
    c. vegetables, except corn and lentils
    d. fruits, except cranberries, plums, and prunes
20. An example of nitrogenous waste found in the urine is
    a. ureter   c. urea
    b. uremia   d. all of these

Case Study 1

Renal Disease

Laura E. had been experiencing a frequent need to urinate the past few days. When she did urinate, she felt a burning sensation that was getting progressively worse. On the fifth day she felt severely ill, experiencing chills and fever, and called her doctor. Examination revealed Laura was febrile; her serum white blood count was severely elevated at 21,000 mm^3; and urinalysis was positive for occult blood, white blood cells, and nitrates. Her doctor told her she had nephritis and admitted her to the hospital.

Laura was placed on intravenous antibiotics. She began to feel better in a few days and was discharged home on oral antibiotics after seven days.

Case Study Questions Based on Nursing Process

Assess

1. Why did the doctor test Laura's blood and urine daily during her hospital stay?
2. What dietary needs would you expect Laura to have at this time?

Plan

3. Why was there no salt on Laura's meal trays?
4. Why was Laura given a vitamin supplement?
5. What medical and nutritional information should be given to Laura concerning her illness?

Implement

6. Laura's appetite was poor during her hospital stay. Why did the nurse encourage her to eat everything on her plate?
7. The nurse also encouraged Laura to drink her milk. Laura questioned this because when her aunt had been hospitalized with nephrosclerosis, she had been allowed only low-sodium milk. How would you explain this to Laura?

Evaluate

8. Judging from Laura's rapid recovery, what probably was the cause of her nephritis?
9. Could Laura help prevent future episodes of nephritis? Explain.
10. What should the range of Laura's white blood count be to indicate recovery? What would her urinalysis show?

Case Study 2

Transplant Patient

Norman had recovered well from his kidney transplant. His chief complaint was that the hospital food was not satisfying in quantity or quality. He told the doctor that if only there were more food, he'd soon be back to his pre-illness weight of 250 pounds. His doctor smiled, but told him that his current 180 pounds was just right for his 5'8" frame.

He convinced his friend, Gordon, to bring him a box of chocolates. As Norman was unwrapping the chocolates, the doctor walked into the room and voiced disapproval.

Study Questions Based on the Nursing Process

Assess

1.   Why did the doctor disapprove of the chocolates?
2.   What nutrients do chocolates primarily contain?

Plan

3.   Would potato chips have been a better treat? Explain.
4.   What food would have been a better treat for Norman?

Implement

5.   What might you have said to Norman if you had been the nurse on duty in his room when Gordon arrived with the chocolates.
6.   How could one gain Norman's cooperation in planning his new diet?

Evaluate

7.   What actions would indicate Norman's acceptance of his new dietary regimen?

CHAPTER 22

DIET AND GASTROINTESTINAL PROBLEMS

OBJECTIVES

After studying this chapter, you should be able to
- Explain the uses of diet therapy in the gastrointestinal disturbances discussed here
- Identify the foods allowed/disallowed in the therapeutic diets discussed
- Adapt normal diets to meet the requirements of patients with these conditions

The gastrointestinal tract is where digestion and absorption of food occur.

The primary organs include the mouth, esophagus, stomach, and the small and large intestine. The liver, gallbladder, and pancreas are accessory organs that are also involved in these processes.

Numerous disorders of the gastrointestinal system cause countless individuals distress and consequently affect the nation's economy because they keep so many people home from work. Some problems are physiologically caused; others can be psychological in origin. It is some-

times difficult to determine the cause or causes of a "GI" problem. Consequently, controversy exists in some cases about proper treatment.

DISORDERS OF THE PRIMARY ORGANS

Dyspepsia

Dyspepsia or indigestion is a condition of discomfort in the digestive tract that can be physical or psychological in origin. Symptoms include "heartburn," bloating, pain, and sometimes, regurgitation. If the cause is physical, it can be due to rushed eating, over-rich foods, or it may be a symptom of another problem, such as appendicitis, kidney, gallbladder, or colon diseases and, possibly, cancer. If the problem is organic in origin, treatment of the underlying cause will be the normal procedure.

Psychological stress can affect stomach secretions and trigger dyspepsia. Treatment should include counseling to help the patient

- find relief from the underlying stress
- allow sufficient time to relax and enjoy meals
- learn to improve eating habits

Hiatal Hernia

Hiatal hernia is a condition in which a part of the stomach protrudes through the **diaphragm** (a muscular sheet separating the abdominal cavity from the chest cavity) into the thoracic cavity. (See figure 22-1.) This prevents the food from moving normally along the digestive tract, although it does mix somewhat with the gastric juices. Sometimes the food will move back into the esophagus, creating a burning sensation ("heartburn"), and sometimes food will be regurgitated into the mouth. This condition can be very uncomfortable.

The problem can sometimes be alleviated by serving small, frequent meals (from a well-balanced diet) so the amount of food in the stomach is never large. If the patient is obese, weight loss may be recommended to reduce pressure on the abdomen. It may also be helpful if patients avoid lying down soon after eating. When they do lie down, they may be more comfortable sleeping with their heads and upper torso somewhat elevated. If discomfort cannot be controlled, surgery may be necessary.

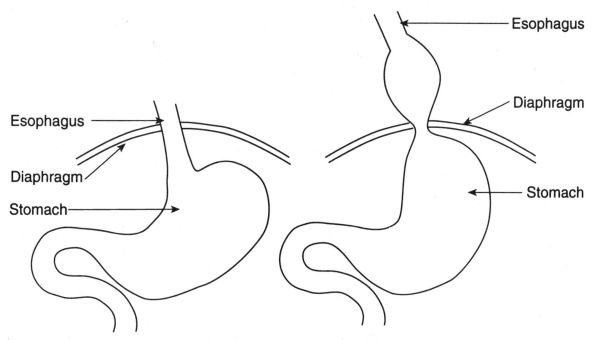

A. Normal position of stomach   B. Hiatal hernia

Figure 22-1 A hiatal hernia prevents food from moving through the diaphragm into the thoracic cavity.

Peptic Ulcers

An ulcer is an erosion of the mucous membrane. **Peptic ulcers** may occur in the stomach (**gastric ulcer**) or the duodenum (**duodenal ulcer**). The specific cause of ulcers is not clear, but some physicians believe that a number of factors including genetic predisposition, abnormally high **secretion** of hydrochloric acid by the stomach, anxiety, excessive use of aspirin or ibuprofen (analgesics), cigarette smoking, and possibly a bacteria may contribute to their development.

Symptoms include gastric pain that is sometimes described as "burning" and, in some cases, hemorrhage. The pain is typically relieved with food or antacids. A hemorrhage usually requires surgery.

Ulcers are generally treated with drugs such as cimetidine, which inhibit acid secretion in the stomach and thus help to heal the ulcer. Antacids can also be prescribed to neutralize any excess acid. Rest and counseling to help the patient learn to deal with pressure and stress are also useful in the treatment of ulcers.

In the past, diet therapy typically began with the **Sippy Diet,** which originally included hourly servings of milk and cream only, and was later liberalized to include some soft foods. It is rarely used today because while whole milk does initially neutralize the gastric acid, the protein it contains stimulates the stomach to secrete additional acid. When it is used, whole or skim milk are now advised because of the danger of atherosclerosis from the cream. Generally, the diet therapy for peptic ulcers has been vastly liberalized and the effectiveness of soft or bland diets has become controversial.

A **bland diet** includes foods that are simply prepared, have little fiber, are mild flavored, and are not known to increase the production of stomach acid. Such a diet should not irritate the gastrointestinal tract chemically or mechanically.

It is seldom used. The soft diet is discussed in Chapter 17.

Sufficient protein should be provided, but not in excess because of its ability to stimulate gastric acid secretion. It is recommended that patients receive no less than 0.8 gram of protein per kilogram of body weight. However, if there has been blood loss, this may be increased to 1 or 1.5 grams per kilogram of body weight. Vitamin and mineral supplements, especially iron if there has been hemorrhage, may be prescribed.

Although fat inhibits gastric secretions, because of the danger of atherosclerosis, the amount of fat in the diet should not be excessive. Carbohydrates have little effect on gastric acid secretion.

While coarse foods were previously prohibited ulcer patients because it was thought that the roughage irritated the ulcer, this is no longer the case. Generally, caffeine and alcohol are to be avoided. Spicy foods may be eaten as tolerated.

Coffee, tea, or anything containing caffeine stimulates gastric secretion. Alcohol and aspirin irritate the **mucous membrane** of the stomach, and cigarette smoking decreases the secretion of the **pancreas** that buffers gastric acid in the duodenum.

Currently, a well-balanced diet of three meals a day consisting of foods that do not irritate the patient is generally recommended.

Diverticulosis/Diverticulitis

Diverticulosis is an intestinal disorder characterized by little pockets in the sides of the intestines. When food collects in these pockets instead of moving on through the intestines, bacteria may breed, and inflammation and pain can result, causing **diverticulitis.** If a diverticulum ruptures, surgery may be needed. This condition is thought to be caused by diet lacking in sufficient fiber. A high-fiber diet is commonly recommended for patients with diverticulosis.

Diet therapy for diverticulitis may begin with a clear liquid diet (see Chapter 17), followed by a low-residue or even minimum-residue diet, and very gradually (over several weeks) progress to a high-fiber diet. The bulk provided by the high-fiber diet increases stool volume, reduces the pressure in the colon, and shortens the time the food is in the intestine, giving bacteria less time to grow.

RESIDUE-CONTROLLED DIETS

Fiber is indigestible carbohydrate found in plants. **Residue** is the solid part of feces. Residue is made up of all the undigested and unabsorbed parts of food (including fiber), connective tissue in meat, dead cells, and intestinal bacteria and their products. Most of this residue is composed of fiber.

Dietary fiber refers to the nondigestible carbohydrates present in a food when it is eaten. Examples are corn kernels, strawberry seeds, and celery strings. **Crude fiber** is the amount of fiber remaining in a plant food after it has been treated with various acids and alkalies in the laboratory. In this process, much of the dietary fiber is destroyed. Therefore, crude fiber is not an accurate measurement of fiber in food. Dietary fiber should be used.

Diets can be adjusted to increase or decrease fiber and residue. The specific names of these diets vary among health care facilities. The specific foods allowed and, thus, the amount of fiber and residue allowed, will depend on the physician's experience and the patient's condition.

The High-Fiber Diet

High-fiber diets are believed to help prevent diverticulosis, constipation, hemorrhoids, and colon cancer. They also are helpful in the treatment of diabetes mellitus (see Chapter 19) and atherosclerosis (see Chapter 20).

It is currently estimated that the normal diet in the United States contains about 20 grams of dietary fiber each day. A high-fiber diet is often 20 to 30 grams and can be as much as 50 grams a day. The recommended foods for this diet include coarse and whole grain breads and cereals, bran, all fruits, vegetables (especially raw), and legumes. Milk, meats, and fats do not contain fiber. (See Table 22-1.) This diet is nutritionally adequate. High-fiber diets must be introduced gradually to prevent the formation of gas and the discomfort that accompanies it.

The Low-Residue Diet

The low-residue diet is intended to reduce the normal work of the intestines by restricting the amount of dietary fiber and reducing food residue. Low-fiber or residue-restricted diets may be used in cases of severe diarrhea, diverticulitis, ulcerative colitis, intestinal blockage, and in preparation for and immediately after intestinal surgery.

In some facilities, these diets consist of foods that provide no more than three grams of fiber a day and that do not increase fecal residue. (See Tables 22-2 and 22-3.) Some foods that do not actually leave residue in the colon are considered "high-residue" foods because they increase stool volume or provide a laxative effect. Milk and prune juice are examples of them. Milk increases stool volume and prune juice acts as a laxative.

The Minimum-Residue Diet

The **minimum-residue diet** is extremely restrictive and can contain no more than one gram of fiber per day. Generally, fruits or vegetables

Table 22-1 Sample Menus for a High-Fiber Diet

Breakfast	Dinner	Lunch or Supper
Stewed Prunes	Baked Pork Chops	Fresh Fruit Cup
Bran Cereal with Milk and Sugar	Baked Potato	Roast Beef Sandwich on Cracked Wheat Bread with Lettuce and Tomato
Whole Wheat Toast with Marmalade	Fresh Corn	Coleslaw
Coffee	Green Salad with Oil and Vinegar Dressing	Carrot Cake
	Whole Grain Bread with Margarine	Skim Milk
	Fresh Pineapple	Coffee or Tea
	Skim Milk	
	Tea	

Table 22-2 Foods to Allow/Avoid on Low-Residue Foods

Foods Allowed in Low-Residue Diet	Foods to be Avoided
milk, buttermilk (limited to two cups daily) if physician allows	fresh or dried fruits and vegetables
cottage cheese and some mild cheeses as flavorings in small amounts	whole grain breads and cereals
butter and margarine	nuts, seeds, legumes, coconut, and marmalade
eggs, except fried	tough meats
tender chicken, fish, sweetbreads, ground beef, and ground lamb (meats must be baked, boiled, or broiled)	rich pastries
soup broth	milk, unless physician allows
cooked, mild-flavored vegetables without coarse fibers; strained fruit juices (except for prune); applesauce; canned fruits including white cherries, peaches, and pears; pureed apricots, ripe banana	meats and fish with tough connective tissue
refined breads and cereals, white crackers, macaroni, spaghetti, and noodles	
custard, sherbet, vanilla ice cream, junket, and *cereal puddings* when considered as part of the 2-cup milk allowance and if physician allows; plain gelatin; angel cake, sponge cake; and plain cookies	
coffee, tea, cocoa, carbonated beverage	
salt, sugar, small amount of spices as permitted by the physician	

Table 22-3 Sample Menus for a Low-Residue Diet

Breakfast	Dinner	Lunch or Supper
Strained Orange Juice	Chicken Broth	Tomato Juice
Cream of Rice Cereal with Milk and Sugar	Ground Beef Patty	Macaroni and Cheese
White Toast with Margarine and Jelly	Boiled Potato	Green Beans
Coffee with Cream and Sugar	Baked Squash	White Bread and Butter
	Gelatin Dessert	Lemon Sherbet
	Milk	Tea with Milk and Sugar

are not allowed except for limited amounts of fruit and vegetable juices (other than prune). Whole grain breads and cereals are not allowed, and milk may be prohibited. (See Table 22-4.)

Because of the severe limitations of foods allowed, this diet may be inadequate in vitamins and minerals. If this diet must be used for a period of time, the physician may prescribe vitamin and mineral supplements. The modifications made for the minimum-residue diet can be seen in Table 22-5.

Inflammatory Bowel Disease

Inflammatory bowel diseases are chronic conditions causing inflammation in the gastrointestinal tract. The inflammation causes malab-

sorption that often leads to malnutrition. The acute phases of these diseases occur at irregular intervals and are followed by periods where patients are relatively free of symptoms. Neither cause nor cure for these conditions is known.

Two examples are **ulcerative colitis** and **Crohn's disease.** Ulcerative colitis causes inflammation and ulceration of the colon, the rectum or, sometimes, the entire large intestine. Chrohn's disease can occur in any part of the gastrointestinal tract. The ulcers can penetrate the entire intestinal wall, and the chronic inflammation can thicken the intestinal wall causing obstruction.

Both conditions cause bloody diarrhea, cramps, nausea, anorexia, malnutrition, and weight loss. Electrolytes, fluids, vitamins, and

Table 22-4 Minimum-Residue Foods

Foods Allowed in a Minimum-Residue Diet		Foods to be Avoided
1 cup or less milk, if allowed	refined breads and cereals, white crackers	fruits and vegetables
cottage cheese, if tolerated and in small amounts	macaroni, spaghetti, and noodles	fried foods
margarine	sherbet, gelatin, plain cake and plain cookies	coarse, whole-grain breads and cereals, quick breads
eggs, except fried	tea, coffee (if physician permits)	fibrous meats
tender chicken and fish; ground beef and lamb	small amounts of salt and sugar	milk, unless permitted by physician
soup broth		nuts, seeds, legumes
vegetable juice		
fruit juice except prune		

Table 22-5 Sample Menus for a Minimum-Residue Diet

Breakfast	Dinner	Lunch or Supper
Strained Orange Juice	Pineapple Juice	Tomato Juice
Poached Egg on White Toast	Ground Beef	Minced White Poached Fish
Coffee or Tea	Buttered Noodles	Macaroni with Butter
	Toast with Butter	White Bread and Butter
	Plain Gelatin	Lemon Sherbet
	Tea	Tea

other minerals are lost in the diarrhea, and the bleeding can cause loss of iron and protein.

Treatment may involve anti-inflammatory drugs plus nutritional therapy. Usually a low-residue diet is required to avoid irritating the inflamed area and to avoid the danger of obstruction. When tolerated, the diet should include about 100 g of protein, additional kcal, vitamins, and minerals.

In severe cases, *total parenteral feeding* (directly into the superior vena cava; see Chapter 24) may be necessary for a period. As the patient begins to regain health, the diet may be increasingly liberalized to suit the patient's tastes while maintaining good nutrition.

Celiac Disease

Celiac disease, also called **non-tropical sprue** or **celiac sprue,** is a disorder characterized by malabsorption. It is thought to be due to heredity.

Symptoms include diarrhea, weight loss, and general malnutrition. Stools are usually foul smelling, light colored, and bulky. The cause is unknown, but it has been found that the elimination of **gluten** (a protein found in grains) from the diet gives relief. Untreated, it leads to decreased absorption of all nutrients, hence the malnutrition and weight loss.

A *gluten-controlled diet* (see Table 22-6) is used in the treatment of celiac disease. All products containing wheat, buckwheat, barley, rye, and oats are disallowed. Rice and corn may be used. A reduction in the fiber content is also frequently recommended. If the patient is underweight, the diet should also be high in kcal, carbohydrates, and protein (Table 22-7). Fat may be restricted until bowel function is normalized. Vitamin and mineral supplements may be prescribed.

The avoidance of food products containing wheat is not a simple thing to do. Breads, cereals, crackers, pasta products, desserts, gravies, white sauces, and beer contain wheat or other cereal grains with gluten. The patient will have to learn to read food labels carefully and to avoid restaurant foods such as breaded meats or fish, meat loaf, creamed vegetables, and cream soups.

DISORDERS OF THE ACCESSORY ORGANS

Cirrhosis and Hepatitis

The liver is of major importance to, and plays many roles in, metabolism. Except for a few of the fatty acids, all nutrients that are absorbed in the intestines are transported to the liver. The liver dismantles some of these nutrients, stores others, and uses some to synthesize other substances.

The liver determines where amino acids are needed and synthesizes some proteins, enzymes, and urea. It changes the simple sugars to glycogen, provides glucose to body cells, and synthesizes glucose from amino acids if needed. It converts fats to lipoproteins and synthesizes cholesterol. It stores iron, copper, zinc, and magnesium as well as the fat-soluble vitamins and B vitamins. The liver synthesizes bile and stores it in the gallbladder. It detoxifies many substances such as barbiturates and morphine.

Liver disease may be acute or chronic. Early treatment can usually lead to recovery.

Cirrhosis is a general term referring to all types of liver disease characterized by cell loss. Alcohol abuse is the most common cause of cirrhosis, but it can also be caused by congenital defects, infections, or other toxic chemicals.

Although the liver does regenerate, the replacement during cirrhosis does not match the

Table 22-6 Sources of Gluten

Food Groups	Foods that Contain Gluten	Foods that may Contain Gluten	Foods that do not Contain Gluten
Beverage	Cereal beverages (e.g., Postum), malt, Ovaltine, beer and ale	Commercial chocolate milk; cocoa mixes; other beverage mixes; dietary supplements	Coffee; tea; decaffeinated coffee; carbonated beverages; chocolate drinks made with pure cocoa powder; wine; distilled liquor
Meat and meat substitutes	Commercially breaded meats	Meat loaf and patties, cold cuts and prepared meats, stuffing, cheese foods and spreads; commercial souffles, omelets, and fondue; soy protein meat substitutes	Pure meat, fish, fowl, egg, cottage cheese, and peanut butter
Fat and oil	Commercial gravies, white and cream sauces	Commercial salad dressing and mayonnaise, non-dairy creamer	Butter, margarine, vegetable oil
Milk	Milk beverages that contain malt	Commercial chocolate milk	Whole, low-fat, and skim milk; buttermilk
Grains and grain products	Bread, crackers, cereal, and pasta that contains wheat, oats, rye, malt, malt flavoring, graham flour, durham flour, pastry flour, bran, or wheat germ; barley; millet; pretzels; communion wafers	Commercial seasoned rice and potato mixes	Specially prepared breads made with wheat starch, rice, potato, or soybean flour or cornmeal; pure corn or rice cereals; hominy grits; white, brown, and wild rice; popcorn; low protein pasta made from wheat starch
Vegetable	Commercially breaded vegetables or vegetables with a cream or cheese sauce	Commercial seasoned vegetable mixes; canned baked beans	All fresh vegetables; plain commercially frozen or canned vegetables
Fruit		Commercial pie fillings	All plain or sweetened fruits; fruit thickened with tapioca or cornstarch

Table 22-6 (*Continued*)

Food Groups	Foods that Contain Gluten	Foods that may Contain Gluten	Foods that do not Contain Gluten
Soup	Most commercial soup and soup mixes; soup that contains barley, wheat pasta; soup thickened with wheat flour or other gluten-containing grains	Broth	Soup thickened with corn-starch, wheat starch, or potato, rice or soybean flour; pure broth
Desserts	Commercial cakes, cookies and pastries; commercial dessert mixes	Commercial ice cream and sherbet, puddings	Gelatin; custard; fruit ice; specially prepared cakes, cookies, and pastries made with gluten-free flour or starch; pudding and fruit filling thickened with tapioca, cornstarch, or arrowroot flour
Sweets		Commercial candies, especially chocolates	
Miscellaneous		Ketchup; prepared mustard; soy sauce; commercially prepared meat sauces and pickles; white vinegar; flavoring syrups (syrups for pancakes or ice cream)	Monosodium glutamate; salt; pepper; pure spices and herbs; yeast; pure baking chocolate or cocoa powder; carob; flavoring extracts; artificial flavoring; cider and wine vinegar

Source: Permission of Mayo Clinic

loss. In addition to the cell loss during cirrhosis, there is fatty infiltration and **fibrosis** (development of tough, stringy tissue). These developments prevent the liver from functioning normally. Blood flow through the liver is upset and a form of hypertension, anemia, and hemorrhage in the esophagus can occur. The normal metabolic processes will also be disturbed to such a degree that in severe cases, death may result.

The dietary treatment of cirrhosis provides at least 35 to 50 kcal or more, and 1 to 1.5 grams of protein per kilogram of weight each day, depending on the patient's condition. If hepatic coma appears imminent, the lower amount is advocated. Supplements of vitamins and minerals are usually needed. In advanced cirrhosis, 50 to 60 percent of the kcal should be from carbohydrates.

In some forms of cirrhosis, patients cannot tolerate fat well, so it is restricted. In another

Table 22-7 High-kcal, High-Protein, Low-Residue Diet Menus

Breakfast	Lunch	Dinner
Orange Juice	Baked Chicken	Ground Beef Patty
Poached Egg	Macaroni	Mashed Potato
White Toast	Pureed Green Beans	Mashed Acorn Squash
Butter and Jelly	Rolls & Butter	Bread & Butter
Coffee with Milk and Sugar	Lemon Chiffon Pie	Apple Sauce with Sponge Cake
	Tea with Milk and Sugar	Coffee with Milk and Sugar
Snack		
Eggnog—If tolerated	**Snack**	**Snack**
	Sugar Cookies	Beef Broth
	Pineapple Juice	Soda Crackers

Contains 3,000 kcal
130 grams protein

form, protein may not be well tolerated so it is restricted to 35 to 40 grams per day. Sometimes cirrhosis causes **ascites** (accumulation of fluid in the abdomen). In such a case, sodium and fluids may be restricted. If there is bleeding in the esophagus, fiber can be restricted to prevent irritation of the tissue. Smaller feedings will be better accepted than larger ones. No alcohol is allowed.

Hepatitis

Hepatitis is an inflammation of the liver. It is caused by viruses or toxic agents such as drugs and alcohol. **Necrosis** (tissue death due to loss of blood supply) occurs, and the liver's normal metabolic activities are constricted. It may be acute or chronic.

In mild cases, the cells can be replaced. In severe cases, the damage can be so extensive that the necrosis leads to liver failure and death. There cn be bile **stasis** (stoppage or slowing) and decreased blood albumin levels. Patients ex-

perience nausea, headache, fever, fatigue, tender and enlarged liver, anorexia and **jaundice** (yellow caste of the skin and eyes). Weight loss can be pronounced.

Treatment is usually bedrest, plenty of fluids, and diet therapy. During early treatment, a full liquid diet (see Chapter 17) may be prescribed. As the patient improves and accepts food, the diet should provide 35 to 40 kcal per kilogram of body weight. Most of these should be provided by carbohydrates; there should be moderate amounts of fat; and, if the necrosis has not been severe, up to 70 to 80 grams of protein for cell regeneration. If the necrosis has been severe and the proteins cannot be properly metabolized, they must be limited to prevent the accumulation of ammonia in the blood. Patients may prefer frequent, small meals rather than three large ones.

Patients with liver disease require a great deal of encouragement because their anorexia and consequent feelings of general malaise can be severe. Their recovery takes patience, rest, and time.

Cholecystitis and Cholelithiasis

The dual function of the **gallbladder** is the concentration and storage of bile. After bile is formed in the liver, the gallbladder concentrates it to several times its original strength, and stores it until needed. Fat in the duodenum triggers the gallbladder to contract and release bile into the common duct for the digestion of fat in the small intestine. If this flow is hindered, there may be pain.

The precise etiology of gallbladder disease is unknown, but hereditary factors may be involved. Women develop gallbladder disease more often than men do. Obesity, **total parenteral nutrition** (TPN—feeding entirely via a vein), the use of estrogen, and various diseases of the small intestine are frequently associated.

Cholecystitis (inflammation of the gallbladder) and **cholelithiasis** (gallstones) may inhibit the flow of bile and cause pain. Cholecystitis can cause changes in the gallbladder tissue which in turn can affect the cholesterol (a constituent of bile), causing it to harden and form stones. It is also thought that chronic overindulgence in fats may contribute to gallstones because the fat stimulates the liver to produce more cholesterol for the bile, which is necessary for the digestion of fat. In addition to pain, which can be severe, there may be indigestion and vomiting, particularly after the ingestion of fatty foods.

Treatment may include medication to dissolve the stones and diet therapy. If medication does not succeed, surgery to remove the gallbladder (**cholecystectomy**) may be indicated.

Diet therapy includes abstinence during the acute phase. This is followed by a clear liquid diet and, gradually, a regular but fat-restricted diet. Amounts of fats allowed run from 20 to 60 grams, with the amount being increased gradually. In chronic cases, fat may be restricted on a permanent basis. For the obese patients, weight loss is recommended in addition to a fat-restricted diet. (For information on fat-restricted diets, see Chapter 20.)

Pancreatitis

In addition to the hormone insulin, the pancreas produces other hormones and enzymes that are important in the digestion of protein, fats, and carbohydrates. When food reaches the duodenum, the pancreas sends its enzymes to the small intestine to aid in digestion.

Pancreatitis is an inflammation of the pancreas. It may be caused by infections, surgery, alcoholism, biliary tract (includes bile ducts and gallbladder) disease, or certain drugs. It may be acute or chronic.

Abdominal pain, nausea, and **steatorrhea** (fat in the stool) are symptoms. Malabsorption (particularly of fat-soluble vitamins), and weight loss occur and, in cases where the islets of Langerhans are destroyed, diabetes mellitus may result.

Diet therapy is intended to reduce pancreatic secretions and bile. Just as fat stimulates the gallbladder to secrete bile, protein and hydrochloric acid stimulate the pancreas to secrete its juices and enzymes. During acute pancreatitis, the patient is nourished strictly parenterally. Later, when the patient can tolerate oral feedings, a liquid diet consisting mainly of carbohydrates is given because, of these three nutrients, carbohydrates have the least stimulatory effect on pancreatic secretions.

As recovery progresses, small, frequent feedings of carbohydrates and protein with little fat or fiber are given. The fat is restricted because of the deficiencies of pancreatic lipase. The patient is gradually returned to a regular diet as tolerated. Vitamin supplements may be given. Alcohol is forbidden in all cases.

CONSIDERATIONS FOR THE HEALTH CARE PROFESSIONAL

Patients with gastrointestinal problems can be particularly sensitive. Their problems can be psychologically caused; they may fear surgery or cancer; and they may suffer nausea, pain, or both. Some will want to eat foods that are disallowed; others will refuse foods they need.

Health care professionals who show respect and understanding for their patients will have the most success in helping them learn what they should and should not eat and why.

In teaching these patients, it is helpful to group foods by types, to draw diagrams or pictures, to use colored paper, and, most of all, to maintain a sense of humor.

SUMMARY

Disturbances of the gastrointestinal tract require a wide variety of therapeutic diets. Peptic ulcers are treated with drugs, and diet therapy generally involves only the avoidance of alcohol and caffeine. Diverticulosis may be treated with a high-fiber diet, while diverticulitis is treated with a gradual progression from clear liquid to the high-fiber diet. Ulcerative colitis may require a low-residue diet combined with high protein and high kcal. Cirrhosis requires a substantial, balanced diet, with occasional restrictions of fat, protein, salt, or fluids. Diet therapy for hepatitis may range from parenteral to a full, well-balanced diet, although protein may be restricted, depending upon the patient's condition. Cholecystitis and cholelithiasis require a fat-restricted diet and, in cases of overweight, a kcal-restricted diet as well. Pancreatitis diet therapy ranges from parenteral to a regular diet, if tolerated.

Discussion Topics

1. Name the accessory organs in the gastrointestinal system and explain their roles in digestion and metabolism.
2. Discuss dyspepsia. Include its probable causes and the suggested therapy for it.
3. Describe hiatal hernia. Name its symptoms and possible treatment.
4. Define ulcers. Where are they found in the gastrointestinal system and how are they treated? Why is the Sippy Diet seldom used? What substances should not be allowed an ulcer patient? Why?
5. Explain the difference between diverticulosis and diverticulitis. How are these conditions treated?
6. Discuss the high-fiber diet. For what conditions might it be used? Compare it to the low- and minimum-residue diets. Why is corn on the cob not allowed on the minimum-residue diet? Name other foods that are not allowed on the minimum-residue diet and tell why they would not be allowed.
7. Discuss ulcerative colitis. What is it? What causes it? How is it treated?

Suggested Activities

1. Hold a panel discussion on the gastrointestinal disturbances included in this chapter and the dietary treatment of them.
2. Make a list of foods eaten yesterday. Circle the foods that would be allowed on a restricted-residue diet.
3. Find recipes for low-residue and minimum-residue diets and add them to the special diet recipe file.
4. Plan a day's menu for a low-residue diet, another for a minimum-residue diet, and another for a high-fiber diet. Evaluate the menus for nutritional value, using the Food Guide Pyramid. Exchange menu plans with a fellow student and evaluate each other's plans in terms of nutrient content, flavor, aroma, color, shape, appearance, texture, and satiety value.
5. Prepare at least one of the meals on each of the above menus. Evaluate each in terms of nutrient content, flavor, aroma, color, shape, appearance, texture, and satiety value.
6. Adapt the following menu to suit a patient on a minimum-residue diet:

Orange Juice
Fried Egg
Bacon
Whole Wheat Toast
with
Butter and Marmalade
Milk
Coffee

7. List ten of your favorite foods. Circle those foods that would not be allowed on a low-residue diet.

Review

Multiple choice. Select the *letter* that precedes the best answer.
1. Dyspepsia
   1. may be an indication of serious gastrointestinal disturbance
   2. is usually psychological in origin
   3. may be overcome with improved eating habits
   4. is caused by high-fiber foods
      a) 1,2   b) 1,2,3   c) 1,3   d) 2,3,4
2. Hiatal hernia
   1. only occurs in the small intestine
   2. can cause regurgitation
   3. causes "heartburn"

    4. patients may be more comfortable with small, frequent meals
       a) 1,3   b) 2,3,4   c) 2,4   d) 2,3

3. Peptic ulcers
    1. occur in the stomach or the duodenum
    2. can be partially caused by anxiety
    3. are always treated with the Sippy Diet
    4. are sometimes treated with a regular diet
       a) 1,2,4   b) 1,2,3   c) 1,2   d) 2,3

4. Protein foods may be somewhat restricted in cases of peptic ulcers because they
    1. contribute to uremia
    2. contain sodium
    3. provide amino acids
    4. stimulate gastric acid secretions
       a) 1,4   b) 4   c) 2,3   d) 3

5. The following should not be allowed an ulcer patient
    1. cola drinks
    2. milkshakes
    3. tea and coffee
    4. beer and wine
       a) 1,3,4   b) 2,3,4   c) 3,4   d) 4

6. Diverticulitis
    1. is the inflammation of diverticula
    2. may be initially treated with a clear-liquid diet
    3. may be prevented with a high-fiber diet
    4. affects the intestines
       a) 1,2,3   b) 2,3,4   c) all   d) 1,3,4

7. Food residue
    1. is ultimately evacuated in the feces
    2. never leaves the stomach
    3. never leaves the intestines
    4. results from incorrect cooking methods
       a) 1   b) 2,3   c) 3,4   d) 4

8. Large amounts of food residue cause
    1. a decrease in fecal matter
    2. an increase in fecal matter
    3. weight gain
    4. diverticulosis
       a) 1   b) 2   c) 2,3   d) 3,4

9. The following foods would not be recommended for the high-fiber diet:
    1. pureed pears

    2. mashed potatoes

    3. rice pudding

    4. bran cereal

      a) 1,2,3   b) 2,3,4   c) 3,4   d) 4

10. The following foods would not be allowed on a low-residue diet:

    1. fresh oranges

    2. corn on the cob

    3. macaroni and cheese

    4. toast with butter

      a) 1,2,3   b) 1,4   c) 1,2   d) 4

11. The following foods would not be allowed on a minimum-residue diet:

    1. corned beef and cabbage

    2. sliced, peeled apples

    3. peas and corn

    4. poached eggs on toast

      a) 1,2,4   b) 1,2   c) 2,3   d) 1,2,3

12. If the minimum-residue diet must be used for a period of time, the physician may

    1. alternate it weekly with the high-iron diet

    2. substitute the full liquid diet from time to time

    3. add fresh fruit juices before each meal

    4. prescribe a vitamin and mineral supplement

      a) 1,2   b) 1,2,3   c) 2,3   d) 4

13. Ulcerative colitis

    1. may affect the colon

    2. always requires parenteral feedings

    3. may be treated with a low-residue diet that is also high in kcal and protein

    4. patients may be malnourished

      a) 1,3,4   b) 2,3,4   c) 3,4   d) 4

14. The following foods would be recommended for an ulcerative colitis patient, provided the patient tolerates milk:

    1. custard with whipped cream

    2. chocolate milkshake

    3. eggnog

    4. cream of tomato soup with crackers

      a) 1,3,4   b) 1,2,3   c) 2,3,4   d) all

15. The liver

    1. plays a major role in metabolism

    2. directs the distribution of amino acids

    3. converts glucose to glycogen

4. stores iron and fat-soluble vitamins
    a) 1,3,4   b) 1,2,3   c) 2,3,4   d) all

16. Cirrhosis
1. is a liver disease characterized by cell loss
2. is always caused by alcoholism
3. inevitably results in death
4. affects the body's ability to tolerate fats
    a) 1,4   b) 1,2,4   c) 1,3,4   d) all

17. Ascites
1. is caused by cirrhosis
2. is an accumulation of fluid in the abdomen
3. may require the restriction of sodium and water
4. is caused by a shortage of iron
    a) 1,4   b) 1,2,3   c) 2,4   d) 4

18. Hepatitis
1. is an inflammation of the liver
2. causes necrosis
3. is always chronic
4. may be caused by viruses or toxic agents
    a) 1,2   b) 1,2,4   c) 2,3   d) 2,3,4

19. Gallbladder problems may require
1. the dietary restriction of fat
2. cholecystectomy
3. loss of weight
4. additional protein in the diet
    a) 1,2,3   b) 1,3,4   c) 1,3   d) 1,4

20. Inflammation of the pancreas
1. is called pancreatitis
2. can cause pain and nausea
3. can require parenteral feeding
4. always signifies cancer
    a) 1,2   b) 1,3   c) 2,3   d) 1,2,3

Case Study 1

Gastrointestinal Disease

Mr. F. was a highly successful man, having reached nearly the top position in his company by the age of 43. He worked long and effectively, taking time for neither breakfast nor lunch unless there was an obligatory business meal. When people asked him how he managed to accomplish so much on so little food, he answered that "black coffee and nervous energy" propelled him.

Since his latest promotion to a situation far from his family, he has worked harder than usual, finding unexpected problems in the new position and at home.

Recently he has felt unusually tired and even faint at times, and occasionally his stool was tarry. He felt he lacked the time to see a doctor.

Last Friday, he decided to work just a bit past 5 P.M., but after the others in the office had left he felt so weak he decided to rest on his couch awhile. The next thing he knew, he was gagging and vomiting blood. The cleaning lady called an ambulance and help soon arrived.

Mr. F. was diagnosed as having a gastric ulcer and was hospitalized. The doctor prescribed an antiulcer medication, rest, and dietary changes. Fluid, electrolyte and hemoglobin tests revealed that he had experienced minimal loss of blood and fluids. Following endoscopy, he was placed on a bland diet with six small feedings.

By the end of the week, Mr. F. felt much better. Experiencing no GI distress, a regular diet was prescribed but he was instructed to avoid alcohol and caffeine. He was discharged, but was not allowed to return to work for several weeks. During that time, he began to evaluate his work habits with the goal of reducing the everyday stress in his life.

Case Study Questions Based on the Nursing Process

Assess

1. What may have been some of the factors leading to the development of Mr. F's ulcer?
2. Did his recent promotion possibly contribute? Explain.
3. What might have happened if Mr. F. had not received emergency help?

Plan

4. What should Mr. F. be taught about the need for changes in his lifestyle?
5. Why is alcohol prohibited in his diet? What can he substitute for alcohol at social events?
6. Why is caffeine restricted in Mr. F's diet plan?

Implement

7. Write a day's menu for Mr. F.
8. Mr. F. is working on a daily menu for himself and states that he will order a cola drink at the bar instead of alcohol. What should he be told about cola drinks?

Evaluate

9. Mr. F. has the choice of the following two menus. Which choice would indicate that he is following his doctor's recommendations?

Menu 1	*Menu 2*
Southern fried chicken	Roast beef
Paprika potatoes	Baked potato
Carrots glazed in sherry	Peas
Tossed salad/poppyseed dress-ing	Cole slaw
Rum cake	Peach pie
Coffee	Herb tea

10. What changes in his lifestyle will indicate that Mr. F. is "taking care of himself"?

Case Study 2

Ulcerative Colitis

Tony J. was a handsome, bright, nervous lawyer who had been a workaholic for all of his 55 years. He had been diagnosed as having ulcerative colitis when he was 40 but, by following his doctor's suggestions carefully, he had managed to control it.

However, on his 55th birthday, he was told his company was cutting back on staff and that he would be let go by the end of the month. He would be paid his regular salary for one more year and would then go on early pension. This meant he would be earning half of his previous salary.

At his birthday party that evening, he ate and drank things he usually never touched—cocktails, champagne, shrimp cocktail, steak, french fries, coleslaw, and cherry nut ice cream cake. That night he was awakened with severe abdominal cramps and bloody diarrhea. He could not go to work or eat properly for several days.

When he returned to work, he felt tired and angry and decided there was no reason not to have some hamburgers with lettuce and tomatoes and beer with the other guys in the department. That night he was again awakened by abdominal cramps and bloody diarrhea, and the next day he was again unable to go to work. He refused to see his physician.

Case Study Questions Based on the Nursing Process

Assess
1. What were contributing factors leading to Tony's changing his diet?
2. If Tony had seen his physician, what information would the doctor probably have given him?

Plan
3. What may the consequences be if Tony continues his current eating trend?
4. What type of nutritional therapy might Tony ultimately face? Why?

Implement
5. If you were Tony's nurse teaching him about his diet, how would you approach him?
6. What information about his overall health and diet needs would you discuss with Tony?

Evaluate
7. What feedback from Tony would indicate that he is taking control of his health?
8. Might Tony benefit from psychological counseling? Why?

VOCABULARY

cachexia
carcinogens
chemotherapy
dysphagia
endometrium
genetic predisposition
hyperglycemia
hypoalbuminemia
malignant
metastasize
neoplasia
neoplasm
oncologist
oncology
resection
xerostomia

DIET AND CANCER

OBJECTIVES

After studying this chapter, you should be able to

- Discuss how nutrition can be related to the development or the prevention of cancer
- State the effects of cancer on the nutritional status of the host
- Describe nutritional problems resulting from the medical treatment of cancer
- Describe nutritional therapy for cancer patients

THE NATURE OF CANCER

Cancer is the second leading cause of death in the United States. It is a disease characterized by abnormal cell growth, and can occur in any organ. In some way the genes lose control of cell growth and reproduction becomes unstructured and excessive. The developing mass caused by the abnormal growth is called a tumor or **neoplasm** (new growth). Cancer is also called **neo-plasia.** Cancerous tumors are **malignant** (life threatening), affecting the structure, and consequently the function of organs. When cancer cells break away from their original site, move through the blood, and spread to a new site, they are said to **metastasize.** The mortality rate for cancer patients is high, but cancer does not always cause death. When it is found early in its development, prompt treatment can irradicate it. **Oncology** is the study of cancer.

THE CAUSES OF CANCER

The precise etiology of cancer is not known, but it is thought that heredity, viruses, environmental **carcinogens** (cancer causing substances), and possibly emotional stress contribute to its development. Cancer is not inherited, but some families appear to have a **genetic predisposition** (inherited tendency) toward it. When such seems to be the case, environmental carcinogens should be carefully avoided and medical checkups made regularly. Environmental carcinogens include radiation (whether from X-rays, sun, or atomic wastes); certain chemicals ingested in food or water; some chemicals that touch the skin regularly; and certain substances that are breathed in, such as tobacco smoke and asbestos.

Carcinogens are not known to cause cancer from one or even a few exposures, but after prolonged exposure. For example, skin cancer does not develop after one sunburn.

RELATIONSHIPS OF FOOD AND CANCER

While the relationships of food and cancer have not been proven, there appear to be associations between them—both good and bad. Certain substances in foods, for example, are thought to be carcinogenic. Nitrites in cured and smoked foods such as bacon and ham can be changed to nitrosamines (carcinogens) during cooking. Regular ingestion of these foods is associated with cancers of the stomach and esophagus. High-fat diets have been associated with cancers of the uterus, breast, prostate, and colon. The regular, excessive intake of kcal is associated with cancers of the gallbladder and **endometrium** (mucous membrane of the uterus). People who smoke and drink alcohol immoderately appear to be at greater risk of cancers of the mouth, pharynx, and esophagus than those who do not.

On the positive side, it is thought that diets high in fiber help to protect against colorectal cancer. Diets containing sufficient amounts of vitamin C-rich foods may protect against cancers of the stomach and esophagus. Diets containing sufficient carotene and vitamin A-rich foods may protect against cancers of the lung, bladder, and larynx. Appropriate amounts of protein foods are essential for the maintenance of a healthy immune system. An immune system that has been damaged—possibly through malnutrition—may be a contributing factor in the development of cancer. Excessive protein intake, however, may be a factor in the development of cancer of the colon.

The obvious bottom line here is *moderation.* An occasional serving of bacon or buttered popcorn or wine is not likely to cause cancer. The regular, excessive use of carcinogenic foods may contribute to cancer. Vitamins that are thought to prevent cancer should be ingested *in foods* that naturally contain them. Excessive intake of vitamin supplements can be harmful. For example, abnormally large amounts of vitamin A can cause bone pain and fragility, hair loss, headaches, and liver and skin problems.

THE EFFECTS OF CANCER

One of the first indications of cancer may be unexplained weight loss. This is because the tumor cells use for their own metabolism and development the nutrients the host has taken in. The host may suffer from weakness, and anorexia may occur, which compounds the weight loss. The weight loss includes the loss of muscle tissue and **hypoalbuminemia** (low albumin [protein] content of the blood), and anemia may develop. The sense of taste and of smell may become abnormal in cancer patients. This may be because of nutrient deficiency. A zinc deficiency, for example, affects the sense of taste. Foods may taste less sweet and more bitter than they would to healthy people. Cancer patients become satiated earlier than normal, possibly because of decreased digestive secretions. Insulin production may be abnormal and **hyperglycemia** (high levels of blood sugar) can delay the stomach's emptying and dull the appetite. Some cancers cause hypercalcemia. If this is chronic, kidney stones and impaired kidney function can occur.

The effect(s) of cancer on the host is/are particularly determined by the location of a tumor. For example, an esophageal or intestinal tumor can cause blockage in the gastorintestinal tract, causing malabsorption as well. If the cancer is untreated, the continued anorexia and weight loss will create a state of malnutrition, which in turn can lead to **cachexia** (severe wasting) and ultimately, death.

THE TREATMENT OF CANCER

Medical treatment of cancer can include surgical removal, radiation, **chemotherapy** (drug), or a combination of these methods. These treatments, unfortunately, have side effects that can further undermine the nutritional status of the patient. The nutritional effects of surgery in general are discussed in Chapter 24. Cancer surgery, however, can have some additional effects. Surgery on the mouth, for example, might well affect the ability to chew or swallow. Gastric or intestinal **resection** (partial removal) can affect absorption and result in nutritional deficiencies. The removal of the pancreas will result in diabetes mellitus.

Radiation can change the senses of taste and smell, particularly if it is done for cancer of the head or neck. It also can cause a decrease in salivary secretions, which causes dry mouth (**xerostomia**) and difficulty in swallowing (**dyspha-**

gia). This reduction in saliva also causes tooth decay and sometimes the loss of teeth. Radiation reduces the amount of absorptive tissue in the small intestine. In addition, it can cause bowel obstruction or diarrhea.

Chemotherapy reduces the ability of the small intestine to regenerate absorptive cells, and it can cause hemorrhagic colitis. Both radiation and chemotherapy depress appetite. They may cause nausea, vomiting, and diarrhea leading to fluid and electrolyte imbalances. This can lead to fluid retention.

However, when the therapy is completed and the patient is able to return to a well-balanced diet, these problems may disappear.

NUTRITIONAL CARE OF THE CANCER PATIENT

The nutrient and kcal needs of the cancer patient are actually greater than they were before the onset of the disease. The cancer causes an increase in the metabolic rate; tissue must be rebuilt; and the nutrients lost to the cancer must be replaced. Patients who can maintain their weight or minimize its loss increase their chances of responding to treatment and, thus, their survival. Patients on high-protein and high-kcal diets tolerate the side effects of therapy and higher doses of drugs better than those who cannot eat normally. And, those patients who can eat will feel better than those who cannot.

Despite their nutritional needs, however, anorexia is a major problem for cancer patients. It is particularly difficult to combat because cancer patients tend to develop strong food aversions that are thought to be caused by the effects of chemotherapy. Patients receiving chemotherapy near mealtime associate the foods at that meal with the nausea caused by the chemotherapy, and often form aversions to those particular foods. These aversions result in limited acceptance of food and contribute further to the patient's malnutrition. It is preferable that chemotherapy be withheld for two to three hours before and after meals. The appetite and absorption usually improve after chemotherapy so the patient can improve nutritional status between chemotherapy treatments.

Obviously, diet plans for cancer patients require special attention. The patient's diet history should be taken, as usual, at the outset of hospitalization. Kcal and nutrient needs must be determined by the diet counselor, and the patient's diet plan made in consultation with the patient. It is essential that favorite foods, prepared in familiar ways and served attractively, be included. Nutritious food beautifully served is useless if the patient refuses it.

If chewing is a problem, a soft diet may be helpful (see Chapter 17). If diarrhea is a problem, a low-residue diet may help (see Chapter 22). Patients should be evaluated continuously, but inconspicuously.

If the patient is scheduled to undergo radiation or chemotherapy, these factors must be included in the diet planning.

High-protein and high-kcal diets may be recommended. Energy demands are high because of the hypermetabolic state often caused by cancer. Kcal needs will vary from patient to patient, but 45 to 50 kcal per kilogram of body weight may be recommended.

Carbohydrates and fat will be needed to provide this energy and spare protein for tissue building and the immune system. Patients with good nutritional status will need from 80 to 100 grams of protein a day. Malnourished patients may need from 100 to 200 grams of protein a day. Vitamins and minerals are essential for metabolism, tissue maintenance, and appetite, and they may be supplied in supplemental form. Fluids are important to help the kidneys eliminate the metabolic wastes and the toxins from drugs.

The patient's food habits can require change if, before the illness, the patient has scrupulously avoided desserts and high kcal foods to maintain normal weight.

Sometimes patients may be willing to eat foods that are brought from home. Some may find cold foods more appealing than hot foods. Meats may taste bitter so milk, cheese, eggs, and fish may be more appealing. If foods taste less sweet to the cancer patient than to the well person, sugar may be added to juices and fruits. This may please the patient and add kcal to the diet.

Supplementation with high-kcal, high-protein, liquid foods between meals may be useful, but should not be used if their consumption reduces the patient's appetite at meals.

If the patient suffers from dry mouth, salad dressings, gravies, sauces, and syrups appropriately served on foods can be helpful. Several small meals may be better tolerated than three large meals. It is preferable to serve the nutritionally richer meals early in the day because the patient is less tired and may have a better appetite at that time. If nausea or pain are a continuous problem, drugs to control them, particularly at mealtimes, may be helpful. While oral feedings are definitely preferred, enteral or parenteral feedings may become necessary if cachexia is extreme. Sometimes an oral diet may be used in conjunction with parenteral feeding (see Chapter 24). As the patient improves, kcal and nutritional content of the diet should be gradually increased.

CONSIDERATIONS FOR THE HEALTH CARE PROFESSIONAL

It is important that the diet counselor establish a good relationship with the patient and that constant reminders to eat be avoided. The patient usually understands the situation and such reminders are only depressing reminders of the cancer.

If and when appropriate, however, it may be helpful to:

1. explain why it is important that the patient eat
2. encourage him or her to eat foods he or she enjoys
3. recommend that he or she avoid eating at the time of day when nausea typically occurs
4. refrain from serving foods that give off odors which contribute to nausea

If the prognosis for the patient is not good, nutritional care will not be as important as the patient's feelings and immediate comfort.

SUMMARY

Cancer is a disease characterized by abnormal cell growth. It can strike any body tissue. Energy needs increase because of the hypermetabolic state and the tumor's needs for energy nutrients at the same time anorexia occurs in the patient. Its cause is not known. It causes severe wasting, blockages, anemia, and various metabolic problems. Treatment of cancer includes surgery, radiation, and chemotherapy. Improving the patient's nutritional state is difficult because of the illness and anorexia. Parenteral or enteral nutrition may be necessary.

Discussion Topics

1. Discuss cancer, telling what it is and how it affects body functions and nutritional status.
2. Discuss the etiology of cancer. Include any current news items that relate to the subject, including their accuracy.
3. Explain why cancer patients lose weight.
4. Discuss current medical treatment of cancer. How does it affect nutritional status?
5. Why is the anorexia of cancer patients especially difficult to combat? What causes it? Are there any ways it can be prevented?
6. How does one attempt to improve the nutritional status of a cancer patient?
7. Are supplemental feedings of liquid foods useful in the nutritional rehabilitation of a cancer patient? Explain.
8. Discuss enteral and parenteral nutrition in relation to cancer patients.

Suggested Activities

1. Invite an **oncologist** (physician specializing in cancer) to speak to the class.
2. Role-play a situation where a nurse is attempting to help a cancer patient with lunch. The patient had chemotherapy an hour after yesterday's lunch and was quite ill afterward.

3. Write an essay giving your feelings if you had just been told that you had a malignant breast tumor.

4. Assume you are chief dietitian in the local hospital. Write your instructions for your assistant who will be making diet plans for a new patient with throat cancer. The patient is seriously malnourished, has xerostomia, and is hospitalized for chemotherapy.

5. Plan a day's menus for a cancer patient who will eat only the following foods:

sweetened orange juice	soda crackers
bananas	milkshakes
applesauce	eggnog
cooked pears	cottage cheese
puffed rice cereal	cream of chicken soup
rice pudding	poached eggs
white toast with currant jelly	bouillon

Review

A. Multiple choice. Select the *letter* that precedes the best answer.

1. Cancer
   1. is characterized by abnormal cell growth
   2. tumor can also be called neoplasm
   3. inevitably causes death
   4. can metastasize
      a) 1,2   b) 1,2,3   c) 1,2,4   d) 4

2. Carcinogens include
   1. viruses
   2. smoke
   3. X-rays
   4. salmonella
      a) 1,2,3   b) 2,3,4   c) 3,4   d) 4

3. Carcinogens
   1. cause cancer after only limited exposure
   2. include some chemical substances
   3. are never found in food or water
   4. should be avoided whenever possible
      a) 1,2   b) 1,3   c) 2,4   d) 3,4

4. Cancer patients
   1. tend to lose weight
   2. may experience a change in their senses of taste and smell

3. seldom suffer from anorexia
4. may suffer from cachexia
    a) 1,2   b) 1,2,3   c) 2,3   d) 1,2,4

5. Radiation and chemotherapy
   1. seldom affect cancer patients' nutritional status
   2. may depress appetite
   3. may cause nausea
   4. may create food aversions
     a) 1,2   b) 1,2,3   c) 2,3   d) 2,3,4

B. Match the items in column I with the definitions in column II.

Column I	Column II
_____ 1. cachexia	a. cancer
_____ 2. carcinogen	b. supports the parasite
_____ 3. chemotherapy	c. high level of blood sugar
_____ 4. genetic predisposition	d. to move from one organ to another
_____ 5. hyperglycemia	e. blockage
_____ 6. hypoalbuminemia	f. cancer-causing substance
_____ 7. malignant	g. etiology
_____ 8. metastasize	h. poor absorption
_____ 9. neoplasia	i. tumor
_____ 10. neoplasm	j. life-threatening
_____ 11. resection	k. severe wasting
_____ 12. xerostomia	l. partial removal
_____ 13. host	m. reduced amounts of protein in the blood
_____ 14. malabsorption	n. inherited tendency
_____ 15. bowel obstruction	o. treatment of cancer with drugs
	p. dry mouth
	q. not inherited

Case Study 1   *Cancer Patient*

The doctor found a lump in Betty G.'s left breast during her annual physical exam and scheduled Betty for mammography that revealed a tumor, which probably was malignant. Betty was scheduled for a biopsy, and was admitted to the hospital the morning of surgery two days after the lump was discovered. The doctor explained that if the tumor were malignant, a radical mastectomy would be performed at that time.

When Betty awoke from anesthesia, she had only one breast. She was depressed but relieved when the doctor told her that she believed all the cancer had been removed.

Betty was offered broth later on the day of surgery, but declined. The next day she was served a clear liquid diet, but could swallow only a bit of gingerale. On the second day, she was served a full liquid diet and on the third day, a soft diet. Betty ate nothing and her depression increased.

Betty's husband, son, daughter-in-law, and friends were very supportive and visited often, frequently bringing homemade cookies, fruit juice, and candy, but Betty could not eat. When her doctor asked her about her appetite, she said she was not eating much. She was being supported with IV solution, but had taken only about 200 kcal of gingerale orally. After four days, the doctor asked the dietitian to consult with Betty. The dietitian did, and afterward Betty began to eat. After eight days, Betty was discharged. She had lost ten pounds.

Case Study Questions Based on the Nursing Process

Assess
1. Why was Betty's biopsy and surgery scheduled so quickly?
2. What factors may have led to Betty's increasing depression during the hospital stay?
3. What symptom(s) of depression did Betty exhibit?

Plan
4. What might you say to Betty to encourage her to express her concerns?
5. What do you think the dietitian asked Betty during their consultation?
6. What are Betty's nutritional needs after discharge?
7. Who could help Betty deal with her depression after discharge?

Implement
8. What referrals should be made for follow-up psychological and physical care? What support groups are available in your area?
9. Plan a menu for Betty that meets her nutritional needs.

Evaluate
10. When she sees her physician for a one-month checkup, Betty discusses her "loss," tells the doctor about the local Cancer Society program she is attending, and has gained two pounds. Do you think Betty's depression is resolved? Explain.

Case Study 2

Diet and Cancer of the Colon

Jimmy had noticed a tarry stool for about one week and, although he wasn't much on "doctoring," decided to see a physician. Tests were completed, and Jimmy was told to call for the results early the following week. When he called, the physician asked Jimmy and his wife, Helen, to come to the office to discuss the test results.

Because Jimmy had mentioned none of this to Helen previously, she was devastated by the news. She was angry, sad, and frightened. Jimmy was angry about her reactions.

The physician explained that Jimmy had a very small area on his colon that indicated cancer and that it should be surgically removed. This was done and, although follow-up tests indicated the cancer had been removed, the doctor ordered chemotherapy and radiation for one year.

Jimmy was extremely tired after returning home from the hospital stay, and had no appetite. When his neighbor, a retired nurse, came to visit him, she brought rice pudding, a known favorite of Jimmy's, and some home-canned peaches. She sat by him and "talked turkey" to him. After her visit, he ate. He continued to eat well during the nausea-free times of the chemotherapy and the radiation treatments. Six years later, Jimmy is cancer-free.

Case Study Questions Based on the Nursing Process

Assess
1. Why do you think Jimmy was "not much on doctoring"?
2. Why did Jimmy tell Helen after the tests were done and not before? Was Helen's reaction one you would expect in such a circumstance? Explain.
3. Why was Jimmy angry at Helen's reaction to his illness?

Plan
4. What did the neighbor probably say to Jimmy? Why did he listen to her?
5. What nutritional needs does Jimmy have postoperatively and through the period of radiation and chemotherapy?

Implement
6. Why did the nurse bring sweet, cold foods for Jimmy to eat?
7. Plan a menu for Jimmy to follow during the radiation and chemotherapy treatments.

Evaluate
8. Do you think Helen could have been as effective as the neighbor, had she "talked turkey" to Jimmy? Explain.
9. What nutritional and other support might be advisable for Jimmy during his recovery?

DIET AND SURGERY, BURNS, AND INFECTIONS

VOCABULARY

AIDS
antibodies
aspirated
aspiration
continuous infusion
dumping syndrome
elective surgery
elemental formulas
endocrine system
enteral nutrition
esophagostomy
fever
gastrostomy
HIV
hemorrhage
homeostasis
hydrolyzed formulas
hypermetabolic
hypoalbuminemia
infectious
intact formulas
jejunostomy
Kaposi's sarcoma
modular formulas
nasogastric tube
opportunistic infections
osmolality
ostomy

parenteral nutrition
peripheral vein
phlebitis
regurgitated
sepsis
thrombosis
total parenteral
   nutrition (TPN)
trauma
tube feedings

DIET AND SURGERY, BURNS, AND INFECTIONS

OBJECTIVES

After studying this chapter, you should be able to
- Describe the body's reactions to stress and relate them to nutrition
- Explain the special dietary needs of surgical and burn patients
- Explain the special dietary needs of patients with fever and infection

Normally, the human body operates in a state of **homeostasis** (balanced, stable condition). When the body experiences the **trauma** (serious physical stress) of surgery, severe burns, or infections, this balance is upset. The body reacts in an attempt to restore itself to homeostasis.

During its response to physical stress, the body signals the **endocrine system,** which activates a self-protective, **hypermetabolic** response. This increases energy output. The intensity of the response depends on the severity of the condition.

Catabolism occurs, causing the rapid breakdown of energy reserves to provide glucose and other substances necessary for the anabolic phase of wound healing and tissue maintenance. Proteins, fats, and minerals are lost in the catabolic phase just when there is an increased need for them to rebuild tissue. When the condition includes **hemorrhage** and vomiting, these losses are compounded.

Sufficient nutrients, fluids, and kcal are required as soon as possible to replace the losses, build and repair tissue, and return the body to

351

homeostasis. Obviously, nutrition plays an important role in the lives of patients undergoing surgery or of those who suffer from burns or infections.

NUTRITIONAL CARE OF SURGERY PATIENTS

Presurgery Nutritional Care

Surgery stresses the patient regardless of whether it is elective or emergency. If **elective,** the patient's nutritional status should be evaluated before surgery, and if improvement is needed, it should be undertaken. A good nutritional status before surgery enhances recovery. A nutritional assessment of the patient before surgery will be helpful to the dietitian in providing foods that will be accepted by the patient after surgery when appetite is poor.

Improvement of nutritional status will usually mean providing extra protein, carbohydrates, vitamins, and minerals. The extra protein is needed for wound healing, tissue building, and blood regeneration. Extra carbohydrates will be converted to glycogen and stored, to help provide energy after surgery, when needs are high, and when patients may be unable to eat normally. The B vitamins are needed for the increased metabolism, vitamins A and C for wound healing, vitamin D for the absorption of calcium, and vitamin K for proper clotting of the blood. Iron is necessary for blood building, calcium and phosphorus for bones, and the other minerals for maintenance of acid-base, electrolyte, and fluid balance in the body.

In cases of overweight, improved nutritional status includes weight reduction before surgery whenever possible. Excess fat is a surgical hazard because the extra tissue increases the chances of infection and fatty tissue tends to retain the anesthetic longer than other tissue.

Food usually is not allowed the patient after the evening meal on the day before surgery. This ensures that the stomach contains no food, which could be **regurgitated** and then **aspirated** (taken into the airway) during surgery. If there is to be gastrointestinal surgery, a low-residue diet may be ordered for a few days before surgery (see Chapter 22). This is intended to reduce intestinal residue.

Postsurgery

The postsurgery diet is intended to provide kcal and nutrients in amounts sufficient to fulfill the patient's increased metabolic needs and to promote healing and subsequent recovery.

In general, for the 24 hours immediately following surgery, most patients will be given intravenous solutions only. These solutions will contain water, 5 to 10 percent dextrose, electrolytes, vitamins, and medications as needed. The maximum number of kcal supplied by them is about 400 to 500 per 24-hour period. The estimated daily kcal requirement for adults after surgery is 35 to 45 per kilogram of body weight. A 110-pound individual would require at least 2000 kcal per day. Obviously, until the patient can take food there will be a considerable kcal deficit each day. Body fat will be used to provide energy and to spare body protein, but the kcal intake must be increased to meet energy demands as soon as possible.

Because protein losses following surgery can be significant and because protein is especially needed then to rebuild tissue, control edema, avoid shock, resist infection, and transport fats, a high-protein diet of 80 to 100 grams a day may be recommended. (See Chapter 21 for high-protein diet.) In addition, extra minerals and vitamins are needed. When peristalsis returns, ice chips may be given and, if they are tolerated, a clear liquid diet can follow. (Peristalsis is evidenced by bowel sounds.)

Normally in postoperative cases, patients proceed from the clear liquid diet to the regular diet. Sometimes this is done directly, and sometimes by way of the full liquid, soft, or residue-restricted diets. It depends on the patient and the type of surgery. (See Chapter 17 for a review of hospital diets and Chapter 22 for residue-restricted diets.)

The average patient will be able to take food within one to four days after surgery. If the patient cannot take food then, parenteral or tube feeding may be necessary.

Sometimes following gastric surgery, **dumping syndrome** occurs within 15 to 30 minutes after eating. This is characterized by dizziness, weakness, cramps, vomiting, and diarrhea. It is caused by food moving too quickly from the stomach into the small intestine.

To prevent dumping syndrome, the diet should be high in protein and fat, and carbohydrates are restricted. Foods should contain little fiber or concentrated sugars and only limited amounts of starch. Complex carbohydrates are gradually reintroduced. This is recommended because carbohydrates leave the stomach faster than do proteins and fats. Fluids should be limited to four ounces at meals, or restricted completely. They can be taken 30 minutes after meals. The total daily food intake may be divided and served as several small meals rather than the usual three meals, in an attempt to avoid overloading the stomach. Some patients do not tolerate milk well after gastric surgery so its inclusion in the diet will depend on the patient's tolerance.

The food habits of the postoperative patient should be closely observed because they will affect recovery. When the patient's appetite fails to improve, the physician and the dietitian should be notified, and efforts made to offer nutritious foods that the patient will eat. The patient should be encouraged to eat and to eat slowly to avoid swallowing air, which can cause abdominal distension and pain.

TUBE FEEDING

The term **enteral nutrition** means the forms of feeding that bring nutrients directly into the digestive tract. Oral feeding is the usual method and should be used whenever possible. When patients cannot or will not take food by mouth, but their gastrointestinal tract is working, they will be given **tube feedings.** Sometimes this may be necessary because of unconsciousness, surgery, stroke, severe malnutrition, or extensive burns.

Usually, for periods that do not exceed three or four weeks, tube feeding is administered through a **nasogastric tube** inserted through the nose and into the stomach or small intestine. When the tube cannot be placed in the nose or when tube feedings will be required for more than four weeks, an opening called an **ostomy** is surgically created into the esophagus (an **esophagostomy**), the stomach (**gastrostomy**), or the intestine (**jejunostomy**).

The tubes used for these feedings are soft, flexible, and as small as they can be and still allow the feeding to pass through. Although some tubes are weighted to help keep them in place in the stomach or intestine, the use of weighted tubes is controversial.

Numerous commercial formulas are available, with varying types and amounts of nutrients. Those patients able to digest and absorb nutrients can be given **intact formulas** containing proteins, carbohydrates, and fats that require digestion. Patients that have limited ability to digest or absorb nutrients may be given **elemental** or **hydrolyzed formulas** that contain the products of digestion of proteins, carbohydrates, and fats. **Modular formulas** can be used as supplements to other formulas, or for developing customized formulas for certain patients.

Tube feedings usually are administered by the **continuous infusion** method with or without a pump. This means the feeding is continuous during a 16 to 24 hour period. Initially, it is usually diluted by half and given at a rate of from 30 to 50 ml per hour. This rate may be increased by about 25 ml every 8 to 24 hours until the desired amount is attained. The strength of the formula also is gradually increased until it reaches full strength.

When patients are ready to return to oral feedings, the transfer must be done gradually.

Problems Associated with Tube Feeding

The **osmolality** of a liquid substance means the number of particles per kilogram of solution. Solutions with more particles (high osmolality) exert more pressure than solutions with fewer particles. Solutions with high osmolality attract water from nearby fluids that contain lower osmolality. When a formula with high osmolality reaches the intestine, the body may draw fluid from the blood to dilute the formula. This can cause weakness and diarrhea in the patient.

Aspiration can occur (some of the formula enters the lung), causing the patient to develop pneumonia. The tube may become clogged, or the patient may pull the tube out.

Obviously, patients requiring tube feeding need a great deal of patience and understanding. They have been deprived of a basic pleasure of life—eating. They may also be fearful, uncomfortable, and apprehensive about the tube.

PARENTERAL NUTRITION

Parenteral nutrition is the provision of nutrients intravenously. It is used if the gastrointestinal tract is not functional or if normal feeding is not adequate for the patient's needs. It can be used alone or as part of a dietary plan that includes oral or tube feeding as well. When parenteral nutrition is used to provide total nutrition, it is called **TPN** for **total parenteral nutrition.**

Nutrient solutions are prescribed by the physician and nutrition specialist and are prepared by a pharmacist. They can be administered via a central vein or, for a period of two weeks or less, a **peripheral** (near the surface) **vein.** Typically, a dextrose/amino acid solution and a separate fat emulsion are given. These two solutions are not combined until just before their entry into the vein because they do not form a stable solution together.

If patients require TPN for extended periods, it is provided via a central vein. When this is done, a catheter is surgically inserted, under sterile conditions, by a physician. It is inserted into the jugular or subclavian vein and then into the superior vena cava. The vena cava is used because the blood flow is high there. This facilitates the quick dilution of the highly-concentrated TPN solution. This reduces the possibility of **phlebitis** (inflammation of a vein) or **thrombosis** (blood clot).

When parenteral nutrition is no longer necessary, the patient must be transferred gradually to an oral diet. Sometimes patients can be given tube feeding before oral feeding as they are weaned from TPN.

Possible Complications Associated with Parenteral Nutrition

Infection can occur at the site of the catheter and enter the bloodstream, causing an infection of the blood called **sepsis.** Bacterial or fungus infections can develop in the solution if it is unrefrigerated for over 12 hours. Abnormal electrolyte levels may develop, as can phlebitis or blood clots. Careful monitoring of the patient is essential.

NUTRITIONAL THERAPY FOR BURN PATIENTS

In cases of serious burns, the loss of skin surface leads to enormous losses of fluids, electrolytes, and proteins. Water moves from other tissues to the burn site in an effort to compensate for the loss, but this only compounds the problem. This fluid loss can reduce the blood volume and thus blood pressure, as well as urine output.

Fluids and electrolytes are replaced by intravenous therapy immediately to prevent shock. Glucose is not included in these fluids for the first two to three days after the burn, because it could cause hyperglycemia.

The hypermetabolic state after a serious burn continues until the skin is largely healed. This means an enormous increase in energy is needed for the healing process. Kcal needs can be more than 3500 because of the increased metabolic rate and to spare protein for tissue building. Protein needs can be as high as 150 g or more. A high-protein, high-kcal diet is used. There is an increased need for vitamin C for healing and B vitamins for the metabolism of the extra nutrients.

Also, it is essential that badly burned patients have sufficient fluids to help the kidneys hold the unusual load of wastes in solution and to replace those lost.

If the patient can and will eat, oral feedings are advisable. Liquid commercial formulas may be used at first, and solid food may be added during the second week following the burn. If the patient cannot or will not eat, tube feedings will be necessary. In some cases, parenteral feeding is required.

The foods served should be those the patient likes, and service should be as attractive as possible. Burn patients need a great deal of encouragement. They may be in pain, worried about disfigurement, and know they face a long, costly, and painful hospital stay with the possibility of surgery.

NUTRITIONAL THERAPY DURING FEVERS AND INFECTIONS

Fever typically accompanies an infection. Fevers and infections may be acute or chronic. **Fever** is a hypermetabolic state in which each degree of fever on the Fahrenheit scale raises the BMR 7 percent. If extra kcal are not provided during fever, the body first uses its supply of glycogen, then its stored fat, and finally its own muscle tissue for energy.

Protein intake should be increased during fever to one or two grams per kilogram of body weight. Protein is needed to replace body tissue and to produce **antibodies** to fight the infection. Minerals are needed to help build and repair body tissue, and to maintain acid-base, electrolyte, and fluid balance. Extra kcal are needed for the increased metabolic rate. Extra vitamins are also necessary for the increased metabolic rate and to help fight the infection causing the fever. Extra liquid is needed to replace that lost through perspiration and possibly vomiting and diarrhea that can accompany the infection.

Patients usually have very poor appetites with fever, but they will often accept ice water, fruit juice, and carbonated beverages. Some will accept bouillon or consommé.

Usually, the diet during fever and infection progresses from the liquid to the regular diet with frequent, small meals recommended. It should be high protein, high kcal, and high vitamin. In some cases, parenteral and enteral feedings are necessary.

NUTRITION FOR AIDS PATIENTS

Acquired immunodeficiency syndrome (**AIDS**) is an **infectious** (contagious) and fatal (resulting in death) disease. It is caused by the human immunodeficiency virus (**HIV**).

This virus affects the T cells which are white blood cells that protect the body from infections. When T cells cannot function normally, the body has no resistance to *opportunistic infections.* **Opportunistic infections** are caused by microorganisms that are present but do not normally affect people with healthy immune systems.

AIDS is transmitted via body fluids:

- through sexual contact
- by transfusions of contaminated blood
- by use of contaminated needles during injection of illegal drugs
- from infected mothers to their infants before birth

Symptoms include fever, swollen lymph nodes, anorexia, diarrhea, and weight loss. Patients can develop infections of the lungs, skin, gastrointestinal and central nervous systems. A type of cancer called **Kaposi's sarcoma,** pneumonia, or severe diarrhea can result in death.

The infections increase the metabolic rate and, thus, nutrient and kcal needs, but decrease the appetite and frequently reduce the body's ability to absorb nutrients. Weight loss, **hypoalbuminemia** (reduced amounts of protein in the blood), and malnutrition result. The immune system is further damaged by insufficient amounts of proteins and kcal.

Feeding Problems

Although a high-kcal/high-protein diet is advisable, the patient may not accept it. The ravages of the disease plus the nausea caused by medications contribute to anorexia.

When possible, medications should be given after meals to reduce the possibility of nausea. Sores in the mouth or esophagus can make eating painful, and soft foods may be better accepted than others. The taste can be affected so spicy or highly acidic foods or foods with extreme temperatures may be rejected. In some cases, it may be useful to discuss nutritional care with the patient.

Frequent small meals and, sometimes, liquid formulas may be helpful. Additional sugar and flavoring may increase the acceptability of liquid formulas. Because of the nausea and diarrhea, sufficient fluids are essential. If the patient has difficulty swallowing or simply cannot eat, tube feeding may be necessary. If the tube causes pain, parenteral nutrition (feeding via the vein) may be necessary. The patient should be helped to eat as much as possible, especially on "good" days.

Some patients may want to try unconventional diets, thinking these diets will help or even cure them. Unless these diets are obviously harmful, they can be used. In some cases, the idea of improvement may help the patient's appetite.

Those patients who will benefit no further from either medication or nutrition can still be helped by the health care professional who shows support, understanding, and respect for them.

CONSIDERATIONS FOR THE HEALTH CARE PROFESSIONAL

Patients who fall within the categories of conditions discussed in this chapter can try the health care professional in many ways. Those recovering from surgery may whine. Those suffering from burns will catch one's heartstrings. Patients suffering from fatal infections can be especially needy, and the health care professional must be particularly alert to protect herself or himself while caring for these patients. Those receiving tube feedings may suffer from frequent diarrhea.

In each of these cases, the health care professional can help herself or himself as well as the patient by thinking positively and showing cheerfulness. Cheerfulness can be contagious, but it is never harmful.

SUMMARY

Surgery, burns, fevers, and infections are traumas that cause the body to react hyper- metabolically. This creates the need for addition- al nutrients at the same time that the injury causes a loss of nutrients. Care must be taken to provide extra fluid, proteins, kcal, vitamins, min- erals, and carbohydrates as needed in these situa- tions. When surgery is elective, nutritional status should be improved before surgery, if necessary. When food cannot be taken orally, tube or paren- teral nutrition should be used.

Discussion Topics

1. Describe the body's reaction to trauma and how nutrition is related to it.
2. Why are extra nutrients needed during trauma?
3. When might surgery be elective?
4. In what ways might a diet history of a presurgical patient be helpful?
5. Explain why a burn patient needs extra protein. What happens when the extra protein is not provided?
6. Why does a surgical patient need extra minerals?
7. Why must a patient's stomach be empty at the time of surgery?
8. Explain why the IV dextrose solutions are not sufficient to fulfill nutritional requirements after surgery.
9. Describe dumping syndrome and tell how it may be alleviated.
10. Describe parenteral nutrition. What is it? How is it delivered? What are some dangers related to it?
11. Could parenteral nutrition be used in the treatment of anorexia nervosa? Explain.

Suggested Activities

1. Ask a doctor or nurse to visit the class and discuss tube feedings, telling why and when they are used and problems associated with them.
2. Invite a nurse from a local hospital to discuss burns and their treatment.
3. Ask if a class member has experienced a trauma as discussed in this chapter. If so, ask that person to describe it, her or his reactions to it, appetite, and recovery.
4. Plan a day's menus for a 175-pound man who requires 100 grams of protein, and 70 kcal per kilogram of body weight.
5. Role-play a situation where a patient is 9 days post surgery, cannot eat, and the nurse is trying to convince her to eat.
6. Role-play a situation between a 10-year-old child and a nurse. The child has rheumatic fever, a temperature of 100°F, and refuses most food.

Review   Multiple choice. Select the *letter* that precedes the best answer.

1. Trauma
   1. can be described as injury
   2. causes a hypermetabolic response in the body
   3. usually increases the body's need for protein
   4. has no relation to nutrition
      a) 1,2   b) 1,2,3   c) 2,3,4   d) 4

2. During trauma, there is usually
   1. reduced need for protein and minerals
   2. a hypermetabolic response in the body
   3. only minor changes in nutritional requirements
   4. an increased need for protein
      a) 1,2   b) 1,3   c) 2,3   d) 2,4

3. Wound healing, tissue building, and blood regeneration all require
   1. extra fat
   2. extra cholesterol
   3. reduced kcal intake
   4. protein
      a) 4   b) 3   c) 3,4   d) 1,2,3

4. Intravenous solutions
   1. sometimes contain vitamins
   2. usually contain dextrose
   3. are usually given following surgery
   4. provide 2000 kcal per day
      a) 1,2,3   b) 1,3   c) 1,4   d) 4

5. Protein is needed to
   1. build tissue
   2. resist infection
   3. control edema
   4. kill bacteria
      a) 1,2   b) 2,3   c) 1,2,3   d) 2,3,4

6. It would not be surprising for TPN to be used in the treatment of
   1. fractured hip
   2. third degree burns over a large part of the patient's body
   3. broken jaw
   4. appendicitis
      a) 1,2   b) 2,3   c) 3,4   d) 4

7. Dumping syndrome is characterized by
   1. migraine headache
   2. hypertension and tremors
   3. vomiting and diarrhea
   4. dizziness and cramps
      a) 1,2   b) 1,2,3   c) 2,3   d) 3,4
8. TPN is given through
   1. a nasogastric tube
   2. a peripheral vein in the ankle
   3. the superior vena cava
   4. an esophagostomy
      a) 1   b) 2   c) 3   d) 4
9. Severely burned patients will need
   1. to replace protein and fluids
   2. to replace electrolytes
   3. intravenous solutions and blood transfusions
   4. a high-protein, high-kcal diet
      a) 1,2   b) 1,2,3   c) 2,3,4   d) all
10. Fever
    1. creates a need for extra kcal
    2. patients have enormous appetites
    3. patients require extra vitamins
    4. patients should be kept on a low-kcal diet
       a) 1,2   b) 1,4   c) 1,3   d) all

Case Study 1

Surgery Patient

Anne was an extremely busy 46-year-old working wife and mother of two teenagers when she fell and fractured her hip. The surgeon performed a hip pinning and bone graft, and instructed her to put no weight on it. During the surgery it was observed that Anne appeared to have early osteoporosis. The surgeon so advised her.

When Anne was in the hospital, the dietitian took a careful diet history and learned that Anne had, in her young adult life, not eaten as she knew she should have. She admitted to having shorted herself on milk all of her adult life. She did eat cheese fairly often, however.

For several days after the surgery, Anne was unable to eat at all. She became extremely depressed. Vitamins were prescribed. As Anne did begin to eat a bit, she felt better and was less depressed. She was discharged after $2\frac{1}{2}$ weeks. When Anne returned home, she weighed 100 pounds and regained her strength slowly. After $3\frac{1}{2}$ months, she went back to work on crutches.

After six months, it became clear that the hip was not healing as the surgeon had hoped, and he advised Anne to have a hip replacement if she were to walk again without crutches. She agreed and a date was set. This time she prepared for surgery. The operation was a success. She suffered no depression, and she was discharged after two weeks. She is walking now without a cane.

Case Study Questions Based on the Nursing Process

Assess
1. What probably contributed to Anne's developing osteoporosis?
2. What relationship is there between Anne's apparent liking for cheese and osteoporosis?
3. What factors contributed to Anne's depression after her first emergency surgery?

Plan
4. How did Anne plan for her second surgery?
5. How did Anne decrease her chances of having postoperative depression after the second surgery?

Implement
6. Describe the diet Anne should be on after surgery.
7. What will you teach Anne to help her prevent the osteoporosis from worsening?

Evaluate
8. What were the major differences affecting the outcome of Anne's first surgery compared with the second?

Case Study 2

AIDS Patient

Peter was a 35-year-old English teacher in Ohio. He liked teaching, and his students enjoyed his classes. Occasionally, he would spend a long weekend in Chicago with friends he'd made during college.

When he was diagnosed with AIDS, he was devastated and, for the first time, felt ashamed of his lifestyle. He was the only child of his widowed mother and dreaded hearing a terrible lecture when he told her of his condition. Instead, she simply cried and hugged him and told him she would care for him. His feelings of shame went away.

He moved in with his mother. She cooked all his favorite foods sometimes serving him four desserts for dinner, watched that he took his medications as prescribed, bathed him when he could no longer care for himself, and never gave up urging him to eat. When he contracted pneumonia, the doctor said she must put him in the hospital, but she would not do so. He died holding her hand.

Case Study Questions Based on the Nursing Process

Assess
1. Why do you think Peter suffered less anorexia than other patients with AIDS?
2. Peter always liked Mexican food but as his condition worsened, he refused it. Why?

Plan
3. Why did Peter's mother sometimes give him four desserts instead of meat or fish and vegetables at dinner? Was this harmful? Explain.
4. What factors did Peter's mother probably consider each time she prepared a meal?

Implement
5. Sometimes Peter's mother would ask him what he would like to eat. Usually, Peter asked her to surprise him. Explain his reasons.
6. What should Peter's mother have been taught about his diet needs when he had pneumonia?

Evaluate
7. At times Peter wanted only fluids for several days. His mother prepared milkshakes and eggnog for him and encouraged him to drink ginger ale as well. Was this appropriate? Explain.
8. What feelings did Peter's mother convey that gave him comfort?
9. How did Peter's mother help him die with dignity?

NUTRITIONAL CARE OF PATIENTS

OBJECTIVES

After studying this chapter, you should be able to
- Describe how illness and surgery can affect the nutrition of patients
- Identify and describe three or more nutrition related health problems that are common among elderly patients needing long-term care
- Demonstrate correct procedures for feeding a bedridden patient
- Explain the importance of adapting the family's meal to suit the patient's nutritional requirements

HOSPITALIZED PATIENTS

Illness and surgery can have devastating effects on nutritional status. Fever, nausea, fear, depression, chemotherapy, and radiation can destroy appetite. Vomiting, diarrhea, chemotherapy, radiation, and some medications can reduce or prevent absorption of nutrients. In addition, food is restricted before surgery and some diagnostic tests. Ironically, this reduced nutrient and kcal intake occurs just at a time when requirements are increased.

Protein-Calorie Malnutrition

When the increased needs for energy and protein are not met by food intake, the body must use its stores of glycogen and fat. When they have been used, the body breaks down its own tissues to provide protein for energy. It has no other "stores" of protein. **Protein-calorie malnutrition,** commonly called **PCM,** is a significant problem among hospitalized patients. It can delay wound healing, contribute to anemia, depress the immune system and, because of the depressed immune system, increase susceptibility to infections. When malnutrition occurs as a result of hospitalization, it is called **iatrogenic malnutrition.** Symptoms of PCM include weight loss and dry, pale skin.

Improving the Patient's Nutritional Status

The importance of improving a patient's nutritional status is obvious. Formal nutritional assessments of patients should be made on a regular basis, but all members of the health care team should be alert to signs of malnutrition every day. The nurse or nursing assistant whom the patient sees regularly is in the best position to help the patient. This person will be most familiar to the patient and will hear the patient's complaints about and see the reactions to the food served. She or he can bring problems to the attention of the dietitian responsible for the patient's nutrition.

The patient may

1. need reassurance about his or her condition
2. need information about nutritional needs
3. need personal attention
4. want other foods

If approved by the dietitian, it can be helpful to invite friends and relatives to bring the patient some of his or her favorite foods.

FEEDING THE PATIENT

In the home, the family menu should serve as the basis of the patient's meal whenever possible. This usually pleases the patient because it makes her or him feel a part of the family. It also reduces food preparation time and costs.

Family meals are easily adapted for the patient by omitting or adding certain foods or by varying the method of preparation. Suppose the patient was to limit fat intake and the family menu was the following:

Fried Hamburgers
Mashed Potatoes with Butter
Buttered Peas
Lettuce
with
French Dressing
Ice Cream
with
Fresh Strawberries
Whole Milk

Broiling the hamburgers instead of frying would help limit the fat content. The patient's mashed potatoes might be served with little or no butter and the peas with only salt and pepper and perhaps a suitable spice, herb, or lemon. The patient could be served lettuce with lemon and for dessert, strawberries without ice cream. Skim milk is a simple substitute for whole milk.

Serving the Meal

To serve a meal at the bedside, the tray should be lined with a pretty cloth or paper liner. Attractive dishes that fit the tray conveniently without crowding it should be used. The food should be arranged attractively on the plate, with a colorful garnish such as a slice of fruit, parsley, a pickle, or vegetable stick. The garnish must fit into the patient's diet plan, however. Utensils must be arranged conveniently. Water should be served as well as another beverage (unless it is prohibited by the physician). Foods must be served at proper temperatures.

When the patient is on complete bedrest, special preparations are required before the meal is served. The patient should be given the opportunity to use the bedpan and to wash before the meal is served. The room can be ventilated and the bedcovers straightened. The patient should be helped to a comfortable position and any unpleasant sights removed before the meal is served. Pleasant conversation during the preparations can improve the patient's mood considerably. Certain topics of conversation can help stimulate the patient's interest in eating. The patient might be told that the family is anticipating the same meal. Perhaps the recipes used will interest some patients. Appropriate remarks on the patient's progress, whenever possible, are helpful.

When the meal preparations are complete, the tray should be placed so it is easy for the patient to feed herself or himself or, if necessary, convenient for someone else to do the feeding. If the patient needs help, the napkin should be opened and placed, the bread spread, the meat cut, the eggs shelled, and the straw offered. The patient should be encouraged to eat and be allowed sufficient time. If the meal is interrupted by the physician, the tray should be removed and the food kept at proper temperatures in the kitchen. It should be served again as soon as the physician leaves.

The tray should be removed and the patient helped to brush her or his teeth when the meal is finished. The kinds and amounts of food refused, the time, the type of diet, and the patient's appetite should be recorded on the patient's chart after each meal. At times, the doctor may request an accurate report of the types and amounts of uneaten food.

Feeding the Disabled Patient

If the patient is unable to feed herself or himself, the person doing the feeding should sit near the side of the bed. Small amounts of food should be placed toward the back of the mouth with a slight pressure on the tongue with the spoon or fork. If the patient is suffering from

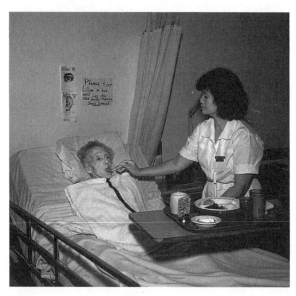

Figure 25-1 Some patients require assistance when eating.

one-sided paralysis, the food and drinking straw must be placed in the nonparalyzed side of the mouth, figure 25-1. The patient must be allowed to help herself or himself as much as possible. If the patient begins to choke, help her or him sit up straight. Do not give food or water while the patient is choking. The patient's mouth should be wiped as needed.

Feeding the Blind Patient

Special care must be taken in serving a meal for a blind patient. An appetizing description of the meal can help create a desire to eat. To help the blind patient feed herself or himself, arrange the food as if the plate were the face of a clock, figure 25-2. The meat might be put at 6 o'clock, vegetables at 9 o'clock, salad at 12, and bread at 3 o'clock. The person who regularly arranges the meal should remember to use the same pattern for all meals. Blind people usually feel better when they can help themselves.

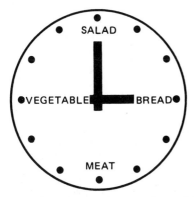

Figure 25-2 To a blind patient, a plate of food can be pictured as the face of a clock.

LONG-TERM CARE OF THE ELDERLY

Because of increased **longevity** (length of life), the number of elderly people requiring long-term care is expected to increase. The changes people undergo with age and that can affect their nutritional status were discussed in Chapter 16.

Physical Problems of the Institutionalized Elderly

It is estimated that the majority of people 85 and over have at least one chronic disease such as arthritis, osteoporosis, diabetes mellitus, cardiovascular disease, or mental disorder. These conditions affect their attitudes, physical activities, appetites and, thus, nutritional status. PCM is a major problem for this population.

Anemia can develop if the patient has too little animal protein in the diet. It can contribute to confusion and depression, but may go unnoticed because one of its major symptoms, fatigue, may be simply thought to be a characteristic of old age. It is helpful to make sure there is sufficient animal protein food and vitamin C (an iron enhancer) in the patient's diet.

Decubitus ulcers (bedsores) can develop in bedridden patients. They develop in areas where there is unrelieved pressure on the skin so the blood cannot bring nutrients and oxygen and remove wastes. Healing requires treatment of the ulcer, relief of the pressure, and high-kcal diet with sufficient protein.

Constipation can be caused by inadequate fiber, fluid or exercise, by medication, reduced peristalsis, or former abuse of laxatives. It can be relieved by increased fluid, fiber, and exercise (if possible).

Diarrhea can be caused by lack of muscle tone in the colon. It will reduce the absorption of nutrients and can contribute to dehydration. A high-kcal/high-protein diet combined with supplemental vitamins and minerals may be helpful.

The *sense of smell* declines with age and diminishes the appetite. A *reduced sense of taste* can be caused by medications, disease, mineral deficiencies, or **xerostomia** (dry mouth). The addition of spices, herbs, salt, and sugar (if allowed) can be helpful. Xerostomia can be caused by disease or medications. Drinking water, frequent small meals, and chewing sugar-free gums or candies may be helpful. The inadequate amount of saliva in these patients contributes to increased tooth decay.

Dysphagia (difficulty swallowing) can result from a stroke or develop in patients with Alzheimer's disease. They may be able to take food as liquid through a bottle with a nipple or possibly as a slightly thickened liquid.

CONSIDERATIONS FOR THE HEALTH CARE PROFESSIONAL

The needs of bedridden patients are nearly total. They are unable to walk, use the bathroom, brush their teeth, or wash their hands without help. The feelings of helplessness they endure are terrible. In addition, they may be embarrassed by their appearance, by vomiting in front of a guest, by needing a bedpan when only a thin curtain separates them from their neighbor's guests. It is helpful to the patient if the health care professional can imagine himself or herself in the place of the patient.

The needs of many elderly patients in nursing homes are also total. They may be arthritic and unable to walk; some may be incontinent; others may forget their names and how to dress; they may wander off the premises unless they are constantly watched; they may need to be fed. Each remains an individual. Each one needs, responds to, and deserves warmth and respect from their caregivers.

SUMMARY

Illness and surgery can have devastating effects on patients' nutritional status. PCM is a significant problem in hospitals. The health care team should work together to improve patients' nutritional status.

A patient's meal should be adapted from the family's meal whenever possible. This saves time and expense, and allows the patient to feel more a part of the family.

A bedridden patient should be given the bedpan and allowed to wash her or his hands before the meal. Patients should be encouraged to feed themselves. However, help should be offered if it is needed. The blind patient can eat more easily if food is arranged in a set pattern on the plate. Pleasant conversation and cheerfulness on the part of the nurse can improve the patient's appetite. The type of diet, time of meal, patient's appetite, type and amount of food eaten should all be recorded on the patient's chart. Elderly patients requiring long-term care may suffer from several nutrition-related health problems that, with proper treatment, can sometimes be relieved.

Discussion Topics

1. How do illness and surgery affect one's nutrition?
2. What is PCM? How does it relate to one's nutritional status?
3. What is iatrogenic malnutrition? How might it develop?
4. In what ways might the nurse help improve the patient's nutrition?
5. When might it be unwise to invite a patient's friends and family to bring foods to the patient? When might it be appropriate? Who would decide?
6. Discuss the following menu in terms of nutrient value and attractiveness. Adapt it to a patient on a low-kcal diet.

Cream of Chicken Soup
Roast Beef with Gravy
Baked Potatoes
Buttered Green Beans
Rolls and Butter
Angel Cake
with
Chocolate Ice Cream

7. Discuss the importance of proper preparation of the patient and room before the meal. What could disturb a patient and affect appetite?
8. How may the appearance of the tray affect the patient's appetite?
9. What is a garnish? Why are some types prohibited?
10. Why should the patient be encouraged to feed herself or himself?
11. Why is it important to remove the tray as soon as the patient has finished the meal?
12. How can the behavior and attitude of the attending person affect the appetite of the patient?
13. Name four chronic diseases that are common to the elderly. Explain why they are called "chronic."
14. Why is anemia so easily overlooked in elderly patients?
15. Discuss how a diminished sense of smell might affect one's appetite.

Suggested Activities

1. Plan a family dinner and adapt it to the needs of a patient who should limit carbohydrate intake.
2. Arrange a tray suitable for serving this meal.
3. Have two students participate in the following role-playing situation. The class should evaluate and discuss the "nurse's" tact and skill in dealing with the "patient."
   Mrs. Jones is a young, active woman with a family. She is recovering from viral pneumonia. Although she is allowed out of bed, she is not supposed to prepare meals or do housework until her condition improves. Dr. Malcolm has told Miss Wilson, the nurse, that it is important for Mrs. Jones to regain her lost weight. One day, before her dinner was served, Mrs. Jones complained to Miss Wilson. She was discouraged about her lack of energy and stated that her family needed her. Miss Wilson noticed that Mrs. Jones had eaten very little for breakfast and lunch. What should she say to Mrs. Jones?
4. Practice feeding each other. Ask the "nurse" to fill in the "patient's" chart.
5. Practice feeding a blindfolded "patient."
6. Invite a gerontologist to speak to the class on nutrition and the elderly.
7. Invite a nurse who works in a nursing home to talk to the class. Ask him or her to describe how these patients are fed.
8. Visit a local nursing home in groups of two or three. Talk to some of the patients. Write a report on your visit.
9. Imagine you are 85 years old, have all your mental faculties, but can no longer shop, cook, clean, do your laundry, or drive. You and your son decide you should go to a nursing home. Write a page or more describing your feelings. Include answers to the following:

a. What would you do with your furniture? Your dishes? Your sheets and towels? Your scrapbooks?
b. What would you do all day?
c. How would you like to be treated in "the home?" What would you do if someone spoke gruffly to you? How would you feel if someone ridiculed you because your hair needed to be cut?
d. What would you do if the food was terrible?

Review

A. A patient on a limited fat intake should avoid foods that are high in fat. Indicate which foods she or he may eat on the following list by writing Y (yes). Write N (no) for the foods to be avoided.

_____ 1. fried hamburger   _____ 6. butter
_____ 2. mashed potatoes   _____ 7. ice cream
_____ 3. peas   _____ 8. fresh strawberries
_____ 4. lettuce   _____ 9. whole milk
_____ 5. French dressing   _____ 10. avocado

B. Briefly answer the following questions.
1. How can the following menu be adapted for a patient who must avoid high-fiber foods?

Fresh Fruit Cup
Roast Turkey
Rice with Peas
Mashed Sweet Potatoes with Pecans
Celery and Carrot Sticks
Whole Wheat Bread
Butter
Cherry-Nut Ice Cream
Milk and Coffee

2. What should be done if the patient's meal is interrupted by a visit from the doctor?

3. What dietary information should be recorded on the patient's chart after a meal?

4. Give two examples of a colorful garnish.

5. How would you like to have your mother or father treated if either were in a nursing home?

Case Study 1

Depression of an Elderly Woman

When Connie's husband died, her only daughter and son-in-law, who lived 1,500 miles away, insisted she move to a nursing home near them. She was only 75, felt fine, and didn't want to leave her brothers and sisters who lived near her. Her daughter and son-in-law insisted and sold all her belongings other than her clothes. She cried.

When she saw her new "home," she cried. The food was bad and many of the residents had Alzheimer's. When her brother and his wife made the long trip to see her, they were shocked at Connie's appearance. She was thin, poorly groomed, and seemed a bit confused. They contacted her daughter who agreed to sign release papers to allow Connie to go home with them.

Connie's sister-in-law was a wonderful cook and within a month Connie had regained some weight and felt like her "old self." She rented her own small apartment near her brother's house and, with his help, made arrangements for her small pension and Social Security checks to be sent to her there.

When her daughter visited her later that year, she admitted she'd made a mistake and was pleased with her mother's progress.

Case Study Questions Based on the Nursing Process

Assess
1. What may have contributed to Connie's confusion at the nursing home?
2. Discuss possible reasons for her weight loss.

Plan
3. What might have happened to Connie if her brother had not "rescued" her?

Implement
4. Along with good food, what other factors helped Connie improve and gain weight?
5. Explain why this particular nursing home was inappropriate for Connie. What appropriate alternatives are available in your area for someone like Connie?

Evaluate
6. What may have helped Connie's confusion clear up?
7. What support services might Connie need to maintain her new independent role?

Case Study 2

Protein-Calorie Malnutrition

Donald was a thin hard-working man who had always planned his life's activities carefully. After selling his successful clothing store at the age of 60, he planned to live a modest life of leisure. Within a year of his retirement, he lost his left arm to bone cancer.

His surgeon believed the surgery was successful and expected Donald to recover. Donald hated the hospital, its food and, most of all, the chemotherapy and radiation he underwent. He suffered terribly from nausea and diarrhea and couldn't eat. He lost a great deal of weight. He was given parenteral nutrition and made a very slow recovery.

Case Study Questions Based on the Nursing Process

Assess

1. The doctor told Donald he had PCM that was threatening his life. How was this possible in a modern hospital?
2. What were contributing factors in Donald's PCM?

Plan

3. How could Donald help overcome his PCM? Is it possible that a psychologist could help Donald? Explain.

Implement

4. What might be one reason the doctor did not order *total* parenteral nutrition for Donald?

Evaluate

5. What could have happened to Donald if the doctor hadn't ordered parenteral nutrition?

SECTION 4

FOOD PREPARATION

EVALUATING AND PRESERVING FOOD QUALITY

OBJECTIVES

After studying this chapter, you should be able to
- State criteria for evaluating the quality of meat, poultry, fish, eggs, vegetables, and fruit
- Describe the proper handling and storage of meat, poultry, and eggs
- Identify the different types of milk and milk products and explain how milk is pasteurized

Because of the wide variety of foods available in supermarkets today, it is essential that the **consumer** (one who buys and uses marketed items) be able to determine the **nutritional value** (nutrient content) and quality of these foods. In addition, the consumer should have a basic knowledge of the appropriate uses and storage of food and the government-regulated grading and inspection policies affecting it.

MEAT, POULTRY, AND FISH

Meat, poultry, and fish (animal products) provide the greatest source of protein in the diet of Americans. They also are rich sources of minerals and vitamins. Many also contain fats and cholesterol. These foods play an important role in the American diet, typically serving as the foundation of meals.

Meat

The muscles and organs of animals provide the various types of *meat* available for human diets. Cattle provide beef and veal, sheep provide lamb, and hogs provide pork. Wild game meats such as **venison** (from deer) or rabbit (sometimes labeled **hare**) are sometimes available. Edible organ meats include liver, kidney, heart, brains, and **sweetbreads** (thymus gland from young cattle). Organ meats are especially rich sources of minerals, but their cholesterol content is very high.

Inspection and Grading

Consumers are assisted in their evaluations of meats by federally regulated inspection and grading systems. Inspection is indicated by a United States Department of Agriculture (USDA) stamp on the outer portion of meat, see figure 26-1. This inspection ensures consumers that the meat has been handled under sanitary conditions and is safe to eat.

Quality grading is not required by law, but many meat producers provide it by listing it on the labels of their packaging. Grades are assigned on the basis of fat content, texture, and color of the lean meat. There are four principal grades for

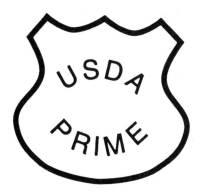

Figure 26-2 USDA Grade Stamp for Meat

meat: *Prime, Choice, Good,* and *Standard.* Grading is indicated by a shield-shaped stamp, figure 26-2. Characteristics of quality are listed in Table 26-1.

Cuts Available

Meats are available in various cuts, figure 26-3. The muscles that the animal uses most are the least tender. Although the less-tender cuts are

Table 26-1 USDA Meat Grades

Characteristics	Grade
Highest quality Highest price Most fat Most tender	Prime
High in quality Abundant supply Tender and juicy Moderate fat	Choice
Lean meat May be tough and dry unless properly cooked Economical	Good
Lowest in quality Used by canners, processors	Standard

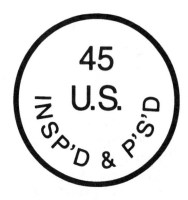

Figure 26-1 USDA Inspection Stamp for Meat

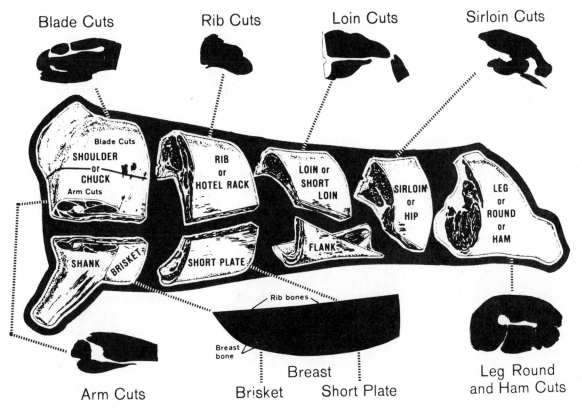

Blade Cuts   Rib Cuts   Loin Cuts   Sirloin Cuts

Blade Cuts
SHOULDER
or
CHUCK
Arm Cuts

RIB
or
HOTEL RACK

LOIN or
SHORT
LOIN

SIRLOIN
or
HIP

LEG
or
ROUND
or
HAM

SHANK   BRISKET

SHORT PLATE

FLANK

Rib bones

Breast
bone

Arm Cuts   Brisket   Breast   Short Plate   Leg Round
and Ham Cuts

Figure 26-3 Seven basic retail cuts are used to prepare veal, lamb, beef, or pork. *(Courtesy of the National Live Stock and Meat Board)*

usually less expensive, the selection should depend on the method of cooking to be used.

Tender cuts may be cooked by **dry heat** methods of cooking such as roasting, broiling, or frying. This means heat is conducted to foods without the use of moisture.

Less tender cuts should be cooked covered, by **moist heat** methods such as **braising** or **stewing.** In these methods, heat is conducted through liquid at low temperatures no higher than 200°F. (See Table 26-2.)

Proteins **coagulate** (thicken) during cooking. Therefore, most protein-rich foods should be cooked at low temperatures to prevent them from becoming tough and shrinking. Exceptions are

tender cuts, which, if cooked to a rare or medium state of doneness, can be cooked at a high temperature for a short time in the broiler or over direct heat. Roasting for a longer time at a low temperature also is recommended for tender cuts.

Purchase, Storage, and Defrosting

Meat is highly perishable and decomposes more readily than carbohydrates and fats. One should always check the *sell by date* on the package to determine the freshness of the meat. If the meat does not have a pleasant odor when the package is held near one's nose, it should not be purchased. Meats in damaged containers should never be purchased.

Table 26-2 Retail Cuts of Meat and Appropriate Cooking Methods

Veal, Lamb, Beef, Pork	Primary Cooking Method

Shoulder or Chuck
   Stew meat
   Cube steaks
   Shoulder roast
	Moist heat

Shank Stew meat	Moist heat
Rib Prime ribs	Dry heat

Short Plate
   Short ribs
   Stew meat
	Moist heat

Loin or Short Loin
   Tenderloin
   T-bone or Porterhouse Steaks
	Dry heat

Sirloin
   Sirloin Steaks
   Roast
	Dry heat

Flank Flank Steak	Moist heat

Leg or Round
   Rump (pot roast)
   Eye of Round
	Moist heat
	Dry heat

Proper storage is essential to maintain the quality and safety of fresh meat. When refrigerated, fresh meats keep well for only two to four days. Ground meats keep only one to two days because so much of their surface area has been exposed to bacteria.

Meat that is to be frozen should be carefully wrapped in freezer paper to prevent freezer burn, labeled, and dated. Frozen meats do not keep indefinitely. There is a recommended *shelf life* of six months for beef, veal, and lamb, and four months for pork. **Shelf life** is the period of time within which a food product should be consumed before a deterioration of quality occurs.

Meats must be defrosted carefully to discourage bacterial growth. Defrosting at room temperature is not advisable unless the meat is immersed in cold water that is changed every 30 minutes. When possible, meat should be defrosted in the refrigerator. Microwaves are also suitable for last minute needs. Thawed meats should not be refrozen before cooking.

Poultry

Common types of poultry available are chicken, turkey, duck, goose, and game hen. Knowledge of proper cooking, handling, and storage is extremely important when working with poultry.

The USDA rules regarding inspection and grading of meat also apply to poultry. Similar stamps of approval are used and are usually found stamped on a paper tag attached to the bird. Poultry quality grades A, B, C (A being the best grade) are based on the shape of the carcass, amount of flesh, fat, blemish, and bruising.

Fresh poultry is highly perishable. Unless it is frozen immediately, it should be refrigerated and used within 24 hours after purchase. Poultry often carries salmonella bacteria that cause salmonellosis, the most common food-borne illness. To prevent salmonellosis, one should:

- Rinse poultry in cold water before cooking to wash away **bacteria.**
- Cook poultry until there is no pink meat.
- Keep cutting boards used to prepare poultry separate from those used to prepare fruit, vegetables, breads, or cheese.
- Wash all utensils used with poultry in the dishwasher if possible. If this is not possi-

ble, they must be thoroughly washed with hot soapy water to avoid contamination of other foods.

- Avoid using a wooden cutting board when preparing poultry. Bacteria can get into the porous wood surface and contaminate other foods.

Poultry is almost always cooked to the well-done stage. The internal temperature tested with a cook's instant read thermometer should be 180°F for a large chicken or turkey. Looseness of joints (a leg will move freely in its socket), clear cavity juices (clear yellow, not pink or red), and a tenderness when touched also will indicate a well-done smaller bird. (See figure 26-4 for storing leftover cooked poultry.)

If the label on the package includes the words *young, broiler,* or *fryer,* the birds should be tender and can be roasted (dry-heat method of

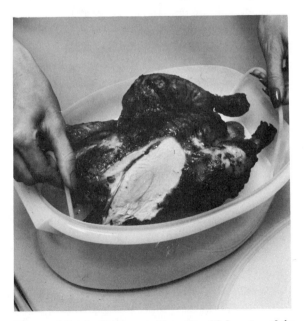

Figure 26-4 Leftover poultry should be stored in the refrigerator in a container with a tight fitting cover. *(Courtesy of Tupperware)*

cooking). If the label says *stewing-hen* or *mature turkey,* the poultry may be tough unless prepared by a moist-heat method of cooking.

Fish and Shellfish

Seafood is divided into two groups: **finfish** (fish with fins and internal skeletons) and **shellfish** (fish with external shells but no internal bones). Seafood can be purchased fresh, canned, frozen, and, sometimes, smoked. It is graded by size and quality, but standards of enforcing the grading are not uniform.

Some common finfish available are cod, flounder, haddock, salmon, tuna, and trout. They are packaged as *round* fish (whole fish with head, bones, and scales), **fillets** (strips of fish free from bone that are cut from the sides of whole fish) and **steaks** (even, crosswise slices).

Shellfish commonly available include shrimp, oysters, mussels, clams, lobster, and crab. Shellfish is usually steamed, boiled, or in some cases sauteed. Oysters and clams can be served raw, on the half shell. Because of pollution in some areas, shellfish may contain viruses or harmful bacteria that can cause illness. Thorough cooking destroys these harmful organisms. The very young, the elderly, pregnant women, and people in poor health should eat their shellfish fully cooked.

MILK AND MILK PRODUCTS

Milk is considered the most nearly perfect food. It is easily digested, and contains complete proteins, carbohydrates, fats, calcium, phosphorus, and vitamins A and B. Milk is low in vitamin C and iron. Most milk sold in the United States has been irradiated with 400 IU of vitamin D per quart, which otherwise is present only in small amounts.

Because bacteria thrive in milk, there are health regulations that must be scrupulously observed by people handling it. Milk that has been handled according to these regulations is **certified.** To ensure its safety, most milk is pasteurized. **Pasteurization** is a process named for Louis Pasteur, its originator. In one method of pasteurization, the milk is heated to at least 62.8°C (145°F) for at least 30 minutes and then immediately cooled to 10°C (50°F). Another method is to heat milk very quickly to 71.7°C (161°F) for at least 15 seconds and then cool it immediately. The pasteurization process kills all harmful bacteria and checks the growth of some harmless bacteria that can cause milk to sour. Milk that has not been pasteurized is called **raw milk.** Raw milk can transmit disease.

Fresh milk is available in containers of various sizes. Usually the larger containers provide the lowest cost per ounce.

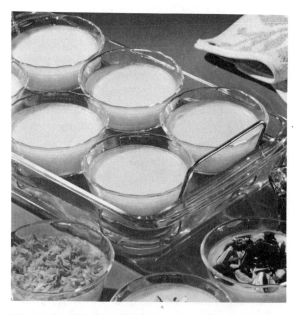

Figure 26-5 Baked custard is one of the many ways in which milk can be added to the diet. *(Courtesy of the National Dairy Council)*

Frequently there is a date on the milk container. Milk should not be purchased after the date indicated because it will not remain fresh for more than a day or two. Milk and milk products should be refrigerated in clean, covered containers to preserve nutrient content and inhibit growth of bacteria. Low temperatures must be used during cooking because milk and its products scorch easily.

Although milk is most often used as a beverage, it is frequently combined with other foods such as soups, gravies, casseroles, baked products, cereals, and desserts, figure 26-5. Milk is available in several forms, some of which are listed in Table 26-3.

Cream

Cream is the fat in milk that rises to the surface. It may also be separated from milk by mechanical means. Cream is classified as light or heavy, depending upon its fat content. The higher the percentage of fat, the heavier the cream. Cream is typically available in one-half pint, pint, and quarter containers and should be kept covered and refrigerated.

Cheese

When milk coagulates, the curd that results is cheese. The hundreds of types available vary according to the kind of milk used, the amount of moisture, types of seasonings, and the method of ripening. *Natural cheese* is commonly classified by moisture content: hard, semisoft, and soft, Table 26-4. Another type of cheese popular in the United States is **process cheese.** It is produced by combining a natural cheese, such as a cheddar, with moisture, seasonings, and sometimes other ingredients to produce a soft, molded cheese, or a cheese spread. American cheese is an example.

Table 26-3 Milk and Milk Products

Dairy Product	Characteristics
Fresh Milk	
Whole	Milk with all its natural nutrients; fat content is 3.3%
Homogenized	Whole milk processed to break the fat into small drops so it does not separate
Skim or non-fat	Milk with all or nearly all fat removed
Low-fat	Milk with fat content of .5 to 3%
Flavored milks	Milk with flavors, such as chocolate, added
Cream	
Whipping cream	Fat content of 30 to 40%
Light cream	Also called coffee cream; 16 to 22% fat
Half and Half	Fat content of 10 to 12%
Fermented Milk Products	
Sour cream	Has been cultured by lactic acid bacteria that make it thick
Yogurt	Milk cultured with harmless bacteria; may have fruit added
Buttermilk	Skim milk, soured by addition of harmless bacteria
Milk Products with Water Removed	
Dried whole or nonfat milk	All water removed
Evaporated	Whole or skim milk with up to 60% of its water removed
Sweetened Condensed	Milk with 60% water removed and heavily sweetened with sugar

Cheese is rich in proteins, vitamins, and the minerals, calcium and phosphorus, but it also contains considerable amounts of sodium, saturated fat, and cholesterol. Cheese is an acceptable meat alternative and is used in sandwiches, casseroles, sauces, salads, and desserts.

Because cheese toughens easily in cooking, low temperatures are recommended. To store cheese, it must be kept tightly wrapped in a cool place. Because the flavor of cheese is most pronounced at room temperature, it should be removed from the refrigerator one hour before serving.

Butter

Butter might be called a byproduct of milk because it is made from the fat in milk. Butter consists of 80 percent milkfat, 16 percent water, some protein, and vitamin A. It is available as sweet butter (no salt has been added) or as lightly salted butter (salt has been added). Butter is available as Grade AA, A, B, and C. The best flavored and most expensive is AA.

Butter must be kept refrigerated and covered because it absorbs other food odors very quickly.

Table 26-4 Natural Cheese Classification According to Moisture Content

Hard	Semisoft	Soft
Parmesan	Mozzarella	Brie
Cheddar	Roquefort	Camembert
Swiss	Blue	Cream
Edam	Gorgonzola	Cottage
Gouda	Muenster	Ricotta

EGGS

Eggs are a good source of proteins, vitamin A, and iron. However, the average egg yolk also contains 6 g of fat and 270 mg of cholesterol. Because the U.S. Committee on Diet and Health suggests that the amount of cholesterol ingested not exceed 300 mg per day, the number of egg yolks should be kept to a minimum, totaling no more than three a week.

Uncooked and undercooked eggs have been known to cause salmonellosis. Therefore, it is advisable to avoid foods such as homemade mayonnaise or eggnog that may contain them. Commercial mayonnaise and eggnog products are safe to eat because they have been pasteurized. The consumer should be careful not to eat eggs with runny yolks or to buy eggs that are cracked or dirty.

Eggs are graded according to size and quality. Large eggs usually cost more per dozen than small, but size has nothing to do with quality. Shell color depends on the hen and has no effect on quality. Brown and white shelled eggs are equally nutritious. When an egg is fresh, it sinks in water; an old egg floats because air has seeped into the shell. Good quality fresh eggs have a thick white that stays together. The whites of eggs that are old or of poor quality are thin and runny.

Grade AA and A eggs are excellent and are recommended when eggs are to be fried, poached, or served whole in some manner. Grade B eggs are seldom available at retail level because they are typically dried or frozen. If available, they are acceptable for combining with other foods. Because their yolks break easily, Grade B eggs are not recommended for use when the whites and yolks must be separated.

Eggs should be stored in their cartons with the small end down because this keeps the air cell at the rounded end and prevents the yolk from slipping out of place. They should be refrigerated until used unless they are to be used in cakes. Because they blend better with other cake ingredients if they are at room temperature, they should be removed from the refrigerator about an hour before the cake is made.

Eggs are a favorite breakfast, lunch, or supper dish and can be prepared in many different ways. They are used in sandwiches, salads, desserts, and baked products. Eggs, like most protein foods, become tough when cooked at high temperatures. They should never be boiled—only simmered.

VEGETABLES

There is a large variety of fresh vegetables available year round in supermarkets today. Most are low in kcal and are good sources of vitamins and the minerals calcium, iron, and potassium, as well as carbohydrates and dietary fiber.

Most vegetables are sold according to grades at the wholesale markets, but few are marked for sale by grade in retail stores. Consequently, it is helpful to be able to recognize good quality fresh vegetables, Table 26-5. Vegetables should be firm, ripe, without **blemish** (bruise spots) and a good, bright color.

Although fresh vegetables are the most nutritious, canned and frozen varieties can be good

Table 26-5 Guide to Purchasing Fresh Vegetables	
Vegetable	**Characteristics of Freshness**
Asparagus	Firm stalks, deep green color
Broccoli	Deep green color; compact, green buds; firm stalks
Carrots	Deep orange color; firm
Cauliflower	White clusters; green leaves
Celery	Crisp stalks; smooth stalks
Corn	Green husks; smooth silk
Greenbeans	Bright green color; firm
Mushrooms	Cream colored; no brown spots
Peppers	Bright color; heavy size; no transparent spots
Potatoes	Firm, smooth skin; no eyes
Spinach	Dark green color; no slime
Tomatoes	Heavy for size; firm; bright red color

substitutes for fresh. Nutrients are better preserved in the frozen than in the canned varieties because some of the minerals and water-soluble vitamins tend to **leach** (separate) into the water in canned vegetables.

Fresh vegetables should be stored in a cool, dry place. Before cooking, they should be carefully washed and, when possible, scrubbed with a vegetable brush.

Fresh vegetables retain most of their nutrients when cooked in their skins for short amounts of time in a small amount of water. Steaming, microwaving, and **stir-frying** (fast cooking at high heat with a small amount of fat added) are recommended methods of cooking vegetables.

FRUITS

Fruit is the fleshy part surrounding the seeds of plants. Fruits are low in kcal and sodium and high in carbohydrates, dietary fiber, vitamins, potassium, and water. Because of the fiber, water,

and fruit acids they contain, they have a laxative effect and are useful in overcoming constipation, figure 26-6.

Fresh fruit should be purchased in amounts that will be eaten within one week. Good fruit should have rich, strong color; firm, smooth skin; heavy weight in relation to its size (this is an indication of juiciness); blemish-free skin; and an absence of mold. (See Table 26-6.) Except for bananas, fruits generally keep best in the refrigerator.

If fruit is to be cooked, it must be done very gently and just until tender. Sugar added at the beginning of the cooking period preserves shape while sugar added later improves flavor.

BREADS AND CEREALS

Cereals are the seeds of grains. As stated previously, these seeds consist of three main parts. The bran contains vitamins, minerals, proteins, and fiber. The endosperm is largely starch,

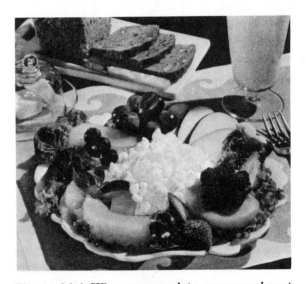

Figure 26-6 When appropriate accompaniment dishes are chosen from the Four Food Groups, a fruit salad may be served as the main course for lunch. *(Courtesy of the National Dairy Council)*

Table 26-6 Guide to Purchasing Good Quality Fresh Fruit

Product	Look For	Avoid
Apples	Firm; well-colored	Soft, mealy flesh, bruised areas
Bananas	Solid yellow skin speckled with yellow	Bruised, soft
Grapes	Plump; firmly attached to stems	Soft; wrinkled grapes
Oranges	Firm and heavy; bright and reasonably smooth skin	Light weight or spongy texture
Cantaloupe	Pale yellow skin; pleasant odor; yields slightly to thumb pressure	Soft rind; mold growth; overly yellow skin color

which is ground and used for flour in various baked products. The germ contains the B vitamins and protein. During **milling** (grinding into flour) some of these vitamins and minerals are lost. Manufacturers restore them to their original nutrient value by adding these same nutrients in synthetic form. After this process, they are known as restored cereals. When these nutrients are added in amounts greater than the grain originally contained, the cereal is called enriched or fortified.

Because cereals are easy to grow, transport, and store, they are inexpensive and popular. Although cereals are easily digested, cooking increases their digestibility. Breakfast cereals, rice, macaroni products, cornmeal, and various flours are the most familiar forms of cereals. Airtight containers preserve their freshness. Soybean flour, because of its fat content, should be stored airtight in a cool, dry place to prevent it from becoming rancid.

Essentially, bread is made from flour, water, and yeast,with sugar, fat, and flavorings added at the discretion of the baker. It is available in countless shapes and flavors. It must be kept airtight to preserve freshness, and may be frozen for long storage. For best nutritional value, it is wise to select whole grain products, the labels of which indicate that the products provide substan-

tial amounts of dietary fiber as well as vitamins and minerals.

BEVERAGES

Beverages are fluids that relieve thirst and provide nourishment. Water is the base of most beverages and is necessary to regulate body processes. Concentrations of 100 percent vegetable and fruit juices are refreshing and provide vitamins, especially vitamin C, potassium, carbohydrates, and water.

Labels should say *100% pure juice, 100% fruit juice blends,* or *100% juice from concentrate.* Fruit juice *drinks* and carbonated beverages can contain less than 5 percent juice and usually provide empty calories and artificial colors and flavors.

Coffee and tea have no food value other than what is present in the added milk, cream, or sugar. People who consume large amounts of the **stimulant caffeine** can experience **insomnia** (difficulty sleeping), irregular heartbeat, diarrhea, headaches, trembling, and nervousness. Children are more vulnerable to caffeine-related problems that makes coffee, tea, and caffeinated beverages (cola drinks, for example) inappropriate for them.

Decaffeinated coffee products have 95 percent or more of their caffeine removed. To preserve flavor, both coffee and tea should be stored tightly covered and coffee should be kept in a cool place.

SUMMARY

Meats are graded and cut to aid the consumer in selecting the level of quality desired. The choice of cut depends on the method of cooking to be used. Milk, which is available in many forms, is one of the most nutritious foods. Cheese is the curd that results from milk coagulation. Natural cheese has three basic forms—soft, semisoft, and hard. Eggs, like cheese, are a suitable meat alternate. Fruits and vegetables usually are most nutritious when eaten raw. If cooking is necessary, using only small amounts of water helps preserve nutritional quality. Breads and cereals are usually restored or enriched and are relatively inexpensive because they are easy to grow, transport, and store. Beverages are fluids necessary to regulate body processes.

Discussion Topics	
1.	Using the meat chart in this chapter, discuss which cuts of meat are tender and which are less tender.
2.	Which methods of cooking are advised for less tender cuts of meat? Why?
3.	How does the grade of eggs relate to their use in the menu? Describe 3 ways of using eggs in the diet.
4.	Discuss various means of including milk in the diet. Why is milk a wise purchase? Why must it be refrigerated?
5.	At what general temperature should meat, milk, eggs, and cheese usually be cooked? Why?
6.	What is a meat alternate? Name some and explain how they might be used in a menu.
7.	Discuss recommended methods of cooking vegetables.
8.	Discuss why fruits are sometimes cooked.
9.	Name 3 vegetables and list 3 characteristics of their freshness.
10.	Discuss the nutritional values of various beverages, especially fruit *drinks* and sodas. As a parent, could you advise your children to drink these beverages? Why?

Suggested Activities	
1.	Organize the class into groups and visit a local supermarket. Each group should make a survey of the various forms and prices of one of the groups of foods discussed in this chapter. Reports should be exchanged and filed for future use in meal preparation.
2.	Using other sources, prepare a report to the class on the diseases caused by bacteria that may be present in raw milk. Find out what precautions are taken by dairy farmers to prevent the contamination of milk.

3. Make an appointment and visit a meat market to observe meatcutters at work. Take notes and discuss the visit when you return to class.
4. Using Table A-5 in the Appendix and other sources, write a short report on meat. Include the following:
   nutritional value
   kcal content
   cholesterol content
   saturated fat content
   cost
   place in the menu
5. Find four recipes for baked products such as cookies or cakes that include no more than one egg. If possible, prepare one and bring it to class for evaluation.
6. Buy and taste a fresh vegetable that is new to you. Describe this experience to the class.

Review

A. Multiple choice. Select the *letter* that precedes the best answer.
1. Milk is an important beverage because it
   1. contains complete protein and calcium
   2. has been pasteurized to increase the amount of vitamin D
   3. contains phosphorus, vitamin A, and riboflavin
   4. contains a stimulant
   5. contains vitamin C and iron
      a) all   b) 1,3,4   c) 1,2,5   d) 1,3
2. The following forms of milk have had some of their natural nutrients removed
   1. homogenized milk
   2. pasteurized milk
   3. skim milk
   4. evaporated milk
   5. raw milk
      a) 1,2,3,4   b) 3,4   c) 2,3,5   d) all
3. Vegetables are essential to a well-balanced diet because they
   1. contain vitamins and minerals
   2. contain large amounts of fat
   3. are the only source of iron
   4. are good sources of dietary fiber
   5. are good sources of complete protein
      a) 1,4   b) 2,3,4   c) 3,4,5   d) all
4. Coffee should be
   1. stored in a cool place

    2. tightly covered for storage

    3. diluted by boiling for 2 minutes

    4. given to children only after the caffeine is removed

    5. added to meals for its food value

       a) 1,2,5   b) 1,2,4   c) 2,4,5   d) 1,2

5. Beverages

    1. help to regulate body processes

    2. provide nourishment

    3. relieve thirst

    4. provide the best source of fat

       a) all   b) 1,2,3   c) 2,3,4   d) 1,3,4

6. A specific cut of meat should be chosen according to its

    1. intended use

    2. protein content

    3. water content

    4. total carbohydrate content

       a) 1,2,4   b) 1   c) 1,4   d) 3,4

7. The best quality of meat

    1. is graded as *choice*

    2. is graded as *prime*

    3. contains more fat than other grades

    4. should never be cooked by dry heat methods

       a) all   b) 1,4   c) 2,3   d) 1,4

8. Less tender cuts of meat

    1. should be roasted or broiled

    2. are best braised or stewed

    3. are from the least used muscles of the animal

    4. are generally less expensive than tender cuts

       a) 1,3   b) 2,3,4   c) 2,4   d) 3

9. Salmonella bacteria

    1. can cause a food-borne illness called salmonellosis

    2. can be carried by fresh poultry

    3. cannot be spread by wooden cutting boards

    4. can be present in uncooked eggs

       a) 1   b) 1,3   c) 1,2,4   d) 3

10. Good quality fresh fruit generally

    1. provides a great deal of sodium

    2. can be stored in the refrigerator indefinitely

    3. should never be cooked

    4. provides dietary fiber and vitamins

       a) 1,3   b) 4   c) 2   d) all

B. Match the items in column I to the correct statement in column II.

Column I	Column II
_____ 1. coagulate	a. milk with fat removed
_____ 2. caffeine	b. person who buys and uses products
_____ 3. pasteurization	c. microorganism
_____ 4. skim milk	d. milk with 60% of water removed
_____ 5. evaporated milk	e. stimulant
_____ 6. bacteria	f. grinding into flour
_____ 7. consumer	g. natural cheese with additional moisture
_____ 8. milling	h. may be intentional or incidental
_____ 9. process cheese	i. thicken
_____ 10. dried milk	j. process of killing harmful bacteria in food
	k. with all water removed
	l. process of breaking up fat in milk

C. Briefly answer the following questions.
1. Why are coffee and tea not advisable for children?

2. How is milk pasteurized?

VOCABULARY

antioxidants
convenience food
daily values
dehydrated
descriptors
emulsifiers
federal Food, Drug, and
    Cosmetic Act
food additives
freeze-dried foods
GRAS list
generic brands
health food
humectants
imitation foods
impulsive shopper
incidental additives
intentional additives
irradiated foods
mandatory
natural foods
organic foods
season

CONSUMER CONCERNS AND TRENDS RELATING TO FOOD

OBJECTIVES

After studying this chapter, you should be able to
- Identify information commonly found on food labels
- Evaluate *organic*, *natural*, and *health* foods
- Describe reasons for and some types of food additives

The wise consumer knows the value of food is measured by its nutritional quality and not its price. Achieving a well-balanced diet does not depend on a large food budget. It does depend on a sound knowledge of nutrition. Despite this knowledge, the appropriate selection of food in today's high-tech world can be challenging.

There are countless varieties of foods available. They have been treated, prepared, and packaged in many different ways, and they carry widely diverging prices. Some are labeled *organic,* a few have been irradiated, others contain additives. The intelligent consumer will want to know the meaning of these and other terms. This chapter briefly covers some of them.

LAWS REGULATING THE UNITED STATES FOOD SUPPLY

There are numerous laws and agencies in the United States that help maintain the safety of the food supply and prevent misleading advertising of food products. The Food and Drugs Act of

1906 was the first "pure food law" in the United States. It was superceded in 1938 by the **federal Food, Drug, and Cosmetic Act.** This has since been amended several times, and additional laws regarding pure food have been passed as well. The federal Food, Drug,.and Cosmetic Act specifies that food must be pure, safe to eat, prepared under sanitary conditions, and honestly packaged and labeled. The Food and Drug Administration (FDA) was established as a result of this law.

The FDA is responsible for the safety of all foods except for meats and poultry. Meats and poultry are monitored by the United States Department of Agriculture (USDA). USDA inspectors examine meats and poultry sold for human consumption and the plants in which they are processed.

The Environmental Protection Agency (EPA) sets the safety standards for tap water in the United States, but the states must enforce them. The FDA regulates bottled water as well as that used in food processing.

The Federal Trade Commission (FTC) regulates advertising of food products.

LABELING

As a result of the passage by Congress of the Nutrition Labeling and Education Act (NLEA) in 1990, new nutrition labeling regulations will be **mandatory** (required) by May 1994 for nearly all processed foods. The new food labels will provide the consumer with more information on the nutrient contents of foods and how those nutrients affect health than current labels provide. Health claims allowed on labels will be limited and set by the FDA. Serving sizes will be determined by the FDA and not by the individual food processor. Descriptive terms used for foods will be **standardized** so that, for example, when a food is described as "low fat" it will mean that each serving contains 3 grams of fat or less.

New Label

The nutrition label will have a new format and will be called *Nutrition Facts,* figure 27-1. It will include required and voluntary information.

The items, with amounts per serving, that must be included on the food label are:

- total calories
- calories from fat
- total fat
- saturated fat
- cholesterol
- sodium
- total carbohydrates
- dietary fiber
- sugars
- protein
- vitamin A
- vitamin C
- calcium
- iron

The food processor can voluntarily include additional information on food products. If a health claim is made about the food or if the food is enriched or fortified with an optional nutrient, then nutrition information about those nutrients becomes required. The standardized serving size is based on amounts of the specified food commonly eaten, and it is given in both English and metric measurements.

Daily values on the label give the consumer the percentage per serving of each nutritional item listed, based on a daily diet of 2000 kcal. For example, Total Fat on figure 27-1 shows 13 g that represent 20 percent of the amount of fat someone on a 2000-kcal diet should have. (Nine kcal per gram times 13 grams equals 117 kcal.)

Nutrition Facts

Serving Size ½ cup (114g)

Servings Per Container 4

Amount Per Serving

Calories 260   Calories from Fat 120

	% Daily Value*
Total Fat 13g	**20%**
Saturated Fat 5g	**25%**
Cholesterol 30mg	**10%**
Sodium 660mg	**28%**
Total Carbohydrate 31g	**11%**
Dietary Fiber 0g	**0%**
Sugars 5g	
Protein 5g	

Vitamin A 4%	•	Vitamin C 2%	
Calcium 15%	•	Iron 4%	

*Percent Daily Values are based on a 2,000 calorie diet. Your daily values may be higher or lower depending on your calorie needs:

	Calories:	2,000	2,500
Total Fat	Less than	65g	80g
Sat Fat	Less than	20g	25g
Cholesterol	Less than	300mg	300mg
Sodium	Less than	2,400mg	2,400mg
Total Carbohydrate		300g	375g
Dietary Fiber		25g	30g

Calories per gram:
Fat 9 • Carbohydrate 4 • Protein 4

Figure 27-1 The New Food Label (*Source:* Federal Register, *Vol. 58, No. 3, Wednesday, January 6, 1993*)

The label also will show the *maximum* amount of a nutrient that should be eaten (for example, fat) or the *minimum* requirement for specified nutrients (for example, carbohydrates) based on a daily diet of 2000 kcal and another based on 2500 kcal. The items included here are the amounts of total fat, saturated fat, cholesterol, sodium, total carbohydrate, and fiber. In addition, the label lists the calories per gram for carbohydrates, proteins, and fats.

Health Claims

Because diet has been implicated as a factor in heart disease, stroke, and cancer, the following *health claims* relating a nutrient to a health-related condition will be allowed on labels. They are intended to help consumers both choose foods that are the most healthful for them and avoid being deceived by false advertisements on the label. The allowed claims are for the relationship between:

- Calcium and *osteoporosis*
- Sodium and *hypertension*
- Diets low in saturated fat and cholesterol and high in fruits, vegetables, and grains containing dietary fiber and *coronary heart disease*
- Diets low in fat and high in fruits and vegetables containing dietary fiber and the antioxidants, vitamins A and C and *cancer*
- Diets low in fat and high in fiber-containing grains, fruits, and vegetables and *cancer*

Terminology

Descriptors (terms used by manufacturers to describe products) found on the new food labels also have been standardized by the FDA. This will help the consumer select the most appropriate and healthful foods. The following are examples:

- *Low calorie* means 40 calories or less per serving.
- *Calorie free* means there are less than 5 calories per serving.
- *Low fat* means a food cannot have more than 3 g per serving or per 100 grams of the food.
- *Fat free* means a food contains less than 0.5 g of fat per serving.
- *Low saturated fat* means 1 g or less per serving.
- *Low cholesterol* means 20 mg or less per serving.
- *Cholesterol free* means less than 2 mg of cholesterol per serving.
- *No added sugar* means no sugar or sweeteners of any kind have been added at any time during the preparation and packaging. When such a term is used, the package must also state that it is not low calorie or calorie reduced (unless it actually is).
- *Low sodium* means less than 140 mg per serving.
- *Very low sodium* means less than 35 mg per serving.

Obviously, the information on food labels is useful to all consumers and especially to those who must select foods for therapeutic diets. Health care professionals should become thoroughly knowledgeable about the new labeling law. On request, many food manufacturers will provide the consumer with additional detailed information about their products.

PACKAGING

The sizes and styles of food packages purchased depend on several factors (see Table 27-1). The size of the family and its members' appetites are important considerations, as are the cooking methods to be used, and the time allowed for cooking. The storage space available also helps determine the size of the package to be purchased. If there is sufficient storage space and the food keeps well, large packages can be economical even for small families. When there is inadequate storage space, small packages may be more practical. One should select the size of the package needed according to its actual weight or volume. The consumer cannot depend on manufacturers' descriptions such as *jumbo, giant,* or *economy* size. All food containers should be checked for breaks or leaks in the packaging and, when appropriate, washed before storing.

CONVENIENCE FOODS

An extremely popular form of food today is the **convenience food** that requires little or no preparation. The term is used to describe cake, bread, and dessert mixes; instant puddings; brown-and-serve breads and pastries; frozen dinners, breads and desserts; and frozen or canned fruits, vegetables, meats, and fish.

Most of these products are good quality, and they do save kitchen work and thus time. In the case of single people, they may be economical as well because they reduce the waste that can occur with leftovers.

With the addition of a fresh vegetable and milk, the frozen dinner can provide a nutritionally balanced meal. Many, however, contain saturated fats, cholesterol, and a great deal of sodium. It may be wise to keep some of these products on hand for unexpected situations, but their use should be occasional and not regular.

Frozen Foods

It is advisable to buy frozen foods in packages that can be used at one time or in a type of package, usually a plastic bag, that allows the cook to remove only as much food as is needed for a meal. Frozen foods are sold according to

Table 27-1 Servings per Package or per Pound

Meat, poultry, and fish

The amount of meat, poultry, and fish to buy varies with the amount of bone, fat, and breading.

	Servings per pound[1]
MEAT	
Much bone or gristle	1 or 2
Medium amounts of bone	2 or 3
Little or no bone	3 or 4
POULTRY (READY-TO-COOK)	
Chicken	2 or 3
Turkey	2 or 3
Duck and goose	2
FISH	
Whole	1 or 2
Dressed or pan-dressed	2 or 3
Portions or steaks	3
Fillets	3 or 4

[1] Three ounces of cooked lean meat, poultry, or fish per serving.

CEREAL PRODUCTS

One serving of a cereal may vary from ½ cup to 1¼ cup. Check package labels.

	Servings per lb.
Flaked corn cereals	18–24
Other flaked cereals	21
Puffed cereals	32–38
Wheat cereals:	
Coarse	12
Fine	16–22
Oatmeal	13
Hominy grits	20
Macaroni, noodles	12
Rice	16
Spaghetti	13

Vegetables and fruits

For this table, a serving of vegetable is ½ cup cooked vegetable unless otherwise noted. A serving of fruit is ½ cup fruit; 1 medium apple, banana, peach, or pear; or 2 apricots or plums. A serving of cooked fresh or dried fruit is ½ cup fruit and liquid.

	Servings per pound[1]
FRESH VEGETABLES	
Asparagus	2 or 3
Beans, lima[2]	2
Beans, snap	5 or 6
Beets, diced[3]	3 or 4
Broccoli	3 or 4
Brussels sprouts	4
Cabbage:	
Raw, shredded	9 or 10
Cooked	4 or 5
Carrots:	
Raw, diced or shredded[3]	5 or 6
Cooked[3]	4
Cauliflower	3
Celery:	
Raw, chopped or diced	5 or 6
Cooked	4
Kale[4]	5 or 6
Okra	4 or 5
Onions, cooked	3 or 4
Parsnips[3]	4
Peas[2]	2
Potatoes	4
Spinach[5]	4
Squash, summer	3 or 4
Squash, winter	2 or 3
Sweetpotatoes	3 or 4
Tomatoes, raw, diced or sliced	4

[1] As purchased.
[2] Bought in pod.
[3] Bought without tops.
[4] Bought untrimmed.
[5] Bought prepackaged.

	Servings per package (9 or 10 oz.)
FROZEN VEGETABLES	
Asparagus	2 or 3
Beans, lima	3 or 4
Beans, snap	3 or 4
Broccoli	2 or 3
Brussels sprouts	3
Cauliflower	3
Corn, whole kernel	3
Kale	2 or 3
Peas	3
Spinach	2 or 3

	Servings per can (16 oz.)
CANNED VEGETABLES	
Most vegetables	3 or 4
Greens, such as kale or spinach	2 or 3

	Servings per pound
DRY VEGETABLES	
Dry beans	11
Dry peas, lentils	10 or 11

	Servings per market unit[1]
FRESH FRUIT	
Apples	
Bananas	
Peaches	3 or 4 per pound
Pears	
Plums	
Apricots	
Cherries, sweet	5 or 6 per pound
Grapes, seedless	
Blueberries	
Raspberries	4 or 5 per pint
Strawberries	5 or 6 per unit

[1] As purchased.

	Servings per package (10 or 12 oz.)
FROZEN FRUIT	
Blueberries	3 or 4
Peaches	2 or 3
Raspberries	2 or 3
Strawberries	2 or 3

	Servings per can (16 oz.)
CANNED FRUIT	
Served with liquid	4
Drained	2 or 3

	Servings per package (8 oz.)
DRIED FRUIT	
Apples	8
Apricots	6
Mixed fruits	5
Peaches	6
Pears	4
Prunes, unpitted	4 or 5

Source: USDA Home and Garden Bulletin No. 1.

weight, serving, or piece. The labels usually indicate the number of servings per package.

While frozen foods can be more expensive than fresh foods, they are sometimes more economical because they contain no waste and are always in season. Also, when they are fully-cooked foods that require only reheating, they are economical in terms of the cook's time. They do not spoil if stored properly and usually take little time to prepare.

Canned Foods

Because canned foods keep well, they are popular and especially useful to someone with limited refrigerator space. There are few foods that are not available in cans. Except for certain meats, canned foods are relatively inexpensive. They are sold in varying can sizes. Sometimes the weights of two different products in identical cans vary because of the different densities of the foods.

Freeze-Dried Foods

Freeze-dried foods are frozen so rapidly their flavors and textures are not noticeably changed. They are then **dehydrated** (have water removed). The consumer purchases them in small packages that may be kept for long periods of time without refrigeration. Directions for preparing freeze-dried foods usually include a specified period of time for soaking in a specified amount of liquid. By soaking, they regain their original moisture content and approach their original appearance. After soaking, they are cooked as if they were fresh foods.

SEASONAL FOODS

Shipping foods from distant locations is expensive and can increase the amount of food bills. For this reason, it is most economical to use foods that are in season. A food's **season** is the period it is normally ripe or ready, and thus, most flavorful and economical. Fruits, vegetables, and certain fish are seasonal. This should be considered when planning menus. When a desired food is not locally in season, canned and frozen foods may be more economical than the fresh.

GENERIC BRANDS

Most large supermarkets have many **generic brands** available. These items do not carry a manufacturer's name or quality grade—only their generic names as, for example, *Peas,* or *Peaches,* or *Napkins.* These items are less expensive than name brands but qualities vary. Where quality is not a concern, they are economical purchases and should not be overlooked.

ECONOMY IN PURCHASING

Economy is a major goal of the concerned shopper. Careful planning is the key to economical food purchasing. Consideration of the following factors should aid the consumer in planning economical food purchases.

Menu Planning

Careful menu planning is essential if one is to make economical food purchases. In addition, such planning saves time. Meals for the week should be planned at one time around the weekly specials advertised in local newspapers. Planning should also include the appropriate use of leftovers. The food marketing list should be made according to the weekly menu and based on the Food Guide Pyramid.

Intended Use

Foods should be selected according to their intended use. For example, less-expensive, small fruit is satisfactory for making peach jam, but if peaches are to be served whole or as halves, the larger, more attractive fruit should be purchased. Less tender cuts of meat are as nutritious and, when prepared appropriately, as appealing as tender cuts. However, the less tender cuts of meat require longer cooking times than the tender cuts. Large cuts of meat are often less expensive per pound than small cuts. Therefore, it is economical to buy large quantities if subsequent meals are planned around leftovers. Leftovers should be properly wrapped and frozen for future use. Sometimes a few portions can be separated from the whole before cooking. The extra portions can then be wrapped and frozen for future use.

Table 27-2 Common Cooking Substitutions

1 square chocolate (ounce)
  3 tablespoons cocoa plus 1 to 3 teaspoons fat

1 cup cake flour
  1 cup all-purpose flour less 2 tablespoons

1 tablespoon cornstarch
  2 tablespoons flour (for thickening)

$\frac{2}{3}$ teaspoon double-action type baking powder
  $\frac{1}{4}$ teaspoon baking soda plus $\frac{1}{2}$ teaspoon cream of tartar

1 cup fresh whole milk
  $\frac{1}{2}$ cup evaporated milk plus $\frac{1}{2}$ cup water
  or
  $\frac{1}{2}$ cup condensed milk plus $\frac{1}{2}$ cup water with reduction of sugar used
  or
  $\frac{1}{4}$ cup powdered whole milk plus 1 cup water
  or
  $\frac{1}{4}$ cup powdered skim milk plus 2 tablespoons butter plus 1 cup water

Substitutions

Cheaper foods can often be substituted for expensive foods without any loss in nutrition. Some examples include fortified margarine in place of butter, and dried milk instead of fresh milk. Such substitutions can substantially lower food costs. Recipes should be carefully checked and substitutions made whenever appropriate. Table 27-2 shows some common cooking substitutions.

Quantities Needed

A person should, of course, purchase only as much food as can be used or properly stored. Because fresh fruits, vegetables, meat, fish, poultry, fats, sugar, and many cereal products are sold according to weight, it is advisable to know the number of servings per pound that each of these foods will yield.

Selection of the Store or Market

The type of store or market can greatly affect the total cost of the food purchased. Typically, the large cash-and-carry supermarkets have lower prices and offer a wider selection of foods than the small neighborhood markets. Small stores sometimes charge higher prices because they are convenient and open more hours than the supermarket.

Large stores use a great deal of advertising that can ruin the budget of the **impulsive shopper** (one who buys because of a momentary desire). The prices of the "super-specials" displayed at prominent places in the markets should be carefully checked against the regular prices of the same article. The actual value of the special should be carefully evaluated by the consumer before the purchase.

FOOD ADDITIVES

Food additives are chemical substances added to food during its growth, processing, or packaging. While all additives are chemicals, it must be remembered that all foods are also chemicals.

There are two basic types of additives—the intentional additives, which are added to perform specific functions in the food; and the incidental additives, which are not intentionally added but that can be found in the foods as a result of some stage of production or packaging.

Intentional Additives

Many **intentional additives** are naturally occurring substances, including vitamin C, thiamin, riboflavin, calcium, and vitamin D. The intentional additives serve four basic purposes:

1. *Enrich nutrient content* by adding vitamins, minerals, or protein. Examples include the addition of vitamin D to milk, which is considered the major reason for the near elimination of rickets in the United States; the addition of the vitamins thiamin, niacin, and riboflavin, and the mineral iron to cereals and breads (it is the addition of niacin that is thought to have virtually eliminated pellagra from the U.S.); and the addition of iodine to salt, which has greatly reduced the incidence of goiter in the U.S.
2. *Preserve freshness and retard spoilage.* Examples include the addition of **humectants** to promote the retention of moisture (sorbitol, a carbohydrate derivative, is often used as a humectant); **antioxidants** to preserve color in fruit and prevent fats from becoming rancid (vitamins E and C are antioxidants); and nitrites that prevent the development of botulism in packaged meats. (Nitrites sometimes combine with amines to form nitrosamines that appear to be carcinogenic in experiments with animals. However, the ingestion of vitamin C at the same time a food containing nitrites is eaten inhibits nitrosamine formation.)
3. *Enhance appearance and texture.* Examples are coloring agents, flavorings, and bleaching agents used in wheat flour.
4. *Facilitate food processing.* Examples include stabilizers, **emulsifiers,** buffers, and thickeners that aid in the maintenance of foods' integrity.

Incidental Additives

Incidental additives are substances that may remain on foods as the result of farmers' use of fertilizers, pesticides, or growth hormones, or from food processing or packaging.

Safety of Additives

There is controversy about the addition of additives to foods. Some people want additives eliminated altogether on grounds that they may cause disease. The food industry maintains that without some additives, foods would not grow or keep as well as they now do and there would be an increase in food spoilage, which could increase food costs.

The FDA requires that the manufacturer provide proof of the safety of food additives before they are used. When such proof has been accepted by the FDA, the substance is added to its **GRAS list.** This is a list of substances *generally regarded as safe.* Even after a substance has been accepted on the GRAS list, its use is still limited. It cannot be used in amounts greater than 1 percent of the amount of the product that was shown to be safe.

Nevertheless, research is ongoing regarding additives, and occasionally the use of one or another is prohibited. Consumers are advised to follow news of controversial additives. When controversy about a particular additive is unresolved, it may be advisable to limit, but not necessarily eliminate, the use of a food product containing it.

ORGANIC, NATURAL, AND HEALTH FOODS

The terms organic, natural, and health food are of great interest today. In evaluating foods, it is advisable that the consumer understand what these terms mean. Actually, organic materials are chemical compounds of various sorts that contain the element carbon, in addition to other elements. *All food is organic.* Carbohydrates, fats, proteins, and vitamins all contain carbon; and minerals are found in foods containing carbon.

Organic foods by current definition are plants that have been grown without the addition of artificial fertilizers or pesticides, and animal foods from animals raised without treatments of antibiotics or hormones and prepared for market without the use of chemicals.

Natural foods are foods that have not been treated or processed in any way. They may or may not have been organically grown. Potatoes and apples are natural foods—provided they have not been waxed or irradiated.

Health food is a general term used to describe foods that some food faddists claim have large quantities of nutrients that prevent, treat, or cure certain diseases. Honey, blackstrap molasses, granola, and wheat germ are often said to be health foods. Honey is considered to be a health food by some because it contains B vitamins, iron, and calcium. It does contain these nutrients but only in traces. Considering the small amounts of honey that one can eat at one time, it does not seem to be a superior source of any nutrient.

Blackstrap molasses is an excellent source of calcium and iron if used in large amounts. However, because molasses is strong-flavored and sweet, the amounts used in the everyday diet would not provide any significant proportion of these nutrients. Some granola cereals provide fewer vitamins and minerals than well-known varieties of the restored or enriched cereals and, in addition, usually contain a great deal of sugar and coconut oil (saturated fat). Among cereals, wheat germ is a good source of protein. It is also a good source of vitamin E but, again, the amounts used are relatively small. Consequently, the nutrient intake from it is also small.

Health foods are frequently overrated regarding their nutrient content and their potential to prevent or cure disease. Many of these so-called health foods are good sources of certain nutrients, but most are nutritionally overrated and, if purchased in health food stores, they are generally overpriced.

Many foods grown or prepared traditionally are equally rich in nutrients. Product labels and prices should be compared before one product is deemed better than another. Most of the *organic, natural,* and *health* foods are no more nutritious, but are far more expensive, than traditional foods.

IMITATION FOODS

There is an ever-increasing number of **imitation (artificial) foods** available. Margarine, of course, has been in existence for many years. Others on, or soon to be on, grocers' shelves include nondairy creamers, imitation fruit juices, artificial sweeteners, imitation fats, meat analogs, and noncaloric flour. When a food is a frank imitation of a real food, this must be stated on its label.

Some of these products serve useful purposes. Margarine is an inexpensive substitute for butter, and contains considerably less saturated fat or cholesterol than butter. Nondairy creamers are convenient when there is no refrigeration. Imitation orange juice is a help to campers. Artificial sweeteners can be useful to diabetics, but millions of Americans are using and abusing these sweeteners. Their use as a sugar substitute for people who are not diabetic does not seem particularly wise. There is no certainty that their continued use will not ultimately cause health problems. They are overused because they are *no-cal* or *low cal*. The irony of the situation is that those-who-would-be-thin use these artificial sweeteners instead of sugar and subsequently eat other high-kcal, high-sugar foods so their daily kcal totals are not reduced at all. For this reason, artificial sweeteners do not appear to contribute to weight loss. Also, these artificial sweeteners cause headache, diarrhea, or nausea in some individuals.

The consumer must be vigilant about nutrient content of artificial foods. Just because the label states "imitation milk" does not necessarily mean the nutrient content of the imitation is the equal of the original. Also, as the number of these products grows, there is the danger that consumers will use them and not real food. This could not only result in nutrient deficiencies, but over time, large amounts of certain of these products in and of themselves could cause health problems.

FOOD IRRADIATION

Food irradiation is a controversial method of food preservation that has been under discussion for many years. In low doses, irradiation kills insects that tend to cause food spoilage or food-borne diseases such as trichinosis and sal-

Figure 27-2 The Irradiation Logo

monella. It can inhibit sprouting of potatoes and onions, and retard mold growth on fruits.

The FDA has approved its use on fruits, vegetables, grains, and spices, but **irradiated foods** must display the irradiation logo, figure 27-2. Some countries have approved its use for certain food products; other countries have banned it.

Irradiation breaks up molecules in the microbes and insects that cause disease and spoilage of food, and causes some breakdown of the processed food itself. Depending on the strength of the dosage, there are some chemical changes in fruits and vegetables treated. The vitamins and minerals may be reduced, and the color of green vegetables changed. These chemical changes can leave compounds that are health hazards. In addition, the use and transport of radioactive materials necessary for food irradiation create additional hazards.

In view of these facts and the knowledge that animal blood tests can determine infected pork, and cold temperatures preserve fresh fruits and vegetables well, the irradiation of food may not be in the best interests of public health.

SUMMARY

Nutritious food can be prepared on a small budget as well as on a large budget. Labels on packaged foods give contents and weight. Consumers who know how a food item will be used can select the appropriate type and size of the package as well as the level of quality needed. Planning menus around weekly specials, buying fresh foods in season, and making nutritionally equal substitutions can reduce food costs. Usually, the large supermarkets offer foods at lower prices than the small stores. Various convenience foods save time and energy, but frequently contain large amounts of sodium and saturated fats.

Food additives are useful, but remain controversial in terms of health. Organic, natural, and health foods are generally nutritionally overrated and overpriced. Some imitation foods can be useful, but consumers should be vigilant concerning their safety and nutrient contents. Food irradiation may not be in the best interests of the consumer.

Discussion Topics

1. Bring grocery advertisements from the newspaper to class.
   a. Compare the prices of the week's specials. Remember to consider the varying qualities of food.
   b. Discuss any new foods that are listed. Ask if anyone in the class has used them.
   c. Discuss the various ways in which one of the meats "on special" can be prepared.
   d. Discuss which foods, if any, are seasonal.
2. What are convenience foods? Name six. Discuss their advantages and disadvantages.
3. Discuss the information found on food packages and how it may or may not affect the purchase and use of some foods. Why is this particularly important to a diabetic patient? To a heart patient? What is nutrition labeling?
4. Discuss food irradiation, including potential benefits and risks.
5. Discuss *organic, health,* and *natural* foods. Are they nutritionally superior to other foods? Explain.
6. Has anyone in class used generic brands? If so, discuss their quality.
7. What is the FDA and what is its purpose?
8. Discuss the Federal Trade Commission's role in relation to food.
9. Discuss what a two-person family could do with a ten-pound loin of beef.
10. Why is it wise to base a shopping list on the Food Guide Pyramid?

Suggested Activities

1. Plan a week's menu for a family of four who have no special dietary needs. Assume the cost of the week's menu is $125.
   a. List some possible changes that would lower the cost, without lowering the nutritional value.
   b. Determine the amounts of food required for the menu. Refer to Table 27-1.

    c. Make a market list for this menu, organized according to the Food Guide Pyramid.

    d. Adapt this menu to suit a single person; to suit a middle-aged couple who have no children.

2. List the fresh fruits and vegetables available at a local supermarket this week. Have the instructor explain the unfamiliar ones. Compare their costs with the identical frozen products and with the canned products. Consider edible portions and waste.

3. List the information printed on the label of a canned food. Define the terms used.

4. Check the local supermarkets to see what freeze-dried foods are available. Buy one and prepare it according to package instructions. Compare it with the same frozen food in regard to flavor, appearance, preparation, and cost.

5. Visit a supermarket and determine the number of different preparations available for each of the following (frozen, fresh, canned, etc.): green peas, potatoes, corn, orange juice, bananas, rice, milk, shrimp, margarine, and yogurt. Evaluate ease of home preparation and cost of each.

6. Have a panel discussion entitled: "Food Additives; Their Advantages and Disadvantages."

7. Invite a microbiologist or chemist to speak to the class on irradiation of food and food additives.

8. Visit a supermarket, a green grocer, a specialty "gourmet" food shop, and a health food store. Compare prices of the same food, say apples or tomatoes or rice cakes.

9. Make a list of all the artificial foods available in the local supermarket. Buy one and evaluate it for taste, nutrient content, and kcal content.

Review

A. Multiple choice. Select the *letter* that precedes the best answer.

  1. The value of food is determined by its

    a. cost   c. ease in preparation

    b. nutritional quality   d. all of these

  2. A foundation of all good food purchasing plans is

    a. the Food Guide Pyramid

    b. nutritional labeling

    c. the federal Food, Drug, and Cosmetic Act

    d. quality grading

  3. A substitute for one cup of fresh milk is

    a. $\frac{1}{4}$ cup dried milk plus 1 cup water

    b. $\frac{1}{2}$ cup sweetened condensed milk plus $\frac{1}{2}$ cup water

    c. both a and b

    d. none of the above

4. The new food labeling regulations
   a. were determined by the FTC
   b. must include the number of kcal per serving
   c. were not determined by an agency of the federal government
   d. do not require the manufacturer to include the amount of cholesterol per serving
5. The size of the food package purchased depends on
   a. family size, appetites, and storage space
   b. its cost alone
   c. its purpose
   d. none of the above
6. It is advisable to plan meals for a period of
   a. one day   c. two weeks
   b. one week   d. one month
7. An example of a convenience food is
   a. frozen dinners   c. bagged coffee beans
   b. fresh picked vegetables   d. Grade AA eggs
8. Because of the NLEA of 1990, food labels
   a. can include no health claims
   b. can include a health claim relating calcium to heart disease
   c. can include a health claim relating fats to cancer
   d. can include health claims as determined by the food producer
9. The nutrition labeling regulations were issued by the
   a. Food and Drug Administration
   b. United States Department of Agriculture
   c. National Research Council
   d. Food and Nutrition Board
10. Organic foods are
    a. the same as natural foods
    b. only animal foods
    c. produced without the use of any chemicals
    d. all of the above

B. Complete the following sentences.
   1. The law requiring that food shipped from one state to another be uncontaminated, safe to eat, and prepared under sanitary conditions is the _____ .
   2. This same law requires that labels on food containers list total calories and calories from _____ .
   3. Health claims on labels relate nutrients to _____ .
   4. Foods that are easy to serve because they are partially prepared are called _____ .

5. Freeze-dried foods have the nutrient, _____ , removed.
6. A food's _____ is the period during which it is usually ripe and at its best.
7. Large cuts of meat usually cost _____ (less, more) per pound than small cuts.
8. A person who buys foods because of a momentary desire is a (an) _____ shopper.
9. A satisfactory substitute for butter is margarine which is _____ .
10. Humectants help to keep foods _____ .

C. Briefly answer the following questions.
   1. Name at least five considerations that help the consumer maintain a well-balanced diet on a low food budget.

   2. What factors determine the size and style of food package to be purchased?

   3. Why are frozen or canned foods sometimes more economical than fresh foods?

CHAPTER 28

Cooking Equipment

OBJECTIVES

After studying this chapter, you should be able to
- Identify frequently used cooking utensils
- Name three practices that can reduce accidents in the kitchen
- Explain how to smother a grease fire
- Describe the proper manual dishwashing procedure

Cooking can be complicated because it involves so many different tools and techniques. It is important to have a working knowledge of the basic **culinary** (relating to the kitchen or cookery) tools and their uses. After studying this chapter, the student should understand the safe and efficient use of standard kitchen equipment and be able to discuss the importance of a clean and well-organized kitchen.

SELECTION OF EQUIPMENT

Equipment is chosen for its **durability, efficiency,** ease with which it can be maintained, and price in relation to these considerations. The appropriate kitchen tools, utensils, and appliances must be available in order to measure, mix, bake, and cook the ingredients as recipes direct. (See figure 28-1 and Table 28-1.)

1. Strainer
2. Food Mill
3. Box Grater
4. Wire Whip
5. Knife Sharpening Steele
6. Sandwich Spreader
7. Meat Thermometer
8. Instant Read Thermometer
9. Rubber Spatula
10. Offset Spatula
11. Pastry Brush
12. Scoop

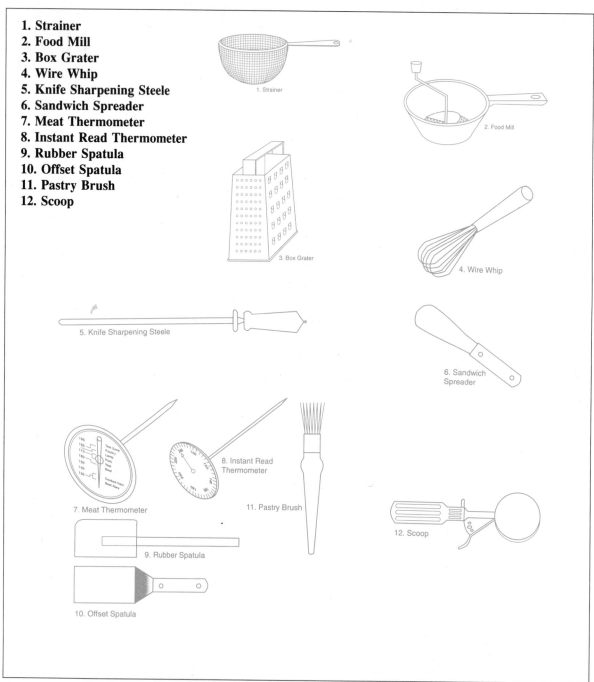

Figure 28-1 Cooking Tools and Equipment

13. **French Knife or Chef's Knife**
14. **Paring Knife**
15. **Boning Knife**
16. **Serrated Knife**
17. **Butcher Knife**
18. **Vegetable Peeler**
19. **Cutting Board**
20. **Saucepan**
21. **Saute Pan**
22. **Liquid Volume Measure**
23. **Nest of Dry Measure Cups**
24. **Measuring Spoons**
25. **Food Processor**

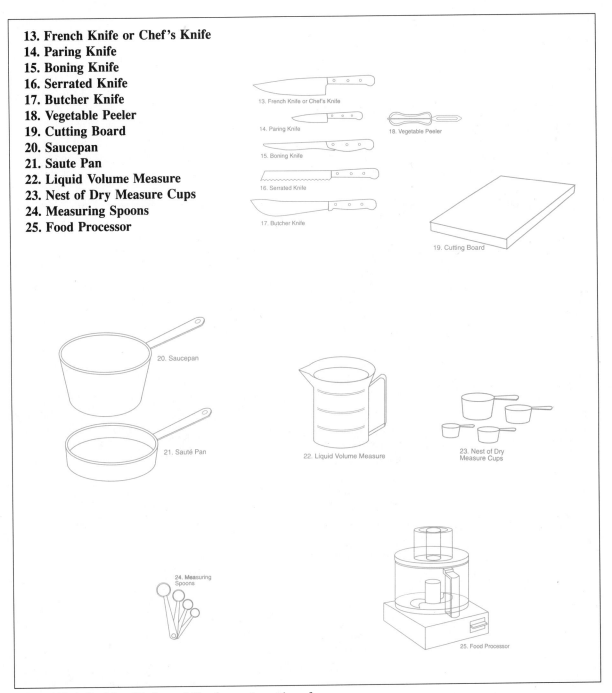

Figure 28-1 Cooking Tools and Equipment *continued*

Table 28-1 List of Essential Tools for Cooking

Item	Description	Function
Strainer	Round-bottomed made of screen type mesh or perforated metal	used for straining pasta or vegetables
Food mill	A tool that forces food through a perforated disc	used for pureeing foods
Box grater	A four-sided metal box with different-sized grids	used for shredding cheese and grating vegetables and citrus rinds
Wire whip	Loops of stainless steel wire	used for general mixing and beating
Knife sharpening steel	An essential part of the knife kit	used for maintaining knife edges
Sandwich spreader	A short spatula	used for spreading sandwich filling and spreads
Meat thermometer	Measures temperatures	indicates internal temperature of meat; left in while cooking
Instant read thermometer	Kept in a chef's jacket pocket	measures internal temperatures in a food product instantly
Rubber spatula	Broad flexible rubber spatula with long handle	used to scrape bowls or pans
Offset spatula	Broad metal blade, bent to keep hand off hot surfaces	used for turning and lifting eggs, pancake, and meats on griddles, grill
Pastry brush	Wooden handled brush w/ natural or synthetic bristles	used to brush food items with egg wash, glaze, etc.
Scoop	Scoops come in many standard sizes and have a lever for mechanical release	used for portioning ice-cream desserts and soft salad spreads
French or chef's knife	Most frequently used knife in the kitchen. Blade length usually 10″–12″	used for general purpose chopping, slicing, dicing, and so on
Paring knife	Small blade approx. 2″–2½″ long	used for trimming and paring vegetables and fruits
Boning knife	Thin blade of different flexibilities	used for boning meats and used for filleting fish
Serrated knife	Has jagged edge	for cutting bread
Butcher knife	Heavy, slightly curved blade	used for cutting and trimming raw meat
Vegetable peeler	Small tool with a swiveling blade	used for peeling vegetables & fruits
Cutting board	Cutting boards are made of wood or plastic to use as a cutting surface with knives	wooden or plastic boards used with knives as a preparation surface for chopping, slicing, or dicing

Table 28-1 (*Continued*)

Item	Description	Function
Saucepan	A small, shallow saucepot.	used for general rangetop cooking
Sauté pan	Slope sided fry pan	used for flipping and tossing of food
Liquid volume measure cups	Have lips for easy pouring	used for liquid measure; sizes are pints, quarts, half gallon and gallon
Dry measure cups (8 oz dry)	1 cup line at top of cup	measuring dry ingredients such as flours and sugars
Measuring spoons	Sets include 1 Tbsp, 1 tsp, $\frac{1}{2}$ tsp and $\frac{1}{4}$ tsp	measuring liquid or dry ingredients
Food processor	A small electric kitchen appliance with various sized blades	used for chopping, slicing, shredding and grating. A fast-work time saver

The use of larger equipment and appliances such as range tops, ovens, microwave ovens, broilers, grills, deep fat fryers, mixers, slicers, steamers, refrigerators, freezers, and dishwashers should be carefully explained and demonstrated by trained personnel. Gas, electric, and microwave cooking equipment have varying types of controls and require special instruction before being used. A reference file of **operating manuals** (books) for all large equipment should be available as part of a well-organized kitchen. Before using the large kitchen equipment, one should observe a demonstration of it and read the manufacturer's instructions carefully.

CLEANING EQUIPMENT AND DISHWASHING

Regular cleaning schedules are essential. Most modern kitchens have electric dishwashers that are used to clean and sanitize most small kitchen equipment. Dishwashers have heating elements or boosters that maintain temperatures at 180°F, the temperature required for fast drying and sanitizing. Items with baked-on food must be scraped, prerinsed, and soaked before being placed in the dishwasher. (See figure 28-2.)

Larger equipment is more complicated to clean and can be dangerous if handled by someone who is unfamiliar with it. It is essential that anyone attempting to clean a piece of large equipment consult an operating manual or trained personnel before beginning the job. Electric equipment must be unplugged before it is cleaned. One could be seriously injured if the equipment is not unplugged and the power button is accidently hit during cleaning.

Dishwashing also can be done **manually** (by hand). Because they cannot fit into the electric dishwasher, some large pieces of equipment must be washed by hand (and be **immersed** to sanitize, see Table 28-2).

The sink should be scoured regularly. Grease should not be poured down the drain as it will clog it. Tables and counter tops should be thoroughly washed with detergent and dried with clean cloths after each use. Storage spaces should

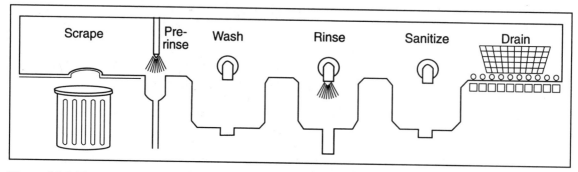

Figure 28-2 Three-compartment manual dishwashing sink

be kept orderly and clean. Practicing good **kitchen hygiene** helps prevent food poisoning and food-borne illness.

KITCHEN SAFETY

It is important to develop safe work habits to prevent accidents in the kitchen. Each year people are injured or killed as a result of careless kitchen habits. All of these incidents are labeled accidents, which means they probably could have been avoided.

Conveniently located fire extinguishers and first-aid kits are essential in every kitchen. Signs showing exits and others listing emergency tele-

phone numbers must be clearly written and posted in obvious places. Knives must be kept sharp and away from the dishwashing area. They should be stored in a safe place and out of the reach of children.

To prevent burns, pot handles must be turned inward on the stove so they do not extend into the aisle. Pot holders must be convenient (but away from the flame of the stove) and used to carry hot pans. Broken glass must be swept up and never picked up by hand. Water should *never* be used to extinguish electric or grease fires. These fires must be smothered with salt, baking soda, or a fire blanket. Water spreads a grease fire. Equipment should not be used by someone who does not understand its operation.

Spills on the floor must be cleaned up immediately to prevent someone from slipping and falling. Spills in the oven must be cleaned up (as soon as the oven is cool enough to do so) to prevent fire the next time the oven is used. Safe ladders and *not* chairs or boxes should be used if it is necessary to climb to reach equipment on high shelves. If it is necessary to move heavy objects or equipment, one should ask for help. A cart should be used to transport heavy objects. Most important, one should always use common sense in the kitchen. For one's own safety, it is important to begin today to develop good work habits.

Table 28-2 Manual Dishwashing

1. Scrape and prerinse. This keeps wash water clean.
2. Wash. Use good quality detergent and have water between 110°F and 120°F.
3. Rinse.
4. Sanitize. Immerse (dip) in hot water (170°F) for 30 seconds.
5. Drain or air dry. Do not use a towel to dry because towels can harbor and thus spread germs.

SUMMARY

Good planning is important in working efficiently in the kitchen. Kitchen equipment is chosen for durability, efficiency, and ease in cleaning. Knowledge of the proper use of equipment is essential in developing efficient kitchen skills. All equipment should be washed, dried, sanitized, and correctly stored after each use.

Discussion Topics

1. Explain why it is important to keep the kitchen clean.
2. Tell why it is especially important to keep school and hospital kitchens clean.
3. Describe the functions of two or three small kitchen utensils and describe why they are considered labor-saving tools.
4. Discuss the importance of proper dishwashing—both manual and automatic. Explain the sanitizing cycle in each.
5. Discuss the importance of a well-organized kitchen. Explain why emergency telephone numbers, fire extinguishers, and a first-aid kit should be available in the kitchen.

Suggested Activities

1. Visit a school, hospital, hotel, or restaurant kitchen and observe a demonstration of the use and care of kitchen equipment. Pay special attention to the dishwashing procedures used. Discuss this later in class.
2. Visit a local supermarket and make a list of the special cleaning products available for specific surfaces such as stainless steel, copper, silver, porcelain, wood, and enamel.
3. Give demonstrations of proper dishwashing, oven cleaning, refrigerator cleaning, and stove-top cleaning.
4. Visit a store that sells cooking equipment such as food processors, knives, saucepans, and fry pans. List the types available. Evaluate the equipment in terms of durability, labor-saving features, and cost.

Review

A. Briefly answer the following questions.
1. What factors should be considered when purchasing kitchen equipment?

2. Describe the five steps in manual dishwashing.

3. Why is it unwise to pour grease in the sink?

4. Why is it especially important to unplug electrical equipment before cleaning it?

5. Why should water *not* be put on a grease fire? What should be used?

6. Name three practices that can reduce accidents in the kitchen.

B. Identify the kitchen utensils sketched below.
   1.
   2.
   3.
   4.
   5.
   6.

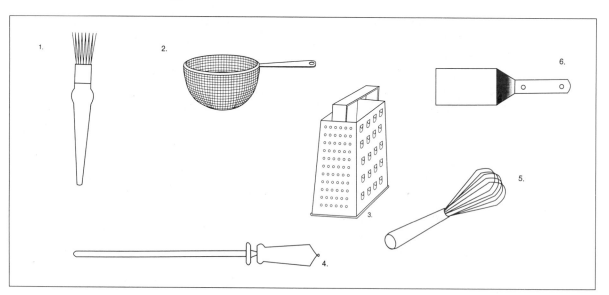

USING RECIPES

OBJECTIVES

After studying this chapter, you should be able to
- Define given cooking terms commonly used in recipes
- Demonstrate the techniques involved in various cooking procedures
- Measure and weigh foods accurately
- State metric equivalents of common household measures

COOKING TERMS

Standard recipes give specific amounts of ingredients and directions for combining them to produce satisfactory and predictable food products. Because the preparation of meals involves the use of recipes, it is important that the cook understand the terms commonly used.

After learning the meaning of cooking terms, the student should observe demonstrations of the techniques defined by these terms and practice them. It is always wise to use tested recipes to avoid disappointing results and waste.

A knowledge of the following terms should make following a recipe a rewarding task.

a la king: served in a white sauce with bits of green pepper and pimento. A common example is chicken a la king.

aspic: highly seasoned jelly made from broth, stock, or tomato juice. An example is tomato aspic.

au gratin: prepared in white sauce with cheese added. Potatoes au gratin are an example.

bake: to cook food by surrounding it with hot, dry air, as done in the oven. Baked bread or potatoes are examples.

barbecue: to cook over coals or wood, basting with spicy sauce, as is done with chicken or ribs, figure 29-1.

baste: to spoon fat over foods during cooking to prevent dryness and promote flavor. This is commonly done when roasting poultry.

beat: to incorporate air by mixing vigorously. Beaten egg whites for a souffle or angel cake are an example, figure 29-3.

blanch: to partially cook in boiling water and then plunge into cold water to stop the cooking. Used to loosen peels from tomatoes or peaches or nuts. Blanched almonds are an example.

blend: to combine ingredients thoroughly, as is done when combining ingredients for cakes and cookies.

boil: to cook in liquid at 100°C (212°F) as is indicated when bubbles break on the surface of the liquid, figure 29-1.

braise: to cook in a covered container with a small amount of liquid, usually after preliminary browning, as is done with less tender cuts of meat. Braised pot roast is an example.

broil: to cook under direct heat, as is done with tender meats and fish, figure 29-1.

casserole: a combination of foods providing a meal in one dish; the container is also called a casserole.

chop: to cut into small, irregular pieces, as is done with onions, celery, hard-cooked eggs, and nuts, figure 29-2.

combine: to mix together.

compote: fruit in syrup; also, the long-stemmed dish in which it may be served.

cream: to mix with beaters or the back of a spoon until mixture is pale, smooth, and creamy in consistency; done when mixing shortening and sugar for cakes and cookies.

croquette: food that has been pureed or finely chopped and combined with a thick sauce, formed into small shapes, breaded, and fried. An example is chicken croquettes.

cube: to dice or cut into small, regular squares, as may be done with cheese.

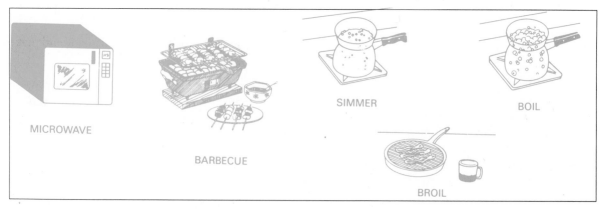

Figure 29-1 Various cooking methods

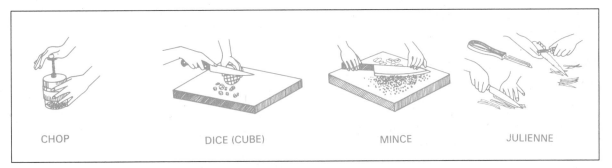

Figure 29-2 Cutting foods into smaller pieces is a process used in many types of cookery.

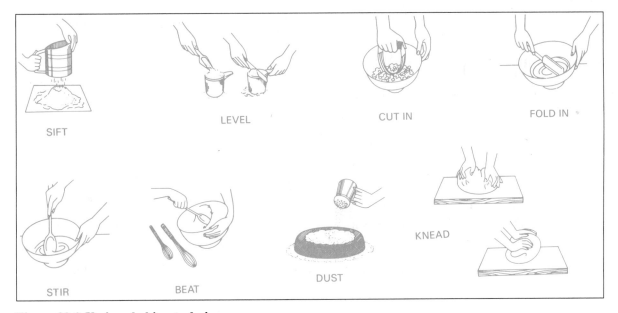

Figure 29-3 Various baking techniques

cut in: to blend shortening with flour using two knives or a pastry blender, figure 29-3.

deep fry: to cook submerged in hot fat. An example is deep fried (French fried) potatoes.

deglaze: to swirl a liquid in a cooking pan to dissolve cooked particles of food remaining on the bottom. The resulting mixture is added to a sauce or gravy for extra flavor.

deviled: highly seasoned. An example might be deviled eggs.

dice: to cube or cut into very small, regular squares, figure 29-2.

dredge: to coat heavily with flour, as is sometimes done before browning meat.

dust: to sprinkle lightly with flour or sugar, as may be done to the top of baked products, figure 29-3.

fillet or *filet:* a boneless tenderloin of meat or a boneless side of fish.

flake: to separate gently with a fork, as may be done to fish before serving.

fold: to blend very gently with a down, across, up and over motion to retain air in a mixture, as is done when combining heavy mixtures with light, whipped ingredients, figure 29-3.

fry: to cook in hot fat, as may be done with potatoes or chicken.

garnish: to trim or decorate food; also, the trimmings. Garnishes should harmonize in color, flavor, and shape with the dishes they decorate. Examples are parsley, egg slices, pickles, carrot curls, olives.

grate: to rub on a rough surface or box grater, producing small particles, as is done with onions, lemons, and oranges.

herbs: the leaves of certain plants used as flavoring. Examples are rosemary, thyme, chervil.

julienne: to cut into thin strips about $\frac{1}{8} \times \frac{1}{8} \times 2\frac{1}{2}''$, as may be done with carrots or meat used in salads, figure 29-2.

knead: to mix by folding and pressing, as in mixing yeast bread doughs, figure 29-3.

leavening agent: ingredient used to make mixtures rise during cooking. Examples include yeast and baking powder.

marinade: distinctive liquid in which some foods are kept for a specified time to alter their original flavors. Usually contains oil, onion, and vinegar, lemon, or wine.

marinate: to let stand in a marinade.

mince: to chop as finely as possible, as may be done with celery, onions, or parsley, figure 29-2.

mocha: combination of coffee and chocolate flavors.

panbroil: to cook uncovered in a saute pan or skillet without fat as done when cooking bacon.

parboil: to cook partially in a boiling or simmering liquid. See also *blanch.*

poach: to cook gently in liquid just below the boiling point, as may be done with eggs, fish, or chicken.

prove: to allow yeast dough to rise before baking.

puree: food that has been mashed or strained to a smooth pulp, or the process of making such a pulp by mashing or straining a food.

reduce: to boil rapidly so moisture is driven off and quantity is decreased; often done to concentrate flavors.

refresh: to immerse blanched vegetables in cold water or to hold them under cold tap water to prevent both further cooking in their own steam and loss of color.

roast: to cook foods by surrounding them with hot, dry air in an oven.

sauce: a flavorful liquid, usually thickened, used to season, flavor, and enhance other foods. An example is broccoli with mornay (cheese) sauce.

saute: to cook quickly in a small amount of fat.

scald: to bring a liquid just to the boiling point and immediately remove it from the heat, as may be done with milk.

score: to make shallow, even cuts on the surface; often done with ham that is to be baked.

sear: to brown the surface quickly at a high temperature, as is sometimes done with meat.

shred: to tear or cut into thin, irregular pieces by the coarse blade of a grater or with a knife. Examples are shredded lettuce or cabbage.

sift: to put dry ingredients through a sieve to remove lumps, as is done with flour, figure 29-3.

simmer: to cook in liquid just below the boiling point; indicated by tiny bubbles breaking just beneath the surface of the liquid, figure 29-1.

skewer: a metal or wooden pick for fastening foods, or to fasten foods with such a pick.

souffle: light, fluffy dish having eggs as the main ingredient. Examples are cheese and chocolate souffles.

steam: to cook in covered container over, but not touching, boiling water; often done with vegetables and shellfish.

steep: to let stand in hot liquid for a specified time, as is done with tea.

stew: to simmer a food or group of foods in a small amount of liquid that is usually served with the food as a sauce.

stock: clear, thin liquid, flavored by meat, fish, vegetables, bones, and seasonings.

sweat: to cook gently, usually in a fat, without browning.

temper: to raise the temperature of a cold mixture by slowly adding hot mixture.

timbale: finely chopped foods combined with eggs and baked in a mold. Examples are chicken timbales.

vinaigrette: dressing or sauce made with oil, vinegar, and flavoring ingredients.

wash: to brush or coat a food with a liquid such as egg wash (egg and milk) or milk, using a pastry brush.

whip: to beat rapidly, introducing air, as may be done to egg whites or heavy cream.

MEASURING AND WEIGHING INGREDIENTS

Accuracy in weighing and measuring ingredients is essential to prepare dishes that are consistent in quality and that fulfill the physician's orders when therapeutic diets are prescribed. A person must be familiar with the systems of weights and measures and know how to use the measuring devices and scales.

Systems of Measurement

The two systems of measurement commonly used are the English and the metric. The **English system** remains the most commonly used in the United States. The units of measurement within it originated in various cultures. It includes many different measuring units such as pints, quarts, and gallons, as well as inch, foot, and yard. It is important for the cook to know the units of measure frequently used in the kitchen, their equivalents, and their abbreviations. (See Table 29-1.)

The **metric system** is an international system of weights and measures based on the number ten. Because a power of ten is common to all its units, conversion within the metric system is simple.

In this system, the basic unit of weight or mass is the **gram.** Length is measured in **meters, volume** is measured in **liters,** and temperature is measured by degrees **Celsius** (instead of Fahrenheit as in the English system.)

Basic unit of *weight* is the *gram* (g)
Basic unit of *volume* is the *liter* (l)
Basic unit of *length* is the *meter* (m)
Temperature is measured in degrees
    Celsius (°C)

The metric units for weight, volume, and length all use the same **prefixes** (beginnings of words), which are based on the number ten. The reader should know the following prefixes and pronunciations:

kilo: (*key*–low) = 1,000
deci: (*dess*–ee) = 0.1 (1/10)
centi: (*sent*–ee) = 0.01 (1/100)
milli: (*mill*–ee) = 0.001 (1/1000)

Table 29-1 Units of Measure in the English System

Unit	Abbreviation	Equivalent
dash		less than $\frac{1}{8}$ teaspoon
few grains	f.g.	less than $\frac{1}{8}$ teaspoon
drop		—
15 drops		—
1 teaspoon	tsp	$\frac{1}{3}$ tablespoon
1 tablespoon	tbsp	3 teaspoons
1 fluid ounce	oz	2 tablespoons
1 cup	c	8 fluid ounces or 16 tablespoons
1 pint	pt	2 cups
1 quart	qt	2 pints or 4 cups
1 gallon	gal	4 quarts
1 peck	pk	2 gallons
1 bushel	bu	4 pecks
1 pound	lb	16 ounces

Table 29-2 Unit Relationships Within the Metric System

Weight	Volume
1000 grams = 1 *kilo*gram	1000 liters = 1 *kilo*liter*
100 grams = 1 *hecto*gram*	100 liters = 1 *hecto*liter*
10 grams = 1 *deka*gram*	10 liters = 1 *deka*liter*
1 gram	1 liter
.1 gram = 1 *deci*gram*	.1 liter = 1 *deci*liter*
.01 gram = 1 *centi*gram*	.01 liter = 1 *centi*liter*
.001 gram = 1 *milli*gram	.001 liter = 1 *milli*liter
.000001 gram = 1 *micro*gram*	.000001 liter = 1 *micro*liter*

*units not commonly used

Table 29-3   Converting from the English System to the Metric System

Convert to Metric	When You Know	Multiply By	To Find
Weight	ounces (oz)	28	grams (g)
	pounds (lb)	0.45	kilograms (kg)
Volume	teaspoons (tsp)	5	milliliters (ml)
	tablespoons (Tbsp)	15	milliliters
	fluid ounces (fl oz)	30	milliliters
	cups (c)	0.24	liters (1)
	pints (pt)	0.47	liters
	quarts (qt)	0.95	liters
	gallons (gal)	3.8	liters
	cubic feet (ft^3)	0.03	cubic meters (m^3)
	cubic yards (yd^3)	0.76	cubic meters
Temperature	Fahrenheit (°F) temperature	5/9 (after subtracting 32)	Celsius (°C) temperature

Source: Adapted from "Some References on Metric Information" by US Dept. of Commerce, National Bureau of Standards

Table 29-4   Converting from the Metric System to the English System

Convert to English	When You Know	Multiply By	To Find
Weight	grams (g)	0.035	ounces (oz)
	kilograms (kg)	2.2	pounds (lb)
	metric tons (1000 kg)	1.1	short tons
Volume	milliliters (ml)	0.03	fluid ounces (fl oz)
	liters (1)	2.1	pints (pt)
	liters	1.06	quarts (qt)
	liters	0.26	gallons (gal)
	cubic meters (m^3)	35	cubic feet (ft^3)
	cubic meters	1.3	cubic yards (yd^3)
Temperature	Celsius (°C) temperature	9/5 (then add 32)	Fahrenheit (°F) temperature

Source: Adapted from "Some References on Metric Information" by US Dept. of Commerce, National Bureau of Standards

Although the metric system is used in many parts of the world, the United States has been slow to accept it. Its use is increasing, however, and consumers will need to know how to use it. In this system, scales will be used to measure dry ingredients (flour and sugar) in grams and kilograms. Liquids will be measured by volume in liters and deciliters. Temperature will be measured in degrees Celsius.

Conversion is not difficult, but it requires practice. See Tables 29-1 through 29-5 for **equiv-**

Table 29-5 Equivalent Weights and Measures

Weight Equivalents

	Milligram	Gram	Kilogram	Grain	Ounce	Pound
1 microgram (μg)	0.001	0.000001				
1 milligram (mg)	1.0	0.001		0.0154		
1 gram (g)	1,000.0	1.0	0.001	15.4	0.035	0.0022
1 kilogram (kg)	1,000,000.0	1,000.0	1.0	15,400.0	35.2	2.2
1 grain (gr)	64.8	0.065		1.0		
1 ounce (oz)		28.3		437.5	1.0	0.063
1 pound (lb)		453.6	0.454		16.0	1.0

Volume Equivalents

	Cubic Millimeter	Cubic Centimeter	Liter	Fluid Ounce	Pint	Quart
1 cubic millimeter (mm³)	1.0	0.001				
1 cubic centimeter (cm³)	1,000.0	1.0	0.001			
1 liter (l)	1,000,000.0	1,000.0	1.0	33.8	2.1	1.06
1 fluid ounce (fl oz)		30.(29.57)	0.03	1.0		
1 pint (pt)		473.0	0.473	16.0	1.0	
1 quart (qt)		946.0	0.946	32.0	2.0	1.0

alents, unit abbreviations, and methods of conversion from one system to the other.

MEASURING DEVICES AND THEIR CORRECT USE

The measuring devices commonly available in the United States are still based on the English system. Measuring spoon sets include ¼ teaspoon, ½ teaspoon, 1 teaspoon, and 1 tablespoon. Measuring cups for solid and dry ingredients include ¼ cup, ⅓ cup, ½ cup, and 1 cup. To use these for dry ingredients, fill them gently, without shaking, and remove the excess with a flat spatula so ingredients are level across the top, figure 29-3. Shaking the measuring cup packs the dry ingredients and results in an excess of the ingredient.

When a solid ingredient such as shortening must be measured or when brown sugar is packed into a cup, air pockets should be pushed out with a slender knife. The substance is leveled by pressing down firmly and then cutting across the top of the cup with a flat spatula.

Liquids are measured in a cup that has marks indicating ¼ cup, ⅓ cup, ½ cup, ⅔ cup, ¾ cup, 1 cup, and sometimes 2 cups, figure 29-4. There is a spill area above the one-cup or two-cup mark and a pouring spout. To use the cup accurately, it must be on a level surface at eye level and the liquid being measured should come exactly to the line of measurement specified. This equipment is inexpensive and is available at most supermarkets or variety stores.

Most food scales measure weight in grams or ounces. It is helpful to remember that one ounce equals approximately 30 grams. Measuring foods and weighing them with the scales should be practiced until it can be done quickly and accurately, figure 29-5. Learning weights and measurements, their equivalents, and their abbreviations becomes easier with practice.

Weight and volume of food depend on its **density.** Therefore, two foods of equal weight may differ in volume. For example, one pound of butter equals 2 cups, but one pound of powdered sugar equals 3¾ cups. When the cook is compar-

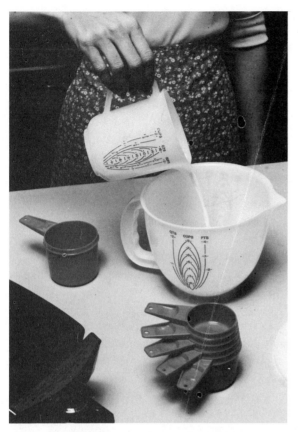

Figure 29-4 Measuring cups are useful in many sizes *(Courtesy of Tupperware)*

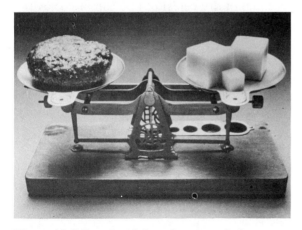

Figure 29-5 Equal weights of meat and cheese can best be determined on a scale. *(Courtesy of Tupperware)*

Table 29-6 Cooking Ingredients Compared in Weight and Volume

Breadcrumbs
4 ounces	¾ cup less 1 tablespoon
100 grams	½ cup

Currants and Raisins
1 pound	2⅜ cups
100 grams	½ cup plus 1 tablespoon

Nuts
4 ounces	⅔ cup, chopped
100 grams	½ cup plus 1 tablespoon (chopped)

Brown sugar
1 pound	2¼ cup
100 grams	½ cup plus 2 tablespoons

Granulated sugar
1 pound	2 cups
100 grams	½ cup less 1 tablespoon

Butter, margarine, solid fats and cheese
1 pound	2 cups
1 ounce	2 tablespoons
100 grams	7 tablespoons

Flour
1 pound	3½ to 4 cups
1 ounce	3 tablespoons
100 grams	¾ cup less 2 tablespoons

Rice, uncooked
1 pound	2 cups

Powdered sugar
1 pound	3¾ cups
100 grams	¾ cup

ing amounts of food, both weight and volume must be considered, Table 29-6.

SUMMARY

A thorough knowledge of the meanings of cooking terms and the ability to use them correctly is essential for efficient meal preparation. Using appropriate equipment correctly is also necessary in applying the techniques described.

Foods must be weighed and measured accurately to maintain quality in cooking and to conform to the physician's prescription when special diets are ordered. There are convenient devices for measuring and weighing foods. The student should be familiar with common weights and measures in both the English and metric systems.

Discussion Topics

1. Why is it important for a cook to know the meaning of cooking terms?
2. Why is it wise to use tested recipes rather than untried recipes?
3. Of what use are the words "serves two" in a recipe?
4. Name five foods frequently used as garnishes. What are some attractive garnishes suitable for egg salad?
5. Why are purees frequently included in hospital menus?
6. Name two ingredients that are frequently folded into other ingredients.
7. Why is it important to measure and weigh foods accurately at home? In the hospital kitchen?
8. Why are liquid measuring cups inappropriate for measuring dry ingredients and vice-versa?
9. Discuss the units of measurement in the English and those in the metric systems. Make comparisons of commonly used units in cooking.
10. Why are there $3\frac{1}{2}$ to 4 cups of flour in one pound, but only two cups of granulated sugar in one pound?
11. Which would weigh more, one cup of dry cereal or one cup of cooked cereal? Why?
12. What is the difference between:
    - fry and pan-broil?
    - dice and julienne?
    - scald and simmer
    - marinate and marinade?
    - mince and grate?
    - whip and fold?
13. Why is it advisable to read through a recipe before preparation?
14. Discuss familiar herbs and their uses.
15. Discuss leavening agents and their uses.

Suggested
Activities

1. Identify the cooking terms in the following recipe and explain them.

Egg Salad

3 eggs	Simmer the eggs 15 minutes. Cool and
1 tbsp grated onion	shell them. Chop the celery and grate
$\frac{1}{2}$ tsp salt	the onion. Cube the eggs and add the
$\frac{1}{4}$ tsp paprika	celery, mayonnaise, salt, paprika, and
$\frac{1}{4}$ c chopped celery	onion. Combine gently. Serve on
$\frac{1}{4}$ c mayonnaise	greens and garnish with tomato
	wedges. Serves two.

2. Organize two teams and have a "spell-down" on the cookery terms and their definitions.

3. Plan a menu that includes aspic, a dish a la king, and a compote. Use cookbooks for reference.

4. Plan a menu that includes a filet, a puree, and a souffle and list some medical conditions for which it would be appropriate.

5. Divide the class into groups and have each group demonstrate one or more of the cooking terms discussed in this chapter.

6. Browse through a cookbook and look for directions that include some of the following terms. Name the recipe in which each is found.

baste	cream	fold	sear
beat	cut in	marinate	sift
blend	deviled	simmer	steam
braise	dredge	saute	whip

7. Prepare a class cookbook composed of favorite recipes from students and teacher. Include sections on appetizers, soups, fish, poultry, meats, vegetables, breads, and desserts. Allow space for additions.

8. Observe demonstrations of measuring sugar, flour, and water. Practice measuring these items. Check each other for accuracy. After the use of scales has been demonstrated, practice weighing one cup each of flour, sugar, and water. Remember to subtract the weight of the measuring cup from the total weight to find the net weight of each item. Write a report of the experiment, listing the items from lightest to heaviest.

9. Weigh a piece of meat with bone before and after cooking. What percentage of the meat is waste? Weigh just the bone. What percentage of the meat was bone? What accounts for the remainder of the waste?

10. Prepare two ground beef patties of equal weight from the same package of ground meat. Fry one patty over medium-low heat until it is cooked through. Fry the second patty over high heat until it has a dark brown crust on the outside. Weigh each again. Is there a difference in the

weights of the two patties? If so, which cooking temperature resulted in the lighter-weight patty? Compare the palatability of the two patties.

Review

A. Briefly answer the following questions.
1.   How many teaspoons are there in one tablespoon?

2.   How many ounces are there in $\frac{1}{2}$ cup of water?

3.   How many cups are there in 1 pint?

4.   How many quarts are there in 1 gallon?

5.   How many cups are there in one gallon?

6.   How many cups are there in 1 pound of butter?

7.   How many cups are there in 1 pound of flour?

8.   How many cups are there in 5 pounds of granulated sugar?

9.   How many grams are there in 2 kilograms?

10.   How many grams are there in 3 ounces?

11.   How many quarts are there in 1 liter?

12.   How many pounds are there in 1 kilogram?

13.   How many grams are there in 1 pound?

14. How many kilograms are there in 4 pounds?

15. On what number is the metric system based?

B. Make the alterations indicated in the following measurements for a brownie recipe.

$\frac{1}{4}$ c butter   1 oz chocolate

1 c sugar $\frac{1}{4}$ c whole milk

1 tsp vanilla   1 c all-purpose flour

2 eggs   1 tsp salt

1. Double the recipe.

2. How many brownie recipes can be prepared from each of the following ingredients?

a. 1 lb of sugar   c. 1 qt of milk

b. 1 lb of butter   d. 1 doz eggs

C. Match the foods listed in column I with the cookery terms commonly used in preparing them, listed in column II. Some choices can be used more than once.

Column I	Column II
_____ 1. egg whites	a. sift
_____ 2. almonds	b. braise
_____ 3. pot roast	c. blanch
_____ 4. lemon rind	d. mince
_____ 5. sirloin steak	e. scald
_____ 6. cookies	f. puree
_____ 7. milk	g. grate
_____ 8. flour	h. whip
_____ 9. bread	i. poach
_____ 10. parsley	j. broil
	k. bake
	l. knead
	m. dice

D. Read the following recipe. In the space provided below the recipe, write definitions of the italicized cookery terms.

Braised Beef

5 pounds top round of beef
3 cups red wine
$\frac{1}{2}$ cup chopped onion
$\frac{1}{2}$ cup diced celery
1 tablespoon minced parsley
$\frac{1}{2}$ cup flour
3 tablespoons margarine
1 cup beef stock

Put the meat in a large bowl. (1) *Chop* the onions, (2) *dice* the celery, (3) *mince* the parsley, and (4) *combine* the vegetables. Place the vegetables on top of, and around the meat. Add the wine. Cover and (5) *marinate* in the refrigerator 24 hours. Discard the (6) *marinade*. Dry the meat and (7) *dredge* with the flour. Melt the margarine in a heavy skillet. Add meat and (8) *sear,* turning as the meat browns. Place the browned meat in a casserole with a tight-fitting cover. Add the (9) beef *stock*. Cover and (10) *braise* over low heat 3 hours or until tender. $1\frac{1}{4}$ hours before serving, add 12 medium white potatoes. Bring to a (11) *boil*. Reduce heat and (12) *simmer* 1 hour. Slice meat. Serve with the potatoes and buttered carrots (13) *julienne*. (14) *Garnish* with parsley.

1.   8.

2.   9.

3.   10.

4.   11.

5.   12.

6.   13.

7.   14.

APPENDIX

Table A-1 Food and Nutrition Board, National Academy of Sciences—National Research Council Recommended Dietary Allowances,[a] Revised 1989

Designed for the maintenance of good nutrition of practically all healthy people in the United States

Category	Age (years) or Condition	Weight[b] (kg)	Weight[b] (lb)	Height[b] (cm)	Height[b] (in)	Protein (g)	Fat-Soluble Vitamins — Vitamin A (µg RE)[c]	Vitamin D (µg)[d]	Vitamin E (mg α-TE)[e]	Vitamin K (µg)	Water-Soluble Vitamins — Vitamin C (mg)	Thiamin (mg)	Riboflavin (mg)	Niacin (mg NE)[f]	Vitamin B₆ (mg)	Folate (µg)	Vitamin B₁₂ (µg)	Minerals — Calcium (mg)	Phosphorus (mg)	Magnesium (mg)	Iron (mg)	Zinc (mg)	Iodine (µg)	Selenium (µg)
Infants	0.0–0.5	6	13	60	24	13	375	7.5	3	5	30	0.3	0.4	5	0.3	25	0.3	400	300	40	6	5	40	10
	0.5–1.0	9	20	71	28	14	375	10	4	10	35	0.4	0.5	6	0.6	35	0.5	600	500	60	10	5	50	15
Children	1–3	13	29	90	35	16	400	10	6	15	40	0.7	0.8	9	1.0	50	0.7	800	800	80	10	10	70	20
	4–6	20	44	112	44	24	500	10	7	20	45	0.9	1.1	12	1.1	75	1.0	800	800	120	10	10	90	20
	7–10	28	62	132	52	28	700	10	7	30	45	1.0	1.2	13	1.4	100	1.4	800	800	170	10	10	120	30
Males	11–14	45	99	157	62	45	1,000	10	10	45	50	1.3	1.5	17	1.7	150	2.0	1,200	1,200	270	12	15	150	40
	15–18	66	145	176	69	59	1,000	10	10	65	60	1.5	1.8	20	2.0	200	2.0	1,200	1,200	400	12	15	150	50
	19–24	72	160	177	70	58	1,000	10	10	70	60	1.5	1.7	19	2.0	200	2.0	1,200	1,200	350	10	15	150	70
	25–50	79	174	176	70	63	1,000	5	10	80	60	1.5	1.7	19	2.0	200	2.0	800	800	350	10	15	150	70
	51+	77	170	173	68	63	1,000	5	10	80	60	1.2	1.4	15	2.0	200	2.0	800	800	350	10	15	150	70
Females	11–14	46	101	157	62	46	800	10	8	45	50	1.1	1.3	15	1.4	150	2.0	1,200	1,200	280	15	12	150	45
	15–18	55	120	163	64	44	800	10	8	55	60	1.1	1.3	15	1.5	180	2.0	1,200	1,200	300	15	12	150	50
	19–24	58	128	164	65	46	800	10	8	60	60	1.1	1.3	15	1.6	180	2.0	1,200	1,200	280	15	12	150	55
	25–50	63	138	163	64	50	800	5	8	65	60	1.1	1.3	15	1.6	180	2.0	800	800	280	15	12	150	55
	51+	65	143	160	63	50	800	5	8	65	60	1.0	1.2	13	1.6	180	2.0	800	800	280	10	12	150	55
Pregnant						60	800	10	10	65	70	1.5	1.6	17	2.2	400	2.2	1,200	1,200	320	30	15	175	65
Lactating	1st 6 months					65	1,300	10	12	65	95	1.6	1.8	20	2.1	280	2.6	1,200	1,200	355	15	19	200	75
	2nd 6 months					62	1,200	10	11	65	90	1.6	1.7	20	2.1	260	2.6	1,200	1,200	340	15	16	200	75

[a] The allowances, expressed as average daily intakes over time, are intended to provide for individual variations among most normal persons as they live in the United States under usual environmental stresses. Diets should be based on a variety of common foods in order to provide other nutrients for which human requirements have been less well defined. See text for detailed discussion of allowances and of nutrients not tabulated.

[b] Weights and heights of Reference Adults are actual medians for the U.S. population of the designated age, as reported by NHANES II. The median weights and heights of those under 19 years of age were taken from Hamill et al. (1979) (see pages 16–17). The use of these figures does not imply that the height-to-weight ratios are ideal.

[c] Retinol equivalents. 1 retinol equivalent = 1 µg retinol or 6 µg β-carotene. See text for calculation of vitamin A activity of diets as retinol equivalents.

[d] As cholecalciferol. 10 µg cholecalciferol = 400 IU of vitamin D.

[e] α-Tocopherol equivalents. 1 mg d-α tocopherol = 1 α-TE. See text for variation in allowances and calculation of vitamin E activity of the diet as α-tocopherol equivalents.

[f] 1 NE (niacin equivalent) is equal to 1 mg of niacin or 60 mg of dietary tryptophan.

Table A-2 1983 Metropolitan Height and Weight Tables. Weights at ages 25–59 based on lowest mortality. Weight in pounds according to frame (in indoor clothing weighing 5 lbs. for men and 3 lbs. for women; shoes with 1″ heels).

Men					Women				
Height		Small Frame	Medium Frame	Large Frame	Height		Small Frame	Medium Frame	Large Frame
Feet	Inches				Feet	Inches			
5	2	128–134	131–141	138–150	4	10	102–111	109–121	118–131
5	3	130–136	133–143	140–153	4	11	103–113	111–123	120–134
5	4	132–138	135–145	142–156	5	0	104–115	113–126	122–137
5	5	134–140	137–148	144–160	5	1	106–118	115–129	125–140
5	6	136–142	139–151	146–164	5	2	108–121	118–132	128–143
5	7	138–145	142–154	149–168	5	3	111–124	121–135	131–147
5	8	140–148	145–157	152–172	5	4	114–127	124–138	134–151
5	9	142–151	148–160	155–176	5	5	117–130	127–141	137–155
5	10	144–154	151–163	158–180	5	6	120–133	130–144	140–159
5	11	146–157	154–166	161–184	5	7	123–136	133–147	143–163
6	0	149–160	157–170	164–188	5	8	126–139	136–150	146–167
6	1	152–164	160–174	168–192	5	9	129–142	139–153	149–170
6	2	155–168	164–178	172–197	5	10	132–145	142–156	152–173
6	3	158–172	167–182	176–202	5	11	135–148	145–159	155–176
6	4	162–176	171–187	181–207	6	0	138–151	148–162	158–179

Source: *Metropolitan Life Insurance Company* Source of basic data 1979 Build Study Society of Actuaries and Association of Life Insurance Medical Directors of America 1980.

Table A-3 Drug-Nutrient Interactions

Drug	Effect
Alcohol	Decreased absorption of thiamin, folic acid, and vitamin B_{12}; increased urinary excretion of magnesium and zinc
Analgesics	
Aspirin (salicylates)	Decreased serum folate level; increased excretion of vitamin C
Colchicine	Decreased absorption of vitamin B_{12}, carotene, fat, lactose, sodium, potassium, protein, and cholesterol
Amphetamines	Decreased appetite and caloric intake; possibly reduced growth
Antacids	
Aluminum hydroxide	Decreased absorption of phosphate
Other antacids	Decreased thiamin and fatty acid absorption
Anticonvulsants	
Barbiturates	Decreased vitamin B_{12} and thiamin absorption; increased excretion of vitamin C; deficiency of folate and vitamin D
Hydantoins	Decreased serum folate, vitamin B_{12}, pyridoxine, calcium, and vitamin D levels; increased excretion of vitamin C
Antidepressants	Increased appetite; weight gain
Antimetabolites	General absorptive decrease secondary to intestinal wall damage and oral mucus break-down; specific malabsorption of B_{12}, folate, fat, and xylose
Antimicrobials	
Chloramphenicol	Increased riboflavin, pyridoxine, and B_{12} requirements
Neomycin	Decreased absorption of fat; carbohydrate; protein; vitamin A, B_{12}, D, and E; calcium; iron; sugar; potassium; sodium, and nitrogen
Penicillin	Increased potassium excretion; inhibition of glutathione
Sulfonamides	Decreased synthesis of folic acid, vitamin K, and B vitamins
Tetracyclines	Decreased absorption of calcium, iron, magnesium, and fat; increased excretion of vitamin C, riboflavin, nitrogen, folic acid, and niacin; decreased vitamin K synthesis
Cathartics	Decreased absorption of calcium, vitamin D, potassium, protein, glucose, and fat
Chelating agents	Increased excretion of zinc, copper, and pyridoxine; depression of appetite
Corticosteroids	Decreased absorption of calcium, phosphorus, and iron; increased excretion of vitamin C, calcium, potassium, zinc, and nitrogen; decreased tolerance of glucose; increased triglyceride and cholesterol absorption; increased vitamin D metabolism; increased appetite
Diuretics	
Furosemide	Increased excretion of calcium, magnesium, and potassium
Mercurials	Increased excretion of thiamin, magnesium, calcium, and potassium
Thiazides	Increased excretion of potassium, magnesium, zinc, and riboflavin
Triamterence	Decreased serum folate and vitamin B_{12} levels
Hypocholesterolemic agent	
Cholestyramine	Decreased absorption of cholesterol; potassium; vitamins A, D, K, and B_{12}; folate, fat; glucose; and iron
Clofibrate	Decreased absorption of vitamin B_{12}, iron, glucose, potassium, and sodium; decreased taste acuity; aftertaste
Hypotensive agents	Increased excretion of pyridoxine
Laxatives	
Mineral oil	Decreased absorption of vitamins A, D, E, and K; calcium; and phosphate
Phenolphthalein	Increased excretion of potassium
Levodopa	Decreased absorption of amino acids; increased use of ascorbic acid and pyridoxine; increased excretion of sodium and potassium
Oral contraceptives	Decreased serum levels of vitamin C, vitamin B_{12}, folate, pyridoxine, riboflavin, magnesium, and zinc; increased absorption of iron; increased serum lipid levels; increased appetite
Potassium chloride	Decreased absorption of vitamin B_{12}
Sedatives	
Glutethimide	Increased metabolism of vitamin D
Sulfonamides	
Azulfidine	Decreased absorption of folate; decreased serum iron level
Other sulfonamides	Decreased synthesis of folate and vitamins B and K
Surfactants	Decreased absorption of fat
Tranquilizers	Increased appetite; weight gain

Source: Green, Marilyn L. and Harry, Joann. *Nutrition in Contemporary Nursing Practice,* Second Edition. New York; John Wiley & Sons, 1987.

Table A-4 Temperature Conversions from Fahrenheit to Celsius

°F	°C	°F	°C	°F	°C	°F	°C
70	21.1	117	47.2	160	71.1	197.6	92
71	21.7	118	47.8	161	71.7	198	92.2
72	22.2	119	48.3	161.6	72	199	92.8
73	22.8	120	48.9	162	72.2	199.4	93
74	23.3	121	49.4	163	72.8	200	93.3
75	23.9	122	50	163.4	73	201	93.9
76	24.4	123	50.6	164	73.3	201.2	94
77	25	124	51.1	165	73.9	202	94.4
78	25.6	125	51.7	165.2	74	203	95
79	26.1	126	52.2	166	74.4	204	95.6
80	26.7	127	52.8	167	75	204.8	96
81	27.2	128	53.3	168	75.6	205	96.1
82	27.8	129	53.9	168.8	76	206	96.7
83	28.3	129.2	54	169	76.1	206.6	97
84	28.9	130	54.4	170	76.7	207	97.2
85	29.4	131	55	170.6	77	208	97.8
86	30	132	55.6	171	77.2	208.4	98
87	30.6	132.8	56	172	77.8	209	98.3
88	31.1	133	56.1	172.4	78	210	98.9
89	31.7	134	56.7	173	78.3	211	99.4
90	32.2	135	57.2	174	78.9	212	100
91	32.8	136	57.8	174.2	79	213	100.6
92	33.3	136.4	58	175	79.4	214	101.1
93	33.9	137	58.3	176	80	215	101.7
94	34.4	138	58.9	177	80.6	215.6	102
95	35	139	59.4	177.8	81	216	102.2
96	35.6	140	60	178	81.1	217	102.8
96.8	36	141	60.6	179	81.7	218	103.3
97	36.1	141.8	61	179.6	82	219	103.9
98	36.7	142	61.1	180	82.2	219.2	104
98.6	37	143	61.7	181	82.8	220	104.4
99	37.2	144	62.2	181.4	83	221	105
100	37.8	145	62.8	182	83.3	225	107.2
100.4	38	145.4	63	183.2	84	230	110
101	38.3	146	63.3	184	84.4	235	112.8
102	38.9	147	63.9	185	85	239	115
102.2	39	147.2	64	186	85.6	240	115.6
103	39.4	148	64.4	186.8	86	245	118.3
104	40	149	65	187	86.1	248	120
105	40.6	150	65.6	188	86.7	250	121.1
105.8	41	150.8	66	188.6	87	255	123.9
106	41.1	151	66.1	189	87.2	257	125
107	41.7	152	66.7	190	87.8	260	126.7
107.6	42	152.6	67	190.4	88	265	129.4
108	42.2	153	67.2	191	88.3	266	130
109	42.8	154	67.8	192	88.9	270	132.2
110	43.3	154.4	68	192.2	89	275	135
111	43.9	155	68.3	193	89.4	280	137.8
112	44.4	156	68.9	194	90	284	140
113	45	156.2	69	195	90.6	285	140.6
114	45.6	157	69.4	195.8	91	290	143.3
115	46.1	158	70	196	91.1	295	146.1
116	46.7	159	70.6	197	91.7	300	148.9
116.6	47	159.8	71				

one day diet analysis

Table A-5 Nutritive Value of the Edible Part of Food

(Tr indicates nutrient present in trace amount.)

Item No.	Foods, approximate measures, units, and weight (weight of edible portion only)			Water	Food energy	Pro-tein	Fat	Fatty acids		
								Satu-rated	Mono-unsatu-rated	Poly-unsatu-rated
			Grams	Per-cent	Cal-ories	Grams	Grams	Grams	Grams	Grams
	Beverages									
	Alcoholic:									
	Beer:									
1	Regular-----------------------	12 fl oz--------	360	92	150	1	0	0.0	0.0	0.0
2	Light-------------------------	12 fl oz--------	355	95	95	1	0	0.0	0.0	0.0
	Gin, rum, vodka, whiskey:									
3	80-proof---------------------	1-1/2 fl oz-----	42	67	95	0	0	0.0	0.0	0.0
4	86-proof---------------------	1-1/2 fl oz-----	42	64	105	0	0	0.0	0.0	0.0
5	90-proof---------------------	1-1/2 fl oz-----	42	62	110	0	0	0.0	0.0	0.0
	Wines:									
6	Dessert----------------------	3-1/2 fl oz-----	103	77	140	Tr	0	0.0	0.0	0.0
	Table:									
7	Red-------------------------	3-1/2 fl oz-----	102	88	75	Tr	0	0.0	0.0	0.0
8	White-----------------------	3-1/2 fl oz-----	102	87	80	Tr	0	0.0	0.0	0.0
	Carbonated:[2]									
9	Club soda----------------------	12 fl oz--------	355	100	0	0	0	0.0	0.0	0.0
	Cola type:									
10	Regular----------------------	12 fl oz--------	369	89	160	0	0	0.0	0.0	0.0
11	Diet, artificially sweetened	12 fl oz--------	355	100	Tr	0	0	0.0	0.0	0.0
12	Ginger ale---------------------	12 fl oz--------	366	91	125	0	0	0.0	0.0	0.0
13	Grape-------------------------	12 fl oz--------	372	88	180	0	0	0.0	0.0	0.0
14	Lemon-lime--------------------	12 fl oz--------	372	89	155	0	0	0.0	0.0	0.0
15	Orange------------------------	12 fl oz--------	372	88	180	0	0	0.0	0.0	0.0
16	Pepper type-------------------	12 fl oz--------	369	89	160	0	0	0.0	0.0	0.0
17	Root beer---------------------	12 fl oz--------	370	89	165	0	0	0.0	0.0	0.0
	Cocoa and chocolate-flavored beverages. See Dairy Products (items 95-98).									
	Coffee:									
18	Brewed------------------------	6 fl oz---------	180	100	Tr	Tr	Tr	Tr	Tr	Tr
19	Instant, prepared (2 tsp powder plus 6 fl oz water)----------	6 fl oz---------	182	99	Tr	Tr	Tr	Tr	Tr	Tr
	Fruit drinks, noncarbonated:									
	Canned:									
20	Fruit punch drink------------	6 fl oz---------	190	88	85	Tr	0	0.0	0.0	0.0
21	Grape drink------------------	6 fl oz---------	187	86	100	Tr	0	0.0	0.0	0.0
22	Pineapple-grapefruit juice drink---------------------	6 fl oz---------	187	87	90	Tr	Tr	Tr	Tr	Tr
	Frozen:									
	Lemonade concentrate:									
23	Undiluted------------------	6-fl-oz can-----	219	49	425	Tr	Tr	Tr	Tr	Tr
24	Diluted with 4-1/3 parts water by volume----------	6 fl oz---------	185	89	80	Tr	Tr	Tr	Tr	Tr
	Limeade concentrate:									
25	Undiluted------------------	6-fl-oz can-----	218	50	410	Tr	Tr	Tr	Tr	Tr
26	Diluted with 4-1/3 parts water by volume----------	6 fl oz---------	185	89	75	Tr	Tr	Tr	Tr	Tr
	Fruit juices. See type under Fruits and Fruit Juices.									
	Milk beverages. See Dairy Products (items 92-105).									
	Tea:									
27	Brewed------------------------	8 fl oz---------	240	100	Tr	Tr	Tr	Tr	Tr	Tr
	Instant, powder, prepared:									
28	Unsweetened (1 tsp powder plus 8 fl oz water)--------	8 fl oz---------	241	100	Tr	Tr	Tr	Tr	Tr	Tr
29	Sweetened (3 tsp powder plus 8 fl oz water)-------------	8 fl oz---------	262	91	85	Tr	Tr	Tr	Tr	Tr

[1]Value not determined.
[2]Mineral content varies depending on water source.

Table A-5 Nutritive Value of the Edible Part of Food *(Continued)*

Nutrients in Indicated Quantity

Cho-les-terol	Carbo-hydrate	Calcium	Phos-phorus	Iron	Potas-sium	Sodium	Vitamin A value		Thiamin	Ribo-flavin	Niacin	Ascorbic acid	Item No
							(IU)	(RE)					
Milli-grams	Grams	Milli-grams	Milli-grams	Milli-grams	Milli-grams	Milli-grams	Inter-national units	Retinol equiva-lents	Milli-grams	Milli-grams	Milli-grams	Milli-grams	
0	13	14	50	0.1	115	18	0	0	0.02	0.09	1.8	0	1
0	5	14	43	0.1	64	11	0	0	0.03	0.11	1.4	0	2
0	Tr	Tr	Tr	Tr	1	Tr	0	0	Tr	Tr	Tr	0	3
0	Tr	Tr	Tr	Tr	1	Tr	0	0	Tr	Tr	Tr	0	4
0	Tr	Tr	Tr	Tr	1	Tr	0	0	Tr	Tr	Tr	0	5
0	8	8	9	0.2	95	9	(1)	(1)	0.01	0.02	0.2	0	6
0	3	8	18	0.4	113	5	(1)	(1)	0.00	0.03	0.1	0	7
0	3	9	14	0.3	83	5	(1)	(1)	0.00	0.01	0.1	0	8
0	0	18	0	Tr	0	78	0	0	0.00	0.00	0.0	0	9
0	41	11	52	0.2	7	18	0	0	0.00	0.00	0.0	0	10
0	Tr	14	39	0.2	7	[3]32	0	0	0.00	0.00	0.0	0	11
0	32	11	0	0.1	4	29	0	0	0.00	0.00	0.0	0	12
0	46	15	0	0.4	4	48	0	0	0.00	0.00	0.0	0	13
0	39	7	0	0.4	4	33	0	0	0.00	0.00	0.0	0	14
0	46	15	4	0.3	7	52	0	0	0.00	0.00	0.0	0	15
0	41	11	41	0.1	4	37	0	0	0.00	0.00	0.0	0	16
0	42	15	0	0.2	4	48	0	0	0.00	0.00	0.0	0	17
0	Tr	4	2	Tr	124	2	0	0	0.00	0.02	0.4	0	18
0	1	2	6	0.1	71	Tr	0	0	0.00	0.03	0.6	0	19
0	22	15	2	0.4	48	15	20	2	0.03	0.04	Tr	[4]61	20
0	26	2	2	0.3	9	11	Tr	Tr	0.01	0.01	Tr	[4]64	21
0	23	13	7	0.9	97	24	60	6	0.06	0.04	0.5	[4]110	22
0	112	9	13	0.4	153	4	40	4	0.04	0.07	0.7	66	23
0	21	2	2	0.1	30	1	10	1	0.01	0.02	0.2	13	24
0	108	11	13	0.2	129	Tr	Tr	Tr	0.02	0.02	0.2	26	25
0	20	2	2	Tr	24	Tr	Tr	Tr	Tr	Tr	Tr	4	26
0	Tr	0	2	Tr	36	1	0	0	0.00	0.03	Tr	0	27
0	1	1	4	Tr	61	1	0	0	0.00	0.02	0.1	0	28
0	22	1	3	Tr	49	Tr	0	0	0.00	0.04	0.1	0	29

[3]Blend of aspartame and saccharin; if only sodium saccharin is used, sodium is 75 mg; if only aspartame is used, sodium is 23 mg.
[4]With added ascorbic acid.

Table A-5 Nutritive Value of the Edible Part of Food *(Continued)*

(Tr indicates nutrient present in trace amount.)

Item No.	Foods, approximate measures, units, and weight (weight of edible portion only)		Water	Food energy	Pro-tein	Fat	Fatty acids Satu-rated	Mono-unsatu-rated	Poly-unsatu-rated
	Dairy Products	Grams	Per-cent	Cal-ories	Grams	Grams	Grams	Grams	Grams
	Butter. See Fats and Oils (items 128-130).								
	Cheese:								
	Natural:								
30	Blue------------------------ 1 oz------------	28	42	100	6	8	5.3	2.2	0.2
31	Camembert (3 wedges per 4-oz container)---------------- 1 wedge---------	38	52	115	8	9	5.8	2.7	0.3
	Cheddar:								
32	Cut pieces---------------- 1 oz------------	28	37	115	7	9	6.0	2.7	0.3
33	1 in³------------	17	37	70	4	6	3.6	1.6	0.2
34	Shredded----------------- 1 cup-----------	113	37	455	28	37	23.8	10.6	1.1
	Cottage (curd not pressed down):								
	Creamed (cottage cheese, 4% fat):								
35	Large curd--------------- 1 cup-----------	225	79	235	28	10	6.4	2.9	0.3
36	Small curd--------------- 1 cup-----------	210	79	215	26	9	6.0	2.7	0.3
37	With fruit-------------- 1 cup-----------	226	72	280	22	8	4.9	2.2	0.2
38	Lowfat (2%)-------------- 1 cup-----------	226	79	205	31	4	2.8	1.2	0.1
39	Uncreamed (cottage cheese dry curd, less than 1/2% fat)-------------------- 1 cup-----------	145	80	125	25	1	0.4	0.2	Tr
40	Cream----------------------- 1 oz------------	28	54	100	2	10	6.2	2.8	0.4
41	Feta----------------------- 1 oz------------	28	55	75	4	6	4.2	1.3	0.2
	Mozzarella, made with:								
42	Whole milk---------------- 1 oz------------	28	54	80	6	6	3.7	1.9	0.2
43	Part skim milk (low moisture)---------------- 1 oz------------	28	49	80	8	5	3.1	1.4	0.1
44	Muenster------------------- 1 oz------------	28	42	105	7	9	5.4	2.5	0.2
	Parmesan, grated:								
45	Cup, not pressed down------ 1 cup-----------	100	18	455	42	30	19.1	8.7	0.7
46	Tablespoon---------------- 1 tbsp----------	5	18	25	2	2	1.0	0.4	Tr
47	Ounce-------------------- 1 oz------------	28	18	130	12	9	5.4	2.5	0.2
48	Provolone------------------ 1 oz------------	28	41	100	7	8	4.8	2.1	0.2
	Ricotta, made with:								
49	Whole milk---------------- 1 cup-----------	246	72	430	28	32	20.4	8.9	0.9
50	Part skim milk------------ 1 cup-----------	246	74	340	28	19	12.1	5.7	0.6
51	Swiss---------------------- 1 oz------------	28	37	105	8	8	5.0	2.1	0.3
	Pasteurized process cheese:								
52	American------------------- 1 oz------------	28	39	105	6	9	5.6	2.5	0.3
53	Swiss---------------------- 1 oz------------	28	42	95	7	7	4.5	2.0	0.2
54	Pasteurized process cheese food, American ------------- 1 oz------------	28	43	95	6	7	4.4	2.0	0.2
55	Pasteurized process cheese spread, American------------- 1 oz------------	28	48	80	5	6	3.8	1.8	0.2
	Cream, sweet:								
56	Half-and-half (cream and milk) 1 cup-----------	242	81	315	7	28	17.3	8.0	1.0
57	1 tbsp----------	15	81	20	Tr	2	1.1	0.5	0.1
58	Light, coffee, or table-------- 1 cup-----------	240	74	470	6	46	28.8	13.4	1.7
59	1 tbsp----------	15	74	30	Tr	3	1.8	0.8	0.1
	Whipping, unwhipped (volume about double when whipped):								
60	Light---------------------- 1 cup-----------	239	64	700	5	74	46.2	21.7	2.1
61	1 tbsp----------	15	64	45	Tr	5	2.9	1.4	0.1
62	Heavy---------------------- 1 cup-----------	238	58	820	5	88	54.8	25.4	3.3
63	1 tbsp----------	15	58	50	Tr	6	3.5	1.6	0.2
64	Whipped topping, (pressurized) 1 cup-----------	60	61	155	2	13	8.3	3.9	0.5
65	1 tbsp----------	3	61	10	Tr	1	0.4	0.2	Tr
66	Cream, sour----------------- 1 cup-----------	230	71	495	7	48	30.0	13.9	1.8
67	1 tbsp----------	12	71	25	Tr	3	1.6	0.7	0.1

Table A-5 Nutritive Value of the Edible Part of Food (Continued)

Cho-les-terol	Carbo-hydrate	Calcium	Phos-phorus	Iron	Potas-sium	Sodium	Vitamin A value (IU)	(RE)	Thiamin	Ribo-flavin	Niacin	Ascorbic acid	Item No.
Milli-grams	Grams	Milli-grams	Milli-grams	Milli-grams	Milli-grams	Milli-grams	Inter-national units	Retinol equiva-lents	Milli-grams	Milli-grams	Milli-grams	Milli-grams	
21	1	150	110	0.1	73	396	200	65	0.01	0.11	0.3	0	30
27	Tr	147	132	0.1	71	320	350	96	0.01	0.19	0.2	0	31
30	Tr	204	145	0.2	28	176	300	86	0.01	0.11	Tr	0	32
18	Tr	123	87	0.1	17	105	180	52	Tr	0.06	Tr	0	33
119	1	815	579	0.8	111	701	1,200	342	0.03	0.42	0.1	0	34
34	6	135	297	0.3	190	911	370	108	0.05	0.37	0.3	Tr	35
31	6	126	277	0.3	177	850	340	101	0.04	0.34	0.3	Tr	36
25	30	108	236	0.2	151	915	280	81	0.04	0.29	0.2	Tr	37
19	8	155	340	0.4	217	918	160	45	0.05	0.42	0.3	Tr	38
10	3	46	151	0.3	47	19	40	12	0.04	0.21	0.2	0	39
31	1	23	30	0.3	34	84	400	124	Tr	0.06	Tr	0	40
25	1	140	96	0.2	18	316	130	36	0.04	0.24	0.3	0	41
22	1	147	105	0.1	19	106	220	68	Tr	0.07	Tr	0	42
15	1	207	149	0.1	27	150	180	54	0.01	0.10	Tr	0	43
27	Tr	203	133	0.1	38	178	320	90	Tr	0.09	Tr	0	44
79	4	1,376	807	1.0	107	1,861	700	173	0.05	0.39	0.3	0	45
4	Tr	69	40	Tr	5	93	40	9	Tr	0.02	Tr	0	46
22	1	390	229	0.3	30	528	200	49	0.01	0.11	0.1	0	47
20	1	214	141	0.1	39	248	230	75	0.01	0.09	Tr	0	48
124	7	509	389	0.9	257	207	1,210	330	0.03	0.48	0.3	0	49
76	13	669	449	1.1	307	307	1,060	278	0.05	0.46	0.2	0	50
26	1	272	171	Tr	31	74	240	72	0.01	0.10	Tr	0	51
27	Tr	174	211	0.1	46	406	340	82	0.01	0.10	Tr	0	52
24	1	219	216	0.2	61	388	230	65	Tr	0.08	Tr	0	53
18	2	163	130	0.2	79	337	260	62	0.01	0.13	Tr	0	54
16	2	159	202	0.1	69	381	220	54	0.01	0.12	Tr	0	55
89	10	254	230	0.2	314	98	1,050	259	0.08	0.36	0.2	2	56
6	1	16	14	Tr	19	6	70	16	0.01	0.02	Tr	Tr	57
159	9	231	192	0.1	292	95	1,730	437	0.08	0.36	0.1	2	58
10	1	14	12	Tr	18	6	110	27	Tr	0.02	Tr	Tr	59
265	7	166	146	0.1	231	82	2,690	705	0.06	0.30	0.1	1	60
17	Tr	10	9	Tr	15	5	170	44	Tr	0.02	Tr	Tr	61
326	7	154	149	0.1	179	89	3,500	1,002	0.05	0.26	0.1	1	62
21	Tr	10	9	Tr	11	6	220	63	Tr	0.02	Tr	Tr	63
46	7	61	54	Tr	88	78	550	124	0.02	0.04	Tr	0	64
2	Tr	3	3	Tr	4	4	30	6	Tr	Tr	Tr	0	65
102	10	268	195	0.1	331	123	1,820	448	0.08	0.34	0.2	2	66
5	1	14	10	Tr	17	6	90	23	Tr	0.02	Tr	Tr	67

Table A-5 Nutritive Value of the Edible Part of Food *(Continued)*

(Tr indicates nutrient present in trace amount.)

Item No.	Foods. approximate measures. units, and weight (weight of edible portion only)			Water	Food energy	Pro-tein	Fat	Fatty acids		
								Satu-rated	Mono-unsatu-rated	Poly-unsatu-rated
	Dairy Products—Con.		Grams	Per-cent	Cal-ories	Grams	Grams	Grams	Grams	Grams
	Cream products, imitation (made with vegetable fat):									
	Sweet:									
	Creamers:									
68	Liquid (frozen)	1 tbsp	15	77	20	Tr	1	1.4	Tr	Tr
69	Powdered	1 tsp	2	2	10	Tr	1	0.7	Tr	Tr
	Whipped topping:									
70	Frozen	1 cup	75	50	240	1	19	16.3	1.2	0.4
71		1 tbsp	4	50	15	Tr	1	0.9	0.1	Tr
	Powdered, made with whole									
72	milk	1 cup	80	67	150	3	10	8.5	0.7	0.2
73		1 tbsp	4	67	10	Tr	Tr	0.4	Tr	Tr
74	Pressurized	1 cup	70	60	185	1	16	13.2	1.3	0.2
75		1 tbsp	4	60	10	Tr	1	0.8	0.1	Tr
76	Sour dressing (filled cream type product, nonbutterfat)	1 cup	235	75	415	8	39	31.2	4.6	1.1
77		1 tbsp	12	75	20	Tr	2	1.6	0.2	0.1
	Ice cream. See Milk desserts, frozen (items 106-111).									
	Ice milk. See Milk desserts, frozen (items 112-114).									
	Milk:									
	Fluid:									
78	Whole (3.3% fat)	1 cup	244	88	150	8	8	5.1	2.4	0.3
	Lowfat (2%):									
79	No milk solids added	1 cup	244	89	120	8	5	2.9	1.4	0.2
80	Milk solids added, label claim less than 10 g of protein per cup	1 cup	245	89	125	9	5	2.9	1.4	0.2
	Lowfat (1%):									
81	No milk solids added	1 cup	244	90	100	8	3	1.6	0.7	0.1
82	Milk solids added, label claim less than 10 g of protein per cup	1 cup	245	90	105	9	2	1.5	0.7	0.1
	Nonfat (skim):									
83	No milk solids added	1 cup	245	91	85	8	Tr	0.3	0.1	Tr
84	Milk solids added, label claim less than 10 g of protein per cup	1 cup	245	90	90	9	1	0.4	0.2	Tr
85	Buttermilk	1 cup	245	90	100	8	2	1.3	0.6	0.1
	Canned:									
86	Condensed, sweetened	1 cup	306	27	980	24	27	16.8	7.4	1.0
	Evaporated:									
87	Whole milk	1 cup	252	74	340	17	19	11.6	5.9	0.6
88	Skim milk	1 cup	255	79	200	19	1	0.3	0.2	Tr
	Dried:									
89	Buttermilk	1 cup	120	3	465	41	7	4.3	2.0	0.3
	Nonfat, instantized:									
90	Envelope, 3.2 oz, net wt.[6]	1 envelope	91	4	325	32	1	0.4	0.2	Tr
91	Cup	1 cup	68	4	245	24	Tr	0.3	0.1	Tr
	Milk beverages:									
	Chocolate milk (commercial):									
92	Regular	1 cup	250	82	210	8	8	5.3	2.5	0.3
93	Lowfat (2%)	1 cup	250	84	180	8	5	3.1	1.5	0.2
94	Lowfat (1%)	1 cup	250	85	160	8	3	1.5	0.8	0.1

[5] Vitamin A value is largely from beta-carotene used for coloring.
[6] Yields 1 qt of fluid milk when reconstituted according to package directions.

Table A-5 Nutritive Value of the Edible Part of Food (Continued)

Cholesterol (Milligrams)	Carbohydrate (Grams)	Calcium (Milligrams)	Phosphorus (Milligrams)	Iron (Milligrams)	Potassium (Milligrams)	Sodium (Milligrams)	Vitamin A value (IU) (International units)	Vitamin A value (RE) (Retinol equivalents)	Thiamin (Milligrams)	Riboflavin (Milligrams)	Niacin (Milligrams)	Ascorbic acid (Milligrams)	Item No
0	2	1	10	Tr	29	12	[5]10	[5]1	0.00	0.00	0.0	0	68
0	1	Tr	8	Tr	16	4	Tr	Tr	0.00	Tr	0.0	0	69
0	17	5	6	0.1	14	19	[5]650	[5]65	0.00	0.00	0.0	0	70
0	1	Tr	Tr	Tr	1	1	[5]30	[5]3	0.00	0.00	0.0	0	71
8	13	72	69	Tr	121	53	[5]290	[5]39	0.02	0.09	Tr	1	72
Tr	1	4	3	Tr	6	3	[5]10	[5]2	Tr	Tr	Tr	Tr	73
0	11	4	13	Tr	13	43	[5]330	[5]33	0.00	0.00	0.0	0	74
0	1	Tr	1	Tr	1	2	[5]20	[5]2	0.00	0.00	0.0	0	75
13	11	266	205	0.1	380	113	20	5	0.09	0.38	0.2	2	76
1	1	14	10	Tr	19	6	Tr	Tr	Tr	0.02	Tr	Tr	77
33	11	291	228	0.1	370	120	310	76	0.09	0.40	0.2	2	78
18	12	297	232	0.1	377	122	500	139	0.10	0.40	0.2	2	79
18	12	313	245	0.1	397	128	500	140	0.10	0.42	0.2	2	80
10	12	300	235	0.1	381	123	500	144	0.10	0.41	0.2	2	81
10	12	313	245	0.1	397	128	500	145	0.10	0.42	0.2	2	82
4	12	302	247	0.1	406	126	500	149	0.09	0.34	0.2	2	83
5	12	316	255	0.1	418	130	500	149	0.10	0.43	0.2	2	84
9	12	285	219	0.1	371	257	80	20	0.08	0.38	0.1	2	85
104	166	868	775	0.6	1,136	389	1,000	248	0.28	1.27	0.6	8	86
74	25	657	510	0.5	764	267	610	136	0.12	0.80	0.5	5	87
9	29	738	497	0.7	845	293	1,000	298	0.11	0.79	0.4	3	88
83	59	1,421	1,119	0.4	1,910	621	260	65	0.47	1.89	1.1	7	89
17	47	1,120	896	0.3	1,552	499	[7]2,160	[7]646	0.38	1.59	0.8	5	90
12	35	837	670	0.2	1,160	373	[7]1,610	[7]483	0.28	1.19	0.6	4	91
31	26	280	251	0.6	417	149	300	73	0.09	0.41	0.3	2	92
17	26	284	254	0.6	422	151	500	143	0.09	0.41	0.3	2	93
7	26	287	256	0.6	425	152	500	148	0.10	0.42	0.3	2	94

[7]With added vitamin A.

Table A-5 Nutritive Value of the Edible Part of Food *(Continued)*

(Tr indicates nutrient present in trace amount.)

Item No.	Foods, approximate measures, units, and weight (weight of edible portion only)			Water	Food energy	Pro-tein	Fat	Fatty acids		
								Satu-rated	Mono-unsatu-rated	Poly-unsatu-rated
			Grams	Per-cent	Cal-ories	Grams	Grams	Grams	Grams	Grams
	Dairy Products—Con.									
	Milk beverages:									
	Cocoa and chocolate-flavored beverages:									
95	Powder containing nonfat dry milk	1 oz	28	1	100	3	1	0.6	0.3	Tr
96	Prepared (6 oz water plus 1 oz powder)	1 serving	206	86	100	3	1	0.6	0.3	Tr
97	Powder without nonfat dry milk	3/4 oz	21	1	75	1	1	0.3	0.2	Tr
98	Prepared (8 oz whole milk plus 3/4 oz powder)	1 serving	265	81	225	9	9	5.4	2.5	0.3
99	Eggnog (commercial)	1 cup	254	74	340	10	19	11.3	5.7	0.9
	Malted milk:									
	Chocolate:									
100	Powder	3/4 oz	21	2	85	1	1	0.5	0.3	0.1
101	Prepared (8 oz whole milk plus 3/4 oz powder)	1 serving	265	81	235	9	9	5.5	2.7	0.4
	Natural:									
102	Powder	3/4 oz	21	3	85	3	2	0.9	0.5	0.3
103	Prepared (8 oz whole milk plus 3/4 oz powder)	1 serving	265	81	235	11	10	6.0	2.9	0.6
	Shakes, thick:									
104	Chocolate	10-oz container	283	72	335	9	8	4.8	2.2	0.3
105	Vanilla	10-oz container	283	74	315	11	9	5.3	2.5	0.3
	Milk desserts, frozen:									
	Ice cream, vanilla:									
	Regular (about 11% fat):									
106	Hardened	1/2 gal	1,064	61	2,155	38	115	71.3	33.1	4.3
107		1 cup	133	61	270	5	14	8.9	4.1	0.5
108		3 fl oz	50	61	100	2	5	3.4	1.6	0.2
109	Soft serve (frozen custard)	1 cup	173	60	375	7	23	13.5	6.7	1.0
110	Rich (about 16% fat), hardened	1/2 gal	1,188	59	2,805	33	190	118.3	54.9	7.1
111		1 cup	148	59	350	4	24	14.7	6.8	0.9
	Ice milk, vanilla:									
112	Hardened (about 4% fat)	1/2 gal	1,048	69	1,470	41	45	28.1	13.0	1.7
113		1 cup	131	69	185	5	6	3.5	1.6	0.2
114	Soft serve (about 3% fat)	1 cup	175	70	225	8	5	2.9	1.3	0.2
115	Sherbet (about 2% fat)	1/2 gal	1,542	66	2,160	17	31	19.0	8.8	1.1
116		1 cup	193	66	270	2	4	2.4	1.1	0.1
	Yogurt:									
	With added milk solids:									
	Made with lowfat milk:									
117	Fruit-flavored[8]	8-oz container	227	74	230	10	2	1.6	0.7	0.1
118	Plain	8-oz container	227	85	145	12	4	2.3	1.0	0.1
119	Made with nonfat milk	8-oz container	227	85	125	13	Tr	0.3	0.1	Tr
	Without added milk solids:									
120	Made with whole milk	8-oz container	227	88	140	8	7	4.8	2.0	0.2
	Eggs									
	Eggs, large (24 oz per dozen):									
	Raw:									
121	Whole, without shell	1 egg	50	75	80	6	6	1.7	2.2	0.7
122	White	1 white	33	88	15	3	Tr	0.0	0.0	0.0
123	Yolk	1 yolk	17	49	65	3	6	1.7	2.2	0.7
	Cooked:									
124	Fried in butter	1 egg	46	68	95	6	7	2.7	2.7	0.8
125	Hard-cooked, shell removed	1 egg	50	75	80	6	6	1.7	2.2	0.7
126	Poached	1 egg	50	74	80	6	6	1.7	2.2	0.7
127	Scrambled (milk added) in butter. Also omelet	1 egg	64	73	110	7	8	3.2	2.9	0.8

[8]Carbohydrate content varies widely because of amount of sugar added and amount and solids content of added flavoring. Consult the label if more precise values for carbohydrate and calories are needed.

Table A-5 Nutritive Value of the Edible Part of Food (Continued)

Nutrients in Indicated Quantity

Cho-les-terol	Carbo-hydrate	Calcium	Phos-phorus	Iron	Potas-sium	Sodium	Vitamin A value (IU)	Vitamin A value (RE)	Thiamin	Ribo-flavin	Niacin	Ascorbic acid	Item No.
Milli-grams	Grams	Milli-grams	Milli-grams	Milli-grams	Milli-grams	Milli-grams	Inter-national units	Retinol equiva-lents	Milli-grams	Milli-grams	Milli-grams	Milli-grams	
1	22	90	88	0.3	223	139	Tr	Tr	0.03	0.17	0.2	Tr	95
1	22	90	88	0.3	223	139	Tr	Tr	0.03	0.17	0.2	Tr	96
0	19	7	26	0.7	136	56	Tr	Tr	Tr	0.03	0.1	Tr	97
33	30	298	254	0.9	508	176	310	76	0.10	0.43	0.3	3	98
149	34	330	278	0.5	420	138	890	203	0.09	0.48	0.3	4	99
1	18	13	37	0.4	130	49	20	5	0.04	0.04	0.4	0	100
34	29	304	265	0.5	500	168	330	80	0.14	0.43	0.7	2	101
4	15	56	79	0.2	159	96	70	17	0.11	0.14	1.1	0	102
37	27	347	307	0.3	529	215	380	93	0.20	0.54	1.3	2	103
30	60	374	357	0.9	634	314	240	59	0.13	0.63	0.4	0	104
33	50	413	326	0.3	517	270	320	79	0.08	0.55	0.4	0	105
476	254	1,406	1,075	1.0	2,052	929	4,340	1,064	0.42	2.63	1.1	6	106
59	32	176	134	0.1	257	116	540	133	0.05	0.33	0.1	1	107
22	12	66	51	Tr	96	44	200	50	0.02	0.12	0.1	Tr	108
153	38	236	199	0.4	338	153	790	199	0.08	0.45	0.2	1	109
703	256	1,213	927	0.8	1,771	868	7,200	1,758	0.36	2.27	0.9	5	110
88	32	151	115	0.1	221	108	900	219	0.04	0.28	0.1	1	111
146	232	1,409	1,035	1.5	2,117	836	1,710	419	0.61	2.78	0.9	6	112
18	29	176	129	0.2	265	105	210	52	0.08	0.35	0.1	1	113
13	38	274	202	0.3	412	163	175	44	0.12	0.54	0.2	1	114
113	469	827	594	2.5	1,585	706	1,480	308	0.26	0.71	1.0	31	115
14	59	103	74	0.3	198	88	190	39	0.03	0.09	0.1	4	116
10	43	345	271	0.2	442	133	100	25	0.08	0.40	0.2	1	117
14	16	415	326	0.2	531	159	150	36	0.10	0.49	0.3	2	118
4	17	452	355	0.2	579	174	20	5	0.11	0.53	0.3	2	119
29	11	274	215	0.1	351	105	280	68	0.07	0.32	0.2	1	120
274	1	28	90	1.0	65	69	260	78	0.04	0.15	Tr	0	121
0	Tr	4	4	Tr	45	50	0	0	Tr	0.09	Tr	0	122
272	Tr	26	86	0.9	15	8	310	94	0.04	0.07	Tr	0	123
278	1	29	91	1.1	66	162	320	94	0.04	0.14	Tr	0	124
274	1	28	90	1.0	65	69	260	78	0.04	0.14	Tr	0	125
273	1	28	90	1.0	65	146	260	78	0.03	0.13	Tr	0	126
282	2	54	109	1.0	97	176	350	102	0.04	0.18	Tr	Tr	127

Table A-5 Nutritive Value of the Edible Part of Food *(Continued)*

(Tr indicates nutrient present in trace amount.)

Item No.	Foods, approximate measures, units, and weight (weight of edible portion only)		Grams	Water Per-cent	Food energy Cal-ories	Pro-tein Grams	Fat Grams	Fatty acids Satu-rated Grams	Mono-unsatu-rated Grams	Poly-unsatu-rated Grams
	Fats and Oils									
	Butter (4 sticks per lb):									
128	Stick	1/2 cup	113	16	810	1	92	57.1	26.4	3.4
129	Tablespoon (1/8 stick)	1 tbsp	14	16	100	Tr	11	7.1	3.3	0.4
130	Pat (1 in square, 1/3 in high; 90 per lb)	1 pat	5	16	35	Tr	4	2.5	1.2	0.2
131	Fats, cooking (vegetable shortenings)	1 cup	205	0	1,810	0	205	51.3	91.2	53.5
132		1 tbsp	13	0	115	0	13	3.3	5.8	3.4
133	Lard	1 cup	205	0	1,850	0	205	80.4	92.5	23.0
134		1 tbsp	13	0	115	0	13	5.1	5.9	1.5
	Margarine:									
135	Imitation (about 40% fat), soft	8-oz container	227	58	785	1	88	17.5	35.6	31.3
136		1 tbsp	14	58	50	Tr	5	1.1	2.2	1.9
	Regular (about 80% fat): Hard (4 sticks per lb):									
137	Stick	1/2 cup	113	16	810	1	91	17.9	40.5	28.7
138	Tablespoon (1/8 stick)	1 tbsp	14	16	100	Tr	11	2.2	5.0	3.6
139	Pat (1 in square, 1/3 in high; 90 per lb)	1 pat	5	16	35	Tr	4	0.8	1.8	1.3
140	Soft	8-oz container	227	16	1,625	2	183	31.3	64.7	78.5
141		1 tbsp	14	16	100	Tr	11	1.9	4.0	4.8
	Spread (about 60% fat): Hard (4 sticks per lb):									
142	Stick	1/2 cup	113	37	610	1	69	15.9	29.4	20.5
143	Tablespoon (1/8 stick)	1 tbsp	14	37	75	Tr	9	2.0	3.6	2.5
144	Pat (1 in square, 1/3 in high; 90 per lb)	1 pat	5	37	25	Tr	3	0.7	1.3	0.9
145	Soft	8-oz container	227	37	1,225	1	138	29.1	71.5	31.3
146		1 tbsp	14	37	75	Tr	9	1.8	4.4	1.9
	Oils, salad or cooking:									
147	Corn	1 cup	218	0	1,925	0	218	27.7	52.8	128.0
148		1 tbsp	14	0	125	0	14	1.8	3.4	8.2
149	Olive	1 cup	216	0	1,910	0	216	29.2	159.2	18.1
150		1 tbsp	14	0	125	0	14	1.9	10.3	1.2
151	Peanut	1 cup	216	0	1,910	0	216	36.5	99.8	69.1
152		1 tbsp	14	0	125	0	14	2.4	6.5	4.5
153	Safflower	1 cup	218	0	1,925	0	218	19.8	26.4	162.4
154		1 tbsp	14	0	125	0	14	1.3	1.7	10.4
155	Soybean oil, hydrogenated (partially hardened)	1 cup	218	0	1,925	0	218	32.5	93.7	82.0
156		1 tbsp	14	0	125	0	14	2.1	6.0	5.3
157	Soybean-cottonseed oil blend, hydrogenated	1 cup	218	0	1,925	0	218	39.2	64.3	104.9
158		1 tbsp	14	0	125	0	14	2.5	4.1	6.7
159	Sunflower	1 cup	218	0	1,925	0	218	22.5	42.5	143.2
160		1 tbsp	14	0	125	0	14	1.4	2.7	9.2
	Salad dressings: Commercial:									
161	Blue cheese	1 tbsp	15	32	75	1	8	1.5	1.8	4.2
	French:									
162	Regular	1 tbsp	16	35	85	Tr	9	1.4	4.0	3.5
163	Low calorie	1 tbsp	16	75	25	Tr	2	0.2	0.3	1.0
	Italian:									
164	Regular	1 tbsp	15	34	80	Tr	9	1.3	3.7	3.2
165	Low calorie	1 tbsp	15	86	5	Tr	Tr	Tr	Tr	Tr
	Mayonnaise:									
166	Regular	1 tbsp	14	15	100	Tr	11	1.7	3.2	5.8
167	Imitation	1 tbsp	15	63	35	Tr	3	0.5	0.7	1.6
168	Mayonnaise type	1 tbsp	15	40	60	Tr	5	0.7	1.4	2.7
169	Tartar sauce	1 tbsp	14	34	75	Tr	8	1.2	2.6	3.9
	Thousand island:									
170	Regular	1 tbsp	16	46	60	Tr	6	1.0	1.3	3.2
171	Low calorie	1 tbsp	15	69	25	Tr	2	0.2	0.4	0.9

[9] For salted butter; unsalted butter contains 12 mg sodium per stick, 2 mg per tbsp, or 1 mg per pat.
[10] Values for vitamin A are year-round average.

Table A-5 Nutritive Value of the Edible Part of Food (Continued)

Nutrients in Indicated Quantity

| Cholesterol | Carbohydrate | Calcium | Phosphorus | Iron | Potassium | Sodium | Vitamin A value (IU) | Vitamin A value (RE) | Thiamin | Riboflavin | Niacin | Ascorbic acid | Item No. |
Milligrams	Grams	Milligrams	Milligrams	Milligrams	Milligrams	Milligrams	International units	Retinol equivalents	Milligrams	Milligrams	Milligrams	Milligrams	
247	Tr	27	26	0.2	29	[9]933	[10]3,460	[10]852	0.01	0.04	Tr	0	128
31	Tr	3	3	Tr	4	[9]116	[10]430	[10]106	Tr	Tr	Tr	0	129
11	Tr	1	1	Tr	1	[9]41	[10]150	[10]38	Tr	Tr	Tr	0	130
0	0	0	0	0.0	0	0	0	0	0.00	0.00	0.0	0	131
0	0	0	0	0.0	0	0	0	0	0.00	0.00	0.0	0	132
195	0	0	0	0.0	0	0	0	0	0.00	0.00	0.0	0	133
12	0	0	0	0.0	0	0	0	0	0.00	0.00	0.0	0	134
0	1	40	31	0.0	57	[11]2,178	[12]7,510	[12]2,254	0.01	0.05	Tr	Tr	135
0	Tr	2	2	0.0	4	[11]134	[12]460	[12]139	Tr	Tr	Tr	Tr	136
0	1	34	26	0.1	48	[11]1,066	[12]3,740	[12]1,122	0.01	0.04	Tr	Tr	137
0	Tr	4	3	Tr	6	[11]132	[12]460	[12]139	Tr	0.01	Tr	Tr	138
0	Tr	1	1	Tr	2	[11]47	[12]170	[12]50	Tr	Tr	Tr	Tr	139
0	1	60	46	0.0	86	[11]2,449	[12]7,510	[12]2,254	0.02	0.07	Tr	Tr	140
0	Tr	4	3	0.0	5	[11]151	[12]460	[12]139	Tr	Tr	Tr	Tr	141
0	0	24	18	0.0	34	[11]1,123	[12]3,740	[12]1,122	0.01	0.03	Tr	Tr	142
0	0	3	2	0.0	4	[11]139	[12]460	[12]139	Tr	Tr	Tr	Tr	143
0	0	1	1	0.0	1	[11]50	[12]170	[12]50	Tr	Tr	Tr	Tr	144
0	0	47	37	0.0	68	[11]2,256	[12]7,510	[12]2,254	0.02	0.06	Tr	Tr	145
0	0	3	2	0.0	4	[11]139	[12]460	[12]139	Tr	Tr	Tr	Tr	146
0	0	0	0	0.0	0	0	0	0	0.00	0.00	0.0	0	147
0	0	0	0	0.0	0	0	0	0	0.00	0.00	0.0	0	148
0	0	0	0	0.0	0	0	0	0	0.00	0.00	0.0	0	149
0	0	0	0	0.0	0	0	0	0	0.00	0.00	0.0	0	150
0	0	0	0	0.0	0	0	0	0	0.00	0.00	0.0	0	151
0	0	0	0	0.0	0	0	0	0	0.00	0.00	0.0	0	152
0	0	0	0	0.0	0	0	0	0	0.00	0.00	0.0	0	153
0	0	0	0	0.0	0	0	0	0	0.00	0.00	0.0	0	154
0	0	0	0	0.0	0	0	0	0	0.00	0.00	0.0	0	155
0	0	0	0	0.0	0	0	0	0	0.00	0.00	0.0	0	156
0	0	0	0	0.0	0	0	0	0	0.00	0.00	0.0	0	157
0	0	0	0	0.0	0	0	0	0	0.00	0.00	0.0	0	158
0	0	0	0	0.0	0	0	0	0	0.00	0.00	0.0	0	159
0	0	0	0	0.0	0	0	0	0	0.00	0.00	0.0	0	160
3	1	12	11	Tr	6	164	30	10	Tr	0.02	Tr	Tr	161
0	1	2	1	Tr	2	188	Tr	Tr	Tr	Tr	Tr	Tr	162
0	2	6	5	Tr	3	306	Tr	Tr	Tr	Tr	Tr	Tr	163
0	1	1	1	Tr	5	162	30	3	Tr	Tr	Tr	Tr	164
0	2	1	1	Tr	4	136	Tr	Tr	Tr	Tr	Tr	Tr	165
8	Tr	3	4	0.1	5	80	40	12	0.00	0.00	Tr	0	166
4	2	Tr	Tr	0.0	2	75	0	0	0.00	0.00	0.0	0	167
4	4	2	4	Tr	1	107	30	13	Tr	Tr	Tr	0	168
4	1	3	4	0.1	11	182	30	9	Tr	Tr	0.0	Tr	169
4	2	2	3	0.1	18	112	50	15	Tr	Tr	Tr	0	170
2	2	2	3	0.1	17	150	50	14	Tr	Tr	Tr	0	171

[11] For salted margarine.
[12] Based on average vitamin A content of fortified margarine. Federal specifications for fortified margarine require a minimum of 15,000 IU per pound.

Table A-5 Nutritive Value of the Edible Part of Food *(Continued)*

(Tr indicates nutrient present in trace amount.)

Item No.	Foods, approximate measures, units, and weight (weight of edible portion only)			Water	Food energy	Pro- tein	Fat	Fatty acids		
								Satu- rated	Mono- unsatu- rated	Poly- unsatu- rated
			Grams	Per- cent	Cal- ories	Grams	Grams	Grams	Grams	Grams
	Fats and Oils—Con.									
	Salad dressings:									
	Prepared from home recipe:									
172	Cooked type[13]	1 tbsp	16	69	25	1	2	0.5	0.6	0.3
173	Vinegar and oil	1 tbsp	16	47	70	0	8	1.5	2.4	3.9
	Fish and Shellfish									
	Clams:									
174	Raw, meat only	3 oz	85	82	65	11	1	0.3	0.3	0.3
175	Canned, drained solids	3 oz	85	77	85	13	2	0.5	0.5	0.4
176	Crabmeat, canned	1 cup	135	77	135	23	3	0.5	0.8	1.4
177	Fish sticks, frozen, reheated, (stick, 4 by 1 by 1/2 in)	1 fish stick	28	52	70	6	3	0.8	1.4	0.8
	Flounder or Sole, baked, with lemon juice:									
178	With butter	3 oz	85	73	120	16	6	3.2	1.5	0.5
179	With margarine	3 oz	85	73	120	16	6	1.2	2.3	1.9
180	Without added fat	3 oz	85	78	80	17	1	0.3	0.2	0.4
181	Haddock, breaded, fried[14]	3 oz	85	61	175	17	9	2.4	3.9	2.4
182	Halibut, broiled, with butter and lemon juice	3 oz	85	67	140	20	6	3.3	1.6	0.7
183	Herring, pickled	3 oz	85	59	190	17	13	4.3	4.6	3.1
184	Ocean perch, breaded, fried[14]	1 fillet	85	59	185	16	11	2.6	4.6	2.8
	Oysters:									
185	Raw, meat only (13-19 medium Selects)	1 cup	240	85	160	20	4	1.4	0.5	1.4
186	Breaded, fried[14]	1 oyster	45	65	90	5	5	1.4	2.1	1.4
	Salmon:									
187	Canned (pink), solids and liquid	3 oz	85	71	120	17	5	0.9	1.5	2.1
188	Baked (red)	3 oz	85	67	140	21	5	1.2	2.4	1.4
189	Smoked	3 oz	85	59	150	18	8	2.6	3.9	0.7
190	Sardines, Atlantic, canned in oil, drained solids	3 oz	85	62	175	20	9	2.1	3.7	2.9
191	Scallops, breaded, frozen, reheated	6 scallops	90	59	195	15	10	2.5	4.1	2.5
	Shrimp:									
192	Canned, drained solids	3 oz	85	70	100	21	1	0.2	0.2	0.4
193	French fried (7 medium)[16]	3 oz	85	55	200	16	10	2.5	4.1	2.6
194	Trout, broiled, with butter and lemon juice	3 oz	85	63	175	21	9	4.1	2.9	1.6
	Tuna, canned, drained solids:									
195	Oil pack, chunk light	3 oz	85	61	165	24	7	1.4	1.9	3.1
196	Water pack, solid white	3 oz	85	63	135	30	1	0.3	0.2	0.3
197	Tuna salad[17]	1 cup	205	63	375	33	19	3.3	4.9	9.2
	Fruits and Fruit Juices									
	Apples:									
	Raw:									
	Unpeeled, without cores:									
198	2-3/4-in diam. (about 3 per lb with cores)	1 apple	138	84	80	Tr	Tr	0.1	Tr	0.1
199	3-1/4-in diam. (about 2 per lb with cores)	1 apple	212	84	125	Tr	1	0.1	Tr	0.2
200	Peeled, sliced	1 cup	110	84	65	Tr	Tr	0.1	Tr	0.1
201	Dried, sulfured	10 rings	64	32	155	1	Tr	Tr	Tr	0.1
202	Apple juice, bottled or canned[19]	1 cup	248	88	115	Tr	Tr	Tr	Tr	0.1
	Applesauce, canned:									
203	Sweetened	1 cup	255	80	195	Tr	Tr	0.1	Tr	0.1
204	Unsweetened	1 cup	244	88	105	Tr	Tr	Tr	Tr	Tr

[13] Fatty acid values apply to product made with regular margarine.
[14] Dipped in egg, milk, and breadcrumbs; fried in vegetable shortening.
[15] If bones are discarded, value for calcium will be greatly reduced.
[16] Dipped in egg, breadcrumbs, and flour; fried in vegetable shortening.

Table A-5 Nutritive Value of the Edible Part of Food *(Continued)*

Nutrients in Indicated Quantity

Cholesterol	Carbohydrate	Calcium	Phosphorus	Iron	Potassium	Sodium	Vitamin A value		Thiamin	Riboflavin	Niacin	Ascorbic acid	Item No.
							(IU)	(RE)					
Milligrams	Grams	Milligrams	Milligrams	Milligrams	Milligrams	Milligrams	International units	Retinol equivalents	Milligrams	Milligrams	Milligrams	Milligrams	
9	2	13	14	0.1	19	117	70	20	0.01	0.02	Tr	Tr	172
0	Tr	0	0	0.0	1	Tr	0	0	0.00	0.00	0.0	0	173
43	2	59	138	2.6	154	102	90	26	0.09	0.15	1.1	9	174
54	2	47	116	3.5	119	102	90	26	0.01	0.09	0.9	3	175
135	1	61	246	1.1	149	1,350	50	14	0.11	0.11	2.6	0	176
26	4	11	58	0.3	94	53	20	5	0.03	0.05	0.6	0	177
68	Tr	13	187	0.3	272	145	210	54	0.05	0.08	1.6	1	178
55	Tr	14	187	0.3	273	151	230	69	0.05	0.08	1.6	1	179
59	Tr	13	197	0.3	286	101	30	10	0.05	0.08	1.7	1	180
75	7	34	183	1.0	270	123	70	20	0.06	0.10	2.9	0	181
62	Tr	14	206	0.7	441	103	610	174	0.06	0.07	7.7	1	182
85	0	29	128	0.9	85	850	110	33	0.04	0.18	2.8	0	183
66	7	31	191	1.2	241	138	70	20	0.10	0.11	2.0	0	184
120	8	226	343	15.6	290	175	740	223	0.34	0.43	6.0	24	185
35	5	49	73	3.0	64	70	150	44	0.07	0.10	1.3	4	186
34	0	[15]167	243	0.7	307	443	60	18	0.03	0.15	6.8	0	187
60	0	26	269	0.5	305	55	290	87	0.18	0.14	5.5	0	188
51	0	12	208	0.8	327	1,700	260	77	0.17	0.17	6.8	0	189
85	0	[15]371	424	2.6	349	425	190	56	0.03	0.17	4.6	0	190
70	10	39	203	2.0	369	298	70	21	0.11	0.11	1.6	0	191
128	1	98	224	1.4	104	1,955	50	15	0.01	0.03	1.5	0	192
168	11	61	154	2.0	189	384	90	26	0.06	0.09	2.8	0	193
71	Tr	26	259	1.0	297	122	230	60	0.07	0.07	2.3	1	194
55	0	7	199	1.6	298	303	70	20	0.04	0.09	10.1	0	195
48	0	17	202	0.6	255	468	110	32	0.03	0.10	13.4	0	196
80	19	31	281	2.5	531	877	230	53	0.06	0.14	13.3	6	197
0	21	10	10	0.2	159	Tr	70	7	0.02	0.02	0.1	8	198
0	32	15	15	0.4	244	Tr	110	11	0.04	0.03	0.2	12	199
0	16	4	8	0.1	124	Tr	50	5	0.02	0.01	0.1	4	200
0	42	9	24	0.9	288	[18]56	0	0	0.00	0.10	0.6	[20]2	201
0	29	17	17	0.9	295	7	Tr	Tr	0.05	0.04	0.2	[20]2	202
0	51	10	18	0.9	156	8	30	3	0.03	0.07	0.5	[20]4	203
0	28	7	17	0.3	183	5	70	7	0.03	0.06	0.5	[20]3	204

[17] Made with drained chunk light tuna, celery, onion, pickle relish, and mayonnaise-type salad dressing.
[18] Sodium bisulfite used to preserve color; unsulfited product would contain less sodium.
[19] Also applies to pasteurized apple cider.
[20] Without added ascorbic acid. For value with added ascorbic acid, refer to label.

Table A-5 Nutritive Value of the Edible Part of Food *(Continued)*

(Tr indicates nutrient present in trace amount.)

Item No.	Foods, approximate measures, units, and weight (weight of edible portion only)		Water	Food energy	Pro-tein	Fat	Fatty acids		
							Satu-rated	Mono-unsatu-rated	Poly-unsatu-rated
		Grams	Per-cent	Cal-ories	Grams	Grams	Grams	Grams	Grams

Fruits and Fruit Juices—Con.

	Apricots:								
205	Raw, without pits (about 12 per lb with pits)	3 apricots	106	86	50	1	Tr	Tr	0.2	0.1
	Canned (fruit and liquid):								
206	Heavy syrup pack	1 cup	258	78	215	1	Tr	Tr	0.1	Tr
207		3 halves	85	78	70	Tr	Tr	Tr	Tr	Tr
208	Juice pack	1 cup	248	87	120	2	Tr	Tr	Tr	Tr
209		3 halves	84	87	40	1	Tr	Tr	Tr	Tr
	Dried:								
210	Uncooked (28 large or 37 medium halves per cup)	1 cup	130	31	310	5	1	Tr	0.3	0.1
211	Cooked, unsweetened, fruit and liquid	1 cup	250	76	210	3	Tr	Tr	0.2	0.1
212	Apricot nectar, canned	1 cup	251	85	140	1	Tr	Tr	0.1	Tr
	Avocados, raw, whole, without skin and seed:								
213	California (about 2 per lb with skin and seed)	1 avocado	173	73	305	4	30	4.5	19.4	3.5
214	Florida (about 1 per lb with skin and seed)	1 avocado	304	80	340	5	27	5.3	14.8	4.5
	Bananas, raw, without peel:								
215	Whole (about 2-1/2 per lb with peel)	1 banana	114	74	105	1	1	0.2	Tr	0.1
216	Sliced	1 cup	150	74	140	2	1	0.3	0.1	0.1
217	Blackberries, raw	1 cup	144	86	75	1	1	0.2	0.1	0.1
	Blueberries:								
218	Raw	1 cup	145	85	80	1	1	Tr	0.1	0.3
219	Frozen, sweetened	10-oz container	284	77	230	1	Tr	Tr	0.1	0.2
220		1 cup	230	77	185	1	Tr	Tr	Tr	0.1
	Cantaloup. See Melons (item 251).								
	Cherries:								
221	Sour, red, pitted, canned, water pack	1 cup	244	90	90	2	Tr	0.1	0.1	0.1
222	Sweet, raw, without pits and stems	10 cherries	68	81	50	1	1	0.1	0.2	0.2
223	Cranberry juice cocktail, bottled, sweetened	1 cup	253	85	145	Tr	Tr	Tr	Tr	0.1
224	Cranberry sauce, sweetened, canned, strained	1 cup	277	61	420	1	Tr	Tr	0.1	0.2
	Dates:								
225	Whole, without pits	10 dates	83	23	230	2	Tr	0.1	0.1	Tr
226	Chopped	1 cup	178	23	490	4	1	0.3	0.2	Tr
227	Figs, dried	10 figs	187	28	475	6	2	0.4	0.5	1.0
	Fruit cocktail, canned, fruit and liquid:								
228	Heavy syrup pack	1 cup	255	80	185	1	Tr	Tr	Tr	0.1
229	Juice pack	1 cup	248	87	115	1	Tr	Tr	Tr	Tr
	Grapefruit:								
230	Raw, without peel, membrane and seeds (3-3/4-in diam., 1 lb 1 oz, whole, with refuse)	1/2 grapefruit	120	91	40	1	Tr	Tr	Tr	Tr
231	Canned, sections with syrup	1 cup	254	84	150	1	Tr	Tr	Tr	0.1
	Grapefruit juice:								
232	Raw	1 cup	247	90	95	1	Tr	Tr	Tr	0.1
	Canned:								
233	Unsweetened	1 cup	247	90	95	1	Tr	Tr	Tr	0.1
234	Sweetened	1 cup	250	87	115	1	Tr	Tr	Tr	0.1
	Frozen concentrate, unsweetened								
235	Undiluted	6-fl-oz can	207	62	300	4	1	0.1	0.1	0.2
236	Diluted with 3 parts water by volume	1 cup	247	89	100	1	Tr	Tr	Tr	0.1

[20] Without added ascorbic acid. For value with added ascorbic acid, refer to label.
[21] With added ascorbic acid.

Table A-5 Nutritive Value of the Edible Part of Food (Continued)

Nutrients in Indicated Quantity

Cholesterol	Carbohydrate	Calcium	Phosphorus	Iron	Potassium	Sodium	Vitamin A value		Thiamin	Riboflavin	Niacin	Ascorbic acid	Item No
							(IU)	(RE)					
Milligrams	Grams	Milligrams	Milligrams	Milligrams	Milligrams	Milligrams	International units	Retinol equivalents	Milligrams	Milligrams	Milligrams	Milligrams	
0	12	15	20	0.6	314	1	2,770	277	0.03	0.04	0.6	11	205
0	55	23	31	0.8	361	10	3,170	317	0.05	0.06	1.0	8	206
0	18	8	10	0.3	119	3	1,050	105	0.02	0.02	0.3	3	207
0	31	30	50	0.7	409	10	4,190	419	0.04	0.05	0.9	12	208
0	10	10	17	0.3	139	3	1,420	142	0.02	0.02	0.3	4	209
0	80	59	152	6.1	1,791	13	9,410	941	0.01	0.20	3.9	3	210
0	55	40	103	4.2	1,222	8	5,910	591	0.02	0.08	2.4	4	211
0	36	18	23	1.0	286	8	3,300	330	0.02	0.04	0.7	[20]2	212
0	12	19	73	2.0	1,097	21	1,060	106	0.19	0.21	3.3	14	213
0	27	33	119	1.6	1,484	15	1,860	186	0.33	0.37	5.8	24	214
0	27	7	23	0.4	451	1	90	9	0.05	0.11	0.6	10	215
0	35	9	30	0.5	594	2	120	12	0.07	0.15	0.8	14	216
0	18	46	30	0.8	282	Tr	240	24	0.04	0.06	0.6	30	217
0	20	9	15	0.2	129	9	150	15	0.07	0.07	0.5	19	218
0	62	17	20	1.1	170	3	120	12	0.06	0.15	0.7	3	219
0	50	14	16	0.9	138	2	100	10	0.05	0.12	0.6	2	220
0	22	27	24	3.3	239	17	1,840	184	0.04	0.10	0.4	5	221
0	11	10	13	0.3	152	Tr	150	15	0.03	0.04	0.3	5	222
0	38	8	3	0.4	61	10	10	1	0.01	0.04	0.1	[21]108	223
0	108	11	17	0.6	72	80	60	6	0.04	0.06	0.3	6	224
0	61	27	33	1.0	541	2	40	4	0.07	0.08	1.8	0	225
0	131	57	71	2.0	1,161	5	90	9	0.16	0.18	3.9	0	226
0	122	269	127	4.2	1,331	21	250	25	0.13	0.16	1.3	1	227
0	48	15	28	0.7	224	15	520	52	0.05	0.05	1.0	5	228
0	29	20	35	0.5	236	10	760	76	0.03	0.04	1.0	7	229
0	10	14	10	0.1	167	Tr	[22]10	[22]1	0.04	0.02	0.3	41	230
0	39	36	25	1.0	328	5	Tr	Tr	0.10	0.05	0.6	54	231
0	23	22	37	0.5	400	2	20	2	0.10	0.05	0.5	94	232
0	22	17	27	0.5	378	2	20	2	0.10	0.05	0.6	72	233
0	28	20	28	0.9	405	5	20	2	0.10	0.06	0.8	67	234
0	72	56	101	1.0	1,002	6	60	6	0.30	0.16	1.6	248	235
0	24	20	35	0.3	336	2	20	2	0.10	0.05	0.5	83	236

[22]For white grapefruit; pink grapefruit have about 310 IU or 31 RE.

Table A-5 Nutritive Value of the Edible Part of Food *(Continued)*

(Tr indicates nutrient present in trace amount.)

Item No.	Foods, approximate measures, units, and weight (weight of edible portion only)			Water	Food energy	Protein	Fat	Fatty acids Saturated	Mono-unsaturated	Poly-unsaturated
			Grams	Percent	Calories	Grams	Grams	Grams	Grams	Grams
	Fruits and Fruit Juices—Con.									
	Grapes, European type (adherent skin), raw:									
237	Thompson Seedless---------------	10 grapes-------	50	81	35	Tr	Tr	0.1	Tr	0.1
238	Tokay and Emperor, seeded types	10 grapes-------	57	81	40	Tr	Tr	0.1	Tr	0.1
	Grape juice:									
239	Canned or bottled---------------	1 cup-----------	253	84	155	1	Tr	0.1	Tr	0.1
	Frozen concentrate, sweetened:									
240	Undiluted--------------------	6-fl-oz can-----	216	54	385	1	1	0.2	Tr	0.2
241	Diluted with 3 parts water by volume--------------------	1 cup-----------	250	87	125	Tr	Tr	0.1	Tr	0.1
242	Kiwifruit, raw, without skin (about 5 per lb with skin)-----	1 kiwifruit-----	76	83	45	1	Tr	Tr	0.1	0.1
243	Lemons, raw, without peel and seeds (about 4 per lb with peel and seeds)--------------------	1 lemon---------	58	89	15	1	Tr	Tr	Tr	0.1
	Lemon juice:									
244	Raw-------------------------	1 cup-----------	244	91	60	1	Tr	Tr	Tr	Tr
245	Canned or bottled, unsweetened	1 cup-----------	244	92	50	1	1	0.1	Tr	0.2
246		1 tbsp----------	15	92	5	Tr	Tr	Tr	Tr	Tr
247	Frozen, single-strength, unsweetened------------------	6-fl-oz can-----	244	92	55	1	1	0.1	Tr	0.2
	Lime juice:									
248	Raw-------------------------	1 cup-----------	246	90	65	1	Tr	Tr	Tr	0.1
249	Canned, unsweetened------------	1 cup-----------	246	93	50	1	1	0.1	0.1	0.2
250	Mangos, raw, without skin and seed (about 1-1/2 per lb with skin and seed)------------------	1 mango---------	207	82	135	1	1	0.1	0.2	0.1
	Melons, raw, without rind and cavity contents:									
251	Cantaloup, orange-fleshed (5-in diam., 2-1/3 lb, whole, with rind and cavity contents)----	1/2 melon-------	267	90	95	2	1	0.1	0.1	0.3
252	Honeydew (6-1/2-in diam., 5-1/4 lb, whole, with rind and cavity contents)----------------	1/10 melon------	129	90	45	1	Tr	Tr	Tr	0.1
253	Nectarines, raw, without pits (about 3 per lb with pits)-----	1 nectarine-----	136	86	65	1	1	0.1	0.2	0.3
	Oranges, raw:									
254	Whole, without peel and seeds (2-5/8-in diam., about 2-1/2 per lb, with peel and seeds)	1 orange--------	131	87	60	1	Tr	Tr	Tr	Tr
255	Sections without membranes-----	1 cup-----------	180	87	85	2	Tr	Tr	Tr	Tr
	Orange juice:									
256	Raw, all varieties-------------	1 cup-----------	248	88	110	2	Tr	0.1	0.1	0.1
257	Canned, unsweetened------------	1 cup-----------	249	89	105	1	Tr	Tr	0.1	0.1
258	Chilled-----------------------	1 cup-----------	249	88	110	2	1	0.1	0.1	0.2
	Frozen concentrate:									
259	Undiluted--------------------	6-fl-oz can-----	213	58	340	5	Tr	0.1	0.1	0.1
260	Diluted with 3 parts water by volume----------------------	1 cup-----------	249	88	110	2	Tr	Tr	Tr	Tr
261	Orange and grapefruit juice, canned-------------------------	1 cup-----------	247	89	105	1	Tr	Tr	Tr	Tr
262	Papayas, raw, 1/2-in cubes-------	1 cup-----------	140	86	65	1	Tr	0.1	0.1	Tr
	Peaches: Raw:									
263	Whole, 2-1/2-in diam., peeled, pitted (about 4 per lb with peels and pits)----	1 peach---------	87	88	35	1	Tr	Tr	Tr	Tr
264	Sliced-----------------------	1 cup-----------	170	88	75	1	Tr	Tr	0.1	0.1
	Canned, fruit and liquid:									
265	Heavy syrup pack-------------	1 cup-----------	256	79	190	1	Tr	Tr	0.1	0.1
266		1 half----------	81	79	60	Tr	Tr	Tr	Tr	Tr
267	Juice pack-------------------	1 cup-----------	248	87	110	2	Tr	Tr	Tr	Tr
268		1 half----------	77	87	35	Tr	Tr	Tr	Tr	Tr

[20]Without added ascorbic acid. For value with added ascorbic acid, refer to label.
[21]With added ascorbic acid.

Table A-5 Nutritive Value of the Edible Part of Food *(Continued)*

Nutrients in Indicated Quantity

Cholesterol	Carbohydrate	Calcium	Phosphorus	Iron	Potassium	Sodium	Vitamin A value		Thiamin	Riboflavin	Niacin	Ascorbic acid	Item No.
							(IU)	(RE)					
Milligrams	Grams	Milligrams	Milligrams	Milligrams	Milligrams	Milligrams	International units	Retinol equivalents	Milligrams	Milligrams	Milligrams	Milligrams	
0	9	6	7	0.1	93	1	40	4	0.05	0.03	0.2	5	237
0	10	6	7	0.1	105	1	40	4	0.05	0.03	0.2	6	238
0	38	23	28	0.6	334	8	20	2	0.07	0.09	0.7	[20]Tr	239
0	96	28	32	0.8	160	15	60	6	0.11	0.20	0.9	[21]179	240
0	32	10	10	0.3	53	5	20	2	0.04	0.07	0.3	[21]60	241
0	11	20	30	0.3	252	4	130	13	0.02	0.04	0.4	74	242
0	5	15	9	0.3	80	1	20	2	0.02	0.01	0.1	31	243
0	21	17	15	0.1	303	2	50	5	0.07	0.02	0.2	112	244
0	16	27	22	0.3	249	[23]51	40	4	0.10	0.02	0.5	61	245
0	1	2	1	Tr	15	[23]3	Tr	Tr	0.01	Tr	Tr	4	246
0	16	20	20	0.3	217	2	30	3	0.14	0.03	0.3	77	247
0	22	22	17	0.1	268	2	20	2	0.05	0.02	0.2	72	248
0	16	30	25	0.6	185	[23]39	40	4	0.08	0.01	0.4	16	249
0	35	21	23	0.3	323	4	8,060	806	0.12	0.12	1.2	57	250
0	22	29	45	0.6	825	24	8,610	861	0.10	0.06	1.5	113	251
0	12	8	13	0.1	350	13	50	5	0.10	0.02	0.8	32	252
0	16	7	22	0.2	288	Tr	1,000	100	0.02	0.06	1.3	7	253
0	15	52	18	0.1	237	Tr	270	27	0.11	0.05	0.4	70	254
0	21	72	25	0.2	326	Tr	370	37	0.16	0.07	0.5	96	255
0	26	27	42	0.5	496	2	500	50	0.22	0.07	1.0	124	256
0	25	20	35	1.1	436	5	440	44	0.15	0.07	0.8	86	257
0	25	25	27	0.4	473	2	190	19	0.28	0.05	0.7	82	258
0	81	68	121	0.7	1,436	6	590	59	0.60	0.14	1.5	294	259
0	27	22	40	0.2	473	2	190	19	0.20	0.04	0.5	97	260
0	25	20	35	1.1	390	7	290	29	0.14	0.07	0.8	72	261
0	17	35	12	0.3	247	9	400	40	0.04	0.04	0.5	92	262
0	10	4	10	0.1	171	Tr	470	47	0.01	0.04	0.9	6	263
0	19	9	20	0.2	335	Tr	910	91	0.03	0.07	1.7	11	264
0	51	8	28	0.7	236	15	850	85	0.03	0.06	1.6	7	265
0	16	2	9	0.2	75	5	270	27	0.01	0.02	0.5	2	266
0	29	15	42	0.7	317	10	940	94	0.02	0.04	1.4	9	267
0	9	5	13	0.2	99	3	290	29	0.01	0.01	0.4	3	268

[23]Sodium benzoate and sodium bisulfite added as preservatives.

Table A-5 Nutritive Value of the Edible Part of Food *(Continued)*

(Tr indicates nutrient present in trace amount.)

Item No.	Foods, approximate measures, units, and weight (weight of edible portion only)		Water	Food energy	Pro-tein	Fat	Fatty acids Satu-rated	Mono-unsatu-rated	Poly-unsatu-rated
		Grams	Per-cent	Cal-ories	Grams	Grams	Grams	Grams	Grams
	Fruits and Fruit Juices—Con.								
	Peaches:								
	Dried:								
269	Uncooked-------------------- 1 cup----------	160	32	380	6	1	0.1	0.4	0.6
270	Cooked, unsweetened, fruit and liquid---------------- 1 cup----------	258	78	200	3	1	0.1	0.2	0.3
271	Frozen, sliced, sweetened------ 10-oz container	284	75	265	2	Tr	Tr	0.1	0.2
272	1 cup----------	250	75	235	2	Tr	Tr	0.1	0.2
	Pears:								
	Raw, with skin, cored:								
273	Bartlett, 2-1/2-in diam. (about 2-1/2 per lb with cores and stems)---------- 1 pear----------	166	84	100	1	1	Tr	0.1	0.2
274	Bosc, 2-1/2-in diam. (about 3 per lb with cores and stems)-------------------- 1 pear----------	141	84	85	1	1	Tr	0.1	0.1
275	D'Anjou, 3-in diam. (about 2 per lb with cores and stems)-------------------- 1 pear----------	200	84	120	1	1	Tr	0.2	0.2
	Canned, fruit and liquid:								
276	Heavy syrup pack------------- 1 cup----------	255	80	190	1	Tr	Tr	0.1	0.1
277	1 half----------	79	80	60	Tr	Tr	Tr	Tr	Tr
278	Juice pack------------------- 1 cup----------	248	86	125	1	Tr	Tr	Tr	Tr
279	1 half----------	77	86	40	Tr	Tr	Tr	Tr	Tr
	Pineapple:								
280	Raw, diced-------------------- 1 cup----------	155	87	75	1	1	Tr	0.1	0.2
	Canned, fruit and liquid:								
	Heavy syrup pack:								
281	Crushed, chunks, tidbits--- 1 cup----------	255	79	200	1	Tr	Tr	Tr	0.1
282	Slices-------------------- 1 slice--------	58	79	45	Tr	Tr	Tr	Tr	Tr
	Juice pack:								
283	Chunks or tidbits---------- 1 cup----------	250	84	150	1	Tr	Tr	Tr	0.1
284	Slices-------------------- 1 slice--------	58	84	35	Tr	Tr	Tr	Tr	Tr
285	Pineapple juice, unsweetened, canned------------------------ 1 cup----------	250	86	140	1	Tr	Tr	Tr	0.1
	Plantains, without peel:								
286	Raw------------------------ 1 plantain------	179	65	220	2	1	0.3	0.1	0.1
287	Cooked, boiled, sliced--------- 1 cup----------	154	67	180	1	Tr	0.1	Tr	0.1
	Plums, without pits:								
	Raw:								
288	2-1/8-in diam. (about 6-1/2 per lb with pits)------ 1 plum----------	66	85	35	1	Tr	Tr	0.3	0.1
289	1-1/2-in diam. (about 15 per lb with pits)-------------- 1 plum----------	28	85	15	Tr	Tr	Tr	0.1	Tr
	Canned, purple, fruit and liquid:								
290	Heavy syrup pack------------- 1 cup----------	258	76	230	1	Tr	Tr	0.2	0.1
291	3 plums--------	133	76	120	Tr	Tr	Tr	0.1	Tr
292	Juice pack------------------- 1 cup----------	252	84	145	1	Tr	Tr	Tr	Tr
293	3 plums--------	95	84	55	Tr	Tr	Tr	Tr	Tr
	Prunes, dried:								
294	Uncooked---------------------- 4 extra large or 5 large prunes	49	32	115	1	Tr	Tr	0.2	0.1
295	Cooked, unsweetened, fruit and liquid-------------------- 1 cup----------	212	70	225	2	Tr	Tr	0.3	0.1
296	Prune juice, canned or bottled--- 1 cup----------	256	81	180	2	Tr	Tr	0.1	Tr
	Raisins, seedless:								
297	Cup, not pressed down---------- 1 cup----------	145	15	435	5	1	0.2	Tr	0.2
298	Packet, 1/2 oz (1-1/2 tbsp)---- 1 packet--------	14	15	40	Tr	Tr	Tr	Tr	Tr
	Raspberries:								
299	Raw-------------------------- 1 cup----------	123	87	60	1	1	Tr	0.1	0.4
300	Frozen, sweetened-------------- 10-oz container	284	73	295	2	Tr	Tr	Tr	0.3
301	1 cup----------	250	73	255	2	Tr	Tr	Tr	0.2

[21] With added ascorbic acid.

Table A-5 Nutritive Value of the Edible Part of Food *(Continued)*

Nutrients in Indicated Quantity

Cholesterol	Carbohydrate	Calcium	Phosphorus	Iron	Potassium	Sodium	Vitamin A value		Thiamin	Riboflavin	Niacin	Ascorbic acid	Item No.
							(IU)	(RE)					
Milligrams	Grams	Milligrams	Milligrams	Milligrams	Milligrams	Milligrams	International units	Retinol equivalents	Milligrams	Milligrams	Milligrams	Milligrams	
0	98	45	190	6.5	1,594	11	3,460	346	Tr	0.34	7.0	8	269
0	51	23	98	3.4	826	5	510	51	0.01	0.05	3.9	10	270
0	68	9	31	1.1	369	17	810	81	0.04	0.10	1.9	[21]268	271
0	60	8	28	0.9	325	15	710	71	0.03	0.09	1.6	[21]236	272
0	25	18	18	0.4	208	Tr	30	3	0.03	0.07	0.2	7	273
0	21	16	16	0.4	176	Tr	30	3	0.03	0.06	0.1	6	274
0	30	22	22	0.5	250	Tr	40	4	0.04	0.08	0.2	8	275
0	49	13	18	0.6	166	13	10	1	0.03	0.06	0.6	3	276
0	15	4	6	0.2	51	4	Tr	Tr	0.01	0.02	0.2	1	277
0	32	22	30	0.7	238	10	10	1	0.03	0.03	0.5	4	278
0	10	7	9	0.2	74	3	Tr	Tr	0.01	0.01	0.2	1	279
0	19	11	11	0.6	175	2	40	4	0.14	0.06	0.7	24	280
0	52	36	18	1.0	265	3	40	4	0.23	0.06	0.7	19	281
0	12	8	4	0.2	60	1	10	1	0.05	0.01	0.2	4	282
0	39	35	15	0.7	305	3	100	10	0.24	0.05	0.7	24	283
0	9	8	3	0.2	71	1	20	2	0.06	0.01	0.2	6	284
0	34	43	20	0.7	335	3	10	1	0.14	0.06	0.6	27	285
0	57	5	61	1.1	893	7	2,020	202	0.09	0.10	1.2	33	286
0	48	3	43	0.9	716	8	1,400	140	0.07	0.08	1.2	17	287
0	9	3	7	0.1	114	Tr	210	21	0.03	0.06	0.3	6	288
0	4	1	3	Tr	48	Tr	90	9	0.01	0.03	0.1	3	289
0	60	23	34	2.2	235	49	670	67	0.04	0.10	0.8	1	290
0	31	12	17	1.1	121	25	340	34	0.02	0.05	0.4	1	291
0	38	25	38	0.9	388	3	2,540	254	0.06	0.15	1.2	7	292
0	14	10	14	0.3	146	1	960	96	0.02	0.06	0.4	3	293
0	31	25	39	1.2	365	2	970	97	0.04	0.08	1.0	2	294
0	60	49	74	2.4	708	4	650	65	0.05	0.21	1.5	6	295
0	45	31	64	3.0	707	10	10	1	0.04	0.18	2.0	10	296
0	115	71	141	3.0	1,089	17	10	1	0.23	0.13	1.2	5	297
0	11	7	14	0.3	105	2	Tr	Tr	0.02	0.01	0.1	Tr	298
0	14	27	15	0.7	187	Tr	160	16	0.04	0.11	1.1	31	299
0	74	43	48	1.8	324	3	170	17	0.05	0.13	0.7	47	300
0	65	38	43	1.6	285	3	150	15	0.05	0.11	0.6	41	301

Table A-5 Nutritive Value of the Edible Part of Food *(Continued)*

(Tr indicates nutrient present in trace amount.)

Item No.	Foods, approximate measures, units, and weight (weight of edible portion only)		Water	Food energy	Pro- tein	Fat	Fatty acids		
							Satu- rated	Mono- unsatu- rated	Poly- unsatu- rated
		Grams	Per- cent	Cal- ories	Grams	Grams	Grams	Grams	Grams
	Fruits and Fruit Juices—Con.								
302	Rhubarb, cooked, added sugar----- 1 cup-----------	240	68	280	1	Tr	Tr	Tr	0.1
	Strawberries:								
303	Raw, capped, whole------------- 1 cup-----------	149	92	45	1	1	Tr	0.1	0.3
304	Frozen, sweetened, sliced------ 10-oz container	284	73	275	2	Tr	Tr	0.1	0.2
305	1 cup-----------	255	73	245	1	Tr	Tr	Tr	0.2
	Tangerines:								
306	Raw, without peel and seeds (2-3/8-in diam., about 4 per lb, with peel and seeds)----- 1 tangerine-----	84	88	35	1	Tr	Tr	Tr	Tr
307	Canned, light syrup, fruit and liquid---------------------- 1 cup-----------	252	83	155	1	Tr	Tr	Tr	0.1
308	Tangerine juice, canned, sweet- ened----------------------- 1 cup-----------	249	87	125	1	Tr	Tr	Tr	0.1
	Watermelon, raw, without rind and seeds:								
309	Piece (4 by 8 in wedge with rind and seeds; 1/16 of 32-2/3-lb melon, 10 by 16 in) 1 piece---------	482	92	155	3	2	0.3	0.2	1.0
310	Diced------------------------ 1 cup-----------	160	92	50	1	1	0.1	0.1	0.3
	Grain Products								
311	Bagels, plain or water, enriched, 3-1/2-in diam.[24] ---------------- 1 bagel---------	68	29	200	7	2	0.3	0.5	0.7
312	Barley, pearled, light, uncooked 1 cup-----------	200	11	700	16	2	0.3	0.2	0.9
	Biscuits, baking powder, 2-in diam. (enriched flour, vege- table shortening):								
313	From home recipe--------------- 1 biscuit-------	28	28	100	2	5	1.2	2.0	1.3
314	From mix---------------------- 1 biscuit-------	28	29	95	2	3	0.8	1.4	0.9
315	From refrigerated dough-------- 1 biscuit-------	20	30	65	1	2	0.6	0.9	0.6
	Breadcrumbs, enriched:								
316	Dry, grated-------------------- 1 cup-----------	100	7	390	13	5	1.5	1.6	1.0
	Soft. See White bread (item 351).								
	Breads:								
317	Boston brown bread, canned, slice, 3-1/4 in by 1/2 in[25] -- 1 slice---------	45	45	95	2	1	0.3	0.1	0.1
	Cracked-wheat bread (3/4 en- riched wheat flour, 1/4 cracked wheat flour):[25]								
318	Loaf, 1 lb------------------- 1 loaf---------	454	35	1,190	42	16	3.1	4.3	5.7
319	Slice (18 per loaf)---------- 1 slice---------	25	35	65	2	1	0.2	0.2	0.3
320	Toasted-------------------- 1 slice---------	21	26	65	2	1	0.2	0.2	0.3
	French or vienna bread, en- riched:[25]								
321	Loaf, 1 lb------------------- 1 loaf---------	454	34	1,270	43	18	3.8	5.7	5.9
	Slice:								
322	French, 5 by 2-1/2 by 1 in 1 slice---------	35	34	100	3	1	0.3	0.4	0.5
323	Vienna, 4-3/4 by 4 by 1/2 in---------------------- 1 slice---------	25	34	70	2	1	0.2	0.3	0.3
	Italian bread, enriched:								
324	Loaf, 1 lb------------------- 1 loaf---------	454	32	1,255	41	4	0.6	0.3	1.6
325	Slice, 4-1/2 by 3-1/4 by 3/4 in---------------------- 1 slice---------	30	32	85	3	Tr	Tr	Tr	0.1
	Mixed grain bread, enriched:[25]								
326	Loaf, 1 lb------------------- 1 loaf---------	454	37	1,165	45	17	3.2	4.1	6.5
327	Slice (18 per loaf)---------- 1 slice---------	25	37	65	2	1	0.2	0.2	0.4
328	Toasted-------------------- 1 slice---------	23	27	65	2	1	0.2	0.2	0.4

[24] Egg bagels have 44 mg cholesterol and 22 IU or 7 RE vitamin A per bagel.
[25] Made with vegetable shortening.

Table A-5 Nutritive Value of the Edible Part of Food *(Continued)*

Nutrients in Indicated Quantity

Cholesterol	Carbohydrate	Calcium	Phosphorus	Iron	Potassium	Sodium	Vitamin A value (IU)	(RE)	Thiamin	Riboflavin	Niacin	Ascorbic acid	Item No.
Milligrams	Grams	Milligrams	Milligrams	Milligrams	Milligrams	Milligrams	International units	Retinol equivalents	Milligrams	Milligrams	Milligrams	Milligrams	
0	75	348	19	0.5	230	2	170	17	0.04	0.06	0.5	8	302
0	10	21	28	0.6	247	1	40	4	0.03	0.10	0.3	84	303
0	74	31	37	1.7	278	9	70	7	0.05	0.14	1.1	118	304
0	66	28	33	1.5	250	8	60	6	0.04	0.13	1.0	106	305
0	9	12	8	0.1	132	1	770	77	0.09	0.02	0.1	26	306
0	41	18	25	0.9	197	15	2,120	212	0.13	0.11	1.1	50	307
0	30	45	35	0.5	443	2	1,050	105	0.15	0.05	0.2	55	308
0	35	39	43	0.8	559	10	1,760	176	0.39	0.10	1.0	46	309
0	11	13	14	0.3	186	3	590	59	0.13	0.03	0.3	15	310
0	38	29	46	1.8	50	245	0	0	0.26	0.20	2.4	0	311
0	158	32	378	4.2	320	6	0	0	0.24	0.10	6.2	0	312
Tr	13	47	36	0.7	32	195	10	3	0.08	0.08	0.8	Tr	313
Tr	14	58	128	0.7	56	262	20	4	0.12	0.11	0.8	Tr	314
1	10	4	79	0.5	18	249	0	0	0.08	0.05	0.7	0	315
5	73	122	141	4.1	152	736	0	0	0.35	0.35	4.8	0	316
3	21	41	72	0.9	131	113	[26]0	[26]0	0.06	0.04	0.7	0	317
0	227	295	581	12.1	608	1,966	Tr	Tr	1.73	1.73	15.3	Tr	318
0	12	16	32	0.7	34	106	Tr	Tr	0.10	0.09	0.8	Tr	319
0	12	16	32	0.7	34	106	Tr	Tr	0.07	0.09	0.8	Tr	320
0	230	499	386	14.0	409	2,633	Tr	Tr	2.09	1.59	18.2	Tr	321
0	18	39	30	1.1	32	203	Tr	Tr	0.16	0.12	1.4	Tr	322
0	13	28	21	0.8	23	145	Tr	Tr	0.12	0.09	1.0	Tr	323
0	256	77	350	12.7	336	2,656	0	0	1.80	1.10	15.0	0	324
0	17	5	23	0.8	22	176	0	0	0.12	0.07	1.0	0	325
0	212	472	962	14.8	990	1,870	Tr	Tr	1.77	1.73	18.9	Tr	326
0	12	27	55	0.8	56	106	Tr	Tr	0.10	0.10	1.1	Tr	327
0	12	27	55	0.8	56	106	Tr	Tr	0.08	0.10	1.1	Tr	328

[26]Made with white cornmeal. If made with yellow cornmeal, value is 32 IU or 3 RE.

Table A-5 Nutritive Value of the Edible Part of Food *(Continued)*

(Tr indicates nutrient present in trace amount.)

Item No.	Foods, approximate measures, units, and weight (weight of edible portion only)		Water	Food energy	Pro-tein	Fat	Fatty acids Satu-rated	Mono-unsatu-rated	Poly-unsatu-rated
		Grams	Per-cent	Cal-ories	Grams	Grams	Grams	Grams	Grams
	Grain Products—Con.								
	Breads:								
	Oatmeal bread, enriched:[25]								
329	Loaf, 1 lb	1 loaf	454	37	1,145	38	20	3.7	7.1	8.2
330	Slice (18 per loaf)	1 slice	25	37	65	2	1	0.2	0.4	0.5
331	Toasted	1 slice	23	30	65	2	1	0.2	0.4	0.5
332	Pita bread, enriched, white, 6-1/2-in diam.	1 pita	60	31	165	6	1	0.1	0.1	0.4
	Pumpernickel (2/3 rye flour, 1/3 enriched wheat flour):[25]								
333	Loaf, 1 lb	1 loaf	454	37	1,160	42	16	2.6	3.6	6.4
334	Slice, 5 by 4 by 3/8 in	1 slice	32	37	80	3	1	0.2	0.3	0.5
335	Toasted	1 slice	29	28	80	3	1	0.2	0.3	0.5
	Raisin bread, enriched:[25]								
336	Loaf, 1 lb	1 loaf	454	33	1,260	37	18	4.1	6.5	6.7
337	Slice (18 per loaf)	1 slice	25	33	65	2	1	0.2	0.3	0.4
338	Toasted	1 slice	21	24	65	2	1	0.2	0.3	0.4
	Rye bread, light (2/3 enriched wheat flour, 1/3 rye flour):[25]								
339	Loaf, 1 lb	1 loaf	454	37	1,190	38	17	3.3	5.2	5.5
340	Slice, 4-3/4 by 3-3/4 by 7/16 in	1 slice	25	37	65	2	1	0.2	0.3	0.3
341	Toasted	1 slice	22	28	65	2	1	0.2	0.3	0.3
	Wheat bread, enriched:[25]								
342	Loaf, 1 lb	1 loaf	454	37	1,160	43	19	3.9	7.3	4.5
343	Slice (18 per loaf)	1 slice	25	37	65	2	1	0.2	0.4	0.3
344	Toasted	1 slice	23	28	65	3	1	0.2	0.4	0.3
	White bread, enriched:[25]								
345	Loaf, 1 lb	1 loaf	454	37	1,210	38	18	5.6	6.5	4.2
346	Slice (18 per loaf)	1 slice	25	37	65	2	1	0.3	0.4	0.2
347	Toasted	1 slice	22	28	65	2	1	0.3	0.4	0.2
348	Slice (22 per loaf)	1 slice	20	37	55	2	1	0.2	0.3	0.2
349	Toasted	1 slice	17	28	55	2	1	0.2	0.3	0.2
350	Cubes	1 cup	30	37	80	2	1	0.4	0.4	0.3
351	Crumbs, soft	1 cup	45	37	120	4	2	0.6	0.6	0.4
	Whole-wheat bread:[25]								
352	Loaf, 1 lb	1 loaf	454	38	1,110	44	20	5.8	6.8	5.2
353	Slice (16 per loaf)	1 slice	28	38	70	3	1	0.4	0.4	0.3
354	Toasted	1 slice	25	29	70	3	1	0.4	0.4	0.3
	Bread stuffing (from enriched bread), prepared from mix:								
355	Dry type	1 cup	140	33	500	9	31	6.1	13.3	9.6
356	Moist type	1 cup	203	61	420	9	26	5.3	11.3	8.0
	Breakfast cereals:								
	Hot type, cooked:								
	Corn (hominy) grits:								
357	Regular and quick, enriched	1 cup	242	85	145	3	Tr	Tr	0.1	0.2
358	Instant, plain	1 pkt	137	85	80	2	Tr	Tr	Tr	0.1
	Cream of Wheat®:								
359	Regular, quick, instant	1 cup	244	86	140	4	Tr	0.1	Tr	0.2
360	Mix'n Eat, plain	1 pkt	142	82	100	3	Tr	Tr	Tr	0.1
361	Malt-O-Meal®	1 cup	240	88	120	4	Tr	Tr	Tr	0.1
	Oatmeal or rolled oats:								
362	Regular, quick, instant, nonfortified	1 cup	234	85	145	6	2	0.4	0.8	1.0
	Instant, fortified:								
363	Plain	1 pkt	177	86	105	4	2	0.3	0.6	0.7
364	Flavored	1 pkt	164	76	160	5	2	0.3	0.7	0.8

[25] Made with vegetable shortening.
[27] Nutrient added.
[28] Cooked without salt. If salt is added according to label recommendations, sodium content is 540 mg.
[29] For white corn grits. Cooked yellow grits contain 145 IU or 14 RE.
[30] Value based on label declaration for added nutrients.

Table A-5 Nutritive Value of the Edible Part of Food *(Continued)*

Nutrients in Indicated Quantity

Cholesterol	Carbohydrate	Calcium	Phosphorus	Iron	Potassium	Sodium	Vitamin A value (IU)	Vitamin A value (RE)	Thiamin	Riboflavin	Niacin	Ascorbic acid	Item No.
Milligrams	Grams	Milligrams	Milligrams	Milligrams	Milligrams	Milligrams	International units	Retinol equivalents	Milligrams	Milligrams	Milligrams	Milligrams	
0	212	267	563	12.0	707	2,231	0	0	2.09	1.20	15.4	0	329
0	12	15	31	0.7	39	124	0	0	0.12	0.07	0.9	0	330
0	12	15	31	0.7	39	124	0	0	0.09	0.07	0.9	0	331
0	33	49	60	1.4	71	339	0	0	0.27	0.12	2.2	0	332
0	218	322	990	12.4	1,966	2,461	0	0	1.54	2.36	15.0	0	333
0	16	23	71	0.9	141	177	0	0	0.11	0.17	1.1	0	334
0	16	23	71	0.9	141	177	0	0	0.09	0.17	1.1	0	335
0	239	463	395	14.1	1,058	1,657	Tr	Tr	1.50	2.81	18.6	Tr	336
0	13	25	22	0.8	59	92	Tr	Tr	0.08	0.15	1.0	Tr	337
0	13	25	22	0.8	59	92	Tr	Tr	0.06	0.15	1.0	Tr	338
0	218	363	658	12.3	926	3,164	0	0	1.86	1.45	15.0	0	339
0	12	20	36	0.7	51	175	0	0	0.10	0.08	0.8	0	340
0	12	20	36	0.7	51	175	0	0	0.08	0.08	0.8	0	341
0	213	572	835	15.8	627	2,447	Tr	Tr	2.09	1.45	20.5	Tr	342
0	12	32	47	0.9	35	138	Tr	Tr	0.12	0.08	1.2	Tr	343
0	12	32	47	0.9	35	138	Tr	Tr	0.10	0.08	1.2	Tr	344
0	222	572	490	12.9	508	2,334	Tr	Tr	2.13	1.41	17.0	Tr	345
0	12	32	27	0.7	28	129	Tr	Tr	0.12	0.08	0.9	Tr	346
0	12	32	27	0.7	28	129	Tr	Tr	0.09	0.08	0.9	Tr	347
0	10	25	21	0.6	22	101	Tr	Tr	0.09	0.06	0.7	Tr	348
0	10	25	21	0.6	22	101	Tr	Tr	0.07	0.06	0.7	Tr	349
0	15	38	32	0.9	34	154	Tr	Tr	0.14	0.09	1.1	Tr	350
0	22	57	49	1.3	50	231	Tr	Tr	0.21	0.14	1.7	Tr	351
0	206	327	1,180	15.5	799	2,887	Tr	Tr	1.59	0.95	17.4	Tr	352
0	13	20	74	1.0	50	180	Tr	Tr	0.10	0.06	1.1	Tr	353
0	13	20	74	1.0	50	180	Tr	Tr	0.08	0.06	1.1	Tr	354
0	50	92	136	2.2	126	1,254	910	273	0.17	0.20	2.5	0	355
67	40	81	134	2.0	118	1,023	850	256	0.10	0.18	1.6	0	356
0	31	0	29	[27]1.5	53	[28]0	[29]0	[29]0	[27]0.24	[27]0.15	[27]2.0	0	357
0	18	7	16	[27]1.0	29	343	0	0	[27]0.18	[27]0.08	[27]1.3	0	358
0	29	[30]54	[31]43	[30]10.9	46	[31,32]5	0	0	[30]0.24	[30]0.07	[30]1.5	0	359
0	21	[30]20	[30]20	[30]8.1	38	241	[30]1,250	[30]376	[30]0.43	[30]0.28	[30]5.0	0	360
0	26	5	[30]24	[30]9.6	31	[33]2	0	0	[30]0.48	[30]0.24	[30]5.8	0	361
0	25	19	178	1.6	131	[34]2	40	4	0.26	0.05	0.3	0	362
0	18	[27]163	133	[27]6.3	99	[27]285	[27]1,510	[27]453	[27]0.53	[27]0.28	[27]5.5	0	363
0	31	[27]168	148	[27]6.7	137	[27]254	[27]1,530	[27]460	[27]0.53	[27]0.38	[27]5.9	Tr	364

[31] For regular and instant cereal. For quick cereal, phosphorus is 102 mg and sodium is 142 mg.
[32] Cooked without salt. If salt is added according to label recommendations, sodium content is 390 mg.
[33] Cooked without salt. If salt is added according to label recommendations, sodium content is 324 mg.
[34] Cooked without salt. If salt is added according to label recommendations, sodium content is 374 mg.

Table A-5 Nutritive Value of the Edible Part of Food *(Continued)*

(Tr indicates nutrient present in trace amount.)

Item No.	Foods, approximate measures, units, and weight (weight of edible portion only)			Water	Food energy	Pro-tein	Fat	Fatty acids		
								Satu-rated	Mono-unsatu-rated	Poly-unsatu-rated
	Grain Products—Con.		Grams	Per-cent	Cal-ories	Grams	Grams	Grams	Grams	Grams
	Breakfast cereals:									
	Ready to eat:									
365	All-Bran® (about 1/3 cup)----	1 oz------------	28	3	70	4	1	0.1	0.1	0.3
366	Cap'n Crunch® (about 3/4 cup)	1 oz------------	28	3	120	1	3	1.7	0.3	0.4
367	Cheerios® (about 1-1/4 cup)--	1 oz------------	28	5	110	4	2	0.3	0.6	0.7
	Corn Flakes (about 1-1/4 cup):									
368	Kellogg's®----------------	1 oz------------	28	3	110	2	Tr	Tr	Tr	Tr
369	Toasties®-----------------	1 oz------------	28	3	110	2	Tr	Tr	Tr	Tr
	40% Bran Flakes:									
370	Kellogg's® (about 3/4 cup)	1 oz------------	28	3	90	4	1	0.1	0.1	0.3
371	Post® (about 2/3 cup)------	1 oz------------	28	3	90	3	Tr	0.1	0.1	0.2
372	Froot Loops® (about 1 cup)---	1 oz------------	28	3	110	2	1	0.2	0.1	0.1
373	Golden Grahams® (about 3/4									
	cup)--------------------	1 oz------------	28	2	110	2	1	0.7	0.1	0.2
374	Grape-Nuts® (about 1/4 cup)--	1 oz------------	28	3	100	3	Tr	Tr	Tr	0.1
375	Honey Nut Cheerios® (about									
	3/4 cup)-----------------	1 oz------------	28	3	105	3	1	0.1	0.3	0.3
376	Lucky Charms® (about 1 cup)--	1 oz------------	28	3	110	3	1	0.2	0.4	0.4
377	Nature Valley® Granola (about									
	1/3 cup)-----------------	1 oz------------	28	4	125	3	5	3.3	0.7	0.7
378	100% Natural Cereal (about									
	1/4 cup)-----------------	1 oz------------	28	2	135	3	6	4.1	1.2	0.5
379	Product 19® (about 3/4 cup)--	1 oz------------	28	3	110	3	Tr	Tr	Tr	0.1
	Raisin Bran:									
380	Kellogg's® (about 3/4 cup)	1 oz------------	28	8	90	3	1	0.1	0.1	0.3
381	Post® (about 1/2 cup)------	1 oz------------	28	9	85	3	1	0.1	0.1	0.3
382	Rice Krispies® (about 1 cup)	1 oz------------	28	2	110	2	Tr	Tr	Tr	0.1
383	Shredded Wheat (about 2/3									
	cup)--------------------	1 oz------------	28	5	100	3	1	0.1	0.1	0.3
384	Special K® (about 1-1/3 cup)	1 oz------------	28	2	110	6	Tr	Tr	Tr	Tr
385	Super Sugar Crisp® (about 7/8									
	cup)--------------------	1 oz------------	28	2	105	2	Tr	Tr	Tr	0.1
386	Sugar Frosted Flakes,									
	Kellogg's® (about 3/4 cup)	1 oz------------	28	3	110	1	Tr	Tr	Tr	Tr
387	Sugar Smacks® (about 3/4 cup)	1 oz------------	28	3	105	2	1	0.1	0.1	0.2
388	Total® (about 1 cup)---------	1 oz------------	28	4	100	3	1	0.1	0.1	0.3
389	Trix® (about 1 cup)---------	1 oz------------	28	3	110	2	Tr	0.2	0.1	0.1
390	Wheaties® (about 1 cup)------	1 oz------------	28	5	100	3	Tr	0.1	Tr	0.2
391	Buckwheat flour, light, sifted---	1 cup-----------	98	12	340	6	1	0.2	0.4	0.4
392	Bulgur, uncooked-------------	1 cup-----------	170	10	600	19	3	1.2	0.3	1.2
	Cakes prepared from cake mixes with enriched flour:[35]									
	Angelfood:									
393	Whole cake, 9-3/4-in diam. tube cake------------------	1 cake----------	635	38	1,510	38	2	0.4	0.2	1.0
394	Piece, 1/12 of cake----------	1 piece---------	53	38	125	3	Tr	Tr	Tr	0.1
	Coffeecake, crumb:									
395	Whole cake, 7-3/4 by 5-5/8 by 1-1/4 in---------------	1 cake----------	430	30	1,385	27	41	11.8	16.7	9.6
396	Piece, 1/6 of cake----------	1 piece---------	72	30	230	5	7	2.0	2.8	1.6
	Devil's food with chocolate frosting:									
397	Whole, 2-layer cake, 8- or 9-in diam.-----------------	1 cake----------	1,107	24	3,755	49	136	55.6	51.4	19.7
398	Piece, 1/16 of cake----------	1 piece---------	69	24	235	3	8	3.5	3.2	1.2
399	Cupcake, 2-1/2-in diam.-------	1 cupcake-------	35	24	120	2	4	1.8	1.6	0.6
	Gingerbread:									
400	Whole cake, 8 in square------	1 cake----------	570	37	1,575	18	39	9.6	16.4	10.5
401	Piece, 1/9 of cake----------	1 piece---------	63	37	175	2	4	1.1	1.8	1.2

[27] Nutrient added.
[30] Value based on label declaration for added nutrients.

Table A-5 Nutritive Value of the Edible Part of Food (*Continued*)

Nutrients in Indicated Quantity

Cholesterol	Carbohydrate	Calcium	Phosphorus	Iron	Potassium	Sodium	Vitamin A value (IU)	Vitamin A value (RE)	Thiamin	Riboflavin	Niacin	Ascorbic acid	Item No.
Milligrams	Grams	Milligrams	Milligrams	Milligrams	Milligrams	Milligrams	International units	Retinol equivalents	Milligrams	Milligrams	Milligrams	Milligrams	
0	21	23	264	[30]4.5	350	320	[30]1,250	[30]375	[30]0.37	[30]0.43	[30]5.0	[30]15	365
0	23	5	36	[27]7.5	37	213	[30]40	[30]4	[27]0.50	[27]0.55	[27]6.6	[30]0	366
0	20	48	134	[30]4.5	101	307	[30]1,250	[30]375	[30]0.37	[30]0.43	[30]5.0	[30]15	367
0	24	1	18	[30]1.8	26	351	[30]1,250	[30]375	[30]0.37	[30]0.43	[30]5.0	[30]15	368
0	24	1	12	[27]0.7	33	297	[30]1,250	[30]375	[30]0.37	[30]0.43	[30]5.0	0	369
0	22	14	139	[30]8.1	180	264	[30]1,250	[30]375	[30]0.37	[30]0.43	[30]5.0	0	370
0	22	12	179	[30]4.5	151	260	[30]1,250	[30]375	[30]0.37	[30]0.43	[30]5.0	0	371
0	25	3	24	[30]4.5	26	145	[30]1,250	[30]375	[30]0.37	[30]0.43	[30]5.0	[30]15	372
Tr	24	17	41	[30]4.5	63	346	[30]1,250	[30]375	[30]0.37	[30]0.43	[30]5.0	[30]15	373
0	23	11	71	1.2	95	197	[30]1,250	[30]375	[30]0.37	[30]0.43	[30]5.0	0	374
0	23	20	105	[30]4.5	99	257	[30]1,250	[30]375	[30]0.37	[30]0.43	[30]5.0	[30]15	375
0	23	32	79	[30]4.5	59	201	[30]1,250	[30]375	[30]0.37	[30]0.43	[30]5.0	[30]15	376
0	19	18	89	0.9	98	58	20	2	0.10	0.05	0.2	0	377
Tr	18	49	104	0.8	140	12	20	2	0.09	0.15	0.6	0	378
0	24	3	40	[30]18.0	44	325	[30]5,000	[30]1,501	[30]1.50	[30]1.70	[30]20.0	[30]60	379
0	21	10	105	[30]3.5	147	207	[30]960	[30]288	[30]0.28	[30]0.34	[30]3.9	0	380
0	21	13	119	[30]4.5	175	185	[36]1,250	[30]375	[30]0.37	[30]0.43	[30]5.0	0	381
0	25	4	34	[30]1.8	29	340	[30]1,250	[30]375	[30]0.37	[30]0.43	[30]5.0	[30]15	382
0	23	11	100	1.2	102	3	0	0	0.07	0.08	1.5	0	383
Tr	21	8	55	[30]4.5	49	265	[30]1,250	[30]375	[30]0.37	[30]0.43	[30]5.0	[30]15	384
0	26	6	52	[30]1.8	105	25	[30]1,250	[30]375	[30]0.37	[30]0.43	[30]5.0	0	385
0	26	1	21	[30]1.8	18	230	[30]1,250	[30]375	[30]0.37	[30]0.43	[30]5.0	[30]15	386
0	25	3	31	[30]1.8	42	75	[30]1,250	[30]375	[30]0.37	[30]0.43	[30]5.0	[30]15	387
0	22	48	118	[30]18.0	106	352	[30]5,000	[30]1,501	[30]1.50	[30]1.70	[30]20.0	[30]60	388
0	25	6	19	[30]4.5	27	181	[30]1,250	[30]375	[30]0.37	[30]0.43	[30]5.0	[30]15	389
0	23	43	98	[30]4.5	106	354	[30]1,250	[30]375	[30]0.37	[30]0.43	[30]5.0	[30]15	390
0	78	11	86	1.0	314	2	0	0	0.08	0.04	0.4	0	391
0	129	49	575	9.5	389	7	0	0	0.48	0.24	7.7	0	392
0	342	527	1,086	2.7	845	3,226	0	0	0.32	1.27	1.6	0	393
0	29	44	91	0.2	71	269	0	0	0.03	0.11	0.1	0	394
279	225	262	748	7.3	469	1,853	690	194	0.82	0.90	7.7	1	395
47	38	44	125	1.2	78	310	120	32	0.14	0.15	1.3	Tr	396
598	645	653	1,162	22.1	1,439	2,900	1,660	498	1.11	1.66	10.0	1	397
37	40	41	72	1.4	90	181	100	31	0.07	0.10	0.6	Tr	398
19	20	21	37	0.7	46	92	50	16	0.04	0.05	0.3	Tr	399
6	291	513	570	10.8	1,562	1,733	0	0	0.86	1.03	7.4	1	400
1	32	57	63	1.2	173	192	0	0	0.09	0.11	0.8	Tr	401

[35] Excepting angelfood cake, cakes were made from mixes containing vegetable shortening and frostings were made with margarine.

Table A-5 Nutritive Value of the Edible Part of Food *(Continued)*

(Tr indicates nutrient present in trace amount.)

Item No.	Foods, approximate measures, units, and weight (weight of edible portion only)			Water	Food energy	Pro-tein	Fat	Fatty acids		
								Satu-rated	Mono-unsatu-rated	Poly-unsatu-rated
	Grain Products—Con.		Grams	Per-cent	Cal-ories	Grams	Grams	Grams	Grams	Grams
	Cakes prepared from cake mixes with enriched flour:[35]									
	Yellow with chocolate frosting:									
402	Whole, 2-layer cake, 8- or 9-in diam.	1 cake	1,108	26	3,735	45	125	47.8	48.8	21.8
403	Piece, 1/16 of cake	1 piece	69	26	235	3	8	3.0	3.0	1.4
	Cakes prepared from home recipes using enriched flour:									
	Carrot, with cream cheese frosting:[36]									
404	Whole cake, 10-in diam. tube cake	1 cake	1,536	23	6,175	63	328	66.0	135.2	107.5
405	Piece, 1/16 of cake	1 piece	96	23	385	4	21	4.1	8.4	6.7
	Fruitcake, dark:[36]									
406	Whole cake, 7-1/2-in diam., 2-1/4-in high tube cake	1 cake	1,361	18	5,185	74	228	47.6	113.0	51.7
407	Piece, 1/32 of cake, 2/3-in arc	1 piece	43	18	165	2	7	1.5	3.6	1.6
	Plain sheet cake:[37]									
	Without frosting:									
408	Whole cake, 9-in square	1 cake	777	25	2,830	35	108	29.5	45.1	25.6
409	Piece, 1/9 of cake	1 piece	86	25	315	4	12	3.3	5.0	2.8
	With uncooked white frosting:									
410	Whole cake, 9-in square	1 cake	1,096	21	4,020	37	129	41.6	50.4	26.3
411	Piece, 1/9 of cake	1 piece	121	21	445	4	14	4.6	5.6	2.9
	Pound:[38]									
412	Loaf, 8-1/2 by 3-1/2 by 3-1/4 in	1 loaf	514	22	2,025	33	94	21.1	40.9	26.7
413	Slice, 1/17 of loaf	1 slice	30	22	120	2	5	1.2	2.4	1.6
	Cakes, commercial, made with en-riched flour:									
	Pound:									
414	Loaf, 8-1/2 by 3-1/2 by 3 in	1 loaf	500	24	1,935	26	94	52.0	30.0	4.0
415	Slice, 1/17 of loaf	1 slice	29	24	110	2	5	3.0	1.7	0.2
	Snack cakes:									
416	Devil's food with creme filling (2 small cakes per pkg)	1 small cake	28	20	105	1	4	1.7	1.5	0.6
417	Sponge with creme filling (2 small cakes per pkg)	1 small cake	42	19	155	1	5	2.3	2.1	0.5
	White with white frosting:									
418	Whole, 2-layer cake, 8- or 9-in diam.	1 cake	1,140	24	4,170	43	148	33.1	61.6	42.2
419	Piece, 1/16 of cake	1 piece	71	24	260	3	9	2.1	3.8	2.6
	Yellow with chocolate frosting:									
420	Whole, 2-layer cake, 8- or 9-in diam.	1 cake	1,108	23	3,895	40	175	92.0	58.7	10.0
421	Piece, 1/16 of cake	1 piece	69	23	245	2	11	5.7	3.7	0.6
	Cheesecake:									
422	Whole cake, 9-in diam.	1 cake	1,110	46	3,350	60	213	119.9	65.5	14.4
423	Piece, 1/12 of cake	1 piece	92	46	280	5	18	9.9	5.4	1.2
	Cookies made with enriched flour:									
	Brownies with nuts:									
424	Commercial, with frosting, 1-1/2 by 1-3/4 by 7/8 in	1 brownie	25	13	100	1	4	1.6	2.0	0.6
425	From home recipe, 1-3/4 by 1-3/4 by 7/8 in[36]	1 brownie	20	10	95	1	6	1.4	2.8	1.2
	Chocolate chip:									
426	Commercial, 2-1/4-in diam., 3/8 in thick	4 cookies	42	4	180	2	9	2.9	3.1	2.6

[35] Excepting angelfood cake, cakes were made from mixes containing vegetable shortening and frostings were made with margarine.
[36] Made with vegetable oil.

Table A-5 Nutritive Value of the Edible Part of Food *(Continued)*

Nutrients in Indicated Quantity

Cho-les-terol	Carbo-hydrate	Calcium	Phos-phorus	Iron	Potas-sium	Sodium	Vitamin A value (IU)	Vitamin A value (RE)	Thiamin	Ribo-flavin	Niacin	Ascorbic acid	Item No.
Milli-grams	Grams	Milli-grams	Milli-grams	Milli-grams	Milli-grams	Milli-grams	Inter-national units	Retinol equiva-lents	Milli-grams	Milli-grams	Milli-grams	Milli-grams	
576	638	1,008	2,017	15.5	1,208	2,515	1,550	465	1.22	1.66	11.1	1	402
36	40	63	126	1.0	75	157	100	29	0.08	0.10	0.7	Tr	403
1183	775	707	998	21.0	1,720	4,470	2,240	246	1.83	1.97	14.7	23	404
74	48	44	62	1.3	108	279	140	15	0.11	0.12	0.9	1	405
640	783	1,293	1,592	37.6	6,138	2,123	1,720	422	2.41	2.55	17.0	504	406
20	25	41	50	1.2	194	67	50	13	0.08	0.08	0.5	16	407
552	434	497	793	11.7	614	2,331	1,320	373	1.24	1.40	10.1	2	408
61	48	55	88	1.3	68	258	150	41	0.14	0.15	1.1	Tr	409
636	694	548	822	11.0	669	2,488	2,190	647	1.21	1.42	9.9	2	410
70	77	61	91	1.2	74	275	240	71	0.13	0.16	1.1	Tr	411
555	265	339	473	9.3	483	1,645	3,470	1,033	0.93	1.08	7.8	1	412
32	15	20	28	0.5	28	96	200	60	0.05	0.06	0.5	Tr	413
1100	257	146	517	8.0	443	1,857	2,820	715	0.96	1.12	8.1	0	414
64	15	8	30	0.5	26	108	160	41	0.06	0.06	0.5	0	415
15	17	21	26	1.0	34	105	20	4	0.06	0.09	0.7	0	416
7	27	14	44	0.6	37	155	30	9	0.07	0.06	0.6	0	417
46	670	536	1,585	15.5	832	2,827	640	194	3.19	2.05	27.6	0	418
3	42	33	99	1.0	52	176	40	12	0.20	0.13	1.7	0	419
609	620	366	1,884	19.9	1,972	3,080	1,850	488	0.78	2.22	10.0	0	420
38	39	23	117	1.2	123	192	120	30	0.05	0.14	0.6	0	421
2053	317	622	977	5.3	1,088	2,464	2,820	833	0.33	1.44	5.1	56	422
170	26	52	81	0.4	90	204	230	69	0.03	0.12	0.4	5	423
14	16	13	26	0.6	50	59	70	18	0.08	0.07	0.3	Tr	424
18	11	9	26	0.4	35	51	20	6	0.05	0.05	0.3	Tr	425
5	28	13	41	0.8	68	140	50	15	0.10	0.23	1.0	Tr	426

[37]Cake made with vegetable shortening; frosting with margarine.
[38]Made with margarine.

Table A-5 Nutritive Value of the Edible Part of Food *(Continued)*

(Tr indicates nutrient present in trace amount.)

Item No.	Foods, approximate measures, units, and weight (weight of edible portion only)		Water	Food energy	Protein	Fat	Fatty acids Saturated	Monounsaturated	Polyunsaturated
		Grams	Percent	Calories	Grams	Grams	Grams	Grams	Grams
	Grain Products—Con.								
	Cookies made with enriched flour:								
	Chocolate chip:								
427	From home recipe, 2-1/3-in diam.[25]	4 cookies-------	40	3	185	2	11	3.9	4.3	2.0
428	From refrigerated dough, 2-1/4-in diam., 3/8 in thick	4 cookies-------	48	5	225	2	11	4.0	4.4	2.0
429	Fig bars, square, 1-5/8 by 1-5/8 by 3/8 in or rectangular, 1-1/2 by 1-3/4 by 1/2 in	4 cookies-------	56	12	210	2	4	1.0	1.5	1.0
430	Oatmeal with raisins, 2-5/8-in diam., 1/4 in thick----------	4 cookies-------	52	4	245	3	10	2.5	4.5	2.8
431	Peanut butter cookie, from home recipe, 2-5/8-in diam.[25] -----	4 cookies-------	48	3	245	4	14	4.0	5.8	2.8
432	Sandwich type (chocolate or vanilla), 1-3/4-in diam., 3/8 in thick---------------	4 cookies-------	40	2	195	2	8	2.0	3.6	2.2
	Shortbread:								
433	Commercial--------------------	4 small cookies	32	6	155	2	8	2.9	3.0	1.1
434	From home recipe[38] -----------	2 large cookies	28	3	145	2	8	1.3	2.7	3.4
435	Sugar cookie, from refrigerated dough, 2-1/2-in diam., 1/4 in thick-----------------------	4 cookies-------	48	4	235	2	12	2.3	5.0	3.6
436	Vanilla wafers, 1-3/4-in diam., 1/4 in thick-----------------	10 cookies------	40	4	185	2	7	1.8	3.0	1.8
437	Corn chips-----------------------	1-oz package----	28	1	155	2	9	1.4	2.4	3.7
	Cornmeal:								
438	Whole-ground, unbolted, dry form---------------------	1 cup-----------	122	12	435	11	5	0.5	1.1	2.5
439	Bolted (nearly whole-grain), dry form---------------	1 cup-----------	122	12	440	11	4	0.5	0.9	2.2
	Degermed, enriched:								
440	Dry form--------------------	1 cup-----------	138	12	500	11	2	0.2	0.4	0.9
441	Cooked---------------------	1 cup-----------	240	88	120	3	Tr	Tr	0.1	0.2
	Crackers:[39]								
	Cheese:								
442	Plain, 1 in square-----------	10 crackers-----	10	4	50	1	3	0.9	1.2	0.3
443	Sandwich type (peanut butter)	1 sandwich------	8	3	40	1	2	0.4	0.8	0.3
444	Graham, plain, 2-1/2 in square	2 crackers------	14	5	60	1	1	0.4	0.6	0.4
445	Melba toast, plain-------------	1 piece--------	5	4	20	1	Tr	0.1	0.1	0.1
446	Rye wafers, whole-grain, 1-7/8 by 3-1/2 in	2 wafers--------	14	5	55	1	1	0.3	0.4	0.3
447	Saltines[40] ---------------------	4 crackers------	12	4	50	1	1	0.5	0.4	0.2
448	Snack-type, standard-----------	1 round cracker	3	3	15	Tr	1	0.2	0.4	0.1
449	Wheat, thin--------------------	4 crackers------	8	3	35	1	1	0.5	0.5	0.4
450	Whole-wheat wafers--------------	2 crackers------	8	4	35	1	2	0.5	0.6	0.4
451	Croissants, made with enriched flour, 4-1/2 by 4 by 1-3/4 in--	1 croissant-----	57	22	235	5	12	3.5	6.7	1.4
	Danish pastry, made with enriched flour:								
	Plain without fruit or nuts:								
452	Packaged ring, 12 oz-------	1 ring----------	340	27	1,305	21	71	21.8	28.6	15.6
453	Round piece, about 4-1/4-in diam., 1 in high-----------	1 pastry--------	57	27	220	4	12	3.6	4.8	2.6
454	Ounce------------------------	1 oz-----------	28	27	110	2	6	1.8	2.4	1.3
455	Fruit, round piece-------------	1 pastry--------	65	30	235	4	13	3.9	5.2	2.9
	Doughnuts, made with enriched flour:								
456	Cake type, plain, 3-1/4-in diam., 1 in high-----------	1 doughnut------	50	21	210	3	12	2.8	5.0	3.0
457	Yeast-leavened, glazed, 3-3/4-in diam., 1-1/4 in high------	1 doughnut------	60	27	235	4	13	5.2	5.5	0.9
458	English muffins, plain, enriched	1 muffin--------	57	42	140	5	1	0.3	0.2	0.3
459	Toasted---------------------------	1 muffin--------	50	29	140	5	1	0.3	0.2	0.3

[25]Made with vegetable shortening.
[38]Made with margarine.

Table A-5 Nutritive Value of the Edible Part of Food *(Continued)*

Nutrients in Indicated Quantity

Cho-les-terol	Carbo-hydrate	Calcium	Phos-phorus	Iron	Potas-sium	Sodium	Vitamin A value		Thiamin	Ribo-flavin	Niacin	Ascorbic acid	Item No.
							(IU)	(RE)					
Milli-grams	Grams	Milli-grams	Milli-grams	Milli-grams	Milli-grams	Milli-grams	Inter-national units	Retinol equiva-lents	Milli-grams	Milli-grams	Milli-grams	Milli-grams	
18	26	13	34	1.0	82	82	20	5	0.06	0.06	0.6	0	427
22	32	13	34	1.0	62	173	30	8	0.06	0.10	0.9	0	428
27	42	40	34	1.4	162	180	60	6	0.08	0.07	0.7	Tr	429
2	36	18	58	1.1	90	148	40	12	0.09	0.08	1.0	0	430
22	28	21	60	1.1	110	142	20	5	0.07	0.07	1.9	0	431
0	29	12	40	1.4	66	189	0	0	0.09	0.07	0.8	0	432
27	20	13	39	0.8	38	123	30	8	0.10	0.09	0.9	0	433
0	17	6	31	0.6	18	125	300	89	0.08	0.06	0.7	Tr	434
29	31	50	91	0.9	33	261	40	11	0.09	0.06	1.1	0	435
25	29	16	36	0.8	50	150	50	14	0.07	0.10	1.0	0	436
0	16	35	52	0.5	52	233	110	11	0.04	0.05	0.4	1	437
0	90	24	312	2.2	346	1	620	62	0.46	0.13	2.4	0	438
0	91	21	272	2.2	303	1	590	59	0.37	0.10	2.3	0	439
0	108	8	137	5.9	166	1	610	61	0.61	0.36	4.8	0	440
0	26	2	34	1.4	38	0	140	14	0.14	0.10	1.2	0	441
6	6	11	17	0.3	17	112	20	5	0.05	0.04	0.4	0	442
1	5	7	25	0.3	17	90	Tr	Tr	0.04	0.03	0.6	0	443
0	11	6	20	0.4	36	86	0	0	0.02	0.03	0.6	0	444
0	4	6	10	0.1	11	44	0	0	0.01	0.01	0.1	0	445
0	10	7	44	0.5	65	115	0	0	0.06	0.03	0.5	0	446
4	9	3	12	0.5	17	165	0	0	0.06	0.05	0.6	0	447
0	2	2	6	0.1	4	30	Tr	Tr	0.01	0.01	0.1	0	448
0	5	3	15	0.3	17	69	Tr	Tr	0.04	0.03	0.4	0	449
0	5	3	22	0.2	31	59	0	0	0.02	0.03	0.4	0	450
13	27	20	64	2.1	68	452	50	13	0.17	0.13	1.3	0	451
292	152	360	347	6.5	316	1,302	360	99	0.95	1.02	8.5	Tr	452
49	26	60	58	1.1	53	218	60	17	0.16	0.17	1.4	Tr	453
24	13	30	29	0.5	26	109	30	8	0.08	0.09	0.7	Tr	454
56	28	17	80	1.3	57	233	40	11	0.16	0.14	1.4	Tr	455
20	24	22	111	1.0	58	192	20	5	0.12	0.12	1.1	Tr	456
21	26	17	55	1.4	64	222	Tr	Tr	0.28	0.12	1.8	0	457
0	27	96	67	1.7	331	378	0	0	0.26	0.19	2.2	0	458
0	27	96	67	1.7	331	378	0	0	0.23	0.19	2.2	0	459

[39] Crackers made with enriched flour except for rye wafers and whole-wheat wafers.
[40] Made with lard.

Table A-5 Nutritive Value of the Edible Part of Food *(Continued)*

(Tr indicates nutrient present in trace amount.)

Item No.	Foods, approximate measures, units, and weight (weight of edible portion only)		Water	Food energy	Pro-tein	Fat	Satu-rated	Mono-unsatu-rated	Poly-unsatu-rated
		Grams	Per-cent	Cal-ories	Grams	Grams	Grams	Grams	Grams
	Grain Products—Con.								
460	French toast, from home recipe--- 1 slice---------	65	53	155	6	7	1.6	2.0	1.6
	Macaroni, enriched, cooked (cut lengths, elbows, shells):								
461	Firm stage (hot)--------------- 1 cup-----------	130	64	190	7	1	0.1	0.1	0.3
	Tender stage:								
462	Cold------------------------ 1 cup-----------	105	72	115	4	Tr	0.1	0.1	0.2
463	Hot------------------------- 1 cup-----------	140	72	155	5	1	0.1	0.1	0.2
	Muffins made with enriched flour, 2-1/2-in diam., 1-1/2 in high:								
	From home recipe:								
464	Blueberry [25]----------------- 1 muffin--------	45	37	135	3	5	1.5	2.1	1.2
465	Bran [36] ---------------------- 1 muffin--------	45	35	125	3	6	1.4	1.6	2.3
466	Corn (enriched, degermed cornmeal and flour) [25] ------ 1 muffin--------	45	33	145	3	5	1.5	2.2	1.4
	From commercial mix (egg and water added):								
467	Blueberry-------------------- 1 muffin--------	45	33	140	3	5	1.4	2.0	1.2
468	Bran------------------------ 1 muffin--------	45	28	140	3	4	1.3	1.6	1.0
469	Corn------------------------ 1 muffin--------	45	30	145	3	6	1.7	2.3	1.4
470	Noodles (egg noodles), enriched, cooked------------------------ 1 cup-----------	160	70	200	7	2	0.5	0.6	0.6
471	Noodles, chow mein, canned------- 1 cup-----------	45	11	220	6	11	2.1	7.3	0.4
	Pancakes, 4-in diam.:								
472	Buckwheat, from mix (with buck-wheat and enriched flours), egg and milk added----------- 1 pancake-------	27	58	55	2	2	0.9	0.9	0.5
	Plain:								
473	From home recipe using enriched flour------------- 1 pancake-------	27	50	60	2	2	0.5	0.8	0.5
474	From mix (with enriched flour), egg, milk, and oil added--------------------- 1 pancake-------	27	54	60	2	2	0.5	0.9	0.5
	Piecrust, made with enriched flour and vegetable shorten-ing, baked:								
475	From home recipe, 9-in diam.--- 1 pie shell-----	180	15	900	11	60	14.8	25.9	15.7
476	From mix, 9-in diam.----------- Piecrust for 2-crust pie-----	320	19	1,485	20	93	22.7	41.0	25.0
	Pies, piecrust made with enriched flour, vegetable shortening, 9-in diam.:								
	Apple:								
477	Whole----------------------- 1 pie-----------	945	48	2,420	21	105	27.4	44.4	26.5
478	Piece, 1/6 of pie------------ 1 piece---------	158	48	405	3	18	4.6	7.4	4.4
	Blueberry:								
479	Whole----------------------- 1 pie-----------	945	51	2,285	23	102	25.5	44.4	27.4
480	Piece, 1/6 of pie------------ 1 piece---------	158	51	380	4	17	4.3	7.4	4.6
	Cherry:								
481	Whole----------------------- 1 pie-----------	945	47	2,465	25	107	28.4	46.3	27.4
482	Piece, 1/6 of pie------------ 1 piece---------	158	47	410	4	18	4.7	7.7	4.6
	Creme:								
483	Whole----------------------- 1 pie-----------	910	43	2,710	20	139	90.1	23.7	6.4
484	Piece, 1/6 of pie------------ 1 piece---------	152	43	455	3	23	15.0	4.0	1.1
	Custard:								
485	Whole----------------------- 1 pie-----------	910	58	1,985	56	101	33.7	40.0	19.1
486	Piece, 1/6 of pie------------ 1 piece---------	152	58	330	9	17	5.6	6.7	3.2
	Lemon meringue:								
487	Whole----------------------- 1 pie-----------	840	47	2,140	31	86	26.0	34.4	17.6
488	Piece, 1/6 of pie------------ 1 piece---------	140	47	355	5	14	4.3	5.7	2.9
	Peach:								
489	Whole----------------------- 1 pie-----------	945	48	2,410	24	101	24.6	43.5	26.5
490	Piece, 1/6 of pie------------ 1 piece---------	158	48	405	4	17	4.1	7.3	4.4

[25] Made with vegetable shortening.

Table A-5 Nutritive Value of the Edible Part of Food *(Continued)*

Nutrients in Indicated Quantity

Cho-les-terol	Carbo-hydrate	Calcium	Phos-phorus	Iron	Potas-sium	Sodium	Vitamin A value (IU)	Vitamin A value (RE)	Thiamin	Ribo-flavin	Niacin	Ascorbic acid	Item No.
Milli-grams	Grams	Milli-grams	Milli-grams	Milli-grams	Milli-grams	Milli-grams	Inter-national units	Retinol equiva-lents	Milli-grams	Milli-grams	Milli-grams	Milli-grams	
112	17	72	85	1.3	86	257	110	32	0.12	0.16	1.0	Tr	460
0	39	14	85	2.1	103	1	0	0	0.23	0.13	1.8	0	461
0	24	8	53	1.3	64	1	0	0	0.15	0.08	1.2	0	462
0	32	11	70	1.7	85	1	0	0	0.20	0.11	1.5	0	463
19	20	54	46	0.9	47	198	40	9	0.10	0.11	0.9	1	464
24	19	60	125	1.4	99	189	230	30	0.11	0.13	1.3	3	465
23	21	66	59	0.9	57	169	80	15	0.11	0.11	0.9	Tr	466
45	22	15	90	0.9	54	225	50	11	0.10	0.17	1.1	Tr	467
28	24	27	182	1.7	50	385	100	14	0.08	0.12	1.9	0	468
42	22	30	128	1.3	31	291	90	16	0.09	0.09	0.8	Tr	469
50	37	16	94	2.6	70	3	110	34	0.22	0.13	1.9	0	470
5	26	14	41	0.4	33	450	0	0	0.05	0.03	0.6	0	471
20	6	59	91	0.4	66	125	60	17	0.04	0.05	0.2	Tr	472
16	9	27	38	0.5	33	115	30	10	0.06	0.07	0.5	Tr	473
16	8	36	71	0.7	43	160	30	7	0.09	0.12	0.8	Tr	474
0	79	25	90	4.5	90	1,100	-0	0	0.54	0.40	5.0	0	475
0	141	131	272	9.3	179	2,602	0	0	1.06	0.80	9.9	0	476
0	360	76	208	9.5	756	2,844	280	28	1.04	0.76	9.5	9	477
0	60	13	35	1.6	126	476	50	5	0.17	0.13	1.6	2	478
0	330	104	217	12.3	945	2,533	850	85	1.04	0.85	10.4	38	479
0	55	17	36	2.1	158	423	140	14	0.17	0.14	1.7	6	480
0	363	132	236	9.5	992	2,873	4,160	416	1.13	0.85	9.5	0	481
0	61	22	40	1.6	166	480	700	70	0.19	0.14	1.6	0	482
46	351	273	919	6.8	796	2,207	1,250	391	0.36	0.89	6.4	0	483
8	59	46	154	1.1	133	369	210	65	0.06	0.15	1.1	0	484
1010	213	874	1,028	9.1	1,247	2,612	2,090	573	0.82	1.91	5.5	0	485
169	36	146	172	1.5	208	436	350	96	0.14	0.32	0.9	0	486
857	317	118	412	8.4	420	2,369	1,430	395	0.59	0.84	5.0	25	487
143	53	20	69	1.4	70	395	240	66	0.10	0.14	0.8	4	488
0	361	95	274	11.3	1,408	2,533	6,900	690	1.04	0.95	14.2	28	489
0	60	16	46	1.9	235	423	1,150	115	0.17	0.16	2.4	5	490

[36] Made with vegetable oil.

Table A-5 Nutritive Value of the Edible Part of Food *(Continued)*

(Tr indicates nutrient present in trace amount.)

Item No.	Foods, approximate measures, units, and weight (weight of edible portion only)		Grams	Water	Food energy	Pro-tein	Fat	Satu-rated	Mono-unsatu-rated	Poly-unsatu-rated
			Grams	Per-cent	Cal-ories	Grams	Grams	Grams	Grams	Grams
	Grain Products—Con.									
	Pies, piecrust made with enriched flour, vegetable shortening, 9-inch diam.:									
	Pecan:									
491	Whole------------------------	1 pie-----------	825	20	3,450	42	189	28.1	101.5	47.0
492	Piece, 1/6 of pie------------	1 piece---------	138	20	575	7	32	4.7	17.0	7.9
	Pumpkin:									
493	Whole------------------------	1 pie-----------	910	59	1,920	36	102	38.2	40.0	18.2
494	Piece, 1/6 of pie------------	1 piece---------	152	59	320	6	17	6.4	6.7	3.0
	Pies, fried:									
495	Apple------------------------	1 pie-----------	85	43	255	2	14	5.8	6.6	0.6
496	Cherry-----------------------	1 pie-----------	85	42	250	2	14	5.8	6.7	0.6
	Popcorn, popped:									
497	Air-popped, unsalted-----------	1 cup-----------	8	4	30	1	Tr	Tr	0.1	0.2
498	Popped in vegetable oil, salted	1 cup-----------	11	3	55	1	3	0.5	1.4	1.2
499	Sugar syrup coated-------------	1 cup-----------	35	4	135	2	1	0.1	0.3	0.6
	Pretzels, made with enriched flour:									
500	Stick, 2-1/4 in long----------	10 pretzels-----	3	3	10	Tr	Tr	Tr	Tr	Tr
501	Twisted, dutch, 2-3/4 by 2-5/8 in-------------------------	1 pretzel-------	16	3	65	2	1	0.1	0.2	0.2
502	Twisted, thin, 3-1/4 by 2-1/4 by 1/4 in--------------------	10 pretzels-----	60	3	240	6	2	0.4	0.8	0.6
	Rice:									
503	Brown, cooked, served hot------	1 cup-----------	195	70	230	5	1	0.3	0.3	0.4
	White, enriched:									
	Commercial varieties, all types:									
504	Raw-----------------------	1 cup-----------	185	12	670	12	1	0.2	0.2	0.3
505	Cooked, served hot---------	1 cup-----------	205	73	225	4	Tr	0.1	0.1	0.1
506	Instant, ready-to-serve, hot	1 cup-----------	165	73	180	4	0	0.1	0.1	0.1
	Parboiled:									
507	Raw-----------------------	1 cup-----------	185	10	685	14	1	0.1	0.1	0.2
508	Cooked, served hot---------	1 cup-----------	175	73	185	4	Tr	Tr	Tr	0.1
	Rolls, enriched:									
	Commercial:									
509	Dinner, 2-1/2-in diam., 2 in high----------------------	1 roll----------	28	32	85	2	2	0.5	0.8	0.6
510	Frankfurter and hamburger (8 per 11-1/2-oz pkg.)---------	1 roll----------	40	34	115	3	2	0.5	0.8	0.6
511	Hard, 3-3/4-in diam., 2 in high----------------------	1 roll----------	50	25	155	5	2	0.4	0.5	0.6
512	Hoagie or submarine, 11-1/2 by 3 by 2-1/2 in------------	1 roll----------	135	31	400	11	8	1.8	3.0	2.2
	From home recipe:									
513	Dinner, 2-1/2-in diam., 2 in high----------------------	1 roll----------	35	26	120	3	3	0.8	1.2	0.9
	Spaghetti, enriched, cooked:									
514	Firm stage, "al dente," served hot-------------------------	1 cup-----------	130	64	190	7	1	0.1	0.1	0.3
515	Tender stage, served hot-------	1 cup-----------	140	73	155	5	1	0.1	0.1	0.2
516	Toaster pastries-----------------	1 pastry--------	54	13	210	2	6	1.7	3.6	0.4
517	Tortillas, corn------------------	1 tortilla------	30	45	65	2	1	0.1	0.3	0.6
	Waffles, made with enriched flour, 7-in diam.:									
518	From home recipe--------------	1 waffle--------	75	37	245	7	13	4.0	4.9	2.6
519	From mix, egg and milk added---	1 waffle--------	75	42	205	7	8	2.7	2.9	1.5
	Wheat flours:									
	All-purpose or family flour, enriched:									
520	Sifted, spooned--------------	1 cup-----------	115	12	420	12	1	0.2	0.1	0.5
521	Unsifted, spooned------------	1 cup-----------	125	12	455	13	1	0.2	0.1	0.5
522	Cake or pastry flour, enriched, sifted, spooned--------------	1 cup-----------	96	12	350	7	1	0.1	0.1	0.3
523	Self-rising, enriched, unsifted, spooned-----------	1 cup-----------	125	12	440	12	1	0.2	0.1	0.5
524	Whole-wheat, from hard wheats, stirred---------------------	1 cup-----------	120	12	400	16	2	0.3	0.3	1.1

Table A-5 Nutritive Value of the Edible Part of Food *(Continued)*

Nutrients in Indicated Quantity

Cho-les-terol	Carbo-hydrate	Calcium	Phos-phorus	Iron	Potas-sium	Sodium	Vitamin A value		Thiamin	Ribo-flavin	Niacin	Ascorbic acid	Item No.
							(IU)	(RE)					
Milli-grams	Grams	Milli-grams	Milli-grams	Milli-grams	Milli-grams	Milli-grams	Inter-national units	Retinol equiva-lents	Milli-grams	Milli-grams	Milli-grams	Milli-grams	
569	423	388	850	27.2	1,015	1,823	1,320	322	1.82	0.99	6.6	0	491
95	71	65	142	4.6	170	305	220	54	0.30	0.17	1.1	0	492
655	223	464	628	8.2	1,456	1,947	22,480	2,493	0.82	1.27	7.3	0	493
109	37	78	105	1.4	243	325	3,750	416	0.14	0.21	1.2	0	494
14	31	12	34	0.9	42	326	30	3	0.09	0.06	1.0	1	495
13	32	11	41	0.7	61	371	190	19	0.06	0.06	0.6	1	496
0	6	1	22	0.2	20	Tr	10	1	0.03	0.01	0.2	0	497
0	6	3	31	0.3	19	86	20	2	0.01	0.02	0.1	0	498
0	30	2	47	0.5	90	Tr	30	3	0.13	0.02	0.4	0	499
0	2	1	3	0.1	3	48	0	0	0.01	0.01	0.1	0	500
0	13	4	15	0.3	16	258	0	0	0.05	0.04	0.7	0	501
0	48	16	55	1.2	61	966	0	0	0.19	0.15	2.6	0	502
0	50	23	142	1.0	137	0	0	0	0.18	0.04	2.7	0	503
0	149	44	174	5.4	170	9	0	0	0.81	0.06	6.5	0	504
0	50	21	57	1.8	57	0	0	0	0.23	0.02	2.1	0	505
0	40	5	31	1.3	0	0	0	0	0.21	0.02	1.7	0	506
0	150	111	370	5.4	278	17	0	0	0.81	0.07	6.5	0	507
0	41	33	100	1.4	75	0	0	0	0.19	0.02	2.1	0	508
Tr	14	33	44	0.8	36	155	Tr	Tr	0.14	0.09	1.1	Tr	509
Tr	20	54	44	1.2	56	241	Tr	Tr	0.20	0.13	1.6	Tr	510
Tr	30	24	46	1.4	49	313	0	0	0.20	0.12	1.7	0	511
Tr	72	100	115	3.8	128	683	0	0	0.54	0.33	4.5	0	512
12	20	16	36	1.1	41	98	30	8	0.12	0.12	1.2	0	513
0	39	14	85	2.0	103	1	0	0	0.23	0.13	1.8	0	514
0	32	11	70	1.7	85	1	0	0	0.20	0.11	1.5	0	515
0	38	104	104	2.2	91	248	520	52	0.17	0.18	2.3	4	516
0	13	42	55	0.6	43	1	80	8	0.05	0.03	0.4	0	517
102	26	154	135	1.5	129	445	140	39	0.18	0.24	1.5	Tr	518
59	27	179	257	1.2	146	515	170	49	0.14	0.23	0.9	Tr	519
0	88	18	100	5.1	109	2	0	0	0.73	0.46	6.1	0	520
0	95	20	109	5.5	119	3	0	0	0.80	0.50	6.6	0	521
0	76	16	70	4.2	91	2	0	0	0.58	0.38	5.1	0	522
0	93	331	583	5.5	113	1,349	0	0	0.80	0.50	6.6	0	523
0	85	49	446	5.2	444	4	0	0	0.66	0.14	5.2	0	524

Table A-5 Nutritive Value of the Edible Part of Food (Continued)

(Tr indicates nutrient present in trace amount.)

Item No.	Foods, approximate measures, units, and weight (weight of edible portion only)		Grams	Water Per-cent	Food energy Cal-ories	Pro-tein Grams	Fat Grams	Saturated Grams	Mono-unsaturated Grams	Poly-unsaturated Grams
	Legumes, Nuts, and Seeds									
	Almonds, shelled:									
525	Slivered, packed---------------	1 cup-----------	135	4	795	27	70	6.7	45.8	14.8
526	Whole-------------------------	1 oz-----------	28	4	165	6	15	1.4	9.6	3.1
	Beans, dry:									
	Cooked, drained:									
527	Black-----------------------	1 cup-----------	171	66	225	15	1	0.1	0.1	0.5
528	Great Northern---------------	1 cup-----------	180	69	210	14	1	0.1	0.1	0.6
529	Lima------------------------	1 cup-----------	190	64	260	16	1	0.2	0.1	0.5
530	Pea (navy)-------------------	1 cup-----------	190	69	225	15	1	0.1	0.1	0.7
531	Pinto-----------------------	1 cup-----------	180	65	265	15	1	0.1	0.1	0.5
	Canned, solids and liquid:									
	White with:									
532	Frankfurters (sliced)------	1 cup-----------	255	71	365	19	18	7.4	8.8	0.7
533	Pork and tomato sauce------	1 cup-----------	255	71	310	16	7	2.4	2.7	0.7
534	Pork and sweet sauce-------	1 cup-----------	255	66	385	16	12	4.3	4.9	1.2
535	Red kidney-------------------	1 cup-----------	255	76	230	15	1	0.1	0.1	0.6
536	Black-eyed peas, dry, cooked (with residual cooking liquid)	1 cup-----------	250	80	190	13	1	0.2	Tr	0.3
537	Brazil nuts, shelled-------------	1 oz-----------	28	3	185	4	19	4.6	6.5	6.8
538	Carob flour-------------------	1 cup-----------	140	3	255	6	Tr	Tr	0.1	0.1
	Cashew nuts, salted:									
539	Dry roasted--------------------	1 cup-----------	137	2	785	21	63	12.5	37.4	10.7
540		1 oz-----------	28	2	165	4	13	2.6	7.7	2.2
541	Roasted in oil----------------	1 cup-----------	130	4	750	21	63	12.4	36.9	10.6
542		1 oz-----------	28	4	165	5	14	2.7	8.1	2.3
543	Chestnuts, European (Italian), roasted, shelled---------------	1 cup-----------	143	40	350	5	3	0.6	1.1	1.2
544	Chickpeas, cooked, drained-------	1 cup-----------	163	60	270	15	4	0.4	0.9	1.9
	Coconut:									
	Raw:									
545	Piece, about 2 by 2 by 1/2 in	1 piece---------	45	47	160	1	15	13.4	0.6	0.2
546	Shredded or grated-----------	1 cup-----------	80	47	285	3	27	23.8	1.1	0.3
547	Dried, sweetened, shredded-----	1 cup-----------	93	13	470	3	33	29.3	1.4	0.4
548	Filberts (hazelnuts), chopped----	1 cup-----------	115	5	725	15	72	5.3	56.5	6.9
549		1 oz-----------	28	5	180	4	18	1.3	13.9	1.7
550	Lentils, dry, cooked-------------	1 cup-----------	200	72	215	16	1	0.1	0.2	0.5
551	Macadamia nuts, roasted in oil, salted------------------------	1 cup-----------	134	2	960	10	103	15.4	80.9	1.8
552		1 oz-----------	28	2	205	2	22	3.2	17.1	0.4
	Mixed nuts, with peanuts, salted:									
553	Dry roasted--------------------	1 oz-----------	28	2	170	5	15	2.0	8.9	3.1
554	Roasted in oil----------------	1 oz-----------	28	2	175	5	16	2.5	9.0	3.8
555	Peanuts, roasted in oil, salted--	1 cup-----------	145	2	840	39	71	9.9	35.5	22.6
556		1 oz-----------	28	2	165	8	14	1.9	6.9	4.4
557	Peanut butter-------------------	1 tbsp----------	16	1	95	5	8	1.4	4.0	2.5
558	Peas, split, dry, cooked---------	1 cup-----------	200	70	230	16	1	0.1	0.1	0.3
559	Pecans, halves-------------------	1 cup-----------	108	5	720	8	73	5.9	45.5	18.1
560		1 oz-----------	28	5	190	2	19	1.5	12.0	4.7
561	Pine nuts (pinyons), shelled-----	1 oz-----------	28	6	160	3	17	2.7	6.5	7.3
562	Pistachio nuts, dried, shelled---	1 oz-----------	28	4	165	6	14	1.7	9.3	2.1
563	Pumpkin and squash kernels, dry, hulled-------------------------	1 oz-----------	28	7	155	7	13	2.5	4.0	5.9
564	Refried beans, canned-----------	1 cup-----------	290	72	295	18	3	0.4	0.6	1.4
565	Sesame seeds, dry, hulled--------	1 tbsp----------	8	5	45	2	4	0.6	1.7	1.9
566	Soybeans, dry, cooked, drained---	1 cup-----------	180	71	235	20	10	1.3	1.9	5.3
	Soy products:									
567	Miso--------------------------	1 cup-----------	276	53	470	29	13	1.8	2.6	7.3
568	Tofu, piece 2-1/2 by 2-3/4 by 1 in-----------------------	1 piece---------	120	85	85	9	5	0.7	1.0	2.9
569	Sunflower seeds, dry, hulled-----	1 oz-----------	28	5	160	6	14	1.5	2.7	9.3
570	Tahini-------------------------	1 tbsp----------	15	3	90	3	8	1.1	3.0	3.5

[41] Cashews without salt contain 21 mg sodium per cup or 4 mg per oz.
[42] Cashews without salt contain 22 mg sodium per cup or 5 mg per oz.
[43] Macadamia nuts without salt contain 9 mg sodium per cup or 2 mg per oz.

Table A-5 Nutritive Value of the Edible Part of Food *(Continued)*

							Vitamin A value						
Cho-les-terol	Carbo-hydrate	Calcium	Phos-phorus	Iron	Potas-sium	Sodium	(IU)	(RE)	Thiamin	Ribo-flavin	Niacin	Ascorbic acid	Item No.
Milli-grams	Grams	Milli-grams	Milli-grams	Milli-grams	Milli-grams	Milli-grams	Inter-national units	Retinol equiva-ients	Milli-grams	Milli-grams	Milli-grams	Milli-grams	
0	28	359	702	4.9	988	15	0	0	0.28	1.05	4.5	1	525
0	6	75	147	1.0	208	3	0	0	0.06	0.22	1.0	Tr	526
0	41	47	239	2.9	608	1	Tr	Tr	0.43	0.05	0.9	0	527
0	38	90	266	4.9	749	13	0	0	0.25	0.13	1.3	0	528
0	49	55	293	5.9	1,163	4	0	0	0.25	0.11	1.3	0	529
0	40	95	281	5.1	790	13	0	0	0.27	0.13	1.3	0	530
0	49	86	296	5.4	882	3	Tr	Tr	0.33	0.16	0.7	0	531
30	32	94	303	4.8	668	1,374	330	33	0.18	0.15	3.3	Tr	532
10	48	138	235	4.6	536	1,181	330	33	0.20	0.08	1.5	5	533
10	54	161	291	5.9	536	969	330	33	0.15	0.10	1.3	5	534
0	42	74	278	4.6	673	968	10	1	0.13	0.10	1.5	0	535
0	35	43	238	3.3	573	20	30	3	0.40	0.10	1.0	0	536
0	4	50	170	1.0	170	1	Tr	Tr	0.28	0.03	0.5	Tr	537
0	126	390	102	5.7	1,275	24	Tr	Tr	0.07	0.07	2.2	Tr	538
0	45	62	671	8.2	774	[41] 877	0	0	0.27	0.27	1.9	0	539
0	9	13	139	1.7	160	[41] 181	0	0	0.06	0.06	0.4	0	540
0	37	53	554	5.3	689	[42] 814	0	0	0.55	0.23	2.3	0	541
0	8	12	121	1.2	150	[42] 177	0	0	0.12	0.05	0.5	0	542
0	76	41	153	1.3	847	3	30	3	0.35	0.25	1.9	37	543
0	45	80	273	4.9	475	11	Tr	Tr	0.18	0.09	0.9	0	544
0	7	6	51	1.1	160	9	0	0	0.03	0.01	0.2	1	545
0	12	11	90	1.9	285	16	0	0	0.05	0.02	0.4	3	546
0	44	14	99	1.8	313	244	0	0	0.03	0.02	0.4	1	547
0	18	216	359	3.8	512	3	80	8	0.58	0.13	1.3	1	548
0	4	53	88	0.9	126	1	20	2	0.14	0.03	0.3	Tr	549
0	38	50	238	4.2	498	26	40	4	0.14	0.12	1.2	0	550
0	17	60	268	2.4	441	[43] 348	10	1	0.29	0.15	2.7	0	551
0	4	13	57	0.5	93	[43] 74	Tr	Tr	0.06	0.03	0.6	0	552
0	7	20	123	1.0	169	[44] 190	Tr	Tr	0.06	0.06	1.3	0	553
0	6	31	131	0.9	165	[44] 185	10	1	0.14	0.06	1.4	Tr	554
0	27	125	734	2.8	1,019	[45] 626	0	0	0.42	0.15	21.5	0	555
0	5	24	143	0.5	199	[45] 122	0	0	0.08	0.03	4.2	0	556
0	3	5	60	0.3	110	75	0	0	0.02	0.02	2.2	0	557
0	42	22	178	3.4	592	26	80	8	0.30	0.18	1.8	0	558
0	20	39	314	2.3	423	1	140	14	0.92	0.14	1.0	2	559
0	5	10	83	0.6	111	Tr	40	4	0.24	0.04	0.3	1	560
0	5	2	10	0.9	178	20	10	1	0.35	0.06	1.2	1	561
0	7	38	143	1.9	310	2	70	7	0.23	0.05	0.3	Tr	562
0	5	12	333	4.2	229	5	110	11	0.06	0.09	0.5	Tr	563
0	51	141	245	5.1	1,141	1,228	0	0	0.14	0.16	1.4	17	564
0	1	11	62	0.6	33	3	10	1	0.06	0.01	0.4	0	565
0	19	131	322	4.9	972	4	50	5	0.38	0.16	1.1	0	566
0	65	188	853	4.7	922	8,142	110	11	0.17	0.28	0.8	0	567
0	3	108	151	2.3	50	8	0	0	0.07	0.04	0.1	0	568
0	5	33	200	1.9	195	1	10	1	0.65	0.07	1.3	Tr	569
0	3	21	119	0.7	69	5	10	1	0.24	0.02	0.8	1	570

[44]Mixed nuts without salt contain 3 mg sodium per oz.
[45]Peanuts without salt contain 22 mg sodium per cup or 4 mg per oz.

Table A-5 Nutritive Value of the Edible Part of Food *(Continued)*

(Tr indicates nutrient present in trace amount.)

Item No.	Foods, approximate measures, units, and weight (weight of edible portion only)			Water	Food energy	Pro- tein	Fat	Fatty acids		
								Satu- rated	Mono- unsatu- rated	Poly- unsatu- rated
			Grams	Per- cent	Cal- ories	Grams	Grams	Grams	Grams	Grams
	Legumes, Nuts, and Seeds—Con.									
	Walnuts:									
571	Black, chopped-----------------	1 cup-----------	125	4	760	30	71	4.5	15.9	46.9
572		1 oz------------	28	4	170	7	16	1.0	3.6	10.6
573	English or Persian, pieces or									
	chips----------------------	1 cup-----------	120	4	770	17	74	6.7	17.0	47.0
574		1 oz------------	28	4	180	4	18	1.6	4.0	11.1
	Meat and Meat Products									
	Beef, cooked:[46]									
	Cuts braised, simmered, or pot roasted:									
	Relatively fat such as chuck blade:									
575	Lean and fat, piece, 2-1/2 by 2-1/2 by 3/4 in-------	3 oz------------	85	43	325	22	26	10.8	11.7	0.9
576	Lean only from item 575----	2.2 oz----------	62	53	170	19	9	3.9	4.2	0.3
	Relatively lean, such as bottom round:									
577	Lean and fat, piece, 4-1/8 by 2-1/4 by 1/2 in-------	3 oz------------	85	54	220	25	13	4.8	5.7	0.5
578	Lean only from item 577----	2.8 oz----------	78	57	175	25	8	2.7	3.4	0.3
	Ground beef, broiled, patty, 3 by 5/8 in:									
579	Lean------------------------	3 oz------------	85	56	230	21	16	6.2	6.9	0.6
580	Regular---------------------	3 oz------------	85	54	245	20	18	6.9	7.7	0.7
581	Heart, lean, braised-----------	3 oz------------	85	65	150	24	5	1.2	0.8	1.6
582	Liver, fried, slice, 6-1/2 by 2-3/8 by 3/8 in[47]-----------	3 oz------------	85	56	185	23	7	2.5	3.6	1.3
	Roast, oven cooked, no liquid added:									
	Relatively fat, such as rib:									
583	Lean and fat, 2 pieces, 4-1/8 by 2-1/4 by 1/4 in	3 oz------------	85	46	315	19	26	10.8	11.4	0.9
584	Lean only from item 583----	2.2 oz----------	61	57	150	17	9	3.6	3.7	0.3
	Relatively lean, such as eye of round:									
585	Lean and fat, 2 pieces, 2-1/2 by 2-1/2 by 3/8 in	3 oz------------	85	57	205	23	12	4.9	5.4	0.5
586	Lean only from item 585----	2.6 oz----------	75	63	135	22	5	1.9	2.1	0.2
	Steak:									
	Sirloin, broiled:									
587	Lean and fat, piece, 2-1/2 by 2-1/2 by 3/4 in-------	3 oz------------	85	53	240	23	15	6.4	6.9	0.6
588	Lean only from item 587----	2.5 oz----------	72	59	150	22	6	2.6	2.8	0.3
589	Beef, canned, corned-------------	3 oz------------	85	59	185	22	10	4.2	4.9	0.4
590	Beef, dried, chipped-------------	2.5 oz----------	72	48	145	24	4	1.8	2.0	0.2
	Lamb, cooked:									
	Chops, (3 per lb with bone):									
	Arm, braised:									
591	Lean and fat---------------	2.2 oz----------	63	44	220	20	15	6.9	6.0	0.9
592	Lean only from item 591----	1.7 oz----------	48	49	135	17	7	2.9	2.6	0.4
	Loin, broiled:									
593	Lean and fat---------------	2.8 oz----------	80	54	235	22	16	7.3	6.4	1.0
594	Lean only from item 593----	2.3 oz----------	64	61	140	19	6	2.6	2.4	0.4
	Leg, roasted:									
595	Lean and fat, 2 pieces, 4-1/8 by 2-1/4 by 1/4 in	3 oz------------	85	59	205	22	13	5.6	4.9	0.8
596	Lean only from item 595------	2.6 oz----------	73	64	140	20	6	2.4	2.2	0.4
	Rib, roasted:									
597	Lean and fat, 3 pieces, 2-1/2 by 2-1/2 by 1/4 in---------	3 oz------------	85	47	315	18	26	12.1	10.6	1.5
598	Lean only from item 597------	2 oz------------	57	60	130	15	7	3.2	3.0	0.5

[46] Outer layer of fat was removed to within approximately 1/2 inch of the lean. Deposits of fat within the cut were not removed.
[47] Fried in vegetable shortening.

Table A-5 Nutritive Value of the Edible Part of Food *(Continued)*

Nutrients in Indicated Quantity

Cho-les-terol	Carbo-hydrate	Calcium	Phos-phorus	Iron	Potas-sium	Sodium	Vitamin A value (IU)	Vitamin A value (RE)	Thiamin	Ribo-flavin	Niacin	Ascorbic acid	Item No
Milli-grams	Grams	Milli-grams	Milli-grams	Milli-grams	Milli-grams	Milli-grams	Inter-national units	Retinol equiva-lents	Milli-grams	Milli-grams	Milli-grams	Milli-grams	
0	15	73	580	3.8	655	1	370	37	0.27	0.14	0.9	Tr	571
0	3	16	132	0.9	149	Tr	80	8	0.06	0.03	0.2	Tr	572
0	22	113	380	2.9	602	12	150	15	0.46	0.18	1.3	4	573
0	5	27	90	0.7	142	3	40	4	0.11	0.04	0.3	1	574
87	0	11	163	2.5	163	53	Tr	Tr	0.06	0.19	2.0	0	575
66	0	8	146	2.3	163	44	Tr	Tr	0.05	0.17	1.7	0	576
81	0	5	217	2.8	248	43	Tr	Tr	0.06	0.21	3.3	0	577
75	0	4	212	2.7	240	40	Tr	Tr	0.06	0.20	3.0	0	578
74	0	9	134	1.8	256	65	Tr	Tr	0.04	0.18	4.4	0	579
76	0	9	144	2.1	248	70	Tr	Tr	0.03	0.16	4.9	0	580
164	0	5	213	6.4	198	54	Tr	Tr	0.12	1.31	3.4	5	581
410	7	9	392	5.3	309	90	[48]30,690	[48]9,120	0.18	3.52	12.3	23	582
72	0	8	145	2.0	246	54	Tr	Tr	0.06	0.16	3.1	0	583
49	0	5	127	1.7	218	45	Tr	Tr	0.05	0.13	2.7	0	584
62	0	5	177	1.6	308	50	Tr	Tr	0.07	0.14	3.0	0	585
52	0	3	170	1.5	297	46	Tr	Tr	0.07	0.13	2.8	0	586
77	0	9	186	2.6	306	53	Tr	Tr	0.10	0.23	3.3	0	587
64	0	8	176	2.4	290	48	Tr	Tr	0.09	0.22	3.1	0	588
80	0	17	90	3.7	51	802	Tr	Tr	0.02	0.20	2.9	0	589
46	0	14	287	2.3	142	3,053	Tr	Tr	0.05	0.23	2.7	0	590
77	0	16	132	1.5	195	46	Tr	Tr	0.04	0.16	4.4	0	591
59	0	12	111	1.3	162	36	Tr	Tr	0.03	0.13	3.0	0	592
78	0	16	162	1.4	272	62	Tr	Tr	0.09	0.21	5.5	0	593
60	0	12	145	1.3	241	54	Tr	Tr	0.08	0.18	4.4	0	594
78	0	8	162	1.7	273	57	Tr	Tr	0.09	0.24	5.5	0	595
65	0	6	150	1.5	247	50	Tr	Tr	0.08	0.20	4.6	0	596
77	0	19	139	1.4	224	60	Tr	Tr	0.08	0.18	5.5	0	597
50	0	12	111	1.0	179	46	Tr	Tr	0.05	0.13	3.5	0	598

[48] Value varies widely.

Table A-5 Nutritive Value of the Edible Part of Food *(Continued)*

(Tr indicates nutrient present in trace amount.)

Item No.	Foods, approximate measures, units, and weight (weight of edible portion only)		Water	Food energy	Pro-tein	Fat	Fatty acids Satu-rated	Mono-unsatu-rated	Poly-unsatu-rated
		Grams	Per-cent	Cal-ories	Grams	Grams	Grams	Grams	Grams
	Meat and Meat Products—Con.								
	Pork, cured, cooked:								
	Bacon:								
599	Regular---------------------- 3 medium slices	19	13	110	6	9	3.3	4.5	1.1
600	Canadian-style--------------- 2 slices--------	46	62	85	11	4	1.3	1.9	0.4
	Ham, light cure, roasted:								
601	Lean and fat, 2 pieces, 4-1/8 by 2-1/4 by 1/4 in--------- 3 oz------------	85	58	205	18	14	5.1	6.7	1.5
602	Lean only from item 601------ 2.4 oz----------	68	66	105	17	4	1.3	1.7	0.4
603	Ham, canned, roasted, 2 pieces, 4-1/8 by 2-1/4 by 1/4 in----- 3 oz------------	85	67	140	18	7	2.4	3.5	0.8
	Luncheon meat:								
604	Canned, spiced or unspiced, slice, 3 by 2 by 1/2 in---- 2 slices--------	42	52	140	5	13	4.5	6.0	1.5
605	Chopped ham (8 slices per 6 oz pkg)-------------------- 2 slices--------	42	64	95	7	7	2.4	3.4	0.9
	Cooked ham (8 slices per 8-oz pkg):								
606	Regular------------------ 2 slices--------	57	65	105	10	6	1.9	2.8	0.7
607	Extra lean--------------- 2 slices--------	57	71	75	11	3	0.9	1.3	0.3
	Pork, fresh, cooked:								
	Chop, loin (cut 3 per lb with bone):								
	Broiled:								
608	Lean and fat---------------- 3.1 oz----------	87	50	275	24	19	7.0	8.8	2.2
609	Lean only from item 608---- 2.5 oz----------	72	57	165	23	8	2.6	3.4	0.9
	Pan fried:								
610	Lean and fat---------------- 3.1 oz----------	89	45	335	21	27	9.8	12.5	3.1
611	Lean only from item 610---- 2.4 oz----------	67	54	180	19	11	3.7	4.8	1.3
	Ham (leg), roasted:								
612	Lean and fat, piece, 2-1/2 by 2-1/2 by 3/4 in----------- 3 oz------------	85	53	250	21	18	6.4	8.1	2.0
613	Lean only from item 612------ 2.5 oz----------	72	60	160	20	8	2.7	3.6	1.0
	Rib, roasted:								
614	Lean and fat, piece, 2-1/2 by 3/4 in-------------------- 3 oz------------	85	51	270	21	20	7.2	9.2	2.3
615	Lean only from item 614------ 2.5 oz----------	71	57	175	20	10	3.4	4.4	1.2
	Shoulder cut, braised:								
616	Lean and fat, 3 pieces, 2-1/2 by 2-1/2 by 1/4 in--------- 3 oz------------	85	47	295	23	22	7.9	10.0	2.4
617	Lean only from item 616------ 2.4 oz----------	67	54	165	22	8	2.8	3.7	1.0
	Sausages (See also Luncheon meats, items 604-607):								
618	Bologna, slice (8 per 8-oz pkg) 2 slices--------	57	54	180	7	16	6.1	7.6	1.4
619	Braunschweiger, slice (6 per 6-oz pkg)-------------------- 2 slices--------	57	48	205	8	18	6.2	8.5	2.1
620	Brown and serve (10-11 per 8-oz pkg), browned----------- 1 link----------	13	45	50	2	5	1.7	2.2	0.5
621	Frankfurter (10 per 1-lb pkg), cooked (reheated)------------ 1 frankfurter---	45	54	145	5	13	4.8	6.2	1.2
622	Pork link (16 per 1-lb pkg), cooked[50] --------------------- 1 link----------	13	45	50	3	4	1.4	1.8	0.5
	Salami:								
623	Cooked type, slice (8 per 8-oz pkg)------------------ 2 slices--------	57	60	145	8	11	4.6	5.2	1.2
624	Dry type, slice (12 per 4-oz pkg)-------------------- 2 slices--------	20	35	85	5	7	2.4	3.4	0.6
625	Sandwich spread (pork, beef)--- 1 tbsp----------	15	60	35	1	3	0.9	1.1	0.4
626	Vienna sausage (7 per 4-oz can) 1 sausage-------	16	60	45	2	4	1.5	2.0	0.3
	Veal, medium fat, cooked, bone removed:								
627	Cutlet, 4-1/8 by 2-1/4 by 1/2 in, braised or broiled------- 3 oz------------	85	60	185	23	9	4.1	4.1	0.6
628	Rib, 2 pieces, 4-1/8 by 2-1/4 by 1/4 in, roasted---------- 3 oz------------	85	55	230	23	14	6.0	6.0	1.0

[49] Contains added sodium ascorbate. If sodium ascorbate is not added, ascorbic acid content is negligible.

Table A-5 Nutritive Value of the Edible Part of Food (Continued)

Nutrients in Indicated Quantity

Cho-les-terol	Carbo-hydrate	Calcium	Phos-phorus	Iron	Potas-sium	Sodium	Vitamin A value		Thiamin	Ribo-flavin	Niacin	Ascorbic acid	Item No
							(IU)	(RE)					
Milli-grams	Grams	Milli-grams	Milli-grams	Milli-grams	Milli-grams	Milli-grams	Inter-national units	Retinol equiva-lents	Milli-grams	Milli-grams	Milli-grams	Milli-grams	
16	Tr	2	64	0.3	92	303	0	0	0.13	0.05	1.4	6	599
27	1	5	136	0.4	179	711	0	0	0.38	0.09	3.2	10	600
53	0	6	182	0.7	243	1,009	0	0	0.51	0.19	3.8	0	601
37	0	5	154	0.6	215	902	0	0	0.46	0.17	3.4	0	602
35	Tr	6	188	0.9	298	908	0	0	0.82	0.21	4.3	[49]19	603
26	1	3	34	0.3	90	541	0	0	0.15	0.08	1.3	Tr	604
21	0	3	65	0.3	134	576	0	0	0.27	0.09	1.6	[49]8	605
32	2	4	141	0.6	189	751	0	0	0.49	0.14	3.0	[49]16	606
27	1	4	124	0.4	200	815	0	0	0.53	0.13	2.8	[49]15	607
84	0	3	184	0.7	312	61	10	3	0.87	0.24	4.3	Tr	608
71	0	4	176	0.7	302	56	10	1	0.83	0.22	4.0	Tr	609
92	0	4	190	0.7	323	64	10	3	0.91	0.24	4.6	Tr	610
72	0	3	178	0.7	305	57	10	1	0.84	0.22	4.0	Tr	611
79	0	5	210	0.9	280	50	10	2	0.54	0.27	3.9	Tr	612
68	0	5	202	0.8	269	46	10	1	0.50	0.25	3.6	Tr	613
69	0	9	190	0.8	313	37	10	3	0.50	0.24	4.2	Tr	614
56	0	8	182	0.7	300	33	10	2	0.45	0.22	3.8	Tr	615
93	0	6	162	1.4	286	75	10	3	0.46	0.26	4.4	Tr	616
76	0	5	151	1.3	271	68	10	1	0.40	0.24	4.0	Tr	617
31	2	7	52	0.9	103	581	0	0	0.10	0.08	1.5	[49]12	618
89	2	5	96	5.3	113	652	8,010	2,405	0.14	0.87	4.8	[49]6	619
9	Tr	1	14	0.1	25	105	0	0	0.05	0.02	0.4	0	620
23	1	5	39	0.5	75	504	0	0	0.09	0.05	1.2	[49]12	621
11	Tr	4	24	0.2	47	168	0	0	0.10	0.03	0.6	Tr	622
37	1	7	66	1.5	113	607	0	0	0.14	0.21	2.0	[49]7	623
16	1	2	28	0.3	76	372	0	0	0.12	0.06	1.0	[49]5	624
6	2	2	9	0.1	17	152	10	1	0.03	0.02	0.3	0	625
8	Tr	2	8	0.1	16	152	0	0	0.01	0.02	0.3	0	626
109	0	9	196	0.8	258	56	Tr	Tr	0.06	0.21	4.6	0	627
109	0	10	211	0.7	259	57	Tr	Tr	0.11	0.26	6.6	0	628

[50] One patty (8 per pound) of bulk sausage is equivalent to 2 links.

Table A-5 Nutritive Value of the Edible Part of Food (Continued)

(Tr indicates nutrient present in trace amount.)

Item No.	Foods, approximate measures, units, and weight (weight of edible portion only)		Water	Food energy	Pro-tein	Fat	Fatty acids		
							Satu-rated	Mono-unsatu-rated	Poly-unsatu-rated
	Mixed Dishes and Fast Foods	Grams	Per-cent	Cal-ories	Grams	Grams	Grams	Grams	Grams
	Mixed dishes:								
629	Beef and vegetable stew, from home recipe	1 cup	245	82	220	16	11	4.4	4.5	0.5
630	Beef potpie, from home recipe, baked, piece, 1/3 of 9-in diam. pie[51]	1 piece	210	55	515	21	30	7.9	12.9	7.4
631	Chicken a la king, cooked, from home recipe	1 cup	245	68	470	27	34	12.9	13.4	6.2
632	Chicken and noodles, cooked, from home recipe	1 cup	240	71	365	22	18	5.1	7.1	3.9
	Chicken chow mein:								
633	Canned	1 cup	250	89	95	7	Tr	0.1	0.1	0.8
634	From home recipe	1 cup	250	78	255	31	10	4.1	4.9	3.5
635	Chicken potpie, from home recipe, baked, piece, 1/3 of 9-in diam. pie[51]	1 piece	232	57	545	23	31	10.3	15.5	6.6
636	Chili con carne with beans, canned	1 cup	255	72	340	19	16	5.8	7.2	1.0
637	Chop suey with beef and pork, from home recipe	1 cup	250	75	300	26	17	4.3	7.4	4.2
	Macaroni (enriched) and cheese:								
638	Canned[52]	1 cup	240	80	230	9	10	4.7	2.9	1.3
639	From home recipe[38]	1 cup	200	58	430	17	22	9.8	7.4	3.6
640	Quiche Lorraine, 1/8 of 8-in diam. quiche[51]	1 slice	176	47	600	13	48	23.2	17.8	4.1
	Spaghetti (enriched) in tomato sauce with cheese:								
641	Canned	1 cup	250	80	190	6	2	0.4	0.4	0.5
642	From home recipe	1 cup	250	77	260	9	9	3.0	3.6	1.2
	Spaghetti (enriched) with meat-balls and tomato sauce:								
643	Canned	1 cup	250	78	260	12	10	2.4	3.9	3.1
644	From home recipe	1 cup	248	70	330	19	12	3.9	4.4	2.2
	Fast food entrees:								
	Cheeseburger:								
645	Regular	1 sandwich	112	46	300	15	15	7.3	5.6	1.0
646	4 oz patty	1 sandwich	194	46	525	30	31	15.1	12.2	1.4
	Chicken, fried. See Poultry and Poultry Products (items 656-659).								
647	Enchilada	1 enchilada	230	72	235	20	16	7.7	6.7	0.6
648	English muffin, egg, cheese, and bacon	1 sandwich	138	49	360	18	18	8.0	8.0	0.7
	Fish sandwich:								
649	Regular, with cheese	1 sandwich	140	43	420	16	23	6.3	6.9	7.7
650	Large, without cheese	1 sandwich	170	48	470	18	27	6.3	8.7	9.5
	Hamburger:								
651	Regular	1 sandwich	98	46	245	12	11	4.4	5.3	0.5
652	4 oz patty	1 sandwich	174	50	445	25	21	7.1	11.7	0.6
653	Pizza, cheese, 1/8 of 15-in diam. pizza[51]	1 slice	120	46	290	15	9	4.1	2.6	1.3
654	Roast beef sandwich	1 sandwich	150	52	345	22	13	3.5	6.9	1.8
655	Taco	1 taco	81	55	195	9	11	4.1	5.5	0.8

[38] Made with margarine.
[51] Crust made with vegetable shortening and enriched flour.

APPENDIX 469

Table A-5 Nutritive Value of the Edible Part of Food (Continued)

Nutrients in Indicated Quantity

Cholesterol	Carbohydrate	Calcium	Phosphorus	Iron	Potassium	Sodium	Vitamin A value (IU)	Vitamin A value (RE)	Thiamin	Riboflavin	Niacin	Ascorbic acid	Item No.
Milligrams	Grams	Milligrams	Milligrams	Milligrams	Milligrams	Milligrams	International units	Retinol equivalents	Milligrams	Milligrams	Milligrams	Milligrams	
71	15	29	184	2.9	613	292	5,690	568	0.15	0.17	4.7	17	629
42	39	29	149	3.8	334	596	4,220	517	0.29	0.29	4.8	6	630
221	12	127	358	2.5	404	760	1,130	272	0.10	0.42	5.4	12	631
103	26	26	247	2.2	149	600	430	130	0.05	0.17	4.3	Tr	632
8	18	45	85	1.3	418	725	150	28	0.05	0.10	1.0	13	633
75	10	58	293	2.5	473	718	280	50	0.08	0.23	4.3	10	634
56	42	70	232	3.0	343	594	7,220	735	0.32	0.32	4.9	5	635
28	31	82	321	4.3	594	1,354	150	15	0.08	0.18	3.3	8	636
68	13	60	248	4.8	425	1,053	600	60	0.28	0.38	5.0	33	637
24	26	199	182	1.0	139	730	260	72	0.12	0.24	1.0	Tr	638
44	40	362	322	1.8	240	1,086	860	232	0.20	0.40	1.8	1	639
285	29	211	276	1.0	283	653	1,640	454	0.11	0.32	Tr	Tr	640
3	39	40	88	2.8	303	955	930	120	0.35	0.28	4.5	10	641
8	37	80	135	2.3	408	955	1,080	140	0.25	0.18	2.3	13	642
23	29	53	113	3.3	245	1,220	1,000	100	0.15	0.18	2.3	5	643
89	39	124	236	3.7	665	1,009	1,590	159	0.25	0.30	4.0	22	644
44	28	135	174	2.3	219	672	340	65	0.26	0.24	3.7	1	645
104	40	236	320	4.5	407	1,224	670	128	0.33	0.48	7.4	3	646
19	24	97	198	3.3	653	1,332	2,720	352	0.18	0.26	Tr	Tr	647
213	31	197	290	3.1	201	832	650	160	0.46	0.50	3.7	1	648
56	39	132	223	1.8	274	667	160	25	0.32	0.26	3.3	2	649
91	41	61	246	2.2	375	621	110	15	0.35	0.23	3.5	1	650
32	28	56	107	2.2	202	463	80	14	0.23	0.24	3.8	1	651
71	38	75	225	4.8	404	763	160	28	0.38	0.38	7.8	1	652
56	39	220	216	1.6	230	699	750	106	0.34	0.29	4.2	2	653
55	34	60	222	4.0	338	757	240	32	0.40	0.33	6.0	2	654
21	15	109	134	1.2	263	456	420	57	0.09	0.07	1.4	1	655

[52]Made with corn oil.

Table A-5 Nutritive Value of the Edible Part of Food *(Continued)*

(Tr indicates nutrient present in trace amount.)

Item No.	Foods, approximate measures, units, and weight (weight of edible portion only)		Water	Food energy	Pro-tein	Fat	Fatty acids Satu-rated	Mono-unsatu-rated	Poly-unsatu-rated
		Grams	Per-cent	Cal-ories	Grams	Grams	Grams	Grams	Grams
	Poultry and Poultry Products								
	Chicken:								
	Fried, flesh, with skin:[53]								
	Batter dipped:								
656	Breast, 1/2 breast (5.6 oz with bones)-------------- 4.9 oz----------		140	52	365	35	18	4.9	7.6	4.3
657	Drumstick (3.4 oz with bones)------------------- 2.5 oz----------		72	53	195	16	11	3.0	4.6	2.7
	Flour coated:								
658	Breast, 1/2 breast (4.2 oz with bones)------------- 3.5 oz----------		98	57	220	31	9	2.4	3.4	1.9
659	Drumstick (2.6 oz with bones)------------------- 1.7 oz----------		49	57	120	13	7	1.8	2.7	1.6
	Roasted, flesh only:								
660	Breast, 1/2 breast (4.2 oz with bones and skin)------- 3.0 oz----------		86	65	140	27	3	0.9	1.1	0.7
661	Drumstick, (2.9 oz with bones and skin)----------------- 1.6 oz----------		44	67	75	12	2	0.7	0.8	0.6
662	Stewed, flesh only, light and dark meat, chopped or diced-- 1 cup-----------		140	67	250	38	9	2.6	3.3	2.2
663	Chicken liver, cooked------------ 1 liver--------		20	68	30	5	1	0.4	0.3	0.2
664	Duck, roasted, flesh only-------- 1/2 duck--------		221	64	445	52	25	9.2	8.2	3.2
	Turkey, roasted, flesh only:								
665	Dark meat, piece, 2-1/2 by 1-5/8 by 1/4 in------------- 4 pieces--------		85	63	160	24	6	2.1	1.4	1.8
666	Light meat, piece, 4 by 2 by 1/4 in---------------------- 2 pieces--------		85	66	135	25	3	0.9	0.5	0.7
	Light and dark meat:								
667	Chopped or diced------------- 1 cup-----------		140	65	240	41	7	2.3	1.4	2.0
668	Pieces (1 slice white meat, 4 by 2 by 1/4 in and 2 slices dark meat, 2-1/2 by 1-5/8 by 1/4 in)-------- 3 pieces--------		85	65	145	25	4	1.4	0.9	1.2
	Poultry food products:								
	Chicken:								
669	Canned, boneless------------- 5 oz------------		142	69	235	31	11	3.1	4.5	2.5
670	Frankfurter (10 per 1-lb pkg) 1 frankfurter---		45	58	115	6	9	2.5	3.8	1.8
671	Roll, light (6 slices per 6 oz pkg)------------------- 2 slices--------		57	69	90	11	4	1.1	1.7	0.9
	Turkey:								
672	Gravy and turkey, frozen----- 5-oz package----		142	85	95	8	4	1.2	1.4	0.7
673	Ham, cured turkey thigh meat (8 slices per 8-oz pkg)---- 2 slices--------		57	71	75	11	3	1.0	0.7	0.9
674	Loaf, breast meat (8 slices per 6-oz pkg)-------------- 2 slices--------		42	72	45	10	1	0.2	0.2	0.1
675	Patties, breaded, battered, fried (2.25 oz)------------ 1 patty---------		64	50	180	9	12	3.0	4.8	3.0
676	Roast, boneless, frozen, sea-soned, light and dark meat, cooked-------------------- 3 oz------------		85	68	130	18	5	1.6	1.0	1.4
	Soups, Sauces, and Gravies								
	Soups:								
	Canned, condensed:								
	Prepared with equal volume of milk:								
677	Clam chowder, New England-- 1 cup-----------		248	85	165	9	7	3.0	2.3	1.1
678	Cream of chicken----------- 1 cup-----------		248	85	190	7	11	4.6	4.5	1.6
679	Cream of mushroom---------- 1 cup-----------		248	85	205	6	14	5.1	3.0	4.6
680	Tomato-------------------- 1 cup-----------		248	85	160	6	6	2.9	1.6	1.1

[53] Fried in vegetable shortening.

Table A-5 Nutritive Value of the Edible Part of Food *(Continued)*

							Vitamin A value						
Cho-les-terol	Carbo-hydrate	Calcium	Phos-phorus	Iron	Potas-sium	Sodium	(IU)	(RE)	Thiamin	Ribo-flavin	Niacin	Ascorbic acid	Item No
Milli-grams	Grams	Milli-grams	Milli-grams	Milli-grams	Milli-grams	Milli-grams	Inter-national units	Retinol equiva-ients	Milli-grams	Milli-grams	Milli-grams	Milli-grams	
119	13	28	259	1.8	281	385	90	28	0.16	0.20	14.7	0	656
62	6	12	106	1.0	134	194	60	19	0.08	0.15	3.7	0	657
87	2	16	228	1.2	254	74	50	15	0.08	0.13	13.5	0	658
44	1	6	86	0.7	112	44	40	12	0.04	0.11	3.0	0	659
73	0	13	196	0.9	220	64	20	5	0.06	0.10	11.8	0	660
41	0	5	81	0.6	108	42	30	8	0.03	0.10	2.7	0	661
116	0	20	210	1.6	252	98	70	21	0.07	0.23	8.6	0	662
126	Tr	3	62	1.7	28	10	3,270	983	0.03	0.35	0.9	3	663
197	0	27	449	6.0	557	144	170	51	0.57	1.04	11.3	0	664
72	0	27	173	2.0	246	67	0	0	0.05	0.21	3.1	0	665
59	0	16	186	1.1	259	54	0	0	0.05	0.11	5.8	0	666
106	0	35	298	2.5	417	98	0	0	0.09	0.25	7.6	0	667
65	0	21	181	1.5	253	60	0	0	0.05	0.15	4.6	0	668
88	0	20	158	2.2	196	714	170	48	0.02	0.18	9.0	3	669
45	3	43	48	0.9	38	616	60	17	0.03	0.05	1.4	0	670
28	1	24	89	0.6	129	331	50	14	0.04	0.07	3.0	0	671
26	7	20	115	1.3	87	787	60	18	0.03	0.18	2.6	0	672
32	Tr	6	108	1.6	184	565	0	0	0.03	0.14	2.0	0	673
17	0	3	97	0.2	118	608	0	0	0.02	0.05	3.5	[54]0	674
40	10	9	173	1.4	176	512	20	7	0.06	0.12	1.5	0	675
45	3	4	207	1.4	253	578	0	0	0.04	0.14	5.3	0	676
22	17	186	156	1.5	300	992	160	40	0.07	0.24	1.0	3	677
27	15	181	151	0.7	273	1,047	710	94	0.07	0.26	0.9	1	678
20	15	179	156	0.6	270	1,076	150	37	0.08	0.28	0.9	2	679
17	22	159	149	1.8	449	932	850	109	0.13	0.25	1.5	68	680

[54]If sodium ascorbate is added, product contains 11 mg ascorbic acid.

Table A-5 Nutritive Value of the Edible Part of Food *(Continued)*

(Tr indicates nutrient present in trace amount.)

Item No.	Foods, approximate measures, units, and weight (weight of edible portion only)		Water	Food energy	Pro- tein	Fat	Satu- rated	Mono- unsatu- rated	Poly- unsatu- rated
		Grams	Per- cent	Cal- ories	Grams	Grams	Grams	Grams	Grams
	Soups, Sauces, and Gravies—Con.								
	Soups:								
	Canned, condensed:								
	Prepared with equal volume of water:								
681	Bean with bacon----------- 1 cup----------	253	84	170	8	6	1.5	2.2	1.8
682	Beef broth, bouillon, consomme--------------- 1 cup----------	240	98	15	3	1	0.3	0.2	Tr
683	Beef noodle--------------- 1 cup----------	244	92	85	5	3	1.1	1.2	0.5
684	Chicken noodle------------ 1 cup----------	241	92	75	4	2	0.7	1.1	0.6
685	Chicken rice-------------- 1 cup----------	241	94	60	4	2	0.5	0.9	0.4
686	Clam chowder, Manhattan---- 1 cup----------	244	90	80	4	2	0.4	0.4	1.3
687	Cream of chicken---------- 1 cup----------	244	91	115	3	7	2.1	3.3	1.5
688	Cream of mushroom--------- 1 cup----------	244	90	130	2	9	2.4	1.7	4.2
689	Minestrone---------------- 1 cup----------	241	91	80	4	3	0.6	0.7	1.1
690	Pea, green---------------- 1 cup----------	250	83	165	9	3	1.4	1.0	0.4
691	Tomato-------------------- 1 cup----------	244	90	85	2	2	0.4	0.4	1.0
692	Vegetable beef------------ 1 cup----------	244	92	80	6	2	0.9	0.8	0.1
693	Vegetarian---------------- 1 cup----------	241	92	70	2	2	0.3	0.8	0.7
	Dehydrated:								
	Unprepared:								
694	Bouillon------------------ 1 pkt----------	6	3	15	1	1	0.3	0.2	Tr
695	Onion--------------------- 1 pkt----------	7	4	20	1	Tr	0.1	0.2	Tr
	Prepared with water:								
696	Chicken noodle------------ 1 pkt (6-fl-oz)	188	94	40	2	1	0.2	0.4	0.3
697	Onion--------------------- 1 pkt (6-fl-oz)	184	96	20	1	Tr	0.1	0.2	0.1
698	Tomato vegetable---------- 1 pkt (6-fl-oz)	189	94	40	1	1	0.3	0.2	0.1
	Sauces:								
	From dry mix:								
699	Cheese, prepared with milk--- 1 cup----------	279	77	305	16	17	9.3	5.3	1.6
700	Hollandaise, prepared with water--------------------- 1 cup----------	259	84	240	5	20	11.6	5.9	0.9
701	White sauce, prepared with milk--------------------- 1 cup----------	264	81	240	10	13	6.4	4.7	1.7
	From home recipe:								
702	White sauce, medium [55] -------- 1 cup----------	250	73	395	10	30	9.1	11.9	7.2
	Ready to serve:								
703	Barbecue------------------- 1 tbsp----------	16	81	10	Tr	Tr	Tr	0.1	0.1
704	Soy----------------------- 1 tbsp----------	18	68	10	2	0	0.0	0.0	0.0
	Gravies:								
	Canned:								
705	Beef--------------------- 1 cup----------	233	87	125	9	5	2.7	2.3	0.2
706	Chicken------------------ 1 cup----------	238	85	190	5	14	3.4	6.1	3.6
707	Mushroom----------------- 1 cup----------	238	89	120	3	6	1.0	2.8	2.4
	From dry mix:								
708	Brown-------------------- 1 cup----------	261	91	80	3	2	0.9	0.8	0.1
709	Chicken------------------ 1 cup----------	260	91	85	3	2	0.5	0.9	0.4
	Sugars and Sweets								
	Candy:								
710	Caramels, plain or chocolate--- 1 oz------------	28	8	115	1	3	2.2	0.3	0.1
	Chocolate:								
711	Milk, plain------------------ 1 oz------------	28	1	145	2	9	5.4	3.0	0.3
712	Milk, with almonds---------- 1 oz------------	28	2	150	3	10	4.8	4.1	0.7
713	Milk, with peanuts---------- 1 oz------------	28	1	155	4	11	4.2	3.5	1.5
714	Milk, with rice cereal------- 1 oz------------	28	2	140	2	7	4.4	2.5	0.2
715	Semisweet, small pieces (60 per oz)-------------------- 1 cup or 6 oz---	170	1	860	7	61	36.2	19.9	1.9
716	Sweet (dark)---------------- 1 oz------------	28	1	150	1	10	5.9	3.3	0.3
717	Fondant, uncoated (mints, candy corn, other)------------ 1 oz------------	28	3	105	Tr	0	0.0	0.0	0.0
718	Fudge, chocolate, plain-------- 1 oz------------	28	8	115	1	3	2.1	1.0	0.1
719	Gum drops--------------------- 1 oz------------	28	12	100	Tr	Tr	Tr	Tr	0.1

[55] Made with enriched flour, margarine, and whole milk.

Table A-5 Nutritive Value of the Edible Part of Food *(Continued)*

							Vitamin A value						
Cho-les-terol	Carbo-hydrate	Calcium	Phos-phorus	Iron	Potas-sium	Sodium	(IU)	(RE)	Thiamin	Ribo-flavin	Niacin	Ascorbic acid	Item No.
Milli-grams	Grams	Milli-grams	Milli-grams	Milli-grams	Milli-grams	Milli-grams	Inter-national units	Retinol equiva-lents	Milli-grams	Milli-grams	Milli-grams	Milli-grams	
3	23	81	132	2.0	402	951	890	89	0.09	0.03	0.6	2	681
Tr	Tr	14	31	0.4	130	782	0	0	Tr	0.05	1.9	0	682
5	9	15	46	1.1	100	952	630	63	0.07	0.06	1.1	Tr	683
7	9	17	36	0.8	55	1,106	710	71	0.05	0.06	1.4	Tr	684
7	7	17	22	0.7	101	815	660	66	0.02	0.02	1.1	Tr	685
2	12	34	59	1.9	261	1,808	920	92	0.06	0.05	1.3	3	686
10	9	34	37	0.6	88	986	560	56	0.03	0.06	0.8	Tr	687
2	9	46	49	0.5	100	1,032	0	0	0.05	0.09	0.7	1	688
2	11	34	55	0.9	313	911	2,340	234	0.05	0.04	0.9	1	689
0	27	28	125	2.0	190	988	200	20	0.11	0.07	1.2	2	690
0	17	12	34	1.8	264	871	690	69	0.09	0.05	1.4	66	691
5	10	17	41	1.1	173	956	1,890	189	0.04	0.05	1.0	2	692
0	12	22	34	1.1	210	822	3,010	301	0.05	0.05	0.9	1	693
1	1	4	19	0.1	27	1,019	Tr	Tr	Tr	0.01	0.3	0	694
Tr	4	10	23	0.1	47	627	Tr	Tr	0.02	0.04	0.4	Tr	695
2	6	24	24	0.4	23	957	50	5	0.05	0.04	0.7	Tr	696
0	4	9	22	0.1	48	635	Tr	Tr	0.02	0.04	0.4	Tr	697
0	8	6	23	0.5	78	856	140	14	0.04	0.03	0.6	5	698
53	23	569	438	0.3	552	1,565	390	117	0.15	0.56	0.3	2	699
52	14	124	127	0.9	124	1,564	730	220	0.05	0.18	0.1	Tr	700
34	21	425	256	0.3	444	797	310	92	0.08	0.45	0.5	3	701
32	24	292	238	0.9	381	888	1,190	340	0.15	0.43	0.8	2	702
0	2	3	3	0.1	28	130	140	14	Tr	Tr	0.1	1	703
0	2	3	38	0.5	64	1,029	0	0	0.01	0.02	0.6	0	704
7	11	14	70	1.6	189	117	0	0	0.07	0.08	1.5	0	705
5	13	69	69	1.1	259	1,373	880	264	0.04	0.10	1.1	0	706
0	13	17	36	1.6	252	1,357	0	0	0.08	0.15	1.6	0	707
2	14	66	47	0.2	61	1,147	0	0	0.04	0.09	0.9	0	708
3	14	39	47	0.3	62	1,134	0	0	0.05	0.15	0.8	3	709
1	22	42	35	0.4	54	64	Tr	Tr	0.01	0.05	0.1	Tr	710
6	16	50	61	0.4	96	23	30	10	0.02	0.10	0.1	Tr	711
5	15	65	77	0.5	125	23	30	8	0.02	0.12	0.2	Tr	712
5	13	49	83	0.4	138	19	30	8	0.07	0.07	1.4	Tr	713
6	18	48	57	0.2	100	46	30	8	0.01	0.08	0.1	Tr	714
0	97	51	178	5.8	593	24	30	3	0.10	0.14	0.9	Tr	715
0	16	7	41	0.6	86	5	10	1	0.01	0.04	0.1	Tr	716
0	27	2	Tr	0.1	1	57	0	0	Tr	Tr	Tr	0	717
1	21	22	24	0.3	42	54	Tr	Tr	0.01	0.03	0.1	Tr	718
0	25	2	Tr	0.1	1	10	0	0	0.00	Tr	Tr	0	719

Table A-5 Nutritive Value of the Edible Part of Food *(Continued)*
(Tr indicates nutrient present in trace amount.)

Item No.	Foods, approximate measures, units, and weight (weight of edible portion only)		Water	Food energy	Pro-tein	Fat	Fatty acids		
							Satu-rated	Mono-unsatu-rated	Poly-unsatu-rated
		Grams	Per-cent	Cal-ories	Grams	Grams	Grams	Grams	Grams
	Sugars and Sweets—Con.								
	Candy:								
720	Hard------------------------ 1 oz------------	28	1	110	0	0	0.0	0.0	0.0
721	Jelly beans------------------ 1 oz------------	28	6	105	Tr	Tr	Tr	Tr	0.1
722	Marshmallows------------------ 1 oz------------	28	17	90	1	0	0.0	0.0	0.0
723	Custard, baked------------------ 1 cup-----------	265	77	305	14	15	6.8	5.4	0.7
724	Gelatin dessert prepared with gelatin dessert powder and water------------------------ 1/2 cup--------	120	84	70	2	0	0.0	0.0	0.0
725	Honey, strained or extracted----- 1 cup-----------	339	17	1,030	1	0	0.0	0.0	0.0
726	1 tbsp----------	21	17	65	Tr	0	0.0	0.0	0.0
727	Jams and preserves--------------- 1 tbsp----------	20	29	55	Tr	Tr	0.0	Tr	Tr
728	1 packet--------	14	29	40	Tr	Tr	0.0	Tr	Tr
729	Jellies------------------------ 1 tbsp----------	18	28	50	Tr	Tr	Tr	Tr	Tr
730	1 packet--------	14	28	40	Tr	Tr	Tr	Tr	Tr
731	Popsicle, 3-fl-oz size----------- 1 popsicle------	95	80	70	0	0	0.0	0.0	0.0
	Puddings:								
	Canned:								
732	Chocolate-------------------- 5-oz can--------	142	68	205	3	11	9.5	0.5	0.1
733	Tapioca--------------------- 5-oz can--------	142	74	160	3	5	4.8	Tr	Tr
734	Vanilla--------------------- 5-oz can--------	142	69	220	2	10	9.5	0.2	0.1
	Dry mix, prepared with whole milk:								
	Chocolate:								
735	Instant-------------------- 1/2 cup--------	130	71	155	4	4	2.3	1.1	0.2
736	Regular (cooked)----------- 1/2 cup--------	130	73	150	4	4	2.4	1.1	0.1
737	Rice----------------------- 1/2 cup--------	132	73	155	4	4	2.3	1.1	0.1
738	Tapioca-------------------- 1/2 cup--------	130	75	145	4	4	2.3	1.1	0.1
	Vanilla:								
739	Instant-------------------- 1/2 cup--------	130	73	150	4	4	2.2	1.1	0.2
740	Regular (cooked)----------- 1/2 cup--------	130	74	145	4	4	2.3	1.0	0.1
	Sugars:								
741	Brown, pressed down------------ 1 cup-----------	220	2	820	0	0	0.0	0.0	0.0
	White:								
742	Granulated------------------- 1 cup-----------	200	1	770	0	0	0.0	0.0	0.0
743	1 tbsp----------	12	1	45	0	0	0.0	0.0	0.0
744	1 packet--------	6	1	25	0	0	0.0	0.0	0.0
745	Powdered, sifted, spooned into cup------------------- 1 cup-----------	100	1	385	0	0	0.0	0.0	0.0
	Syrups:								
	Chocolate-flavored syrup or topping:								
746	Thin type------------------- 2 tbsp----------	38	37	85	1	Tr	0.2	0.1	0.1
747	Fudge type------------------ 2 tbsp----------	38	25	125	2	5	3.1	1.7	0.2
748	Molasses, cane, blackstrap----- 2 tbsp----------	40	24	85	0	0	0.0	0.0	0.0
749	Table syrup (corn and maple)--- 2 tbsp----------	42	25	122	0	0	0.0	0.0	0.0
	Vegetables and Vegetable Products								
750	Alfalfa seeds, sprouted, raw----- 1 cup-----------	33	91	10	1	Tr	Tr	Tr	0.1
751	Artichokes, globe or French, cooked, drained--------------- 1 artichoke-----	120	87	55	3	Tr	Tr	Tr	0.1
	Asparagus, green:								
	Cooked, drained:								
	From raw:								
752	Cuts and tips-------------- 1 cup-----------	180	92	45	5	1	0.1	Tr	0.2
753	Spears, 1/2-in diam. at base-------------------- 4 spears--------	60	92	15	2	Tr	Tr	Tr	0.1
	From frozen:								
754	Cuts and tips-------------- 1 cup-----------	180	91	50	5	1	0.2	Tr	0.3
755	Spears, 1/2-in diam. at base-------------------- 4 spears--------	60	91	15	2	Tr	0.1	Tr	0.1
756	Canned, spears, 1/2-in diam. at base-------------------- 4 spears--------	80	95	10	1	Tr	Tr	Tr	0.1
757	Bamboo shoots, canned, drained--- 1 cup-----------	131	94	25	2	1	0.1	Tr	0.2

[56] For regular pack; special dietary pack contains 3 mg sodium.

Table A-5 Nutritive Value of the Edible Part of Food *(Continued)*

Nutrients in Indicated Quantity

| Cho-les-terol | Carbo-hydrate | Calcium | Phos-phorus | Iron | Potas-sium | Sodium | Vitamin A value | | Thiamin | Ribo-flavin | Niacin | Ascorbic acid | Item No. |
| | | | | | | | (IU) | (RE) | | | | | |
Milli-grams	Grams	Milli-grams	Milli-grams	Milli-grams	Milli-grams	Milli-grams	Inter-national units	Retinol equiva-lents	Milli-grams	Milli-grams	Milli-grams	Milli-grams	
0	28	Tr	2	0.1	1	7	0	0	0.10	0.00	0.0	0	720
0	26	1	1	0.3	11	7	0	0	0.00	Tr	Tr	0	721
0	23	1	2	0.5	2	25	0	0	0.00	Tr	Tr	0	722
278	29	297	310	1.1	387	209	530	146	0.11	0.50	0.3	1	723
0	17	2	23	Tr	Tr	55	0	0	0.00	0.00	0.0	0	724
0	279	17	20	1.7	173	17	0	0	0.02	0.14	1.0	3	725
0	17	1	1	0.1	11	1	0	0	Tr	0.01	0.1	Tr	726
0	14	4	2	0.2	18	2	Tr	Tr	Tr	0.01	Tr	Tr	727
0	10	3	1	0.1	12	2	Tr	Tr	Tr	Tr	Tr	Tr	728
0	13	2	Tr	0.1	16	5	Tr	Tr	Tr	0.01	Tr	1	729
0	10	1	Tr	Tr	13	4	Tr	Tr	Tr	Tr	Tr	1	730
0	18	0	0	Tr	4	11	0	0	0.00	0.00	0.0	0	731
1	30	74	117	1.2	254	285	100	31	0.04	0.17	0.6	Tr	732
Tr	28	119	113	0.3	212	252	Tr	Tr	0.03	0.14	0.4	Tr	733
1	33	79	94	0.2	155	305	Tr	Tr	0.03	0.12	0.6	Tr	734
14	27	130	329	0.3	176	440	130	33	0.04	0.18	0.1	1	735
15	25	146	120	0.2	190	167	140	34	0.05	0.20	0.1	1	736
15	27	133	110	0.5	165	140	140	33	0.10	0.18	0.6	1	737
15	25	131	103	0.1	167	152	140	34	0.04	0.18	0.1	1	738
15	27	129	273	0.1	164	375	140	33	0.04	0.17	0.1	1	739
15	25	132	102	0.1	166	178	140	34	0.04	0.18	0.1	1	740
0	212	187	56	4.8	757	97	0	0	0.02	0.07	0.2	0	741
0	199	3	Tr	0.1	7	5	0	0	0.00	0.00	0.0	0	742
0	12	Tr	Tr	Tr	Tr	Tr	0	0	0.00	0.00	0.0	0	743
0	6	Tr	Tr	Tr	Tr	Tr	0	0	0.00	0.00	0.0	0	744
0	100	1	Tr	Tr	4	2	0	0	0.00	0.00	0.0	0	745
0	22	6	49	0.8	85	36	Tr	Tr	Tr	0.02	0.1	0	746
0	21	38	60	0.5	82	42	40	13	0.02	0.08	0.1	0	747
0	22	274	34	10.1	1,171	38	0	0	0.04	0.08	0.8	0	748
0	32	1	4	Tr	7	19	0	0	0.00	0.00	0.0	0	749
0	1	11	23	0.3	26	2	50	5	0.03	0.04	0.2	3	750
0	12	47	72	1.6	316	79	170	17	0.07	0.06	0.7	9	751
0	8	43	110	1.2	558	7	1,490	149	0.18	0.22	1.9	49	752
0	3	14	37	0.4	186	2	500	50	0.06	0.07	0.6	16	753
0	9	41	99	1.2	392	7	1,470	147	0.12	0.19	1.9	44	754
0	3	14	33	0.4	131	2	490	49	0.04	0.06	0.6	15	755
0	2	11	30	0.5	122	[56]278	380	38	0.04	0.07	0.7	13	756
0	4	10	33	0.4	105	9	10	1	0.03	0.03	0.2	1	757

Table A-5 Nutritive Value of the Edible Part of Food *(Continued)*

(Tr indicates nutrient present in trace amount.)

Item No.	Foods, approximate measures, units, and weight (weight of edible portion only)			Water	Food energy	Pro-tein	Fat	Fatty acids		
								Satu-rated	Mono-unsatu-rated	Poly-unsatu-rated
			Grams	Per-cent	Cal-ories	Grams	Grams	Grams	Grams	Grams
	Vegetables and Vegetable Products—Con.									
	Beans:										
	Lima, immature seeds, frozen, cooked, drained:										
758	Thick-seeded types (Ford-hooks)--------------------	1 cup-----------	170	74	170	10	1	0.1	Tr	0.3
759	Thin-seeded types (baby limas)-----------	1 cup-----------	180	72	190	12	1	0.1	Tr	0.3
	Snap:										
	Cooked, drained:										
760	From raw (cut and French style)-------------------	1 cup-----------	125	89	45	2	Tr	0.1	Tr	0.2
761	From frozen (cut)----------	1 cup-----------	135	92	35	2	Tr	Tr	Tr	0.1
762	Canned, drained solids (cut)	1 cup-----------	135	93	25	2	Tr	Tr	Tr	0.1
	Beans, mature. See Beans, dry (items 527-535) and Black-eyed peas, dry (item 536).										
	Bean sprouts (mung):										
763	Raw-------------------------	1 cup-----------	104	90	30	3	Tr	Tr	Tr	0.1
764	Cooked, drained----------------	1 cup-----------	124	93	25	3	Tr	Tr	Tr	Tr
	Beets:										
	Cooked, drained:										
765	Diced or sliced--------------	1 cup----------	170	91	55	2	Tr	Tr	Tr	Tr
766	Whole beets, 2-in diam.------	2 beets---------	100	91	30	1	Tr	Tr	Tr	Tr
767	Canned, drained solids, diced or sliced--------------------	1 cup----------	170	91	55	2	Tr	Tr	Tr	0.1
768	Beet greens, leaves and stems, cooked, drained----------------	1 cup-----------	144	89	40	4	Tr	Tr	0.1	0.1
	Black-eyed peas, immature seeds, cooked and drained:										
769	From raw----------------------	1 cup----------	165	72	180	13	1	0.3	0.1	0.6
770	From frozen-------------------	1 cup----------	170	66	225	14	1	0.3	0.1	0.5
	Broccoli:										
771	Raw--------------------------	1 spear---------	151	91	40	4	1	0.1	Tr	0.3
	Cooked, drained:										
	From raw:										
772	Spear, medium--------------	1 spear---------	180	90	50	5	1	0.1	Tr	0.2
773	Spears, cut into 1/2-in pieces--------------------	1 cup----------	155	90	45	5	Tr	0.1	Tr	0.2
	From frozen:										
774	Piece, 4-1/2 to 5 in long--	1 piece--------	30	91	10	1	Tr	Tr	Tr	Tr
(775)	Chopped--------------------	1 cup----------	185	91	50	6	Tr	Tr	Tr	0.1
	Brussels sprouts, cooked, drained:										
776	From raw, 7-8 sprouts, 1-1/4 to 1-1/2-in diam.------------	1 cup-----------	155	87	60	4	1	0.2	0.1	0.4
777	From frozen-------------------	1 cup-----------	155	87	65	6	1	0.1	Tr	0.3
	Cabbage, common varieties:										
778	Raw, coarsely shredded or sliced-----------------------	1 cup-----------	70	93	15	1	Tr	Tr	Tr	0.1
779	Cooked, drained----------------	1 cup-----------	150	94	30	1	Tr	Tr	Tr	0.2
	Cabbage, Chinese:										
780	Pak-choi, cooked, drained------	1 cup-----------	170	96	20	3	Tr	Tr	Tr	0.1
781	Pe-tsai, raw, 1-in pieces------	1 cup-----------	76	94	10	1	Tr	Tr	Tr	0.1
782	Cabbage, red, raw, coarsely shredded or sliced-------------	1 cup-----------	70	92	20	1	Tr	Tr	Tr	0.1
783	Cabbage, savoy, raw, coarsely shredded or sliced------------	1 cup-----------	70	91	20	1	Tr	Tr	Tr	Tr

[57] For green varieties; yellow varieties contain 101 IU or 10 RE.
[58] For green varieties; yellow varieties contain 151 IU or 15 RE.
[59] For regular pack; special dietary pack contains 3 mg sodium.

Table A-5 Nutritive Value of the Edible Part of Food (Continued)

Nutrients in Indicated Quantity

Cholesterol	Carbohydrate	Calcium	Phosphorus	Iron	Potassium	Sodium	Vitamin A value (IU)	Vitamin A value (RE)	Thiamin	Riboflavin	Niacin	Ascorbic acid	Item No
Milligrams	Grams	Milligrams	Milligrams	Milligrams	Milligrams	Milligrams	International units	Retinol equivalents	Milligrams	Milligrams	Milligrams	Milligrams	
0	32	37	107	2.3	694	90	320	32	0.13	0.10	1.8	22	758
0	35	50	202	3.5	740	52	300	30	0.13	0.10	1.4	10	759
0	10	58	49	1.6	374	4	[57]830	[57]83	0.09	0.12	0.8	12	760
0	8	61	32	1.1	151	18	[58]710	[58]71	0.06	0.10	0.6	11	761
0	6	35	26	1.2	147	[59]339	[60]470	[60]47	0.02	0.08	0.3	6	762
0	6	14	56	0.9	155	6	20	2	0.09	0.13	0.8	14	763
0	5	15	35	0.8	125	12	20	2	0.06	0.13	1.0	14	764
0	11	19	53	1.1	530	83	20	2	0.05	0.02	0.5	9	765
0	7	11	31	0.6	312	49	10	1	0.03	0.01	0.3	6	766
0	12	26	29	3.1	252	[61]466	20	2	0.02	0.07	0.3	7	767
0	8	164	59	2.7	1,309	347	7,340	734	0.17	0.42	0.7	36	768
0	30	46	196	2.4	693	7	1,050	105	0.11	0.18	1.8	3	769
0	40	39	207	3.6	638	9	130	13	0.44	0.11	1.2	4	770
0	8	72	100	1.3	491	41	2,330	233	0.10	0.18	1.0	141	771
0	10	205	86	2.1	293	20	2,540	254	0.15	0.37	1.4	113	772
0	9	177	74	1.8	253	17	2,180	218	0.13	0.32	1.2	97	773
0	2	15	17	0.2	54	7	570	57	0.02	0.02	0.1	12	774
0	10	94	102	1.1	333	44	3,500	350	0.10	0.15	0.8	74	775
0	13	56	87	1.9	491	33	1,110	111	0.17	0.12	0.9	96	776
0	13	37	84	1.1	504	36	910	91	0.16	0.18	0.8	71	777
0	4	33	16	0.4	172	13	90	9	0.04	0.02	0.2	33	778
0	7	50	38	0.6	308	29	130	13	0.09	0.08	0.3	36	779
0	3	158	49	1.8	631	58	4,370	437	0.05	0.11	0.7	44	780
0	2	59	22	0.2	181	7	910	91	0.03	0.04	0.3	21	781
0	4	36	29	0.3	144	8	30	3	0.04	0.02	0.2	40	782
0	4	25	29	0.3	161	20	700	70	0.05	0.02	0.2	22	783

[60] For green varieties; yellow varieties contain 142 IU or 14 RE.
[61] For regular pack; special dietary pack contains 78 mg sodium.

Table A-5 Nutritive Value of the Edible Part of Food *(Continued)*

(Tr indicates nutrient present in trace amount.)

Item No.	Foods, approximate measures, units, and weight (weight of edible portion only)		Grams	Water	Food energy	Pro-tein	Fat	Fatty acids		
								Satu-rated	Mono-unsatu-rated	Poly-unsatu-rated
	Vegetables and Vegetable Products—Con.		Grams	Per-cent	Cal-ories	Grams	Grams	Grams	Grams	Grams
	Carrots:									
	Raw, without crowns and tips, scraped:									
784	Whole, 7-1/2 by 1-1/8 in, or strips, 2-1/2 to 3 in long	1 carrot or 18 strips	72	88	30	1	Tr	Tr	Tr	0.1
785	Grated	1 cup	110	88	45	1	Tr	Tr	Tr	0.1
	Cooked, sliced, drained:									
786	From raw	1 cup	156	87	70	2	Tr	0.1	Tr	0.1
787	From frozen	1 cup	146	90	55	2	Tr	Tr	Tr	0.1
788	Canned, sliced, drained solids	1 cup	146	93	35	1	Tr	0.1	Tr	0.1
	Cauliflower:									
789	Raw, (flowerets)	1 cup	100	92	25	2	Tr	Tr	Tr	0.1
	Cooked, drained:									
790	From raw (flowerets)	1 cup	125	93	30	2	Tr	Tr	Tr	0.1
791	From frozen (flowerets)	1 cup	180	94	35	3	Tr	0.1	Tr	0.2
	Celery, pascal type, raw:									
792	Stalk, large outer, 8 by 1-1/2 in (at root end)	1 stalk	40	95	5	Tr	Tr	Tr	Tr	Tr
793	Pieces, diced	1 cup	120	95	20	1	Tr	Tr	Tr	0.1
	Collards, cooked, drained:									
794	From raw (leaves without stems)	1 cup	190	96	25	2	Tr	0.1	Tr	0.2
795	From frozen (chopped)	1 cup	170	88	60	5	1	0.1	0.1	0.4
	Corn, sweet:									
	Cooked, drained:									
796	From raw, ear 5 by 1-3/4 in	1 ear	77	70	85	3	1	0.2	0.3	0.5
	From frozen:									
797	Ear, trimmed to about 3-1/2 in long	1 ear	63	73	60	2	Tr	0.1	0.1	0.2
798	Kernels	1 cup	165	76	135	5	Tr	Tr	Tr	0.1
	Canned:									
799	Cream style	1 cup	256	79	185	4	1	0.2	0.3	0.5
800	Whole kernel, vacuum pack	1 cup	210	77	165	5	1	0.2	0.3	0.5
	Cowpeas. See Black-eyed peas, immature (items 769,770), mature (item 536).									
801	Cucumber, with peel, slices, 1/8 in thick (large, 2-1/8-in diam.; small, 1-3/4-in diam.)	6 large or 8 small slices	28	96	5	Tr	Tr	Tr	Tr	Tr
802	Dandelion greens, cooked, drained	1 cup	105	90	35	2	1	0.1	Tr	0.3
803	Eggplant, cooked, steamed	1 cup	96	92	25	1	Tr	Tr	Tr	0.1
804	Endive, curly (including esca-role), raw, small pieces	1 cup	50	94	10	1	Tr	Tr	Tr	Tr
805	Jerusalem-artichoke, raw, sliced	1 cup	150	78	115	3	Tr	0.0	Tr	Tr
	Kale, cooked, drained:									
806	From raw, chopped	1 cup	130	91	40	2	1	0.1	Tr	0.3
807	From frozen, chopped	1 cup	130	91	40	4	1	0.1	Tr	0.3
808	Kohlrabi, thickened bulb-like stems, cooked, drained, diced	1 cup	165	90	50	3	Tr	Tr	Tr	0.1
	Lettuce, raw:									
	Butterhead, as Boston types:									
809	Head, 5-in diam	1 head	163	96	20	2	Tr	Tr	Tr	0.2
810	Leaves	1 outer or 2 inner leaves	15	96	Tr	Tr	Tr	Tr	Tr	Tr
	Crisphead, as iceberg:									
811	Head, 6-in diam	1 head	539	96	70	5	1	0.1	Tr	0.5
812	Wedge, 1/4 of head	1 wedge	135	96	20	1	Tr	Tr	Tr	0.1
813	Pieces, chopped or shredded	1 cup	55	96	5	1	Tr	Tr	Tr	0.1
814	Looseleaf (bunching varieties including romaine or cos), chopped or shredded pieces	1 cup	56	94	10	1	Tr	Tr	Tr	0.1

[62] For regular pack; special dietary pack contains 61 mg sodium.
[63] For yellow varieties; white varieties contain only a trace of vitamin A.

Table A-5 Nutritive Value of the Edible Part of Food *(Continued)*

Nutrients in Indicated Quantity

Cho-les-terol	Carbo-hydrate	Calcium	Phos-phorus	Iron	Potas-sium	Sodium	Vitamin A value		Thiamin	Ribo-flavin	Niacin	Ascorbic acid	Item No.
							(IU)	(RE)					
Milli-grams	Grams	Milli-grams	Milli-grams	Milli-grams	Milli-grams	Milli-grams	Inter-national units	Retinol equiva-lents	Milli-grams	Milli-grams	Milli-grams	Milli-grams	
0	7	19	32	0.4	233	25	20,250	2,025	0.07	0.04	0.7	7	784
0	11	30	48	0.6	355	39	30,940	3,094	0.11	0.06	1.0	10	785
0	16	48	47	1.0	354	103	38,300	3,830	0.05	0.09	0.8	4	786
0	12	41	38	0.7	231	86	25,850	2,585	0.04	0.05	0.6	4	787
0	8	37	35	0.9	261	[62]352	20,110	2,011	0.03	0.04	0.8	4	788
0	5	29	46	0.6	355	15	20	2	0.08	0.06	0.6	72	789
0	6	34	44	0.5	404	8	20	2	0.08	0.07	0.7	69	790
0	7	31	43	0.7	250	32	40	4	0.07	0.10	0.6	56	791
0	1	14	10	0.2	114	35	50	5	0.01	0.01	0.1	3	792
0	4	43	31	0.6	341	106	150	15	0.04	0.04	0.4	8	793
0	5	148	19	0.8	177	36	4,220	422	0.03	0.08	0.4	19	794
0	12	357	46	1.9	427	85	10,170	1,017	0.08	0.20	1.1	45	795
0	19	2	79	0.5	192	13	[63]170	[63]17	0.17	0.06	1.2	5	796
0	14	2	47	0.4	158	3	[63]130	[63]13	0.11	0.04	1.0	3	797
0	34	3	78	0.5	229	8	[63]410	[63]41	0.11	0.12	2.1	4	798
0	46	8	131	1.0	343	[64]730	[63]250	[63]25	0.06	0.14	2.5	12	799
0	41	11	134	0.9	391	[65]571	[63]510	[63]51	0.09	0.15	2.5	17	800
0	1	4	5	0.1	42	1	10	1	0.01	0.01	0.1	1	801
0	7	147	44	1.9	244	46	12,290	1,229	0.14	0.18	0.5	19	802
0	6	6	21	0.3	238	3	60	6	0.07	0.02	0.6	1	803
0	2	26	14	0.4	157	11	1,030	103	0.04	0.04	0.2	3	804
0	26	21	117	5.1	644	6	30	3	0.30	0.09	2.0	6	805
0	7	94	36	1.2	296	30	9,620	962	0.07	0.09	0.7	53	806
0	7	179	36	1.2	417	20	8,260	826	0.06	0.15	0.9	33	807
0	11	41	74	0.7	561	35	60	6	0.07	0.03	0.6	89	808
0	4	52	38	0.5	419	8	1,580	158	0.10	0.10	0.5	13	809
0	Tr	5	3	Tr	39	1	150	15	0.01	0.01	Tr	1	810
0	11	102	108	2.7	852	49	1,780	178	0.25	0.16	1.0	21	811
0	3	26	27	0.7	213	12	450	45	0.06	0.04	0.3	5	812
0	1	10	11	0.3	87	5	180	18	0.03	0.02	0.1	2	813
0	2	38	14	0.8	148	5	1,060	106	0.03	0.04	0.2	10	814

[64] For regular pack; special dietary pack contains 8 mg sodium.
[65] For regular pack; special dietary pack contains 6 mg sodium.

Table A-5 Nutritive Value of the Edible Part of Food *(Continued)*

(Tr Indicates nutrient present in trace amount.)

Item No.	Foods, approximate measures, units, and weight (weight of edible portion only)		Water	Food energy	Pro-tein	Fat	Fatty acids		
							Satu-rated	Mono-unsatu-rated	Poly-unsatu-rated
		Grams	Per-cent	Cal-ories	Grams	Grams	Grams	Grams	Grams
	Vegetables and Vegetable Products—Con.								
	Mushrooms:								
815	Raw, sliced or chopped--------- 1 cup-----------	70	92	20	1	Tr	Tr	Tr	0.1
816	Cooked, drained---------------- 1 cup-----------	156	91	40	3	1	0.1	Tr	0.3
817	Canned, drained solids--------- 1 cup-----------	156	91	35	3	Tr	0.1	Tr	0.2
818	Mustard greens, without stems and midribs, cooked, drained------- 1 cup-----------	140	94	20	3	Tr	Tr	0.2	0.1
819	Okra pods, 3 by 5/8 in, cooked--- 8 pods----------	85	90	25	2	Tr	Tr	Tr	Tr
	Onions:								
	Raw:								
820	Chopped---------------------- 1 cup-----------	160	91	55	2	Tr	0.1	0.1	0.2
821	Sliced----------------------- 1 cup-----------	115	91	40	1	Tr	0.1	Tr	0.1
822	Cooked (whole or sliced), drained---------------------- 1 cup-----------	210	92	60	2	Tr	0.1	Tr	0.1
823	Onions, spring, raw, bulb (3/8-in diam.) and white portion of top 6 onions--------	30	92	10	1	Tr	Tr	Tr	Tr
824	Onion rings, breaded, par-fried, frozen, prepared--------------- 2 rings---------	20	29	80	1	5	1.7	2.2	1.0
	Parsley:								
825	Raw------------------------------ 10 sprigs-------	10	88	5	Tr	Tr	Tr	Tr	Tr
826	Freeze-dried--------------------- 1 tbsp----------	0.4	2	Tr	Tr	Tr	Tr	Tr	Tr
827	Parsnips, cooked (diced or 2 in lengths), drained------------- 1 cup-----------	156	78	125	2	Tr	0.1	0.2	0.1
828	Peas, edible pod, cooked, drained 1 cup-----------	160	89	65	5	Tr	0.1	Tr	0.2
	Peas, green:								
829	Canned, drained solids--------- 1 cup-----------	170	82	115	8	1	0.1	0.1	0.3
830	Frozen, cooked, drained-------- 1 cup-----------	160	80	125	8	Tr	0.1	Tr	0.2
	Peppers:								
831	Hot chili, raw----------------- 1 pepper--------	45	88	20	1	Tr	Tr	Tr	Tr
	Sweet (about 5 per lb, whole), stem and seeds removed:								
832	Raw------------------------- 1 pepper--------	74	93	20	1	Tr	Tr	Tr	0.2
833	Cooked, drained------------- 1 pepper--------	73	95	15	Tr	Tr	Tr	Tr	0.1
	Potatoes, cooked:								
	Baked (about 2 per lb, raw):								
834	With skin------------------- 1 potato--------	202	71	220	5	Tr	0.1	Tr	0.1
835	Flesh only------------------ 1 potato--------	156	75	145	3	Tr	Tr	Tr	0.1
	Boiled (about 3 per lb, raw):								
836	Peeled after boiling-------- 1 potato--------	136	77	120	3	Tr	Tr	Tr	0.1
837	Peeled before boiling------- 1 potato--------	135	77	115	2	Tr	Tr	Tr	0.1
	French fried, strip, 2 to 3-1/2 in long, frozen:								
838	Oven heated----------------- 10 strips-------	50	53	110	2	4	2.1	1.8	0.3
839	Fried in vegetable oil------ 10 strips-------	50	38	160	2	8	2.5	1.6	3.8
	Potato products, prepared:								
	Au gratin:								
840	From dry mix---------------- 1 cup-----------	245	79	230	6	10	6.3	2.9	0.3
841	From home recipe------------ 1 cup-----------	245	74	325	12	19	11.6	5.3	0.7
842	Hashed brown, from frozen------ 1 cup-----------	156	56	340	5	18	7.0	8.0	2.1
	Mashed:								
	From home recipe:								
843	Milk added--------------- 1 cup-----------	210	78	160	4	1	0.7	0.3	0.1
844	Milk and margarine added--- 1 cup-----------	210	76	225	4	9	2.2	3.7	2.5
845	From dehydrated flakes (without milk), water, milk, butter, and salt added---------------------- 1 cup-----------	210	76	235	4	12	7.2	3.3	0.5
846	Potato salad, made with mayonnaise-------------------- 1 cup-----------	250	76	360	7	21	3.6	6.2	9.3
	Scalloped:								
847	From dry mix---------------- 1 cup-----------	245	79	230	5	11	6.5	3.0	0.5
848	From home recipe------------ 1 cup-----------	245	81	210	7	9	5.5	2.5	0.4

[66] For regular pack; special dietary pack contains 3 mg sodium.
[67] For red peppers; green peppers contain 350 IU or 35 RE.
[68] For green peppers; red peppers contain 4,220 IU or 422 RE.

Table A-5 Nutritive Value of the Edible Part of Food (Continued)

Nutrients in Indicated Quantity

Choles-terol	Carbo-hydrate	Calcium	Phos-phorus	Iron	Potas-sium	Sodium	Vitamin A value (IU)	(RE)	Thiamin	Ribo-flavin	Niacin	Ascorbic acid	Item No.
Milli-grams	Grams	Milli-grams	Milli-grams	Milli-grams	Milli-grams	Milli-grams	Inter-national units	Retinol equiva-lents	Milli-grams	Milli-grams	Milli-grams	Milli-grams	
0	3	4	73	0.9	259	3	0	0	0.07	0.31	2.9	2	815
0	8	9	136	2.7	555	3	0	0	0.11	0.47	7.0	6	816
0	8	17	103	1.2	201	663	0	0	0.13	0.03	2.5	0	817
0	3	104	57	1.0	283	22	4,240	424	0.06	0.09	0.6	35	818
0	6	54	48	0.4	274	4	490	49	0.11	0.05	0.7	14	819
0	12	40	46	0.6	248	3	0	0	0.10	0.02	0.2	13	820
0	8	29	33	0.4	178	2	0	0	0.07	0.01	0.1	10	821
0	13	57	48	0.4	319	17	0	0	0.09	0.02	0.2	12	822
0	2	18	10	0.6	77	1	1,500	150	0.02	0.04	0.1	14	823
0	8	6	16	0.3	26	75	50	5	0.06	0.03	0.7	Tr	824
0	1	13	4	0.6	54	4	520	52	0.01	0.01	0.1	9	825
0	Tr	1	2	0.2	25	2	250	25	Tr	0.01	Tr	1	826
0	30	58	108	0.9	573	16	0	0	0.13	0.08	1.1	20	827
0	11	67	88	3.2	384	6	210	21	0.20	0.12	0.9	77	828
0	21	34	114	1.6	294	[66]372	1,310	131	0.21	0.13	1.2	16	829
0	23	38	144	2.5	269	139	1,070	107	0.45	0.16	2.4	16	830
0	4	8	21	0.5	153	3	[67]4,840	[67]484	0.04	0.04	0.4	109	831
0	4	4	16	0.9	144	2	[68]390	[68]39	0.06	0.04	0.4	[69]95	832
0	3	3	11	0.6	94	1	[70]280	[70]28	0.04	0.03	0.3	[71]81	833
0	51	20	115	2.7	844	16	0	0	0.22	0.07	3.3	26	834
0	34	8	78	0.5	610	8	0	0	0.16	0.03	2.2	20	835
0	27	7	60	0.4	515	5	0	0	0.14	0.03	2.0	18	836
0	27	11	54	0.4	443	7	0	0	0.13	0.03	1.8	10	837
0	17	5	43	0.7	229	16	0	0	0.06	0.02	1.2	5	838
0	20	10	47	0.4	366	108	0	0	0.09	0.01	1.6	5	839
12	31	203	233	0.8	537	1,076	520	76	0.05	0.20	2.3	8	840
56	28	292	277	1.6	970	1,061	650	93	0.16	0.28	2.4	24	841
0	44	23	112	2.4	680	53	0	0	0.17	0.03	3.8	10	842
4	37	55	101	0.6	628	636	40	12	0.18	0.08	2.3	14	843
4	35	55	97	0.5	607	620	360	42	0.18	0.08	2.3	13	844
29	32	103	118	0.5	489	697	380	44	0.23	0.11	1.4	20	845
170	28	48	130	1.6	635	1,323	520	83	0.19	0.15	2.2	25	846
27	31	88	137	0.9	497	835	360	51	0.05	0.14	2.5	8	847
29	26	140	154	1.4	926	821	330	47	0.17	0.23	2.6	26	848

[69]For green peppers; red peppers contain 141 mg ascorbic acid.
[70]For green peppers; red peppers contain 2,740 IU or 274 RE.
[71]For green peppers; red peppers contain 121 mg ascorbic acid.

Table A-5 Nutritive Value of the Edible Part of Food (Continued)

(Tr indicates nutrient present in trace amount.)

Item No.	Foods, approximate measures, units, and weight (weight of edible portion only)		Water	Food energy	Pro-tein	Fat	Fatty acids		
							Satu-rated	Mono-unsatu-rated	Poly-unsatu-rated
	Vegetables and Vegetable Products—Con.	Grams	Per-cent	Cal-ories	Grams	Grams	Grams	Grams	Grams
849	Potato chips-------------------- 10 chips--------	20	3	105	1	7	1.8	1.2	3.6
	Pumpkin:								
850	Cooked from raw, mashed-------- 1 cup-----------	245	94	50	2	Tr	0.1	Tr	Tr
851	Canned------------------------- 1 cup-----------	245	90	85	3	1	0.4	0.1	Tr
852	Radishes, raw, stem ends, rootlets cut off---------------- 4 radishes------	18	95	5	Tr	Tr	Tr	Tr	Tr
853	Sauerkraut, canned, solids and liquid------------------------- 1 cup-----------	236	93	45	2	Tr	0.1	Tr	0.1
	Seaweed:								
854	Kelp, raw---------------------- 1 oz------------	28	82	10	Tr	Tr	0.1	Tr	Tr
855	Spirulina, dried--------------- 1 oz------------	28	5	80	16	2	0.8	0.2	0.6
	Southern peas. See Black-eyed peas, immature (items 769,770), mature (item 536).								
	Spinach:								
856	Raw, chopped------------------- 1 cup-----------	55	92	10	2	Tr	Tr	Tr	0.1
	Cooked, drained:								
857	From raw---------------------- 1 cup-----------	180	91	40	5	Tr	0.1	Tr	0.2
858	From frozen (leaf)----------- 1 cup-----------	190	90	55	6	Tr	0.1	Tr	0.2
859	Canned, drained solids--------- 1 cup-----------	214	92	50	6	1	0.2	Tr	0.4
860	Spinach souffle---------------- 1 cup-----------	136	74	220	11	18	7.1	6.8	3.1
	Squash, cooked:								
861	Summer (all varieties), sliced, drained---------------------- 1 cup-----------	180	94	35	2	1	0.1	Tr	0.2
862	Winter (all varieties), baked, cubes------------------------- 1 cup-----------	205	89	80	2	1	0.3	0.1	0.5
	Sunchoke. See Jerusalem-arti-choke (item 805).								
	Sweetpotatoes:								
	Cooked (raw, 5 by 2 in; about 2-1/2 per lb):								
863	Baked in skin, peeled-------- 1 potato--------	114	73	115	2	Tr	Tr	Tr	0.1
864	Boiled, without skin--------- 1 potato--------	151	73	160	2	Tr	0.1	Tr	0.2
865	Candied, 2-1/2 by 2-in piece--- 1 piece---------	105	67	145	1	3	1.4	0.7	0.2
	Canned:								
866	Solid pack (mashed)---------- 1 cup-----------	255	74	260	5	1	0.1	Tr	0.2
867	Vacuum pack, piece 2-3/4 by 1 in---------------------- 1 piece---------	40	76	35	1	Tr	Tr	Tr	Tr
	Tomatoes:								
868	Raw, 2-3/5-in diam. (3 per 12 oz pkg.)-------------------- 1 tomato--------	123	94	25	1	Tr	Tr	Tr	0.1
869	Canned, solids and liquid------ 1 cup-----------	240	94	50	2	1	0.1	0.1	0.2
870	Tomato juice, canned----------- 1 cup-----------	244	94	40	2	Tr	Tr	Tr	0.1
	Tomato products, canned:								
871	Paste------------------------- 1 cup-----------	262	74	220	10	2	0.3	0.4	0.9
872	Puree------------------------- 1 cup-----------	250	87	105	4	Tr	Tr	Tr	0.1
873	Sauce------------------------- 1 cup-----------	245	89	75	3	Tr	0.1	0.1	0.2
874	Turnips, cooked, diced--------- 1 cup-----------	156	94	30	1	Tr	Tr	Tr	0.1
	Turnip greens, cooked, drained:								
875	From raw (leaves and stems)---- 1 cup-----------	144	93	30	2	Tr	0.1	Tr	0.1
876	From frozen (chopped)---------- 1 cup-----------	164	90	50	5	1	0.2	Tr	0.3
877	Vegetable juice cocktail, canned 1 cup-----------	242	94	45	2	Tr	Tr	Tr	0.1
	Vegetables, mixed:								
878	Canned, drained solids--------- 1 cup-----------	163	87	75	4	Tr	0.1	Tr	0.2
879	Frozen, cooked, drained-------- 1 cup-----------	182	83	105	5	Tr	0.1	Tr	0.1
880	Waterchestnuts, canned--------- 1 cup-----------	140	86	70	1	Tr	Tr	Tr	Tr

[1] Value not determined.
[72] With added salt; if none is added, sodium content is 58 mg.
[73] For regular pack; special dietary pack contains 31 mg sodium.
[74] With added salt; if none is added, sodium content is 24 mg.

Table A-5 Nutritive Value of the Edible Part of Food *(Continued)*

Nutrients in Indicated Quantity

Cholesterol	Carbohydrate	Calcium	Phosphorus	Iron	Potassium	Sodium	Vitamin A value (IU)	Vitamin A value (RE)	Thiamin	Riboflavin	Niacin	Ascorbic acid	Item No.
Milligrams	Grams	Milligrams	Milligrams	Milligrams	Milligrams	Milligrams	International units	Retinol equivalents	Milligrams	Milligrams	Milligrams	Milligrams	
0	10	5	31	0.2	260	94	0	0	0.03	Tr	0.8	8	849
0	12	37	74	1.4	564	2	2,650	265	0.08	0.19	1.0	12	850
0	20	64	86	3.4	505	12	54,040	5,404	0.06	0.13	0.9	10	851
0	1	4	3	0.1	42	4	Tr	Tr	Tr	0.01	0.1	4	852
0	10	71	47	3.5	401	1,560	40	4	0.05	0.05	0.3	35	853
0	3	48	12	0.8	25	66	30	3	0.01	0.04	0.1	(1)	854
0	7	34	33	8.1	386	297	160	16	0.67	1.04	3.6	3	855
0	2	54	27	1.5	307	43	3,690	369	0.04	0.10	0.4	15	856
0	7	245	101	6.4	839	126	14,740	1,474	0.17	0.42	0.9	18	857
0	10	277	91	2.9	566	163	14,790	1,479	0.11	0.32	0.8	23	858
0	7	272	94	4.9	740	[72] 683	18,780	1,878	0.03	0.30	0.8	31	859
184	3	230	231	1.3	201	763	3,460	675	0.09	0.30	0.5	3	860
0	8	49	70	0.6	346	2	520	52	0.08	0.07	0.9	10	861
0	18	29	41	0.7	896	2	7,290	729	0.17	0.05	1.4	20	862
0	28	32	63	0.5	397	11	24,880	2,488	0.08	0.14	0.7	28	863
0	37	32	41	0.8	278	20	25,750	2,575	0.08	0.21	1.0	26	864
8	29	27	27	1.2	198	74	4,400	440	0.02	0.04	0.4	7	865
0	59	77	133	3.4	536	191	38,570	3,857	0.07	0.23	2.4	13	866
0	8	9	20	0.4	125	21	3,190	319	0.01	0.02	0.3	11	867
0	5	9	28	0.6	255	10	1,390	139	0.07	0.06	0.7	22	868
0	10	62	46	1.5	530	[73] 391	1,450	145	0.11	0.07	1.8	36	869
0	10	22	46	1.4	537	[74] 881	1,360	136	0.11	0.08	1.6	45	870
0	49	92	207	7.8	2,442	[75] 170	6,470	647	0.41	0.50	8.4	111	871
0	25	38	100	2.3	1,050	[76] 50	3,400	340	0.18	0.14	4.3	88	872
0	18	34	78	1.9	909	[77] 1,482	2,400	240	0.16	0.14	2.8	32	873
0	8	34	30	0.3	211	78	0	0	0.04	0.04	0.5	18	874
0	6	197	42	1.2	292	42	7,920	792	0.06	0.10	0.6	39	875
0	8	249	56	3.2	367	25	13,080	1,308	0.09	0.12	0.8	36	876
0	11	27	41	1.0	467	883	2,830	283	0.10	0.07	1.8	67	877
0	15	44	68	1.7	474	243	18,990	1,899	0.08	0.08	0.9	8	878
0	24	46	93	1.5	308	64	7,780	778	0.13	0.22	1.5	6	879
0	17	6	27	1.2	165	11	10	1	0.02	0.03	0.5	2	880

[75] With no added salt; if salt is added, sodium content is 2,070 mg.
[76] With no added salt; if salt is added, sodium content is 998 mg.
[77] With salt added.

Table A-5 Nutritive Value of the Edible Part of Food *(Continued)*

(Tr indicates nutrient present in trace amount.)

Item No.	Foods, approximate measures, units, and weight (weight of edible portion only)			Water	Food energy	Pro-tein	Fat	Fatty acids		
								Satu-rated	Mono-unsatu-rated	Poly-unsatu-rated
	Miscellaneous Items		Grams	Per-cent	Cal-ories	Grams	Grams	Grams	Grams	Grams
	Baking powders for home use:									
	Sodium aluminum sulfate:									
881	With monocalcium phosphate monohydrate	1 tsp	3	2	5	Tr	0	0.0	0.0	0.0
882	With monocalcium phosphate monohydrate, calcium sulfate	1 tsp	2.9	1	5	Tr	0	0.0	0.0	0.0
883	Straight phosphate	1 tsp	3.8	2	5	Tr	0	0.0	0.0	0.0
884	Low sodium	1 tsp	4.3	1	5	Tr	0	0.0	0.0	0.0
885	Catsup	1 cup	273	69	290	5	1	0.2	0.2	0.4
886		1 tbsp	15	69	15	Tr	Tr	Tr	Tr	Tr
887	Celery seed	1 tsp	2	6	10	Tr	1	Tr	0.3	0.1
888	Chili powder	1 tsp	2.6	8	10	Tr	Tr	0.1	0.1	0.2
	Chocolate:									
889	Bitter or baking	1 oz	28	2	145	3	15	9.0	4.9	0.5
	Semisweet, see Candy, (item 715).									
890	Cinnamon	1 tsp	2.3	10	5	Tr	Tr	Tr	Tr	Tr
891	Curry powder	1 tsp	2	10	5	Tr	Tr	(1)	(1)	(1)
892	Garlic powder	1 tsp	2.8	6	10	Tr	Tr	Tr	Tr	Tr
893	Gelatin, dry	1 envelope	7	13	25	6	Tr	Tr	Tr	Tr
894	Mustard, prepared, yellow	1 tsp or indivi-dual packet	5	80	5	Tr	Tr	Tr	0.2	Tr
	Olives, canned:									
895	Green	4 medium or 3 extra large	13	78	15	Tr	2	0.2	1.2	0.1
896	Ripe, Mission, pitted	3 small or 2 large	9	73	15	Tr	2	0.3	1.3	0.2
897	Onion powder	1 tsp	2.1	5	5	Tr	Tr	Tr	Tr	Tr
898	Oregano	1 tsp	1.5	7	5	Tr	Tr	Tr	Tr	0.1
899	Paprika	1 tsp	2.1	10	5	Tr	Tr	Tr	Tr	0.2
900	Pepper, black	1 tsp	2.1	11	5	Tr	Tr	Tr	Tr	Tr
	Pickles, cucumber:									
901	Dill, medium, whole, 3-3/4 in long, 1-1/4-in diam.	1 pickle	65	93	5	Tr	Tr	Tr	Tr	0.1
902	Fresh-pack, slices 1-1/2-in diam., 1/4 in thick	2 slices	15	79	10	Tr	Tr	Tr	Tr	Tr
903	Sweet, gherkin, small, whole, about 2-1/2 in long, 3/4-in diam.	1 pickle	15	61	20	Tr	Tr	Tr	Tr	Tr
	Popcorn. See Grain Products, (items 497-499).									
904	Relish, finely chopped, sweet	1 tbsp	15	63	20	Tr	Tr	Tr	Tr	Tr
905	Salt	1 tsp	5.5	0	0	0	0	0.0	0.0	0.0
906	Vinegar, cider	1 tbsp	15	94	Tr	Tr	0	0.0	0.0	0.0
	Yeast:									
907	Baker's, dry, active	1 pkg	7	5	20	3	Tr	Tr	0.1	Tr
908	Brewer's, dry	1 tbsp	8	5	25	3	Tr	Tr	Tr	0.0

[1]Value not determined.

Table A-5 Nutritive Value of the Edible Part of Food *(Continued)*

Nutrients In Indicated Quantity

Cho-les-terol	Carbo-hydrate	Calcium	Phos-phorus	Iron	Potas-sium	Sodium	Vitamin A value		Thiamin	Ribo-flavin	Niacin	Ascorbic acid	Item No.
							(IU)	(RE)					
Milli-grams	Grams	Milli-grams	Milli-grams	Milli-grams	Milli-grams	Milli-grams	Inter-national units	Retinol equiva-ients	Milli-grams	Milli-grams	Milli-grams	Milli-grams	
0	1	58	87	0.0	5	329	0	0	0.00	0.00	0.0	0	881
0	1	183	45	0.0	4	290	0	0	0.00	0.00	0.0	0	882
0	1	239	359	0.0	6	312	0	0	0.00	0.00	0.0	0	883
0	1	207	314	0.0	891	Tr	0	0	0.00	0.00	0.0	0	884
0	69	60	137	2.2	991	2,845	3,820	382	0.25	0.19	4.4	41	885
0	4	3	8	0.1	54	156	210	21	0.01	0.01	0.2	2	886
0	1	35	11	0.9	28	3	Tr	Tr	0.01	0.01	0.1	Tr	887
0	1	7	8	0.4	50	26	910	91	0.01	0.02	0.2	2	888
0	8	22	109	1.9	235	1	10	1	0.01	0.07	0.4	0	889
0	2	28	1	0.9	12	1	10	1	Tr	Tr	Tr	1	890
0	1	10	7	0.6	31	1	20	2	0.01	0.01	0.1	Tr	891
0	2	2	12	0.1	31	1	0	0	0.01	Tr	Tr	Tr	892
0	0	1	0	0.0	2	6	0	0	0.00	0.00	0.0	0	893
0	Tr	4	4	0.1	7	63	0	0	Tr	0.01	Tr	Tr	894
0	Tr	8	2	0.2	7	312	40	4	Tr	Tr	Tr	0	895
0	Tr	10	2	0.2	2	68	10	1	Tr	Tr	Tr	0	896
0	2	8	7	0.1	20	1	Tr	Tr	0.01	Tr	Tr	Tr	897
0	1	24	3	0.7	25	Tr	100	10	0.01	Tr	0.1	1	898
0	1	4	7	0.5	49	1	1,270	127	0.01	0.04	0.3	1	899
0	1	9	4	0.6	26	1	Tr	Tr	Tr	0.01	Tr	0	900
0	1	17	14	0.7	130	928	70	7	Tr	0.01	Tr	4	901
0	3	5	4	0.3	30	101	20	2	Tr	Tr	Tr	1	902
0	5	2	2	0.2	30	107	10	1	Tr	Tr	Tr	1	903
0	5	3	2	0.1	30	107	20	2	Tr	Tr	0.0	1	904
0	0	14	3	Tr	Tr	2,132	0	0	0.00	0.00	0.0	0	905
0	1	1	1	0.1	15	Tr	0	0	0.00	0.00	0.0	0	906
0	3	3	90	1.1	140	4	Tr	Tr	0.16	0.38	2.6	Tr	907
0	3	[78]17	140	1.4	152	10	Tr	Tr	1.25	0.34	3.0	Tr	908

[78]Value may vary from 6 to 60 mg.

(Courtesy of United States Department of Agriculture)

GLOSSARY

absorption—taking in of nutrients

abstinence—avoidance

acid-ash foods—foods that leave an acid ash after oxidation: meats, cereals, cranberries, plums, and prunes

acid-base balance—the regulation of hydrogen ions in body fluids

acidosis—condition in which excess acids accumulate or there is a loss of base in the body

acne—pimples

acute—sudden but short-lived

acute renal failure—suddenly occurring failure of the kidneys

ADH—antidiuretic hormone, also called vasopressin, excreted by the pituitary gland

adipose tissue—fatty tissue

adolescent—person between the ages of 13 and 20

AIDS—acquired immunedeficiency syndrome; caused by the human immunodeficiency virus (HIV)

alcoholism—chronic and excessive use of alcohol

aldosterone—hormone secreted by adrenal glands that triggers kidneys to increase amount of sodium being reabsorbed

alkaline—base; capable of neutralizing acids

alkaline-ash foods—foods that leave an alkaline ash after oxidation; fruits, vegetables, milk, and cream

alkalosis—condition in which excess base accumulates in, or acids are lost from, the body

allergen—substance causing allergy

allergic reaction—adverse physical reaction to specific substance(s)

allergy—sensitivity to specific substance(s)

alpha-tocopherol—a form of vitamin E

ambulatory—able to walk

amenorrhea—the stoppage of the monthly menstrual flow

amino acids—nitrogen-containing chemical compounds of which protein is composed

amniocentesis—testing of the baby in utero

amniotic fluid—surrounds fetus in the uterus

amphetamines—drugs intended to inhibit appetite

anabolism—the creation of new compounds during metabolism

analogues—imitations

anemia—condition caused by insufficient number of red blood cells, hemoglobin, or blood volume

angina pectoris—pain in the heart muscle due to inadequate blood supply

anorexia nervosa—psychologically induced lack of appetite

anthropometric measurements—of height, weight, head, chest, skinfold

antibiotic therapy—use of medications to destroy harmful microbes

antibodies—substances produced by body in reaction to foreign substance; neutralize toxins from foreign bodies

anticoagulant—drug used to thin blood

antioxidant—substance preventing damage from oxygen

anxiety—apprehension

arachidonic acid—one of three fatty acids needed by the body; can be synthesized by the body

arteriosclerosis—generic term for thickened arteries

arthritis—chronic disease involving the joints

ascites—abnormal collection of fluid in the abdomen

ascorbic acid—vitamin C

aspartame—artificial sweetener made from protein; does not require insulin for metabolism

aspirated—inhaled or suctioned

asymptomatic—without symptoms

atherosclerosis—a form of arteriosclerosis affecting the intima (inner lining) of the artery walls

average weight—normal weight for a particular size

avitaminosis—without vitamins

bacteria—microorganism that may or may not cause disease

balanced diet—one that includes all the essential nutrients in appropriate amounts

basal metabolism rate (BMR)—the rate at which energy is needed for body maintenance

basic four food groups—simplified method of maintaining a balanced diet that divides foods into 4 groups: meats, vegetables and fruits, diary foods, and breads and cereals

beriberi—deficiency disease caused by a lack of vitamin B_1 (thiamin)

beverage—a drink

biekest—solid or semi-solid food

bile—secretion of the liver, stored in the gallbladder; essential for the digestion of fats

biochemical tests—involving biology and chemistry

biotin—a B vitamin; necessary for metabolism

bland—mild or soothing

bland diet—diet containing only mild-flavored foods with soft textures

blemish—mark

blood plasma—fluid part of the blood

bolus—food in the mouth that is ready to be swallowed

bonding—emotional attachment

bone marrow—soft tissue in the bone center

botulism—deadliest of food poisonings; caused by the bacteria *Clostridium botulinum*

bouillon—clear soup broth

braise—to cook in a covered container with a small amount of liquid, as is done with less tender cuts of meat

bran—outer covering of grain kernels

brine—water/salt solution

broth—liquid part of soup

bubbled—burped, to get rid of stomach gas

buffer—protective system regulating amounts of hydrogen ions in body fluids

bulimia—condition in which patient alternately binges and purges

buttermilk—milk made from the addition of harmless bacteria to skim milk

cachexia—severe malnutrition and body wasting caused by chronic disease

caffeine—stimulant in coffee, tea, and many cola beverages

caliper—mechanical device used to measure percentage of body fat by skinfold measurement

caloric density—energy value; number of kcal in a food

calorie—also known as kcal or kilocalorie; represents the amount of heat needed to raise the temperature of one kilogram of water one degree Celsius (C)

calorimeter—device used to scientifically determine the kcal value of foods

capillaries—tiny blood vessels connecting veins and arteries

carbohydrate—the nutrient providing the major source of energy in the average diet

carboxypeptidase—pancreatic enzyme necessary for protein digestion

carcinogen—cancer-causing substance

cardiovascular—pertaining to the heart and entire circulatory system

cardiovascular disease—disease affecting heart and blood vessels

carotene—provitamin A

carrier—one who is capable of transmitting an infectious organism

catabolism—the breakdown of compounds during metabolism

catalyst—a substance that causes another substance to react

cataracts—a clouding of the lens of the eye, obstructing sight

celiac sprue—disorder characterized by malabsorption; causes diarrhea, weight loss, and malnutrition; elimination of gluten provides relief

cell membrane—outer covering

cellular edema—swelling of body cells caused by inadequate amount of sodium in extracellular fluid cellulose—indigestible carbohydrate; provides fiber in the diet

Celsius—metric system of measuring temperature

cerebral hemorrhage—stroke; bleeding in the brain

cerebrospinal fluid—of the brain and spinal cord

certified milk—milk that has been handled according to health regulations

cheilosis—condition caused by riboflavin deficiency; characterized by cracks and sores on the lips

chemical digestion—chemical changes in foods during digestion caused by hydrolysis

chemotherapy—treatment of deceased tissue with chemicals

cholecalciferol—the form of vitamin D that is formed in humans from cholesterol in the skin

cholecystectomy—removal of the gallbladder

cholecystitis—inflammation of the gallbladder

cholelithiasis—gallstones

cholesterol—fat-like substance that is a constituent of body cells; it is synthesized in the liver; also available in animal foods

Chrohn's disease—causes inflammation, ulcers, and thickening of intestinal walls, sometimes causing obstruction

chronic—lasting a long time

chronic renal failure—slow development of kidney failure

chyme—the food mass as it has been mixed with gastric juices

chymopepsin—pancreatic enzyme necessary for protein digestion

chymotrypsin—pancreatic enzyme necessary for the digestion of proteins

circulation—the body process whereby the blood is moved throughout the body

cirrhosis—generic term for liver disease characterized by cell loss

clear liquid diet—diet that includes only liquids containing primarily carbohydrates and water; nutritionally inadequate

clinical evaluation—physical observation

coagulate—to thicken

cobalamin—organic compound known as vitamin B_{12}

coenzyme—an active part of an enzyme

collagen—protein substance that holds body cells together

compensated heart disease—heart disease in which the heart is able to maintain circulation to all body parts

complementary proteins—incomplete proteins that when combined provide all nine essential amino acids

complete protein—proteins that contain all nine essential amino acids

condiment—"extra" food such as catsup, pickles, relish, etc.

congestive heart failure—a form of decompensated heart disease

consistency—texture

constipation—difficulty in evacuating feces; characterized by dry, hard stool

constituent—part

consumer—one who makes purchases and uses commercial products

continuous infusion—enteral nutrition administered continuously during a 16 to 24 hour period

convalescent—in a state of recovery; the convalescent diet is also called the "light" diet

convenience food—food that has been partially prepared commercially and consequently is quickly and easily completed at home

crash reducing diets—fad-type diets intended to reduce weight very quickly; in fact they reduce water, not fat tissue

craving—abnormal desire

creatinine—an end (waste) product of protein metabolism

cretinism—stunted physical and mental development of fetus

crude fiber—amount of fiber in plant foods after treatment with acids and alkalies in a laboratory; not an accurate measure of actual fiber in food

cuisine—style of cooking or preparing food

culinary—referring to cooking

cultural—relating to one's background

curd—solid part resulting when milk is turned into cheese; liquid part is the curd

cystine—a nonessential amino acid

cysts—growths

daily values—represent percentage per serving of each nutritional item listed on new food labels based on daily intake of 2000 kcal

decaffeinated—having had caffeine removed almost completely

decompensated heart disease—heart disease in which the heart cannot maintain circulation to all body parts

decubitus ulcer—bedsore

deficiency disease—disease caused by the lack of a specific nutrient

dehydrated—having lost large amounts of water

dehydration—loss of water

demineralization—loss of mineral or minerals

density—compactness; the mass of substance per unit of volume

dental caries—decayed areas on teeth; cavities

depression—an indentation; or feelings of sadness

dermatitis—inflammation of the skin

descriptors—terms used to describe something

desensitize—to gradually reduce the body's sensitivity (allergic reaction) to specific items

dextrin—the intermediate product in starch digestion; before it changes to maltose and, ultimately, glucose

dextrose—glucose

diabetes insipidus—caused by damaged pituitary gland

diabetes mellitus—chronic disease in which the body lacks the normal ability to metabolize glucose

diabetic coma—unconsciousness caused by a state of acidosis due to too much sugar or too little insulin

dialysis—mechanical filtration of the blood; used when the kidneys are no longer able to perform normally

diaphragm—thin membrane or partition

diarrhea—loose bowel movement

diastolic pressure—blood pressure measured when the heart is at rest

dietary assessment—evaluation of food habits

dietary fiber—indigestible parts of plants; absorbs water in large intestine, helping to create soft, bulky stool; some is believed to bind cholesterol in the colon, helping to rid cholesterol from the body; some is believed to lower blood glucose levels.

dietary laws—rules to be followed in meal planning in some religions

dietitian—person planning therapeutic diets

diet therapy—treatment of a disease through diet

digestion—breakdown of food in the body in preparation for absorption

disaccharides—double sugars that are reduced by hydrolysis to monosaccharides. Examples are sucrose, maltose, and lactose.

diuretics—substances used to increase the amount of urine excreted

diverticulitis—inflammation of the diverticula

diverticulosis—intestinal disorder characterized by little pockets forming in the sides of the intestines; pockets are called diverticula

dried milk—milk with water removed

dry heat—cooking without the addition of liquid; examples are roasting, broiling and frying

dumping syndrome—nausea and diarrhea caused by food moving too quickly from the stomach to the small intestine

duodenal ulcer—ulcer occurring in the duodenum

duodenum—first (and smallest) section of the small intestine

durability—strength

dysentery—disease caused by microorganism; characterized by diarrhea

dyspepsia—gastrointestinal discomfort of vague origin

dysphagia—difficulty swallowing

eclamptic stage—convulsive stage of toxemia

economic status—status as determined by income

eczema—inflamed and scaly condition of skin

edema—the abnormal retention of fluid and sodium by the body

efficiency—effective use of time and energy

elective surgery—surgery performed at patient's choice

electrolyte—chemical compound that in water breaks up into electrically charged atoms called ions

elemental formulas—those formulas containing products of digestion of proteins, carbohydrates, and fats; also called hydrolyzed formulas

elimination—evacuation of wastes

elimination diets—limited diets in which only certain foods are allowed; intended to find the food allergen causing reaction

embolus—blood clot in an artery

embryo—the developing fetus

emotional stress—strain caused by anxiety

emotional trauma—extremely stressful occurrence

empty-calorie foods—foods that provide large amounts of kcal in the form of carbohydrates and fats, but very few vitamins, minerals, or proteins

emulsified fats—finely divided fat, held in suspension by another liquid

emulsifiers—help maintain emulsions (the combination of oil and water)

endocardium—the lining of the heart

endocrine system—the ductless glands

endogenous insulin—insulin produced within the body

endometrium—mucous membrane of uterus

endosperm—the inner part of the kernel of grain; contains the carbohydrate

energy balance—occurs when the number of kcal ingested equals the number of kcal expended

energy imbalance—eating either too much or too little for the amount of energy expended

energy requirement—number of kcal required by the body each day

energy value—the kcal content of specific foods

English systems of weights and measures—includes inch, foot, yard, cup, pound, quart, etc., as opposed to the metric system which is based on the number 10

enriched foods—foods to which nutrients, usually B vitamins and iron, have been added to improve their nutritional value

enteral nutrition—feeding by tube directly into the patient's stomach or intestine

environment—surroundings

enzyme—organic substance that causes changes in other substances

equivalent—equal

ergocalciferol—the form of vitamin D found in plants

erythrocytes—red blood cells

esophagastomy—surgically-created opening into esophagus; intended for tube feedings

esophagus—tube leading from the mouth to the stomach; part of the gastrointestinal system

essential hypertension—high blood pressure with unknown cause; also called primary hypertension

estrogen—hormone secreted by the ovaries

etiology—cause

evaporated milk—milk that has had 60 percent of its water removed

exchange lists—lists of foods with interchangeable nutrient and kcal contents; used in specific forms of diet therapy

exogenous insulin—insulin injected into the body

extracellular—outside the cell

fad diets—currently popular weight reducing diets; usually nutritionally inadequate and not useful, permanent, methods of weight reduction

fast foods—restaurant food that is ready to serve before orders are taken

fat cell theory—belief that fat cells have a natural drive to regain any weight lost

fats—highest kcal energy nutrient

fat soluble—can be dissolved in fat

fatty acids—a component of fats that determines the classification of the fat

fecal matter—solid waste from large intestine

feces—solid waste from the large intestine

Federal Food, Drug, and Cosmetic Act—law requiring that food shipped from one state to another be pure, safe to eat, and prepared under sanitary conditions. It also requires that ingredients and weight be listed on the label

fermentation—changing of sugars and starches to alcohol

fetal alcohol syndrome—subnormal physical and mental development caused by mother's excessive use of alcohol during pregnancy

fetal malformations—physical abnormalities of the fetus

fetus—infant in utero

fever—hypermetabolic state with raised body temperature; commonly due to infection

fiber—indigestible, edible parts of plants

fibrosis—development of tough, stringy tissue

fillet—thin strip of meat or fish

filtrate—the substance to be filtered

finfish—fish with fins and internal skeletons

flatulence—gas in the intestinal tract

folate-deficiency anemia—form of megaloblastic anemia; characterized by too few red blood cells that are large and immature

folic acid—a form of vitamin B, also called folacin; essential for metabolism

food additives—chemical substances added to foods during processing

food customs—food habits

food deprivation—lack of food

food diary—written record of all food and drink ingested in specified period

food faddists—people who have certain beliefs about particular foods or diets

Food Guide Pyramid—outline for making food selections based on Dietary Guidelines

food residue—that part of the food that is indigestible

fortified foods—foods that have had vitamins and minerals added

freeze-dried foods—foods that have been frozen rapidly and then dehydrated

fructose—the simple sugar (monosaccharide) found in fruit and honey

full liquid diet—diet consisting of liquids and food that is liquid at body temperature

fundus (of the stomach)—upper part of the stomach

galactose—the simple sugar (monosaccharide) to which lactose is broken down during digestion

galactosemia—inherited error in metabolism that prevents normal metabolism of lactose

galactosuria—galactose in the urine

gallbladder—the organ located next to the liver; stores the bile produced by the liver and subsequently releases it as needed for the digestion of fats

gastric bypass—surgical reduction of the stomach area

gastric juices—the digestive secretions of the stomach

gastric lipase—enzyme secreted by the stomach to aid in the digestion of fats

gastric ulcer—ulcer in the stomach

gastrointestinal—pertaining to the digestive system

gastrostomy—opening created by the surgeon directly into the stomach for enteral nutrition

generic brands—products without specific brand names

genetic predisposition—inherited tendency

geriatrics—the branch of medicine involved with diseases of the elderly

germ—embryo or tiny life center of each kernel of grain

gerontology—the study of aging

gestational diabetes—diabetes occurring during pregnancy; usually disappears after delivery of the infant

gingivitis—inflammation of the gums

glomerular filtration rate (GFR)—the rate at which the kidneys filter the blood

glomerulonephritis—inflammation of the glomeruli of the kidneys

glomerulus—filtering unit in the kidneys

glossitis—inflammation of the tongue

glucagon—hormone from alpha cells of pancreas; helps cells release energy

glucose—the simple sugar to which carbohydrate must be broken down for absorption; also known as *dextrose*

gluten—protein found in grains

glycerol—a component of fat

glycogen—glucose as stored in the liver and muscles

glycogen loading—process in which the muscle stores of glycogen is maximized; also called "carboloading"

glycosuria—excess sugar in the urine

goiter—enlarged tissue of the thyroid gland due to a deficiency of iodine

grams—small unit of measurement of weight in the metric system; 30 grams equal one ounce

GRAS list—FDA's list of substances "generally regarded as safe"

gross deficiency—extreme lack

hare—rabbit

health foods—said by food faddists to have special health-giving characteristics

hematuria—blood in the urine

heme iron—part of hemoglobin molecule in animal foods

hemochromatosis—condition caused by inborn error of metabolism resulting in excessive absorption of iron

hemoglobin—the red coloring matter in the blood

hemolysis—the destruction of red blood cells

hemorrhage—unusually heavy bleeding

hepatitis—inflammation of the liver caused by viruses, drugs, and alcohol

hiatal hernia—condition wherein part of the stomach protrudes through the diaphragm into the chest cavity

high-density lipoproteins (HDL)—lipoproteins that carry cholesterol from tissues to liver for eventual excretion

HIV—human immunodeficiency virus; causes AIDS

homeostasis—state of physical balance; stable condition

homogenized milk—whole milk processed to break fat into small drops that do not separate

homous—form of serving chick peas common to Middle Easterners

hormone—substance secreted by the endocrine glands

humectants—additives to retain moisture in food

hydrochloric acid—gastric secretion necessary for the digestion of proteins and some minerals

hydrogenation—the combining of fat with hydrogen, thereby making it a saturated fat

hydrolysis—the addition of water resulting in the breakdown of the molecule

hydrolyzed formulas—contain products of digestion of proteins, carbohydrates, and fats; also called elemental formulas; used for patients who have difficulty digesting food

hypercholesteremia—unusually high levels of cholesterol in blood; also known as *high serum cholesterol*

hyperemesis gravidarum—nausea so severe as to be life threatening

hyperglycemia—excessive amounts of sugar in the blood

hyperkalemia—excessive amounts of potassium in the blood

hyperlipidemia—excessive amounts of fats in the blood

hypermetabolic—higher than normal rate of metabolism

hypersensitivity—abnormally strong sensitivity to certain substance(s)

hypertension—higher than normal blood pressure

hyperthyroidism—condition in which the thyroid gland secretes too much thyroxine and T_3; the body's rate of metabolism is unusually high

hypervitaminosis—condition caused by excessive ingestion of one or more vitamins

hypoalbuminemia—abnormally low amounts of protein in the blood

hypocalcemia—abnormally low amount of calcium in the blood

hypoglycemia—subnormal levels of blood sugar

hypoglycemic agents—oral drugs that stimulate the pancreas to produce insulin

hypogonadism—subnormal development of male sex organs

hypokalemia—low level of potassium in the blood

hypoproteinemia—low amounts of protein in the blood

hypothalamus—area at base of brain that regulates appetite and thirst

hypothyroidism—condition in which the thyroid gland secretes too little thyroxine and T_3; body metabolism is slower than normal

iatrogenic malnutrition—malnutrition occurring as a result of hospitalization

IDDM—insulin-dependent diabetes mellitus

ileum—last part of the small intestine

imitation foods—manmade; intended to resemble natural foods

immerse—dip

immunity—ability to resist certain diseases

impulsive shopper—one who buys in accordance with the desires of the moment

inborn errors of metabolism—congenital disabilities preventing normal metabolism

incidental additives—those additives remaining on a food product as a result of farmers' use of fertilizers, pesticides, etc.

incomplete protein—protein that does not contain all of the nine essential amino acids

infarct—dead tissue resulting from blocked artery

infectious—contagious; communicable

inflammatory bowel disease—chronic condition causing inflammation in the gastrointestinal tract

ingest—take in orally

insecticide—chemical used to kill insects

insomnia—inability to sleep

insulin—secretion of the Islets of Langerhans in the pancreas gland, essential for the proper metabolism of glucose

insulin coma—unconsciousness caused by too much insulin or too little food

insulin reaction—hypoglycemia leading to insulin coma caused by too much insulin or too little food

intact formulas—contain proteins, carbohydrates, and fats that require digestion

intentional additives—those additives that are added to perform specific functions in food, such as antioxidants to preserve color

International Units (IU)—units of measurement of some vitamins

interstitial fluid—fluid between tissues

intima—lining of arteries

intracellular—within the cell

intracranial hemorrhage—bleeding within the head

intrinsic factor—secretion of stomach mucosa essential for B_{12} absorption

invisible fats—fats that are not immediately noticeable such as those in egg yolk, cheese, cream, salad dressings, etc.

iodized salts—salt that has had the mineral iodine added for the prevention of goiter

ions—electrically charged atoms resulting from chemical reactions

iron—mineral essential to the blood

iron-deficiency anemia—condition resulting from inadequate amount of iron in the diet, reducing the amount of oxygen carried by the blood to the cells

iron enhancer—assists in absorption of iron

irradiate—expose to ultraviolet light

irradiated foods—exposed to gamma radiation from cobalt source; to retard spoilage

ischemia—reduced blood flow causing inadequate supply of nutrients, oxygen, and wastes to and from tissues

islets of Langerhans—part of the pancreas gland from which insulin is secreted

isoleucine—amino acid

jaundice—yellow cast of the skin and eyes

jejunoileal bypass—surgical procedure in which the jejunum of the small intestine is attached to a small section of the ileum in an effort to reduce the amount of absorptive surface

jejunostomy—opening created by the surgeon in the intestine for parenteral nutrition

jejunum—the middle section comprising about two-fifths of the small intestine

junket—milk pudding

Kaposi's sarcoma—type of cancer common to AIDS patients

kcal—the unit used to measure the fuel value of foods

kcal intake—number of kcal taken in

kcal requirement—number of kcal required daily to meet energy needs

Keshan disease—condition causing abnormalities in the heart muscle

ketones—substances to which fatty acids are broken down in the liver

ketonuria—ketone bodies in the urine

ketosis—condition in which ketones collect in the blood; caused by insufficient glucose available for energy

kilocalorie—*see* kcal

kilojoule—unit used to measure the energy value of food in the metric system; 4.184 kilojoules equal 1 kcal

kitchen hygiene—cleanliness

Krebs cycle—the complete oxidation of carbohydrates, proteins, and fats

kwashiorkor—deficiency disease caused by extreme lack of protein

lactase—enzyme secreted by the small intestine for the digestion of lactose

lactation—the period during which the mother is nursing the baby

lacteals—lymphatic vessels in the small intestine that absorb fatty acids and glycerol

lacto-ovo vegetarian—vegetarians who will eat dairy products and eggs but no meat, poultry, or fish

lactose—the sugar in milk; a disaccharide

lactose intolerance—inability to digest lactose because of a lack of the enzyme, lactase; causes abdominal cramps and diarrhea

lacto-vegetarians—vegetarians who eat dairy products

leach—to dissolve out of a substance

lean body mass—percentage of muscle tissue

leavened bread—bread that contains a leavening agent

lecithin—fatty substance found in plant and animal foods; a natural emulsifier that helps transport fats in the bloodstream; used commercially to make food products smooth

legumes—plant food that is grown in a pod, for example, beans and peas

lesions—a sore; tissue damage

leucine—an amino acid

leukocytes—white blood cells

light diet—also called the convalescent diet; very close to the regular diet but more advanced than the soft diet

linoleic acid—only fatty acid essential for humans; cannot be synthesized by the body

linolenic acid—one of three fatty acids needed by the body; can be synthesized by the body

lipid—fat

lipoproteins—carriers of fat in the blood

liquid diets—diets that contain foods that are liquid at body temperature

liter—unit of volume measurement in the metric system; the approximate equivalent of one quart in the English system

Lofenalac—commercial infant formula with 95 percent of phenylalanine removed

longevity—length of life

low-density lipoproteins (LDL)—carry blood cholesterol to the cells

lumen—the hollow area in a tube

macrosomia—birthweight over 9 pounds

major minerals—those minerals required in amounts greater than 100 mg a day

malignant—life threatening

malnutrition—poor nutrition

maltase—enzyme secreted by the small intestine essential for the digestion of maltose

maltose—the double sugar (disaccharide) occurring as a result of the digestion of grain

manually—by hand, not machine

maple syrup urine disease (MSUD)—disease caused by an inborn error of metabolism in which the body cannot metabolize certain amino acids

marasmus—severe wasting caused by lack of protein and all nutrients, or faulty absorption; PCM

meat analogues—substances made to imitate meat; usually of soybean origin

mechanical digestion—the part of digestion that requires certain mechanical movement such as chewing, swallowing, and peristalsis

mechanical-soft diet—soft diet for people who cannot chew; all meats are ground and fruits and vegetables are pureed

megadose—extraordinarily large amount

megaloblastic anemia—anemia in which the red blood cells are unusually large and are not completely mature

menadione—synthetic vitamin K

menaquinones—the form of vitamin K found in bacteria, animals, and humans

mental retardation—below normal intellectual capacity

metabolism—the use of the food by the body after digestion which results in energy

metastasize—movement of cancer cells through the blood from one organ to another

meter—metric unit of measurement of length; 39 inches

metric system—system of measurement based on the number 10

microorganisms—microscopic organisms such as bacteria or viruses

milling—the grinding of grain

mineral—one of many inorganic substances essential to life and classified generally as minerals

minimum-residue diet—diet severely restricted in food residue; nutritionally inadequate

modification—change

modular formulas—formulas used as supplements for other formulas or for developing customized formulas

moist heat—cooking with the addition of liquid; examples are braising or stewing

monosaccharides—simplest carbohydrates; sugars that cannot be further reduced by hydrolysis. Examples are glucose, fructose, and galactose.

monounsaturated fats—fats that are neither saturated nor polyunsaturated and are thought to play little part in atherosclerosis

morbid—damaging to health

morning sickness—early morning nausea common to some pregnancies

mortality rate—rate of death

MSG—monosodium glutamate; a form of spice containing large amounts of sodium

mucous membrane—lining of body passages that open to the outside such as the alimentary, genitourinary, and respiratory tracts

mutations—changes in the genes

myelin—lipoprotein essential for the protection of nerves

myocardial infarction—heart attack; caused by the blockage of an artery leading to the heart

myocardium—middle muscular layer of the heart wall

myoglobin—protein compound in muscle that provides oxygen to cells

myxedema—hypothyroidism

nasogastric tube—tube leading from the nose to the stomach for tube feeding

natural foods—unchanged; contain no additives

nausea—the urge to vomit

necrosis—tissue death due to lack of blood supply

negative nitrogen balance—more nitrogen lost than taken in

neoplasia—cancer

neoplasm—new growth; refers to cancerous tumors

nephritis—inflammatory disease of the kidneys

nephrolithiasis—kidney stones

nephron—unit of the kidney containing a glomerulus

nephrosclerosis—hardening of renal arteries

neuropathy—nerve damage

niacin—B vitamin

niacin equivalent (NE)—unit of measuring niacin; 1 NE equals 1 mg niacin or 60 mg tryptophan

NIDDM—non-insulin dependent diabetes mellitus

nitrogen—chemical element found in protein; essential to life

nitrogen balance—comparison of nitrogen intake with outgo

nonheme iron—iron from animal foods that is not part of the hemoglobin molecule; and all iron from plant foods

non-tropical sprue—*see* celiac sprue

norepinephrine—neurotransmitter of vasoconstrictor that helps the body cope with stressful conditions

normal weight—average weight for size and age

nourishing—foods or beverages that provide substantial amounts of essential nutrients

nutrient—chemical substance found in food that is necessary for good health

nutrient-dense foods—foods that contain many nutrients but few kcal

nutrient density—nutrient value of foods compared with number of kcal

nutrient requirement—amount of specific nutrient needed by the body

nutrition—the result of those processes whereby the body takes in and uses food for growth, development, and the maintenance of health

nutritional anemia—anemia caused by insufficient iron in the diet

nutritional assessment—evaluation of nutritional status

nutritional edema—edema caused by lack of protein in the diet

nutritionally adequate—contains recommended amounts of essential nutrients

nutritional status—one's physical condition as determined by diet

nutritional value—the nutrient content of foods or beverages

nutritious—foods or beverages containing substantial amounts of essential nutrients

obesity—excessive body fat, 20 percent above average

obstetrician—doctor who cares for the mother during pregnancy and delivery

occlusions—blockages

omega-3 fatty acids—polyunsaturated fatty acids found in fish oil; may contribute to reduction of coronary artery disease

oncologist—doctor specializing in study of cancer

oncology—the study of cancer

on demand—feeding infants as they desire

opaque—neither transparent nor translucent

operating manual—instruction book for machines

opportunistic infections—common to AIDS patients; caused by microorganisms that are present but that do not normally affect people with healthy immune systems

organic foods—grown without synthetic fertilizer and produced without additives

organ meats—liver, kidney, brains, sweetbreads

osmolality—number of particles per kilogram of solution; solutions with high osmolality exert more pressure than do those with fewer particles

osmosis—movement of a substance through a semipermeable membrane

osteomalacia—a condition in which bones become soft, usually in older people, because of calcium loss

osteoporosis—condition in which bones become brittle because there have been insufficient mineral deposits, especially calcium

ostomy—surgically-created opening into an organ of the gastrointestinal tract

overweight—weight 10–20 percent above average

ovo-lacto-vegetarians—vegetarians who will eat dairy products and eggs

oxidation—the process of combining substances with oxygen

pallor—paleness of the skin

panacea—supposed cure for all physical problems

pancreas—gland that secretes enzymes essential for digestion, and insulin which is essential for glucose metabolism

pancreatic amylase—the enzyme secreted by the pancreas gland that is essential for the digestion of starch

pancreatic lipase (steapsin)—the enzyme secreted by the pancreas gland that is essential for the digestion of fat

pancreatic protease—the enzyme secreted by the pancreas that is essential for the digestion of protein

pancreatitis—inflammation of the pancreas

pantothenic acid—a B vitamin

paralysis—inability to move

parasite—organism that is completely dependent on another organism for its existence

parenteral—feeding through a blood vessel

parenteral nutrition—nutrition provided via a vein

pasteurization—process in which harmful microorganisms are killed

PCM—protein calorie malnutrition; marasmus

pediatrician—doctor specializing in the health problems of children

peer group—group of people approximately one's own age

peer pressure—pressure of one's friends and colleagues of the same age

pellagra—deficiency disease caused by a lack of niacin

pepsin—an enzyme secreted by the stomach that is essential for the digestion of proteins

peptic ulcers—ulcer of the stomach or duodenum

peptidases—enzymes secreted by the small intestine that are essential for the digestion of protein

Perfringens—type of bacteria that can cause food poisoning

pericardium—outer covering of the heart

periodontal disease—disease of the mouth and gums

peripheral vascular disease—narrowed arteries some distance from the heart

peripheral vein—a vein that is near the surface of the skin

peristalsis—rhythmical movement of the intestinal tract, moving the chyme along

pernicious anemia—severe, chronic anemia caused by a deficiency of vitamin B_{12}; usually due to the body's inability to absorb B_{12}

pH—symbol for the degree of acid or alkali in a solution

phenylalanine—amino acid

phenylalanine hydroxylase—liver enzyme necessary to metabolize the amino acid, phenylalanine

phenylketonuria—condition caused by an inborn error of metabolism in which the infant lacks an enzyme necessary to metabolize the amino acid, phenylalanine

phenylpropanolamine—constituent of diet pills; can damage blood vessels

phlebitis—inflammation of a vein

phylloquinone—vitamin K as found in green plants

physical stress—bodily strain

physical trauma—extreme physical stress

physiological—relating to bodily functions

pica—abnormal craving for non-food substance

pigmentation—coloring matter in the skin

placenta—organ in the uterus that links blood supplies of mother and infant

plaque—fatty deposits on interior of artery walls

plateau period—period in which there is no change

polycystic kidney disease—rare, hereditary kidney disease causing cysts or growths on the kidneys that can ultimately cause kidney failure in middle age

polydipsia—abnormal thirst

polypeptides—partially digested proteins

polyphagia—abnormally increased appetite

polysaccharides—complex carbohydrates containing combinations of monosaccharides. Examples include starch, dextrin, cellulose, and glycogen

polyunsaturated fats—fats whose carbon atoms contain only limited amounts of hydrogen and consequently do not contribute to heart disease

polyuria—excessive secretion of urine

positive nitrogen balance—nitrogen intake exceeds outgo

positive water balance—condition occurring when more water is taken in than is used or excreted

postoperative—after surgery

postprandial—after meals

posture—body position

precursor—something that comes before something else; in vitamins it is also called a provitamin, something from which the body can synthesize the specific vitamin

prefix—first syllable of word

pregnancy-induced hypertension—typically occurs during late pregnancy; characterized by high blood pressure, albumin in the urine, and edema

primary hypertension—high blood pressure resulting from an unknown cause

process cheese—made from natural cheese, spices, and liquid

prohormone—substance that precedes the hormone and from which the body can synthesize the hormone

proteases—enzymes secreted by the pancreas gland; essential for digestion of proteins

protein calorie malnutrition—*see* PCM

proteins—the only one of six essential nutrients containing nitrogen

proteinuria—protein in the urine

prothrombin—substance that permits clotting of the blood

protozoa—type of microorganism that can cause dysentery

provitamin—*see* precursor

psychological development—development of the psyche

psychosocial development—relating to both psychological and social development

ptyalin—also called *salivary amylase;* it is the digestive secretion of the salivary glands

purines—end products of nucleoprotein metabolism

pylorus—the end of the stomach nearest the intestine

pyridoxal—*see* pyridoxine

pyridoxamine—*see* pyridoxine

pyridoxine—one of the three vitaminers of vitamin B_6

raw milk—milk that has not been processed in any way; may contain harmful microorganisms

RDAs—recommended daily dietary allowances as determined by the Food and Nutrition Board of the National Academy of Sciences—National Research Council

REE—resting energy expenditure; the rate at which the body expends energy just for its maintenance; comparable to the basal metabolism rate (BMR)

refined foods—foods that have been processed to remove most or all naturally occurring fiber

regular diet—normal diet, based on the Food Guide Pyramid

regurgitation—vomiting

renal calculi—kidney stones

renal threshold—kidney's capacity

rennin—enzyme secreted by the stomach necessary for the digestion of proteins in milk

resection—reduction

residue—solid part of feces

resorb—taken back; reabsorbed

respiration—breathing

restored foods—those foods to which manufacturers have returned the naturally occurring nutrients

retardation—slowing

retinol—the preformed vitamin A

Retinol Equivalent (RE)—the equivalent of 3.33 IU of vitamin A

riboflavin—the name for Vitamin B$_2$

rickets—deficiency disease caused by the lack of vitamin D; causes malformed bones and pain in infants

saccharin—artificial sweetener

saliva—secretion of the salivary glands

salivary amylase—also called *ptyalin;* it is the enzyme secreted by the salivary glands to act on starch

salmonella—bacteria causing a form of food poisoning called salmonellosis

sanitation—cleanliness

satiety—feeling of satisfaction; fullness

saturated fats—fats whose carbon atoms contain all of the hydrogen atoms they can; considered a contributory factor in atherosclerosis

scurvy—a deficiency disease caused by a lack of vitamin C

seasonal—sold as the product is ripe, according to the growing season

secondary diabetes mellitus—caused by certain drugs or disease of pancreas; rare disease

secondary hypertension—high blood pressure caused by another condition such as kidney disease

secretions—liquid emissions

self-esteem—feelings of self-worth

sepsis—infection of the blood

serum cholesterol—cholesterol in the blood

set point theory—belief that everyone has a natural weight ("set point") at which the body is most comfortable

shelf life—period of time within which a food product should be consumed before deterioration of quality occurs

shellfish—fish with external shells but no internal bones

shoyu—Japanese form of soy sauce

Sippy Diet—conservative treatment of peptic ulcers; not commonly used, contains only milk and antacids

skeletal system—body's bone structure

skim milk—milk with fat removed

skin tests—allergy tests using potential allergens on scratches on the skin

social status—one's social class

sodium chloride—table salt

soft diet—one of the basic hospital diets; contains only foods with soft textures

solute—the substance dissolved in a solution

solvent—liquid part of a solution

somatostatin—hormone produced by delta cells of pancreas and hypothalamus

sphygmomanometer—instrument used to measure blood pressure

spontaneous abortion—occurring naturally; miscarriage

stamina—strength

standard diets—basic diets used by most hospitals; can be modified in texture, kcal, and nutrient content

standard weight—average weight for height and age

staphylococcus—form of bacteria causing food poisoning called "staph" or "staphylococcal poisoning"

staple food—foods commonly used and kept on hand, such as flour, potatoes, or rice

starch—polysaccharide found in grains and vegetables

stasis—stoppage or slowing

steak—cut of meat or fish across the flesh of the animal

steatorrhea—abnormal amounts of fat in the feces

sterile—free of infectious organisms

stew—to cook slowly in liquid or a mixture of meat and vegetables cooked by this method. An example is beef and vegetable stew

stimulant—substance that increases heart rate, such as caffeine

stir-frying—fast cooking at high heat with small amount of fat added

sucrase—enzyme secreted by the small intestine to aid in digestion of sucrose

sucrose—a double sugar or disaccharide; examples are granulated, powdered, or brown sugar

sweetbreads—edible animal glands

sweetened condensed milk—milk that has had water removed and sugar added

synthesize—to make a substance from other substances

synthetic—human-made

systolic pressure—blood pressure taken as the heart contracts

tachycardia—abnormally rapid heartbeat

tamales—Mexican bread made of cornmeal

tempura—fried foods, Japanese style

terminal—situation in which death is unavoidable

tetany—involuntary muscle movement

texture—consistency

textured protein—meat analogues; imitation meat products

therapeutic diets—diets used in treatment of disease

thiamin—vitamin B_1

thrombosis—blockage, as a blood clot

thyroid gland—controls body metabolism; secretes thyroxine and T_3

thyroxine—secretion of the thyroid gland

tocopherols—vitaminers of vitamin E

tocotrienols—a form of vitamin E

tortillas—Mexican bread made of cornmeal

total parenteral nutrition—*see* TPN

toxic—poisonous

toxicity—poisonousness

toxin—poison

TPN—total parenteral nutrition

trace elements—minerals that are essential, but only in very small amounts

transferase—a liver enzyme necessary for the metabolism of galactose

trauma—stress to the body

trichinosis—disease caused by the parasite, Trichinella spiralis; can be transmitted through undercooked pork

triglycerides—combinations of fatty acids and glycerol

triiodothyronine (T_3)—secretion of the thyroid gland

trimester—three-month period; commonly used to denote periods of pregnancy

trypsin—pancreatic enzyme; helps digest proteins

tryptophan—an amino acid and a precursor of niacin

tube feeding—feeding by tube directly into the stomach or intestine or via a vein

Type I diabetes mellitus—insulin dependent

Type II diabetes mellitus—noninsulin dependent

ulcerative colitis—disease characterized by inflammation and ulceration of the colon, rectum, and sometimes entire large intestine

underweight—weight that is 10–15 percent below average

urea—chief nitrogenous waste product of protein metabolism

uremia—condition in which protein wastes are circulating in the blood

ureters—tubes leading from the kidneys to the bladder

uric acid—one of the nitrogenous waste products of protein metabolism

urticaria—hives; common allergic reaction

valine—amino acid

vascular dilation—expansion of blood vessels

vascular disease—disease of the blood vessels

vascular system—circulatory system

vasopressin—antidiuretic hormone also called ADH

vegans—vegetarians who avoid all animal foods

venison—meat from deer

very low density lipoproteins (VLDL)—carry triglycerides to liver; they are converted to LDL in liver

villi—the tiny, hair-like structures in the small intestines through which nutrients are absorbed

visible fats—fats in foods that are easily seen, such as on meat, or butter or margarine

vitamers—different chemical forms of a vitamin that serve the same purpose in the body

vitamins—organic substances necessary for life although they do not, independently, provide energy

vitamin supplements—concentrated forms of vitamins; may be in tablet or liquid form

volume—amount in terms of space consumed

water soluble—soluble in water

weaning—training an infant to drink from the cup instead of the nipple

whey—liquid part resulting when milk is formed into cheese; solid part is the curd

whole milk—milk with neither fat nor water removed

wok—common form of round bottomed frying pan used for Oriental cooking

xerophthalmia—serious eye disease characterized by dry mucous membranes of the eye, caused by a deficiency of vitamin A

xerostomia—sore, dry mouth caused by a reduction of salivary secretions. May be caused by radiation for treatment of cancer

yo-yo effect—refers to crash diets; the dieter's weight goes up and down over short periods because these diets do not change eating habits

BIBLIOGRAPHY

BOOKS

Albert, M. B., & Callaway, C. W. (1992). *Clinical nutrition for the house officer.* Baltimore: Williams & Wilkins.

Berning, J. R., & Steen, S. N. (Eds.). (1991). *Sports nutrition for the 90s. The health professional's handbook.* Gaithersburg, MD: Aspen Publishers.

Bradley, J., & Nass, S. (1988). *Nutrition of the cancer patient.* Dallas: Nutritional Research Consultants.

Bruch, H. (1979). *The golden cage.* New York: Vintage Books.

Bruch, H. (1988). In D. Czyzewski & M. A. Suhr (Eds.), *Conversations with anorexics.* New York: Basic Books.

Burtis, G., Davis, J., & Martin, S. (1988). *Applied nutrition and diet therapy.* Philadelphia: WB Saunders.

Cataldo, C. B., Nyenhuis, J. R., & Whitney, E. N. (1989). *Nutrition and diet therapy: Principles & practice* (2nd ed.). St. Paul, MN: West Publishing.

Clayman, C. B. (Ed.). (1989). *The American Medical Association's home medical encyclopedia.* New York: Random House.

Christian, J. L., & Greger, J. L. (1988). *Nutrition for living* (3rd ed.). Menlo Park, CA: The Benjamin Cummings Publishing.

Culinary Institute of America. (1991). *The new professional chef* (5th ed.). L. G. Conway (Ed.). New York: Van Nostrand Reinhold.

Eschleman, M. M. (1991). *Introductory nutrition and diet therapy* (2nd ed.). Philadelphia: JB Lippincott.

Feldman, E. B. (1988). *Essentials of clinical nutrition.* Philadelphia: FA Davis.

Frankle, R. T., & Yang, M-U. (1988). *Obesity and weight control.* Gaithersburg, MD: Aspen Publishers.

Gershoff, S. (1990). *The Tufts University guide to total nutrition.* New York: Harper & Row.

Gisslen, W. (1989). *Professional cooking* (2nd ed.). New York: John Wiley & Sons.

Govoni, L. E., & Hayes, J. E. (1985). *Drugs and nursing implications* (5th ed.). Norwalk, CT: Appleton-Century-Crofts.

Gray, H. (1977). *Gray's anatomy.* New York: Bounty Books.

Guthrie, H. A. (1989). *Introductory nutrition.* St. Louis: Times Mirror/Mosby College Publishing.

Halpern, S. (1987). *Clinical nutrition* (2nd ed.). Philadelphia: JB Lippincott.

Hamilton, E. M. N., Whitney, E. N., & Sizer, F. S. (1991). *Nutrition concepts and controversies* (5th ed.). St. Paul, MN: West Publishing.

Hegarty, V. (1988). *Decisions in nutrition.* St. Louis: Times Mirror/Mosby College Publishing.

Horton, E. S., & Terping, R. L. (Eds.). (1988). *Exercise, nutrition, and energy metabolism.* New York: Macmillan.

Hunt, S. M., & Graff, J. L. (1990). *Advanced nutrition and human metabolism.* St. Paul, MN: West Publishing.

Iyer, P. W., Taptich, B. J., & Bernocchi-Losey, D. (1991). *Nursing process and nursing diagnosis.* Philadelphia: WB Saunders.

Jacobson, M. F., Lefferts, L. Y., & Garland, A. W. (1991). Center for Science in the Public Interest. *Safe food: Eating wisely in a risky world*. Los Angeles: Living Planet Press.

Kemp, N., & Richardson, E. (1990). *Quality assurance in nursing practice*. London: Butterworth-Heinemann.

Linder, M. C. (Ed.). (1991). *Nutritional biochemistry and metabolism with clinical applications*. Elsevier, NY: Science Publishing.

Mahan, L. K., & Arlin, M. (1992). *Krause's food, nutrition and diet therapy* (8th ed.). Philadelphia: WB Saunders.

Mayo Clinic, Rochester Methodist Hospital, & St. Mary's Hospital. (1988). *Mayo clinic diet manual, a handbook of dietary practices* (6th ed.). Philadelphia: WB Saunders.

Munro, H., & Schlierf, G. (Eds.). (1992). *Nutrition of the elderly*. (Nestle Nutrition Workshop Series, Vol. 29). New York: Raven Press.

National Research Council. (1989). *Diet and health. Implications for reducing chronic disease risk*. Committee on Diet and Health. Washington, DC: National Academy Press.

National Research Council, National Academy of Sciences. (1989). *Recommended dietary allowances* (10th ed.). Washington, DC.

Peckham, G., & Freelond-Graves, J. (1989). *Foundations of food preparation*. New York: John Wiley & Sons.

Perkin, J. E. (1990). *Food allergies and adverse reactions*. Gaithersburg, MD: Aspen Publishers.

Picciano, M. F., & Lonnerdal, B. (Eds.). (1992). *Contemporary issues in clinical nutrition. Mechanisms regulating lactation and infant nutrient utilization*. New York: John Wiley & Sons.

Pipes, P. L. (1989). *Nutrition in infancy and childhood* (4th ed.). St. Louis: Times Mirror/Mosby College Publishers.

Poleman, C. M., & Peckenpaugh, N. J. (1991). *Nutrition essentials and diet therapy* (6th ed.). Philadelphia: WB Saunders.

Roe, D. A. (1992). *Geriatric nutrition* (3rd ed.). Englewood Cliffs, NJ: Prentice-Hall.

Rolfes, S. R., & DeBruyne, L. K. (1990). In E. R. Whitney, (Ed.), *Life span nutrition. Conception through life*. St. Paul, MN: West Publishing.

Rombeau, J. L., & Caldwell, M. D. (1990). *Clinical nutrition: Enteral and tube feeding* (2nd ed.). Philadelphia: WB Saunders.

Shils, M. E., & Young, V. E. (1988). *Modern nutrition in health and disease* (7th ed.). Philadelphia: Lea & Febiger.

U.S. Department of Agriculture. (1976–1986). *Composition of foods*. Washington, DC: U.S. Government Printing Office.

Whitney, E. N., & Sizer, F. S. (1990). *Nutrition—concepts and controversies*. St. Paul, MN: West Publishing.

Whitney, E. N., Cataldo, C. B., & Rolfes, S. R. (1991). *Understanding normal and clinical nutrition* (3rd ed.). St. Paul, MN: West Publishing.

Whitney, E. N., Hamilton, E. M. N., & Rolfes, S. R. (1990). *Understanding nutrition* (5th ed.). St. Paul, MN: West Publishing.

Williams, S. R. (1992). *Basic nutrition and diet therapy* (9th ed.). St. Louis: Mosby-Year Book.

Williams, S. R. (1990). *Essentials of nutrition and diet therapy* (5th ed.). St. Louis: Times Mirror/Mosby College Publishers.

Williams, S. R. (1989). *Nutrition and diet therapy* (6th ed.). St. Louis: Times Mirror/Mosby College Publishers.

Williams, S. R. (Ed.). (1988). *Nutrition throughout the life cycle*. St. Louis: Times Mirror/Mosby College Publishers.

Winick, M. (Ed.). (1988). *The Columbia encyclopedia of nutrition*. The Institute of Human Nutrition, Columbia University College of Physicians and Surgeons. New York: GP Putnam's Sons.

Zeman, F. J., & Ney, D. M. (1988). *Applications of clinical nutrition*. Englewood Cliffs, NJ: Prentice Hall.

Zeman, F. J. (1991). *Clinical nutrition and dietetics* (2nd ed.). New York: Macmillan.

PERIODICALS AND PUBLICATIONS

American Heart Association. (1969). *Your mild sodium-restricted diet* (revised). Dallas.

American Heart Association. (1969). *Your 1000 milligram sodium diet* (revised). Dallas.

American Heart Association. (1968). *Your 500 milligram sodium diet* (revised). Dallas.

American Heart Association. (1989). *Cholesterol and your heart.* Dallas.

American Heart Association. (1985). *The American Heart Association diet.* Dallas.

American Heart Association. (1969). *Your mild sodium-restricted diet.* Dallas.

American Heart Association. (1986). *Dietary guidelines for healthy American adults.* Dallas.

American Heart Association. *About high blood pressure.* Dallas.

American Nurses Association. (1987). *Standards and scope of gerontological nursing practice.* Kansas City.

Center for science in the public interest. *Shopping smart.* (1988). Washington, DC.

Department of Health and Human Services. (1990). *Weighing food safety risks.* (DHHS Publication No. [FDA] 90-2231). Washington, DC: U.S. Government Printing Office.

Department of Health and Human Services. (1989). *Eating to lower your high blood pressure.* (NIH Publication No. 89-2220). Bethesda, MD.

Department of Health and Human Services. (1987). *Non-insulin dependent diabetes.* (NIH Publication No. 86-241). Bethesda, MD.

Department of Health and Human Services. (1987). *Planning a diet for a healthy heart.* (HHS Publication No. [FDA] 87-2220). Rockville, MD.

Department of Health and Human Services. (1987). *Diet, nutrition & cancer prevention: A guide to food choices.* (NIH Publication No. 87-2878). Bethesda, MD.

Department of Health and Human Services. (1987). *Diet, nutrition, & cancer prevention: The good news.* (NIH Publication No. 87-2878). Bethesda, MD.

Office of the Federal Register, National Archives and Record Services, General Services Administration. (1993). *Federal Register.* (Volume 58, Number 3). Washington, D.C.

U.S. Department of Agriculture. (1990). *Dietary guidelines for Americans* (3rd ed.). (Home & Garden Bulletin No. 232). Washington, DC: U.S. Government Printing Office.

U.S. Department of Agriculture. (1987). *Meat and poultry labels wrap it up.* (Home & Garden Bulletin No. 238). Washington, DC: U.S. Government Printing Office.

U.S. Department of Agriculture. (1990). *Preventing foodborne illness. A guide to safe food handling.* Food Safety and Inspection Service. (Home & Garden Bulletin No. 247). Washington, DC: U.S. Government Printing Office.

U.S. Department of Agriculture. (1990). *A quick consumer guide to safe food handling.* Food Safety and Inspection Service. (Home & Garden Bulletin No. 248). Washington, DC: U.S. Government Printing Office.

U.S. Department of Agriculture. (1990). *Bacteria that cause foodborne illness.* Food Safety and Inspection Service. Washington, DC: U.S. Government Printing Office.

U.S. Department of Agriculture. (1986). *The sodium content of your food.* (Home & Garden Bulletin No. 233). Washington, DC: U.S. Government Printing Office.

U.S. Department of Agriculture. (1989). *Nutritive value of foods.* (Home & Garden Bulletin No. 72). Washington, DC: U.S. Government Printing Office.

U.S. Department of Agriculture. (1986). *Dietary guidelines and your diet.* (Home & Garden Bulletin No. 232-1-7). Washington, DC: U.S. Government Printing Office.

U.S. Department of Agriculture. (1989). *Preparing foods and planning menus using the dietary guidelines.* (Home & Garden Bulletin No. 232-8). Washington, DC: U.S. Government Printing Office.

U.S. Department of Agriculture. (1989). *Making bag lunches, snacks, and desserts using the dietary guidelines.* (Home & Garden Bulletin No. 232-9). Washington, DC: U.S. Government Printing Office.

U.S. Department of Agriculture. (1989). *Shopping for food and making meals in minutes using the dietary guidelines.* (Home & Garden Bulletin No.

232-10). Washington, DC: U.S. Government Printing Office.

U.S. Department of Agriculture. (1989). *Eating better when eating out using the dietary guidelines.* (Home & Garden Bulletin No. 232-11). Washington, DC: U.S. Government Printing Office.

U.S. Department of Agriculture. (1989). *Good sources of nutrients.* (Home & Garden Bulletin Fact Sheets). Washington, DC: U.S. Government Printing Office.

U.S. Department of Agriculture. (1988, revised). *Fast foods.* (Home & Garden Bulletin No. 8-21). Washington, DC: U.S. Government Printing Office.

Belizan, J. M., et al. (1991). Calcium supplementation to prevent hypertensive disorders of pregnancy. *New England Journal of Medicine, 325*(20), pp. 1399–1405.

Bouchard, C. (1991). Is weight fluctuation a risk factor? *New England Journal of Medicine, 324*(26), pp. 1887–1888.

Ferris, T. F. (1991). Pregnancy, preeclampsia, and the endothelial cell. *New England Journal of Medicine, 325*(20), pp. 1439–1440.

Hirsch, J. (1991). Oral anticoagulant drugs. *New England Journal of Medicine, 324*(26), pp. 1865–1873.

Lissner, L. (1991). Variability of body weight and health outcomes in the Framingham population. *New England Journal of Medicine, 324*(26), pp. 1839–1843.

Roberts, C. for the Massachusetts Medical Society Committee on Nutrition. (1989). Sounding board. Fast food Fare. Consumer guidelines. *New England Journal of Medicine, 321*(11), pp. 752–755.

Sacks, F. M., & Willett, W. W. (1991). More on chewing the fat: The good fat and the good cholesterol. *New England Journal of Medicine, 325*(24), pp. 1740–1741.

Trier, J. S. (1991). Celiac sprue. *New England Journal of Medicine, 325*(24), pp. 1709–1716.

INDEX